The
Baby Book

Sears Parenting Library

The A.D.D. Book
The Attachment Parenting Book
The Baby Book
The Birth Book
The Breastfeeding Book
The Discipline Book
The Family Nutrition Book
The Fussy Baby Book
The Pregnancy Book
The Successful Child

Sears Children's Library

Baby on the Way
Eat Healthy, Feel Great
What Baby Needs
You Can Go to the Potty

The Baby Book

Everything You Need to Know
About Your Baby—From Birth to Age Two

William Sears, M.D., and Martha Sears, R.N., with Robert Sears, M.D., and James Sears, M.D.

LITTLE, BROWN AND COMPANY
New York • Boston

Little, Brown and Company
Time Warner Book Group
1271 Avenue of the Americas, New York, NY 10020
Visit our Web site at www.twbookmark.com

Second Edition

All the medications named in this book were thoroughly checked by the authors for safety and efficacy at the time of writing. However, after years of a drug's use, new studies may show that it is either ineffective or unsafe for babies. In addition, procedures and recommendations in this book are not intended to replace regular visits to a health care professional. For this reason, check the safety and efficacy of all medications and procedures with your doctor before using them.

Library of Congress Cataloging-in-Publication Data

The baby book : everything you need to know about your baby — from birth to age two / William Sears . . . [et al.]. — Rev. ed.
    p. cm.
    Previous ed. cataloged under the m.e. Sears, William.
    Includes index.
    ISBN 0-316-77800-1
        1. Infants (Newborn) — Care.   2. Infants — Care.   3. Infants — Development.
I. Sears, William, M.D.

RJ61.S44178 2003
649'.122 — dc21   2002016142

RRD-IN

10   9   8   7   6   5   4   3

Drawings by Deborah Maze

PRINTED IN THE UNITED STATES OF AMERICA

To our "babies"

James

Robert

Peter

Hayden

Erin

Matthew

Stephen

Lauren

and

To our grandbabies

Andrew

Lea

Alex

Jonathan

Joshua

—W. S. and M. S.

Contents

A Word from Dr. Bill and Martha

We have not only written this book — we have *lived* it. In *The Baby Book* we share with you our experience in parenting eight children and caring for thousands of others during thirty years in pediatric practice. As we learned to become keen baby and parent watchers, we kept track of what works for most parents most of the time. Each day in our office we gleaned from successful parents practical advice on baby care. You will find these tips scattered throughout the book. We realize that love for your baby and the desire to be a good parent makes you susceptible to any baby-rearing advice. But children are too valuable and parents too vulnerable for any author to offer unresearched information. We take responsibility for our teachings seriously. Every statement has been thoroughly researched and has stood the test of time.

We also make allowances for the busy lifestyles of today's parents. We too juggle the spontaneous needs of our children and the duties of our professional lives. In our book we present basic tools to help you become a sensitive nurturer as you arrive at a parenting approach that meets the needs of your baby and fits with your life-style. We advise a high-touch style of parenting to balance the high-tech life of the new millennium. In *The Baby Book* you will find a way of caring that brings out the best in you and your baby.

Since its first edition in 1993, *The Baby Book* has been dubbed the "baby bible" by millions of parents. We are so pleased that our advice has made baby care more enjoyable for new parents throughout the world. In this new edition, we add many new topics based on reader feedback and also include updates that have occurred over the past ten years in the fields of parenting and pediatrics.

Besides new material, we have added new authors to this new edition. Dr. James and Dr. Robert Sears, new partners with their mom and dad in the Sears Family Pediatric Practice, have helped update the medical information throughout this book. It gives us great joy to know that by our family advice in this book we have become in some small way part of your family.

William and Martha Sears
San Clemente, California
January 2003

VISIT DR. SEARS ONLINE

www.AskDrSears.com

Now you can access thousands of pages of pediatric medical and parenting information. Our comprehensive online resource, personally written by the Doctors Sears, expands on many of the topics discussed in *The Baby Book*. We continuously update the health information on our website to provide you with the latest in parenting and health care issues. AskDrSears.com offers valuable insights on such topics as Pregnancy and Childbirth, Infant Feeding, Family Nutrition, Discipline and Behavior, Fussy Babies, and Sleep Problems.

Our website also includes these unique features:

- Dr. Sears's Medicine Cabinet, a comprehensive guide to over-the-counter medications, including specific dose information
- Childhood Illnesses, detailed medical information on many common, and not-so-common, child and family illnesses
- Monthly Pediatric Health News Updates
- Seasonal Pediatric Health Alerts
- Valuable month-by-month parenting and medical advice to complement your child's regular checkups
- Frequently Asked Questions answered
- Personal words of encouragement and humor from the daily lives of the Doctors Sears
- *The Baby Book* updates. We will post any significant changes to *The Baby Book* (and all our books) to provide you with the most accurate and up-to-date medical information.

I

Getting Started:
Baby-Care Basics

There is really no such thing as one best way to parent a baby, just as there are no perfect babies and, would you believe, no perfect parents — only people who have studied babies and people who have more experience than you. Being a parent requires on-the-job training. Too much advice from "experts" can actually interfere with the beginning parents' intuition and block their ability to learn as they grow. We are going to show you how to become your own baby experts. Our goal for this book is to help you and your baby fit. *This tiny word economically describes what parenting is all about.*

Let's get started!

1

Getting Attached: What It Means

Parenting, in a nutshell, is giving your children the tools to succeed in life. Every other baby book is missing a chapter that would be entitled "Parenting *Your* Baby." Now, together with you, the expectant couple or new parents, we are going to construct this chapter.

From my experience as a pediatrician, Martha's as a nurse, and our mutual experience as parents of eight, we believe that the best way to achieve the proper fit between parents and child is to practice a parenting style we call *attachment parenting.** This style is a way of caring that brings out the best in parents and their babies. Attachment parenting has been around as long as there have been mothers and babies. It is, in fact, only recently that this style of parenting has needed a name at all, for it is basically the commonsense parenting we all would do if left to our own healthy resources.

Throughout this book, unless stated otherwise, "I" refers to Dr. Bill Sears; "Martha," naturally, refers to Martha Sears.

PARENTING *YOUR* BABY

Thirty years ago, when I began pediatric practice, I had already trained in the two top pediatric hospitals in the world, and I thought I knew everything about babies. In fact, our friends used to tell Martha how fortunate she was to be married to a pediatrician, to which she would reply, "He only knows about sick babies." My first week in practice was really a shock. Mothers kept asking me all sorts of nonmedical questions: "Should I let my baby cry?" "Are we going to spoil her if we pick her up too much?" "Is it all right to sleep with our baby?" I didn't know the answers to any of these questions, but parents were relying on me to be the expert. These were not medical questions, but questions about parenting style. I knew what we did with our own two babies, but I didn't think this made me an expert. So I read baby books, just as you are doing now. The books were confusing. They seemed to be based on the authors' opinions rather than on actual research. Most authors either lacked common sense, refused to take a stand, or preached only what was popular at the time — whether or not it worked.

I decided to consult the true experts — experienced parents in my practice who appeared to have a handle on parenting: parents who seemed to be in harmony with their children, who were able to read their babies' cues, and who responded intuitively and appropriately; parents who enjoyed parenting and whose children seemed to be turning out well. These parents and their children became my teachers, and I became an astute listener and a keen baby watcher, keeping careful notes about which parenting styles they practiced. I accumulated a "what works" list. Martha worked with me in those early years (until our fourth child, Hayden, came along), and she is still active as a parenting adviser and breastfeeding consultant. My practice was our field research, and we had our own growing "laboratory" at home.

After nine years of listening and learning and three children of our own, we began to draw some conclusions about parenting. From an array of parenting styles we selected what worked for most parents most of the time. We taught these concepts to the parents in my practice and have used them in parenting our own eight children. Over the years, Martha and I have modified our approach to fit our changing life-style and to meet the individual needs of our children (and we're still learning). In this short chapter you are hearing the essence of what took us thirty years of practicing pediatrics, parenting eight children, and counseling thousands of parents to learn.

Don't expect to learn everything at once. Parenting is a learn-as-you-go profession. It takes hands-on experience. Our suggestions are just starter tips. From these basics you will grow and develop your own style, one that best fits your baby's temperament and your personality. Also, there is no way you can completely decide on a parenting style before you have a baby. You have no idea what a baby will do to you and how drastically baby will change your outlook. Determining how much to hold your baby, what you will do when your baby wakes up at 3:00 A.M., and how long you will breastfeed requires on-the-job training. Reserve these decisions until you see what your baby is like. But there are some parenting-style ideas to consider before the job begins.

Before we plunge into Parenting 101, let's make a deal. A few of the ideas we will share with you may initially sound strange and different from advice you have heard elsewhere. But please do not close your mind. Enter your parenting career with an open mind, or you may set yourselves up for a lot of frustration. The easy baby you are expecting may not be the baby you get. *Stay open to new ideas,* and then select what best fits your family. In return, be assured that everything we discuss has been well researched.

THE SEVEN BABY B'S OF ATTACHMENT PARENTING

There are three goals that we see as important for beginning parents:

- to know your child
- to help your child feel right
- to enjoy parenting

The style of parenting we discuss helps you achieve these goals. Here are the seven concepts that make up attachment parenting.

1. Birth Bonding — Connect with Your Baby Early

The way baby and parents get started with one another often sets the tone of how this early attachment unfolds. Take an active role in orchestrating the birth you want. Take responsibility for your birth, educate yourself, and work out a birthing philosophy with your obstetrician or birth attendant. A traumatic birth or an unnecessary surgical birth resulting in the separation of mother and baby is not the ideal way to begin parenting. In this case, part of the energy that would be directed toward getting to know your baby is temporarily diverted toward healing yourself. Feeling good about your baby's birth carries over into feeling good about your baby. (Read Chapter 2, "Ten Tips for Having a Safe and Satisfying Birth," to understand the connection between birthing and bonding and how to lower your chances of having a difficult, traumatic birth or even an unnecessary surgical birth. Also see page 67 for tips on catch-up attachment, in case a medical complication does result in temporary mother-baby separation. For an explanation of why having your baby with you in your hospital room is important, see page 48.)

The early weeks and months are a sensitive period when mother and baby need to be together. Early closeness allows the natural attachment-promoting behaviors of a baby and the intuitive, biological caregiving of a mother to unfold. Early closeness gets the pair off to the right start at a time when the baby is most needy and the mother is most eager to nurture. Of course, the process of falling in love with your baby, feeling attached or bonded, begins long before the day of birth and continues long afterward. (For practical suggestions on birth bonding

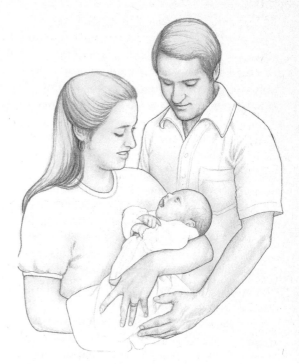

Attachment parenting is all about helping you and your baby fit.

and getting attached with your baby in the postpartum period, see Chapter 4, "Getting the Right Start with Your Newborn," and Chapter 5, "Postpartum Family Adjustments.")

2. Belief in Your Baby's Cries — Read and Respond to Your Baby's Cues

One of your earliest challenges is to figure out what your baby wants and needs from moment to moment. This can be very frustrating and lead to "I'm not a good parent" attacks.

Relax! Your baby will help you learn to be a good cue reader. Researchers used to believe that babies were only passive players in the caretaking game. Now we know that babies actively shape their parents' responses. Here's how: *Babies come wired with attachment-promoting behaviors* (APBs), magnetlike behaviors so irresistible they draw the parent to the baby, in language so penetrating it must be heard. Some APBs are hard to miss — for example, your baby's cries, smiles, and clinging gestures; others are subtle cues, like eye contact and body language. All parents, especially mothers, have a built-in intuitive system with which they listen and respond to the cues of their baby. Like a transmitter-receiver network, mother and baby, through practice, fine-tune their communication until the reception is clear. How quickly this communication network develops varies among mother-baby pairs. Some babies give clearer cues; some parents are more intuitive cue readers. But good connections will happen. They will happen more easily if you remember to be *open and responsive.* Even an occasional "incorrect" response (for example, offering to feed a baby who wants only to be held) is better than no response, because it encourages your baby to keep working with you.

Pick up your baby when he cries. As simple as this sounds, there are many parents who have been told to let their babies cry it out, for the reason that they must not reward "bad" behavior. But newborns don't misbehave; they just communicate the only way nature allows them to. Imagine how you would feel if you were completely uncoordinated — unable to do anything for yourself — and your cries for help went unheeded. A baby whose cries are not answered does not become a "good" baby (though he may become quiet); he does become a discouraged baby. He learns the one thing you don't want him to: that he

can't communicate or trust his needs will be met.

It's easy for someone else to advise you to let *your* baby cry. Unless he or she is a very sensitive person, nothing happens to his or her body chemistry when your baby cries. Let's get a bit technical for a minute. Your baby's cry will bother you; it's supposed to. This is especially true for mothers. If we were to put a mother and baby together in a laboratory and attach blood-flow-measuring instruments to the mother's breasts, here's what would happen: When mother heard her baby cry, the blood flow to her breasts would increase, accompanied by an overwhelming urge to pick up and comfort her baby. Your baby's cry is powerful language designed for the survival and development of the baby and the responsiveness of the parents. Respond to it. (See pages 48 and 343 for more detailed information about the crying-communication network.)

Meeting your baby's needs in the early months means solid communication patterns will develop. With time you can gradually delay your response and gradually your baby will learn to accept waiting a little bit as she learns noncrying language and develops self-

---

THE SEVEN BABY B'S OF ATTACHMENT PARENTING

1. birth bonding
2. belief in the signal value of your baby's cries
3. breastfeeding
4. babywearing
5. bedding close to baby
6. balance and boundaries
7. beware of baby trainers

help mechanisms. If nothing else, consider responding to your baby's needs an investment in the future; you'll be glad for good communication when she gets older and her problems are bigger than being fed or getting off to sleep.

3. Breastfeed Your Baby

Fathers often say, *"We're* going to breastfeed." Breastfeeding is indeed a family affair. The most successful breastfeeding mothers and babies we have seen are those that have a supportive husband and father. The benefits of breastfeeding in enhancing baby's health and development are enormous, but what is not fully appreciated are the magnificent effects of breastfeeding on the mother. Here's what's in it for you: Every time your baby

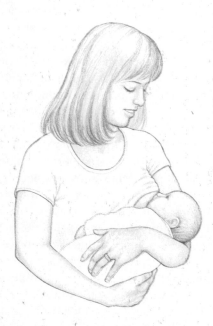

Breastfeeding offers great benefits for babies and mothers.

feeds, hormones (prolactin and oxytocin) enter your system. These "mothering hormones" help form the chemical basis for what is called mother's intuition. As you will learn in greater detail in later chapters, the same hormones that help make milk make mothering easier. And, as you will learn in Chapter 8, new studies show that breastfed babies turn out to be smarter children.

4. Babywearing — Carry Your Baby a Lot

This is the most exciting parenting concept to hit the Western world in years. As we were doing our parenting-style research, we attended an international parenting conference where we noticed that mothers in other cultures wear their babies in slinglike carriers as part of their native dress. Impressed by how content the babies were and how attentive their mothers were, we asked these mothers why they carried their babies. They volunteered two simple but profound reasons: *It's good for the baby, and it makes life easier for the mother.* That's it! That's what all parents want: to do something good for their babies and make life easier for themselves.

A baby carrier will be one of your most indispensable infant-care items. You won't want to leave home without it. This is not to say you must carry your baby *all* the time, but it may mean changing your mind-set about babies. Most people imagine babies lying quietly in their cribs, gazing at dangling mobiles and being picked up only long enough to be fed, changed, played with briefly, and then put down again "where they belong"; that holding periods are just dutiful intervals to calm and cuddle babies so they can be put

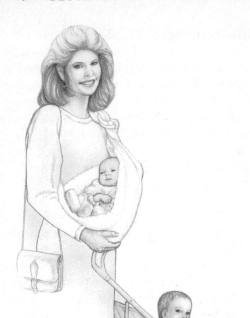

Babywearing makes caring for two babies easier.

you are. (For your personal course on baby-wearing and how it does good things for babies and makes life easier for parents, see Chapter 14, "Babywearing: The Art and Science of Carrying Your Baby.")

5. Bedding Close to Baby

Very early in your parenting career you will learn that the only babies who always sleep through the night are in books or belong to other people. Be prepared for some night-time juggling until you find where baby and you sleep best. Some babies sleep best in their own room, some in the parents' room, and some sleep best snuggled right next to mother. *Wherever you and your baby sleep best is the right arrangement for you, and it's a very personal decision.* Be open to try-ing various sleeping arrangements, including welcoming your baby into your bed — a nighttime parenting style we call sharing sleep.

down again. Babywearing reverses this view. Young babies are carried, or worn, most of the time by parents or substitute caregivers and put down only when sound asleep or when caregivers must attend to their own needs.

Good things happen to carried babies and their parents. Most noticeably, carried babies cry less, as if they forget to fuss. Besides being happier, carried babies develop better, possibly because the energy they would have wasted on crying is diverted into growth. Also, a baby learns much in the arms of a busy parent. Babywearing benefits you because it fits in nicely with busy life-styles. It allows you to take your baby with you wherever you go. You don't have to feel house-bound; home to your baby is where

Sharing sleep seems to evoke more contro-versy than any other feature of attachment parenting, and we don't understand why. We are amazed that such a beautiful custom, so natural for ages, is suddenly "wrong" for mod-ern society. Most babies the world over sleep with their parents. Even in our own culture more and more parents enjoy this sleeping arrangement — they just don't tell their doc-tors or their relatives about it. Try this experi-ment: Next time you're around a lot of new parents, mention one-on-one that you are considering sleeping with your baby. You'll be surprised how many of these people are doing just that, at least some of the time. Don't worry about your child never leaving your bed. He will. For the child who needs nighttime closeness, the time in your bed is

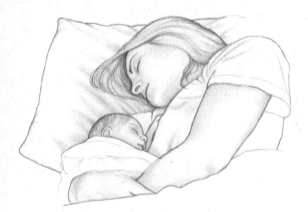

Try sharing sleep with your baby.

relatively short — and the benefits last a lifetime. (For a detailed explanation of how sleeping with your baby makes nighttime parenting easier and enhances the development of your baby, as well as the latest research on this controversial topic, see Chapter 15, "Nighttime Parenting: How to Get Your Baby to Sleep.")

6. Balance and Boundaries

In your zeal to give your baby everything she needs it's tempting to try to give baby everything she wants. This can result in mother burnout. Since a new baby in your home can absolutely turn previously predictable schedules and couple time upside down, it's easy to neglect your own needs and those of your marriage while meeting the needs of your baby. Throughout this book we will show you how to be *appropriately responsive* to your baby, which means knowing when to say yes and when to say no, and also having the wisdom to say yes to your own needs. When mom and dad are doing well, baby will also do well. One day Martha, in exaspera-

tion, said to me, "I don't have time to take a shower, my baby needs me so much!" I lovingly reminded her, "What our baby needs is a happy, rested mother." Remember, while attachment parenting is not the easiest style of parenting, if practiced properly it should be the most joyful one.

7. Beware of Baby Trainers

Because you love your baby so much and want to do the best, you are vulnerable to all kinds of advice. Be prepared to be the target of well-meaning advisers who will shower you with detachment advice, such as: "Let her cry it out," "Get her on a schedule," "You shouldn't still be nursing her!," and "Don't pick her up so much, you're spoiling her!" If carried to the extreme, baby training is a lose-lose situation: Baby loses trust in the signal value of her cues, and parents lose trust in their ability to read and respond to baby's cues. As a result, a distance can develop between baby and parent, which is just the opposite of the closeness that develops with attachment parenting. Whereas attachment parenting is based on sensitivity, baby training requires insensitivity. Attachment parenting helps you get to know and read your baby better. Baby training interferes with this. The basis of baby training is to help babies become more "convenient." It is based upon the misguided assumption that babies cry to manipulate, not to communicate. Baby-training books and classes teach mothers to go against their basic drive to respond to the cues of their baby. Eventually they will lose sensitivity and their trust in their own intuition. Before trying any of these baby-training methods, compare them with your intuitive feelings.

Attachment parenting is an ideal. Because of medical situations, life-style differences, or just plain rough times, you may not be able to practice all of these attachment tips all the time. Parenting is too individual and baby is too complex for there to be only one way. But these seven attachment concepts provide the basic tools from which you can develop a parenting style that works best for you. Some of the Baby B's, especially babywearing and belief in your baby's cries, can be practiced not only by parents but by substitute care-givers. Teaching your subs these two impor-tant Baby B's increases the likelihood that your baby will get attachment-*cared for* dur-ing your absence.

The important point is to *get connected to your baby.* Take advantage of all the valuable things that attachment parenting does for par-ents and babies. Once connected, stick with what is working and modify what is not. You will ultimately arrive at your own style. This is how you and your baby bring out the best in one another.

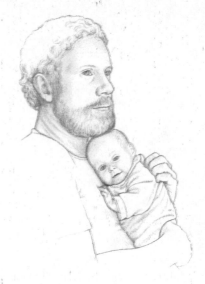

Fathers are nurturers too.

ATTACHMENT PARENTING INCLUDES FATHERS

The seven Baby B's work best with an involved and nurturing dad. While a prefer-ence for mother is natural for babies in the early years, fathers are indispensable. Father creates a supportive environment that allows mother to devote her energy to the baby. Attachment mothers are prone to the "My baby needs me so much, I don't have time to take a shower" mind-set. It's the father's job to nurture the mother so that she can nurture the baby. A mother of a particularly energy-draining baby once confided to me, "I couldn't have survived without the help of my husband." Take breastfeeding, for example, which is the only infant care fathers can't do. Fathers can indirectly feed their babies by supporting and encouraging the mother. As one involved husband boasted, "I can't breastfeed, but I can create an environ-ment that helps my wife breastfeed better." A happier mom makes for a happier baby.

Fathers have more than a supporting role in baby tending. They are more than substi-tute mothers, pinch-hitting while mom is away. Dads make their own unique contribu-tion to the development of their baby. Your baby will not love you less than he does his mother, or more. He or she will love you *dif-ferently.* Nothing matures a man like becom-ing an involved father. (See pages 44 and 291 for unique father-infant relationships and special nurturing tips for dad.)

SOME QUESTIONS YOU MAY HAVE

When we tell parents-to-be about attachment parenting, they react pretty strongly — often with relief. Attachment parenting is, after all, commonsense parenting. But even parents enthusiastic about attachment parenting are often a bit leery, probably because this style of parenting is rather foreign to the fear-of-spoiling mind-set we've all been exposed to. Here are our answers to some of the questions we're asked most often.

Attachment parenting sounds exhausting. Is it one big give-a-thon?

Attachment parenting may sound difficult, but in the long run it's actually the easiest parenting style. Initially, there is a lot of giving. This is a fact of new parent life. Babies are takers, and parents are givers. But a concept we want you to appreciate, and one we emphasize throughout this entire book, is *mutual giving — the more you give to your baby, the more baby gives back to you.* This is how you grow to enjoy your child and feel more competent as a parent. Remember, your baby is not just a passive player in the parenting game. Your infant takes an active part in shaping your attitudes, helping you make wise decisions as you become an astute baby reader.

There is a biological angle to mutual giving, as well. When a mother breastfeeds her baby, she gives nourishment and comfort. The baby's sucking, in turn, stimulates the release of hormones that further enhance mothering behavior, as mentioned previously. The reason that you can breastfeed your baby to sleep is that your milk contains a sleep-inducing substance. Meanwhile, as you suckle your baby,

> ## EARLY ATTACHMENT — LIFELONG MEMORIES
>
> There may be occasions when you wonder if your baby's high-need stage will ever end. It will! The time in your arms, at your breasts, and in your bed is such a relatively short while, but your message of love and availability lasts a lifetime.

you produce more of the hormone prolactin, which has a tranquilizing effect on you. It's as if the mommy puts the baby to sleep, and the baby puts the mommy to sleep.

What is "hard" about parenting is the feeling "I don't know what he wants" or "I just can't seem to get through to her." If you feel you really know your baby and have a handle on the relationship, parenting is easier and more relaxed. There is great comfort in feeling connected to your baby. Attachment parenting is the best way we know to get connected. True, this style of parenting takes tremendous amounts of patience and stamina, but it's worth it! Attachment parenting early on makes later parenting easier, not only in infancy but in childhood and in your child's teenage years. The ability to read and respond to your baby carries over to the ability to get inside your growing child and see things from his or her point of view. When you truly know your child, parenting is easier at all ages.

Won't holding our baby a lot, responding to cries, breastfeeding on cue, and even sleeping with baby create a spoiled and overly dependent child?

No! Both experience and research have shown the opposite to be true. Attachment fosters independence. Attachment parenting implies responding *appropriately* to your baby; spoiling suggests responding *inappropriately.* The spoiling theory began in the 1920s when experts invaded the realm of child rearing. They scoffed at parental intuition and advocated restraint and detachment. They felt that holding a baby a lot, feeding on cue, and responding to cries would create a clingy, dependent child. There was no scientific basis for this spoiling theory, just unwarranted fears and opinions.

We would like to put the spoiling theory on the shelf — to spoil. Studies have proved it wrong. In one study, researchers observed two sets of parents and their children. Group A was securely attached, the product of responsive parenting. Group B babies were parented in a more restrained way: put on schedules and given less intuitive and nurturant responses to their cues. These babies were followed for at least a year. Which group do you think eventually turned out to be more independent? Answer: group A, the securely attached babies. Researchers who have studied the effects of parenting styles on behavior in older children have all concluded that the spoiling theory is utter nonsense. A child must go through a stage of healthy dependence in order to become securely independent later.

How does attachment foster independence?

Studies have shown that infants who develop a secure attachment with their mothers during the first year are better able to tolerate separation from them when they are older. When going from oneness with the mother (which started in the womb) to separateness (an independent child), a growing baby has both a desire to explore and encounter new situations and a continued need for the safety and contentment provided by a parent. In an unfamiliar situation, the securely attached baby looks to mother for a go-ahead message, which provides the confidence to explore and handle the strange situation. The next time the toddler encounters a similar situation, he will have that much more confidence to handle it by himself without enlisting the mother. The consistent availability of the mother or an attached caregiver provides confidence and helps the child learn to trust himself, culminating in the child's developing independence. In essence, the attachment-parented baby learns to trust, and trust fosters healthy independence. (See page 517 for a more detailed discussion of this.)

Doesn't attachment parenting put the baby in the driver's seat?

The issue is that of parents' being responsive, not of baby's being in control. When a hungry or an upset baby cries, he cries to be fed or comforted, not to control. This concern is a carryover from the old spoiling and fear-of-manipulation mind-sets that didn't understand what babies are like. For example, the feeding practice of rigid scheduling (which we now know can be harmful to a baby's nutrition and self-esteem) resulted from this misunderstanding. The baby who has a need signals to the person he trusts will meet that need. The person responds. That's communication, not control. By responding, the parents are teaching their baby to trust them, which ultimately makes it easier for the parents to be in charge. When your baby cries, respond from your heart. Forget the mental gymnastics: Should I pick her up? Will I spoil her? Has she manipulated me? Just pick her up! With time you will better perceive why your baby is crying and how immediate your response should be.

This style should not develop into "martyr mothering": Baby pulls mommy's string, and she jumps. Because of the mutual sensitivity that develops between attached parents and their attached children, parents' response time can gradually lengthen as mother enables the older baby to discover that he does not need instant gratification. Nor does attachment parenting mean overindulgence or possessiveness. The possessive parent or "hover mother" keeps the child from doing what he needs to do because of her own insecurities. Attachment differs from dependency. Attachment enhances development; inappropriate dependency hinders it. There is a beautiful *balance* to attachment parenting.

What does attachment parenting do for my relationship with my child?

Attachment mothers speak of a *flow* between themselves and their babies, a flow of thought and feelings that helps them pull from their many options the right choice at the right time when confronted with the daily "What do I do now?" baby-care decisions. The flexibility of this style helps you adjust your parenting to the changing moods and maturity of your baby. It's important to make gradual adjustments. For example, the eight-month-old doesn't need the quick cry response that the eight-day-old baby does (unless, of course, he has hurt himself or is frightened). The connected pair *mirrors* each other's feelings. Baby learns about himself through mother's eyes. The mother reflects the baby's value to her, and therefore to himself. The flow of attachment parenting helps you read your child's feelings.

Martha notes: One day I was scolding four-year-old Matthew. I was angry. I noticed the forlorn look on his face and suddenly I knew that he felt I was angry at him as a person rather than at what he did. I knew I had to reassure him, so I said, "I am angry, but I still love you." He said, "Oh! Really?" and his face brightened.*

The other dividend to expect is *mutual sensitivity.* As you become more sensitive to your baby, your baby becomes more sensitive to you. As an example of mutual sensitivity that occurred in our family during the writing of this book, here's Martha again:

Martha notes: In the middle of a particularly busy day I discovered that my kitchen was overrun with ants. This was the last straw and I lost it, verbally and emotionally. But as I continued to rant and rave, I became aware of what was going on between Stephen (then twenty-two months) and me. He watched me, sensing my needs. He looked into my eyes, embraced my knees, not in a frightened way, but as though to say, "It's OK, I love you. I would help you if I could." As Stephen got hold of me, I got hold of myself — a mother calmed by her baby's touch.

OK, so the attachment style helps the parent-infant relationship. What specifically does it do for the baby?

Attachment parenting improves behavior, development, and intelligence. Here is why.

------

*As you journey through our description of infant development, you will notice passages entitled "Martha notes" sprinkled throughout the text. These are based on entries in Martha's baby journals.

Attachment parenting improves behavior. Attached babies cry less. They are less bored, colicky, fussy, whiny, and clingy. A very simple reason lies at the root of this observation: *A baby who feels right, acts right.* An attached baby whose cues are read and responded to feels connected. She feels valued. She trusts. Because of this inner feeling of rightness, baby has less need to fuss.

Attachment parenting improves development. If attached babies cry less, they have more time to grow and learn. For the last thirty years I have watched thousands of mother-infant pairs in action and interaction. I am constantly impressed with how content babies are who are worn in a sling, breastfed on cue, and responded to sensitively. They seem to feel better, behave better, and grow better. I believe this is because attachment parenting promotes a state of *quiet alertness* (also called interactive quiet or attentive stillness). A baby in the quiet alert stage is more receptive to interaction with and learning from his environment. He is not bored. The quiet alert state also promotes an inner organization that allows the physiological systems of the body to work better. Baby diverts the energy that he would have spent on fussing into growing, developing, and interacting with his environment.

In essence, attached babies *thrive*, meaning that your baby grows to her full potential. Researchers have long realized the association between good growth and good parenting.

Attachment parenting improves intelligence. Attachment parenting is good food for the brain. Many studies now show that the most powerful enhancers of brain development are the quality of the parent-infant attachment and the response of the caregiving environment to the cues of the infant. I believe that attachment parenting promotes brain development by feeding the brain the right kind of information at a time in the child's life when the brain needs the most

BENEFITS OF ATTACHMENT PARENTING

Baby	Parents	Relationship
• is more trusting	• become more confident	Parents and baby experience:
• feels more competent	• are more sensitive	• mutual sensitivity
• grows better	• can read baby's cues	• mutual giving
• feels right, acts right	• respond intuitively	• mutual shaping of behavior
• is better organized	• flow with baby's	• mutual trust
• learns language more	temperament	• feelings of connectedness
easily	• find discipline easier	• more flexibility
• establishes healthy	• become keen observers	• more lively interactions
independence	• know baby's competen-	• bringing out the best in
• learns intimacy	cies and preferences	one another
• learns to give and	• know which advice to take	
receive love	and which to disregard	

nourishment. By encouraging the behavior state of quiet alertness, attachment parenting creates the conditions that help baby learn.

If you are beginning to feel very important, you are! What parents do with babies makes them smarter. In the keynote address at the 1986 annual meeting of the American Academy of Pediatrics, infant development specialist Dr. Michael Lewis reviewed studies of factors that enhance infant development. This presentation was in response to the overselling of the superbaby phenomenon that emphasized the use of programs and kits rather than the parents' being playful companions and sensitive nurturers. Lewis concluded that the *single most important* influence on a child's intellectual development was the responsiveness of the mother to the cues of her baby. In caring for your baby, keep in mind that relationships, not things, make better babies. (For a discussion of how babywearing aids development, see page 301; for an in-depth discussion of how attachment parenting influences growth and development, see page 444.)

Help! How are we ever going to get our baby on a schedule this way?

I would like to replace the rigid idea of a schedule with the more flexible concept of a *routine* or even with the more flowing experience described by the word "harmony." The more you listen and respond to your baby, the simpler it will be to ease him into a routine that suits both of you.

Won't a mother feel tied down by constant baby tending?

Mothers do need baby breaks. This is why shared parenting by the father and other trusted caregivers is important. But with attachment parenting, instead of feeling tied down, mothers feel tied together with their babies. Attachment mothers we interviewed described their feelings:

"I feel so connected with my baby."

"I feel right when with her, and not right when we're apart."

"I feel fulfilled."

Remember, too, that attachment parenting, by mellowing a child's behavior, makes it easier to go places with your child. You don't have to feel tied down to your house or apartment and a life-style that includes only babies.

Attachment parenting sets high standards. What if I mess up? Am I setting myself up for a real guilt trip?

We all mess up, but when attachment parents mess up, the effect is minimal because their basic relationship with their child is solid. Also, attached children are *resilient,* and this helps take the pressure off parents. The attachment style of parenting is not a list of things you must do to have a bright and well-behaved child. The seven attachment concepts are like foundation blocks, the first steps in building your own parenting style. They are very basic, intuitive, commonsense ways of caring for a baby. Using these starter blocks of attachment parenting, you can *create your own* parenting style according to your individual life-style and the need level of your baby. Also, there may be medical, social, or economic reasons that you may not wish to or be able to practice all of the attachment concepts all the time with each child. Do as much as you can, when you can.

Yes, you will feel guilty at times. Parenting is a guilt-ridden profession. Love for your baby makes you vulnerable to feeling you are not doing enough. But take note. The feeling of guilt can be healthy; guilt is an inner warning system, a sort of alarm that goes off when we behave in ways we are not supposed to. Part of maturing as a person and as a parent is recognizing healthy guilt and using it to make good decisions. Attachment parenting develops your sensitivity, an inner signal that helps you make important baby-care decisions.

Does it mean I'm not a good mother if I don't breastfeed or sleep with my baby?

No, it does not! Becoming attached to your child is a gradual process. There are many interactions that lead to a strong parent-child bond. The seven attachment tips we advise simply give your relationship a head start. There may be medical or domestic circumstances making breastfeeding difficult. And for some parents and babies, sharing sleep is neither desirable nor necessary.

Does attachment parenting require a full-time at-home mother? What about the mother who chooses to or has to return to work?

Attachment parenting is easier for a full-time mother, but a full-time at-home mother is not a requirement for attachment parenting. In fact, this style of parenting is especially helpful for mothers who are separated from their babies for part of the day. Attachment parenting makes the most of your time with your baby and helps you reconnect with your baby after separation. It prevents a distance from developing between you and your baby as you learn to combine employment and parenting. (See Chapter 17, "Working and Parenting," for an in-depth discussion of how to keep attached while working.)

I believe that attachment parenting will be right for our family, but my confidence gets shaky when I read books or talk to people who feel differently.

As new parents you will be bombarded with advice. Attachment parenting is a real confidence builder, enabling you to listen to advice, learn from some of it, and discount the rest. You will check what the "experts" and casual advisers have to say against your own instincts and wisdom. Learn to confide in people who can be supportive. Nothing divides people like different opinions about child rearing, so you will naturally gravitate toward like-minded friends. You don't have to defend your style to others. Just say, "It works for us."

Are there special family situations in which attachment parenting is most needed?

This style of infant and child care gives a boost to any parent who has a special-needs child or a family situation that requires an extra bit of parental intuition. By being able to read their child's behavior, single parents especially profit from any style of parenting that makes discipline easier.

The real payoff occurs with the *high-need baby,* the one who, as it were, at birth says: "Hi, mom and dad! You've been blessed with an above-average baby and I need above-average parenting. If you give it to me, we're going to get along; if not, we're going to have a bit of trouble down the road." This style of parenting helps you match the giving level of the parent with the need level of the baby. The result is that you bring out the best in each other. Matching a high-need child with unconnected parents often brings out the worst.

How do attachment-parented children turn out? What type of people do they become?

Parents should not be too quick to take all the blame or the credit for the person their child becomes. There are many factors that contribute to the eventual person. Attachment parenting during the early formative years just increases the chances of a good outcome.

Early in my years of practice I studied the long-term effects of parenting styles. Parents who were into restraint parenting (scheduling, letting their baby cry it out, fear of spoiling, and so on) got a red dot on their baby's chart. Parents who practiced attachment parenting got a blue dot. Blue dot parents who practiced all seven of the Baby B's (see page 6) plus father involvement got an extra dot. This simple system was not meant to judge parenting styles or the degree of "goodness" of the parents. It was simply to gather information from which I could draw conclusions. It was not very scientific, nor was there a perfect correlation between what parents did and how their children turned out, but I was able to draw some general conclusions.

Not only did attachment-parented children show long-term benefits, good things were happening to the parents too. First, the attachment parents developed confidence sooner. They used the basic tools of attachment parenting, but felt confident and free enough to branch out into their own style until they found what worked for them, their baby, and their life-style. During well-baby checkups I often asked, "Is it working?" I advised parents to periodically take inventory of what worked and discard what didn't. What works at one stage of development may not work at another. For example, some babies initially sleep better in bed with their

THE LONG-TERM EFFECTS OF ATTACHMENT PARENTING

In our experience of caring for families over the past thirty years in pediatric practice and in our review of scientific studies, we have found that attachment-parented children are likely to be:

- smarter
- healthier
- more sensitive
- more empathetic
- easier to discipline
- more bonded to people than to things

parents but become restless later on, necessitating a change of sleeping arrangements. Other babies initially sleep better alone but need to share sleep with their parents in later months. These parents used themselves and their baby as the barometer of their parenting style, not the norms of the neighborhood.

Attachment parents also seemed to *enjoy* parenting more; they got closer to their babies sooner. As a result they orchestrated their life-styles and working schedules to incorporate their baby. Parenting, work, travel, recreation, and social life all revolved around and included baby — because they wanted it that way.

As the years went on I noticed one quality that distinguished attachment parents and their children — *sensitivity*. This sensitivity carried over into other aspects of life: marriage, job, social relationships, and play. In m... experience, sensitivity (in parent and chi... the most outstanding effect of attach... parenting.

As they got older, these connected children were deeply bothered by situations that weren't right. They were compassionate when other children cried and were quickly there to comfort. As teenagers they were bothered by social injustices and did something to correct them. These kids cared! Because they were so firmly rooted in their inner sensitivity, they were willing to swim upstream against the current. These children will become the movers and shakers and leaders and shapers of a better world to come.

A capacity for *intimacy* is another quality I noticed in attachment-parented children. These children learn to bond to people, not things. They become high-touch persons even in a high-tech world. The infant who grows up "in arms" is accustomed to relating to and being fulfilled from interpersonal relationships. This infant is more likely to become a child who forms meaningful attachments with peers, and in adulthood is more likely to develop deep intimacy with a mate. The attached child had learned to give and receive love.

Attachment parenting is contemporary. Today's children are being bombarded with more and more electronic influences, especially from video and computer games. Because this high-tech trend is likely to continue, the best parents can hope for is to provide speed bumps along the way. Attachment parenting gives children a high-touch start to help them be better prepared to survive the high-tech world. These kids are more likely to grow up to prefer bonding to people rather than to things.

Are attachment-parented children easier to discipline?

Discipline — that magic word you've been waiting for — *is* easier for attachment parents and their children. The sensitivity that attachment-style parents develop enables them intuitively to get behind the eyes of their child to see situations from his or her viewpoint. For example, one of the most common problems that parents dread in the toddler years is the tantrum that can develop when a child is asked to stop a play activity because "it's time to go." So many times I have heard parents say, "He just won't listen to me." Over the years I have watched how Martha handles this problem with our toddlers. Because her sensitivity prompts her to see things from her child's perspective, she understands why separation hassles occur and why a child throws a tantrum when asked to stop playing before he is ready. She handles this by a routine she calls *closure:* A few minutes before it is time to leave a play activity, Martha gets down to the toddler's level and asks him to say "Bye-bye" to each one of the toys and the children in the play group. This sensitive understanding gives him the ability to close out his own play activity. Attachment parenting makes life with a toddler easier.

Discipline is not something you do *to* a child. It is something you do *with* a child. In a nutshell, discipline begins with knowing your child and helping your child feel right. A child who feels right is more likely to act right and eventually operates from a set of inner controls rather than from an external force. Parents who can read their child are able to pick up on the real meaning of a child's actions and channel these into desirable behavior. The connected child desires to please. Discipline is a relationship between parent and child that can be summed up in one word — *trust*. The child who trusts his authority figure is easier to discipline. The authority person who can read the child gives better discipline. Attachment parents are better able to convey what behavior they expect of their children, and attached children are better able to perceive what behavior is expected of them. Connected kids are easier to discipline.

One day in my office, I observed a mother caring for her baby. She sensitively nurtured her baby, breastfed him on cue, comforted him when he was upset, and played with him when he was in a playful mood. Mother and baby seemed to be in harmony. I couldn't resist saying to her, "You're a good disciplinarian."

Difficult discipline situations occur when a distance develops between parent and child. The distant parent becomes frustrated by the "nothing's working" feeling and approaches discipline as a trial-and-error list of somebody else's methods — many of which promote an even greater distance between them. Disconnected children are more difficult to discipline because they operate from a basis of anger rather than trust.

The real payoff of this high-touch style of parenting is the ability to read your child. Getting attached is how discipline begins.

One of the most important long-term effects of attachment parenting comes from the concept of *modeling*. Keep in mind that you are bringing up someone's future husband or wife, father or mother. The parenting style that the child learns from you is the one he or she is more likely to follow when becoming a parent. Children pick up nurturing attitudes at a young age, and those early impressions stay with them. One day a mother brought her newborn, Aaron, into my office for a checkup accompanied by her three-year-old daughter, Tiffany, the product of attachment parenting. As soon as Aaron started to fuss, Tiffany pulled at her mother's skirt, saying with much emotion, "Mommy, Aaron's crying. Pick up,

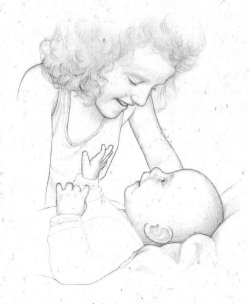

Your parenting style is a model for your children to follow.

rock, rock, nurse!" What do you imagine Tiffany will do when she becomes a parent and her own baby cries? She won't call her doctor, and she won't look it up in a book. She will intuitively pick up, rock, rock, and nurse.

Even teenagers pick up on parenting styles. One day Martha and I were sitting in our family room when we heard our daughter Erin, then nine months old, begin to cry in our bedroom, where she was napping. As we approached the door, the cry stopped. Curious, we looked in to see why Erin had stopped crying, and what we saw left a warm feeling in our hearts. Jim, our sixteen-year-old son (now Dr. Jim, pediatrician and partner in the Sears Family Pediatric Practice), was lying next to Erin, stroking her and gentling her. Why did Jim do this? Because he was following our model that when babies cry, adults listen.

MORE RESOURCES FOR ATTACHMENT PARENTING

If you would like to read more on the new and exciting scientific studies that support attachment parenting, especially those devoted to the long-term effects of this style of parenting on older children and adults, consult our two recent books, *The Attachment Parenting Book* (2001) and *The Successful Child* (2002). See also www.attachmentparenting.org, the website of Attachment Parenting International (API), which provides assistance to individuals who are forming attachment-parenting support groups.

2

Ten Tips for Having a Safe and Satisfying Birth

Parenting begins before birth. Today's mothers-to-be find many birthing options available to them, but along with the opportunity to choose comes the responsibility for making informed decisions. A safe, relaxed birthing experience will go a long way toward helping you get off to a good start with your baby.

We have been in and around the birth scene for a long time. Over the past thirty years I have attended around one thousand births. Martha has been a childbirth educator and has functioned as a labor assistant at births of friends. She has personally experienced birth seven times (our eighth child is adopted).

We have selected from our gallery of birthing-room scenes an overall impression of how birth is designed to happen. True, ideal births are as rare as sleep-through-the-night babies, but there are things you can do to come close to the birth you want. We wish to share with expectant parents the birth plan we have found to work for most mothers most of the time.

1. CHOOSE DR. RIGHT FOR YOURSELF

Mothers, take responsibility for your birth. Select a birth attendant with a dual mind-set. Certainly you owe it to yourself and to your baby to select a birth attendant who is medically competent and experienced enough to deal with unanticipated obstetrical complications during birth. This is the medical/surgical mind-set. But, realistically, only 10 percent of births should fall into this category. The other mind-set that you should expect from your birth attendant goes something like this: "Birth is a healthy process — we will help you create a birthing environment that will allow your birth to progress naturally." In essence you and your attendant enter into a partnership to work out a *birthing philosophy.* You are paying for both the science of obstetrics and the *art* of midwifery. You deserve both.

THE MIDWIVES ARE HERE

The art of midwifery is blending with the science of obstetrics to give a higher standard of care to the laboring mother. A midwife gives routine prenatal care and attends normal births, freeing the doctor to do that for which he or she is trained — caring personally for those mothers who have complications and overseeing the work of the midwives. Certified nurse midwives who have hospital privileges can offer medical pain relief; however, their main goal is to give such good labor support that medication can be avoided.

oversold by the designer showroom appearance of the room. The skills and mind-set of your birth attendants are more important to the well-being of you and your baby.

Birthing rooms are best for mother — best for baby. The LDR birthing environment can minimize pain, help labor progress, and increase your chances of having an uncomplicated birth. (Delivering in the traditional surgical style promotes fear and tension, contributes to that dreaded malady of the laboring mother — failure to progress — and often results in agonizing labors and surgical births.) As an added attraction, baby stays right where he or she belongs — nesting in the room. If your local hospitals do not offer this birthing option, ask for it.

2. CHOOSE THE RIGHT BIRTHING ENVIRONMENT

The birthing option we recommend for most parents is an LDR facility, meaning mother *labors, delivers,* and *recovers* in the same room. This birthing room is more than just a physical facility. It is an atmosphere conducive to giving birth and an attitude that birth is a normal process. This type of birthing room portrays a homelike environment, conveying a "relax while you're here" message. The lighting is soft and adjustable. The windows are large, the lounge chair inviting, and the medical and surgical equipment is efficiently but unobtrusively placed. The bed is adjustable to make birth easier. Visit the birthing room and spend a few moments envisioning labor and birth. Interview the nursing staff, your supporting cast. Does the room give you a nesting feeling? But don't be

3. USE A PROFESSIONAL LABOR ASSISTANT (PLA)

Studies by Dr. Kennell and Dr. Klaus (the same doctors who pioneered the concept of bonding) showed that mothers whose births were attended by a labor assistant had an 8 percent cesarean-section rate versus 18 percent for the matched controls whose births were not attended by one. Studies show that mothers who utilized a professional labor assistant enjoyed shorter labors and needed less medical intervention than mothers who did not avail themselves of professional labor support. Even the babies did better. Only 10 percent of babies in the supported group required extended hospital stays compared with 25 percent of the controls. Science is finally proving what midwives have long known: Babies and mothers do better when women help women give birth.

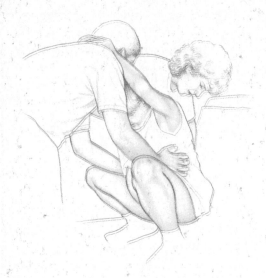

A professional labor assistant, like a choreographer, can help the mother channel her energies toward her goal.

The PLA (also referred to as a *doula* — a Greek word meaning "one who ministers") can be a midwife, childbirth educator, obstetrical nurse, or other qualified person who is trained to support the laboring mother during childbirth. Her role is to help the mother move through labor in harmony with her body, recognizing and acting on her own body's signals, so that labor can progress more comfortably and efficiently.

This special member of the birthing team functions as a *personal* labor assistant, attending to any and all physical, emotional, and mental needs one-on-one. She also acts as a communication liaison between the laboring couple and the medical and nursing staff so that interventions are avoided or decided upon mutually. She is there to provide the experience needed to make decisions wisely. Her fee for this service is worth every penny!

Her role begins by forming a relationship of trust with the couple during pregnancy, and when the mother begins her labor, she comes to her home and assists labor at home as long as the mother is comfortable there. Most women go to the hospital way too soon, even before their labor has actually begun. These false alarms result in either a frustrating trip back home or a premature admission to the hospital, which opens the door for a long list of procedures that might not have been necessary if the mother had labored at home a while longer. Birth at home is not what most couples in this country would choose, but *labor* at home is a wonderful option that many would choose if it were offered to them. A PLA is able to be with the couple at home, monitoring the labor and helping the couple plan the right time to leave for the hospital, neither leaving home too soon nor remaining home too long.

The PLA does not replace the father; rather, she frees him up to do what a man does best — love his wife. Men seldom relate empathetically to the emotional and physical challenges of the laboring woman. It is usually better for the father to leave the technical matters to a professional while he embraces his wife, rubs her back, walks with her, gives her ice chips and fluids, and guards against commotion.

We had a PLA for the birth of our last four babies. She and Martha spoke a woman-to-woman, mother-to-mother language of labor that I did not understand but have grown to respect.

How do you find one of these gems? Ask for one! A list of women available as PLA's may be obtained from your doctor, midwife, hospital, childbirth class, local midwife associations, or friends who have used their services. Mothers in our practice who have had previous traumatic births and those who are attempting a vaginal birth after cesarean (VBAC) have found labor attendants to be indispensable the second time around. For a list of professional labor assistants in your area, see www.dona.org, the website for the Doulas of North America.

4. GET MOVING

Move with the urges of your body. Move when your body says move, and be still when your body says be still. Freely roam around your birthing environment, retreating into a quiet corner when you feel like being alone, embracing your husband when you need a supporting set of arms during labor, and walking around the room or around the halls if this eases your discomfort and helps labor progress. It is important to feel that the environment you are in and the attendants you are with allow you to move with the urges of your body, uninhibited by others' expectations and stereotyped laboring positions.

TEN TIPS FOR HAVING A SAFE AND SATISFYING BIRTH

1. Choose Dr. Right for yourself.
2. Choose the right birthing environment.
3. Use a professional labor assistant.
4. Get moving.
5. Get off your back.
6. Experiment with labor positions.
7. Use technology wisely.
8. Use medical pain relief wisely.
9. Avoid an episiotomy.
10. Formulate your birth plan.

5. GET OFF YOUR BACK

Back birthing makes no medical sense. It is not good for baby, since lying on your back allows the heavy uterus to press on the blood vessels, diminishing blood supply to the uterus and to the baby. This is not good for mother, since back birthing narrows the pelvic outlet and mother is required to push the baby "uphill." (Squatting widens the pelvic outlet for pushing, while vertical birthing allows gravity to aid delivery.) The back position is also more painful and slows the progress of labor. The pelvic muscles, which need to relax during baby's passage through the birth canal, are tensed in the back-lying, feet-up position. Also, this posi-

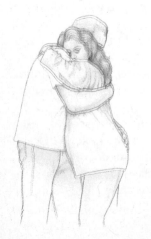

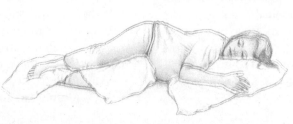

A timely embrace or some well-placed pillows — small things make a big difference during labor.

tion predisposes the mother to tears of the birth canal and unnecessary episiotomies.

6. EXPERIMENT WITH LABOR POSITIONS

Labor in the arms of your husband, sitting up in bed, squatting, leaning forward over the side of the bed, or lying on your side on the bed. Assuming these positions, and going with the urges of your body during labor and delivery, allow gravity to help your baby come down and relax tense muscles. Whatever position works for you, use it, and be ready to change if your body (or your PLA) tells you you need a different position.

7. USE TECHNOLOGY WISELY

Enter a labor room and you will likely see a mother lying on her back with the electronic fetal monitoring (EFM) belt girding her abdomen and attached to a video display terminal. All too often these mothers "fail to progress" in their labor and "need" a cesarean section. Mothers should not be lying on their backs.

Routine continuous EFM for every mother is no longer considered necessary or advisable. Instead, in laboring mothers without any known complications, the birth attendant may choose to periodically monitor the mother for twenty to thirty minutes to obtain information about the well-being of the preborn baby. (Controlled studies have shown that routine continuous EFM has not improved the outcome of babies when compared with intermittent monitoring by a nurse, but EFM mothers have a higher chance of having a cesarean

birth.) If continuous fetal monitoring is medically necessary, it should not restrict the mother's ability to move and change positions during labor. EFM can be done by telemetry, currently available technology that allows the mother to wear the EFM while walking around the delivery area. The monitor tracings are relayed through the air and displayed at a nearby receiving terminal. If an intravenous is necessary, request a heparin lock (a device connected to the needle that allows the IV tubing to be disconnected and permits you to roam without being attached to an IV pole).

8. USE MEDICAL PAIN RELIEF WISELY

The more informed you are about your options for pain relief, the safer and more satisfying your birth is likely to be. In your childbirth class, you will learn about the many options (both natural and medical) that are available to you. Medical pain relief can be a welcome addition to — but not a substitute for — the natural pain-relieving techniques you will learn about in your childbirth classes. No medication can deliver complete pain relief without risks. Overuse of anesthetics, to the extent that you lose all birthing sensations as well as movement, is a setup for a longer labor and possible surgical birth. On the other hand, a drawn-out, agonizing labor is good for neither mother nor baby. Discuss with your birth attendant the use of pain relievers, should they become necessary, that allow you enough sensation and freedom of movement to work with your body to help your labor progress. Whatever it takes to deliver a healthy baby and help you feel good about the process is the right pain package for you. The memories of this birth will last a lifetime.

THE BIG SPLASH — WATER LABOR

Laboring and birthing in water has been practiced in Russia and France for the past thirty years. This natural labor-saving device has now made its way to North America.

Why does water work? Immersion in warm water is a very effective relaxation tool that minimizes the pain and speeds the progress of labor. The buoyancy of water encourages mother to relax and assume her most comfortable labor position. The weightless feeling buoys the mother so that she can more easily support her body and deal with the contractions. Her muscles are less tense because they do not have to support her entire weight. As mother relaxes (without medication), her stress hormones decrease, allowing the natural birth-progressing hormones (oxytocin and endorphins) to flow uninhibited. A study of nearly 1,400 mothers who labored in Jacuzzi-type tubs (body-temperature water; no jets, please) showed better progression of labor and a cesarean-section rate of 10 percent, versus 25–30 percent in traditional hospital births. Some women wind up giving birth in water because of their reluctance to emerge from it in spite of the impending delivery. (This procedure is perfectly safe as long as the baby is brought out of the water right after he is born. The school of water birthing that practices slow emergence, in which the baby is left submerged for an indefinite time, can be dangerous and is not recommended.)

Martha notes: I personally experienced the benefits of water labor with the birth of our seventh baby, Stephen. I typically had fast (one- or two-hour) labors that only became intense a short time before pushing, and then after two or three pushes the baby was born. With baby number seven, however, this pattern changed. After four hours of mild, active labor, I began to experience an intense pain low in front. This was a signal to my body that something

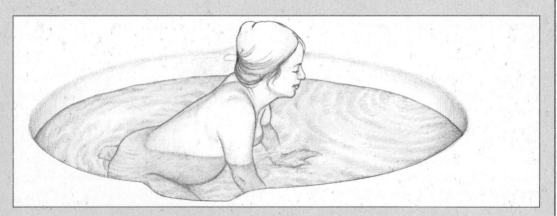

Immersion in warm water is an effective and natural relaxation tool.

needed attention. If it had been pain in my back, the all-fours position would have helped. I tried that position anyway, but it only hurt more. Then my birth attendant suggested I get into the tub. As I slipped into the warm water, I felt my limbs relax. I experimented with different positions and finally found one that allowed me to just let go and float from my shoulders down so that my whole torso and pelvis relaxed as well. At that point of total relaxation, the pain literally melted away — better than Demerol! The buoyancy did for me what I was not able to achieve by myself.

The experience of total release accompanied by total relief was amazing. I stayed in the water for about an hour until I recognized signals of the pushing stage. At that point I decided to get out of the water. I lay down on the bed on my left side and gave birth after two pushes. As the baby emerged we discovered the reason for the pain. The baby's hand was presented alongside his head — two parts coming through at once. My body needed total relaxation to allow my muscles to give way to a larger-than-usual presenting part.

9. AVOID AN EPISIOTOMY

Routine episiotomy for all births is unnecessary. Warm compresses, perineal massage and support, avoiding the rush to push baby out, and correct birthing positions can eliminate the need for episiotomy in most births. Discuss with your birth attendant ways to avoid this procedure. Spending the first week or two healing a painful birth wound while trying to concentrate on baby care is no way to begin life with a baby.

10. FORMULATE YOUR BIRTH PLAN

Birth, like life, is full of surprises, yet the more you plan for your birth, the more likely you are to get what you want. A birth plan will alert your birth attendants to your personal needs. Personalize your plan. Don't

copy it from a class. This is *your* birth, so it must be your plan. Consult our *Birth Book* (Little, Brown, 1994) for step-by-step guidelines on how to compose a personal birth plan.

▶*SPECIAL NOTE: Be flexible. Suppose the birth script does not progress the way you have written it — and some do not. Trust your birth attendant so that both of you can depart from the birth you have planned if it is not working and if it is in the best interest of your baby and yourself to have medical or surgical intervention.*

The reason we stress the importance of a good birthing experience is that birth is where parenting begins. Too often in our practice we see what we term the *poor-start syndrome*, which goes like this: The birth that mother expected is not the birth she gets. She spends the early days and weeks feeling she has failed and diverting most of her energy to healing her birth wounds instead of using that energy to get to know her baby. Also, as a result of a traumatic birth, mother and baby are often separated from each other after birth, at a prime time in their lives when both need to be together. As a result, breastfeeding problems occur, the infant-distress syndrome (fussiness and colic) is more common, and the pair spends most of the time during the early weeks solving problems, many of which could have been avoided.

In the past, birth became a science but lost its art. We see our present time as a blending of art and science toward more safe and satisfying births.

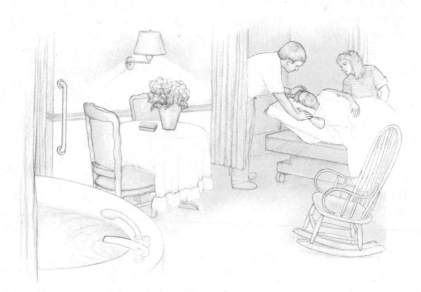

A more relaxed and intimate environment is provided by the LDR (labor, delivery, and recovery) room.

3

Preparing for Baby

Expectant parents visiting our office often begin their prenatal interview, "Doctor, this is a well-researched baby." They have done their homework. Preparing your mind, your body, and your nest helps you get off to the right start. Today's expectant parents have many options. Because of the wide variety of life-styles and parenting styles, they need them.

CHOOSING DR. RIGHT FOR YOUR BABY

Thirty years ago when I began practice, I was told there were three qualities a parent looks for in choosing a doctor for the baby: The doctor must be *able*, *affable*, and *available*. These three *A*'s of doctor choosing haven't changed. Besides hospitals, other physicians, and medical societies, the best references are given by parents themselves. If you are expecting your first baby or are new to a community, ask friends and neighbors about the qualifications of several doctors and interview them prenatally. Here's how to get the

most out of your prenatal interview with the doctor:

- Take a written list of your most important concerns and parenting issues to determine whether your needs are in harmony with your doctor's philosophies.

- If you have a special need, such as "I want to continue breastfeeding even though I'm returning to work," ask if the doctor can help you with this.

- Avoid negative openers. Nothing is more nonproductive than opening the interview with an "I don't want" list — for example, "I don't want my baby to have any bottles in the hospital." It is more productive to ask, "What is your policy about giving bottles to breastfeeding babies in the hospital?" Remember, your purpose for the interview is to determine if you and the prospective pediatrician are on the same wavelength. Negative openers close your mind to the possibility that you may learn something from the doctor's response.

- Keep your interview brief and to the point. Most doctors do not charge for prenatal interviews, and five minutes is usually enough to make a doctor assessment. If you honestly feel you need more time, offer to make a regular appointment so you can pay for the time. Rambling about future behavior worries or trying to cover the whole field of pediatrics, from bed-wetting to vitamins, is not the purpose of your visit.

- Are you and the doctor of a similar mindset? For example, if you are committed to breastfeeding and your doctor is a charter member of the bottlefeeding set, he or she may be Dr. Wrong for you.

- Ask about the availability of special services in your doctor's practice. For example, if you are planning to breastfeed, does your doctor employ the services of a lactation consultant, and how does he or she use the consultant?

- Browse around the office. Either before or after your time with the doctor, here are some observations to consider as you make your reconnaissance. Sit in the waiting room awhile and observe the spirit of the office. Is there a child-considered atmosphere, orderly but friendly and flexible? Is there child-considered furniture that is practical and safe? Is the staff approachable over what may seem to you the silliest of questions?

- Observe the provision for separating sick, possibly contagious children from those who are well. Separate "sick" and "well" waiting rooms, a favorite question on printed sheets handed out at childbirth classes, are impractical. Nobody wants to use the sick waiting room. A more practical method for separating sick and well patients is to immediately shuttle poten-

tially contagious children into an examining room, leaving the waiting room for children who are there for checkups and children who are not contagious.

- Ask the staff for other information: insurance plans, office hours, medical fees, hospital affiliations, availability and coverage when off call, and credentials of medical training. Ask how emergencies are handled, how the office handles phone calls, approximate waiting time, and who does what in the office when you have a question.

Choosing Dr. Right — either a family practitioner or pediatrician — is an investment. Your baby's doctor becomes like another member of the family, an Uncle Harry or Aunt Nancy, who, as your child grows, also grows in the knowledge of your child and family. This is the doctor who examines your newborn fresh after delivery, gets you through those early feeding problems, turns off the runny nose, eases the pain of the middle-of-the-night ear infection, counsels the bed wetter, helps with school problems, and clears the teenage acne. Choose this long-term partner wisely.

CHOOSING OTHER VIPs

In addition to choosing among childbirth options, a birth attendant, a childbirth class, and a baby doctor, there are other choices you will be called upon to make.

Support Groups

Other important members of your extended family before and after birth are support groups of like-minded and experienced parents. The information you receive and the friends you make often carry over into helpful parenting support during your first year as parents. Of the many parenting organizations, the oldest, largest, and the one we most recommend is La Leche League International. You may also find valuable support groups and parent-education classes at your local hospital, YMCA, or church or synagogue. Attend as many of these group meetings as time and energy allow. From each group select the information that best fits your own life-style and the style of parenting you are most comfortable with.

Lactation Consultants

Another very important person for the beginning parent, a lactation consultant is a specialist trained to help the new mother get the right start in her breastfeeding career. Fifteen years ago we tried an experiment with breastfeeding mothers in our practice. Each mother received a one-hour consultation from one of our lactation consultants within forty-eight hours after birth. Results: a 50 percent decline in breastfeeding problems such as sore nipples and insufficient milk. More important, mothers better enjoyed the interaction in which they would be spending the most time — feeding their baby. Obtain the name of a lactation consultant from your birth attendant, hospital, pediatrician's office, or local La Leche League. Look for the credentials IBCLC (International Board of Certified Lactation Consultants). Arrange to have a consultation with her a day or two after birth. Even better, if you are apprehensive about breastfeeding or have nipples inconducive to proper latch-on (see page 124), consult a lactation specialist before birth.

CHOOSING WHETHER TO BREASTFEED OR BOTTLEFEED

By now you probably have decided how to feed your baby. But if you are still on the fence about feeding, consider the following decision-helping tips:

- Remember this is a very personal decision involving individual preferences and life-styles. Don't be discouraged by well-meaning friends who confess, "Breastfeeding didn't work for me." In most of these cases it didn't work because they breastfed in a nonsupportive atmosphere and without early professional help.

- Attend a series of La Leche League meetings before the birth of your baby. Ask other breastfeeding mothers what breastfeeding has done for them and their baby. Breastfeeding is a life-style, not just a method of feeding. Surround yourself with like-minded, supportive mothers. Many women are intellectually convinced that breastfeeding is best but are not prepared for the energy commitments of this style of feeding, and here is where the need for support comes in.

- Read Chapter 8, "Breastfeeding: Why and How," and the section "Formula Facts" (page 200) to learn not only why your milk is best for your baby, but also what's in it for you.

- If you are still undecided by birth time, give breastfeeding a thirty-day trial, using all the right-start tips discussed on page 127. It is easy to go from breast to bottle, but the reverse is very difficult. Many breastfeeding mothers find that after they get over the hump of the first few weeks of learning latch-on and establish a routine, they settle down into a comfortable and lasting breastfeeding relationship. If after the trial period you do not joyfully anticipate most feedings, or if you feel pressured to breastfeed but really do not wish to, consider an alternative method of feeding or a combination. It's important to feed your baby in a way that works for both of you.

CIRCUMCISED OR INTACT?

No part of an infant's body has stirred so much international debate as this tiny half inch of skin. Whole cultures and religious groups circumcise as a ritual and as a right; national organizations, even international conventions, come together to protect the foreskin — and they have appropriate protective titles: Intact, No Circ, and Peaceful Beginnings. Some parents definitely want their son circumcised for religious or cultural reasons, or they just prefer circumcision. A new father once told us, "I want my son to have a maintenance-free penis." Others are adamant, nearly militant, about leaving the penis intact. Some agonize about this decision, feeling, "I'm going to great lengths to bring my baby into the world as gently as possible. Circumcision just doesn't seem to fit the scene." If you are undecided about your son's foreskin, read on.

Circumcision was once considered routine procedure for most newborn males in the United States, but, as with most routine procedures, many parents question if circumcision is really necessary for their babies. The following are the most common questions we are asked about circumcision. The answers are intended to help you make an informed choice.

How is circumcision performed?

Baby is placed on a restraining board, and his hands and feet are secured by straps. A local anesthetic is usually injected into the foreskin of the penis. The tight adhesions between the foreskin and the glans (or head) of the penis are separated with a medical instrument. The foreskin is held in place by metal clamps while a vertical cut is made into the foreskin to about one-third of its length. A metal or plastic bell is placed over the head of the penis to protect the glans, and the foreskin is pulled up over the bell and circumferentially cut. Between one-third and one-half of the skin of the penis (which is what the foreskin is) is removed. A protective lubricant is put on to cover the incision area for a few days. The healing of the circumcised area takes approximately one week, during which time you can expect the circumcision, like most cuts, to go through the usual stages of healing. (See "Care of the Circumcision Site," page 83.)

Is circumcision a safe procedure?

Circumcision is usually a very safe surgical procedure. There are rarely any complications. As with any surgical procedure, however, there are occasional problems such as bleeding, infection, or injury to the penis. If there is a family history of bleeding tendencies or one of your previous newborns bled a lot during circumcision, be sure to inform your doctor of this fact.

Does it hurt?

Yes, it hurts. The skin of the penis of a newborn baby has pain receptors completely sensitive to clamping and cutting. The myth that newborns do not feel pain came from the observation that newborns sometimes withdraw into a deep sleep toward the end of the operation. This *does not mean* that they do not feel pain. Falling into a deep sleep is a retreat mechanism, a withdrawal reaction as a consequence of overwhelming pain. Not only does circumcision cause pain in the penis, the rest of the newborn's overall physiology is upset. During unanesthetized circumcision, stress hormones rise, the heart rate speeds, and valuable blood oxygen diminishes. Sick babies and premature babies should never be subjected to this shock.

A local anesthetic can and should always be used. Painless circumcision should be a birthright. I have used a local anesthesia in nearly a thousand babies over the past twenty years. It is a safe procedure and it works. Sometimes the anesthetic will not remove all the pain, but it certainly helps. Within a few hours, after the anesthetic wears off, some babies exhibit no discomfort; others will fuss for the next twenty-four hours. The most common and effective method is called a dorsal penile nerve block, in which a few drops of Xylocaine (similar to the anesthetic your dentist uses) is injected into the nerves in the skin on each side of the base of the penis.

Does circumcision make the penis easier to keep clean?

Making hygiene easier is often a reason given for performing circumcision. In the adolescent and the adult male the glands of the foreskin secrete a fluid called smegma. These secretions may accumulate beneath the foreskin. Sometimes, though rarely, the penis becomes infected. Removing the foreskin removes the secretions, makes the care of the penis easier, and lessens the risk of infection.

With normal bathing, however, an intact foreskin is quite easy to care for.

What happens if the foreskin is left intact?

Leaving the foreskin intact protects the penis from irritation caused by rubbing on wet and soiled diapers. At birth it is impossible to make a judgment about how tight the foreskin will remain, since almost all boys have tight foreskins for the first year. In about 50 percent of boys the foreskin loosens from the head of the penis and retracts completely by two years. By three years of age, 90 percent of intact boys have fully retractable foreskins. Once the foreskin retracts easily, it becomes a part of normal male hygiene to pull back the foreskin and cleanse beneath it during a bath. While it is true that infections from the secretions beneath the foreskin can more often be a problem in intact males, simple hygiene can prevent this problem.

If the foreskin doesn't retract naturally, will the boy need a circumcision later on?

Circumcision is very rarely necessary for medical reasons, but occasionally the foreskin does not retract, becomes tight and infected, and obstructs the flow of urine. This unusual condition, called phimosis, requires circumcision. If circumcision for phimosis is necessary later on in childhood or adulthood, anesthesia is given, and the boy is involved in the decision.

How do we care for the foreskin if left intact?

Above all, *do not forcibly retract the foreskin,* but allow it to retract naturally over a number of years. Retracting the foreskin before it is time loosens the protective seal between the foreskin and glans and increases the chance of infection. If you choose to leave your baby's foreskin intact, follow these suggestions for its care. In most babies the foreskin is tightly adhered to the underlying head of the penis during the first year. As your baby begins having normal erections, the foreskin gradually loosens itself, but may not fully retract until the second or third year. *Leave the foreskin alone* until it retracts easily, which occurs between six months and three years. The age at which the foreskin begins to retract varies considerably from baby to baby. Respect this difference and *do not allow anyone to prematurely break the seal* between the foreskin and the head of the penis, which may allow secretions to accumulate beneath the foreskin and cause infection. As the foreskin naturally retracts (usually around the third year) gently clean out the secretions that may have accumulated between the foreskin and the glans of the penis. This should be done as part of the child's normal bath routine. Usually by three years of age, when most foreskins are fully retracted, your child can be taught to clean beneath his foreskin as part of his normal bath routine.

If he isn't circumcised, won't he feel different from his friends?

You cannot predict how different your son will feel if he is circumcised or intact. Boys generally have a wider acceptance of these individual differences than adults do. Locker-room comparisons are a bit of a myth. It is difficult to know whether the majority of the boys will be circumcised or intact in the future. The number of circumcisions has been steadily declining in recent years as more parents begin to question routine circumcision. In the western United States around 63 percent of the infant males are being left intact, up from 50 percent in the early 1980s.

My husband is circumcised. Shouldn't my son be the same as his father?

Some fathers have strong feelings that if they are circumcised, their sons should be, and this feeling is only natural. But the "like father, like son" complex alone is not a good reason to choose circumcision, as few fathers and sons compare foreskins. It will be many years before the boy looks like the father anyway. Even some of these fathers (usually because of pressure from their wives) are beginning to question the necessity of routine circumcision.

We have a son who is already circumcised. Should brothers be the same?

Since little boys do sometimes compare the styles of their penis, many parents feel that sameness is important among brothers. Just as you learn a lot from your first birth and may choose a different style for the next, not every male in the family must be circumcised. If you choose to leave your next child intact, your problem will most likely be not in explaining to your intact child why he is intact but rather in explaining to your circumcised child why his foreskin is missing.

Does circumcision prevent any disease?

Circumcision does not prevent cancer of the penis, which is a very rare disease anyway and occurs more frequently in males who do not practice proper hygiene. Cervical cancer, which is not prevented by circumcision, is not more common in the sexual partners of intact males who practice proper hygiene. Circumcision also does not prevent sexually transmitted diseases.

The decision is yours. As you can see from the previous discussion, there is no compelling reason for circumcision. If you are looking to your doctor to be your son's foreskin attorney, you may still be left undecided. In 1999 the American Academy of Pediatrics issued the opinion that current data are "not sufficient to recommend routine circumcision," adding "circumcision is not essential to the child's well-being."

CORD BLOOD STEM CELL BANKING

When a baby is born, stem cells can be collected from the umbilical cord. Stem cells are immature white blood cells that are abundant within the bloodstream of a fetus and newborn. As a baby gets older, these stem cells mature and differentiate into a variety of white blood cell types, which protect the body from infection. Here are some questions you may have about stem cell banking.

What is the purpose of banking, or storing, stem cells?

If a person is diagnosed with leukemia or one of a variety of other cancers of the bloodstream, chemotherapy or radiation is used to kill the cancerous blood cells. Unfortunately, this treatment also kills most of the normal blood cells in the bloodstream and bone marrow, leaving the person extremely vulnerable to infection until the bone marrow regenerates enough white blood cells. Certain people in this situation receive a bone marrow transplant, which is an infusion of a large supply of stem cells from a donor. These cells repopulate the bone marrow. Complications can arise if the donated stem cells are not a perfect match with the patient's own immune system and therefore are rejected. Cord blood stem cell banking provides a perfectly matched supply of stem cells that won't be rejected. They can also be used by another family member whose immune system matches.

How are the stem cells collected?

The long portion of umbilical cord that is still attached to the placenta inside the uterus contains a large amount of the baby's blood that was circulating through the umbilical cord and placenta at the time the cord was cut. The labor attendant drains this blood out of the cord (thus the term "cord blood") by either squeezing the blood into a tube or using a needle to withdraw the blood into a syringe. It is painless and only takes five extra minutes. The blood is not taken from the mom or the baby. If it is not collected for banking, it is thrown away.

How are the stem cells stored?

The cells are filtered out of the whole cord blood and frozen in liquid nitrogen or by another deep-freeze method.

Are there any drawbacks to this procedure?

The only negative aspect is what it does to your bank account. At this writing, cord blood stem cell banking costs approximately $1,500. There is also a yearly storage fee of around $150. You can find advertisements in pregnancy and childbirth magazines for various cord blood stem cell banks. It's necessary to make arrangements for collecting the blood sample well in advance of your due date.

Dr. Bob notes: *There is no right or wrong decision about whether or not you should* *store your baby's cord blood stem cells. The hope is that you will never need the stem cells. Leukemia and other blood cancers are extremely rare. Out of tens of thousands of units of stem cells that have been stored, only a few dozen have been used by donors so far. On the other hand, if the cost is not a hardship, then you may want to consider it. Other medical conditions may be treated with stem cells in the future.*

EXPANDED NEWBORN SCREENING BLOOD TEST

Every newborn gets a blood test twenty-four hours after birth to check for a variety of inherited conditions that could have a significant impact on an infant's health. These include phenylketonuria, or PKU, and hypothyroidism. There is, however, an aspect of this testing that you should consider well in advance of your baby's birth. Currently there is no worldwide or even national standard for deciding what conditions a baby should be tested for. Many states test for only three or four conditions, which is only a fraction of the dozens of genetic and metabolic diseases that can be detected by newborn screening. If these conditions are detected and treated early, in many cases their harmful effects can be prevented. Some states are now offering *expanded* newborn screening tests for dozens of conditions. If you live in a state that does not offer expanded testing, you can order a testing kit from a commercial lab in advance, and the health care provider can collect blood for the expanded testing at the same time the standard test is done. The

cost is usually between $50 and $100. Look for advertisements in pregnancy and childbirth magazines. Many of the cord blood stem cell banks also offer expanded newborn screening.

PREPARING YOUR NEST

You've glanced wishfully through those baby magazines for months, admiring the dazzling colors of designer nurseries, the animal-appliquéd bedding and matching ensembles. Now, with birth only weeks away, you too can design your nest and outfit your baby as plain or as fancy as your imagination and budget allow. Just the thought of your baby-to-be brings back the doll-dressing instinct and the spendthrift in you. Pocket your credit cards. You will be amazed how few items you absolutely have to buy.

Clothing Tips

Buy the basics. Purchase only what you will need for the first couple of weeks. As soon as baby arrives, so do the gifts. Grandparents splurge and gifts come pouring in from baby showers.

Plan now — buy later. Make a list of items you need and items you want. Check off the items that you are given or able to borrow, and purchase the rest as the need arises. Periodically update your list according to baby's developmental needs and your strength to resist the tempting delights in the baby-product catalogs.

Buy large. Plan at least one size ahead. Buy a few three-month-sized outfits, but most of baby's early wardrobe should be size six to nine months. Letting baby live with the baggy look is not only more comfortable but gets more mileage from the clothing.

Buy few. Buy only a few of the clothing basics at each stage of development, as the steady stream of gifts will likely continue. Babies outgrow their clothes long before they outwear them, leaving a closet filled with rows of hanging mementos of a stage that passed too soon.

Buy safe and comfortable. The beads and buttons on a tight knit outfit may look irresistible in the catalog, but will it be safe and comfortable on baby? Buttons are out; snaps are in. Baby can choke on buttons — and besides, who has time for them anymore? Also watch out for loose threads and fringes that could catch and strangle baby's fingers and toes, and avoid strings and ribbons longer than eight inches (twenty centimeters) — they are strangulation hazards.

Choose easy-access clothing. When examining an irresistible outfit, imagine dressing your baby. Does it have easy access to the diaper area? Is the head opening roomy enough, and does it contain neck snaps to make it easy to slip on?

Think cotton. The most comfortable fabric is 100 percent cotton. Many babies find synthetic clothing irritating, yet in order for sleepwear to comply with federal fire codes, it must be flame-retardant. The good news is that this is becoming available in 100 percent cotton.

> ## CO-SLEEPERS
>
> A wonderful innovation to join the crib and cradle selection is a co-sleeper, a bedside bassinette that attaches safely and securely to the side of the parents' bed. A co-sleeper allows you and your baby to have separate sleeping space, yet it keeps baby within arm's reach for easy nursing and comforting. See www.armsreach.com, the website of the Arm's Reach Co-sleeper, or call (800) 954-9353 or (818) 879-9353.

Designing Your Baby's Nursery

The patterns are endless — so is the fun. Hold on to your credit cards as you journey through nursery fantasyland. There is the heirloom look with a four-poster crib that may have housed decades of family babies. You have the country look — a collection of wicker and patchwork quilts. For the delicate, there is the marshmallow motif, the elegance of white with the soft and puffy feel. And in your vision of the perfect nursery, there is mother, sitting peacefully cribside in her padded rocking chair reading Mother Goose. As you take your fantasy walk down nursery lane, dad may throw in a few plain and simple hints, "I can fix up . . . , I can repaint . . . , and remember the garage sales."

Undaunted by your quest for the perfect nest, you continue leafing through baby-furniture magazines imagining how your precious babe will look in each setting. You're not only feeling soft, you're thinking pretty. Then along comes a friend of yours, an infant stimulator (alias a mother, hip on things baby) who puts a new twist in your soft designs. "Pastels are out, black and white is in," she informs. Ms. Stimulator extols the mind-building virtues of contrasting stripes and dots (which have been shown to hold baby's attention longer than pastels). She subscribes to all the right baby magazines. You've become confused as to whether a nursery should help baby think or sleep. The zebra or Dalmation look is not what you envisioned.

By the time you've been through the nursery mill, your mind is filled with visions of every dazzling color and imaginable motif. Just as you are about to reach the end of your designer rope, you meet a group of experienced parents who know the nursery scene. There is your pediatrician, who admonishes you to, above all, think *safety*. Dad runs into a seasoned survivor of the shopping scene who suggests you buy the basics and spend the extra money on the mother. Your psychologist friend warns about the terminal dependency that occurs in babies that sleep with their parents, and your mother reminds you that you were one of those high-need babies who wanted to sleep snuggled next to your mom and dad and who was unwilling to join the crib-and-cradle set. It begins to dawn on you: "What's wrong with these nursery pictures? My baby may not be in any of them. Perhaps we should wait to see what the sleep temperament of our baby is."

By now you're still thinking pretty, but practical. "Perhaps we can borrow a crib and splurge on a king-size bed for us." Finally along comes the fairy godmother to add a happy ending to the nursery tale. She advises, "Have fun with your nursery — that's what it's for."

PREPARING FOR BABY

The following checklists should help you get organized as you prepare to welcome a new member into your family. Don't be overwhelmed by a long shopping list of "things" for baby. Most of what your baby really needs you already have — warm milk, warm hearts, strong arms, and endless patience — and these don't cost any money. (For further information about specific items in the list, consult the index.)

OUTFITTING BABY'S LAYETTE AND NURSERY

First Wardrobe
- [ ] Four terry-cloth sleepers
- [ ] Three pairs of bootees or socks
- [ ] Two receiving blankets
- [ ] Three undershirts
- [ ] Three lightweight tops (kimonos, sacques, and/or gowns)
- [ ] Burp cloths (cloth diapers work well)

As Baby Grows
- [ ] Four rompers (snap-at-the-crotch outfits)
- [ ] Two washable bibs
- [ ] Outing clothes, according to age and occasion

Seasonal Clothes
- [ ] Two hats: sun hat, lightweight with brim; heavier-weight ear-covering hat for cold weather

- ☐ Two sweaters, weight according to season
- ☐ One bunting with attached mitts for cold weather
- ☐ Two blankets, weight according to season

Diapering Needs

- ☐ Package of disposable diapers
- ☐ Three-dozen cloth diapers (we suggest diaper service)
- ☐ Diaper pins or clips
- ☐ Three waterproof diaper covers (or consider all-in-one diapers)
- ☐ Diaper pail (usually supplied by diaper service)
- ☐ Cotton balls, cotton swabs
- ☐ Premoistened disposable baby wipes/washcloths
- ☐ Diaper-rash cream (zinc-oxide type)
- ☐ Black-and-white mobile to hang above changing area

Feeding Supplies

Bottlefeeding Items

- ☐ Four bottles, four-ounce (120-milliliter)
- ☐ Four nipples (see nipple suggestions, page 210)
- ☐ Utensils: tongs, measuring pitchers, spoons, can opener, bottle brush, sterilizing pot

Breastfeeding Helpers

- ☐ Three nursing bras
- ☐ Breast pads, no plastic lining
- ☐ Nursing blouses and dresses
- ☐ Baby sling
- ☐ Footstool to prop feet while feeding
- ☐ Extra pillows, or a nursing pillow

Bedding Supplies

- ☐ Two rubber-backed waterproof pads
- ☐ Three crib or bassinet sheets
- ☐ Soft comforter
- ☐ Bassinet blankets, weight according to season

Bathing Supplies

- ☐ Two soft washcloths
- ☐ Two terry-cloth towels with hoods
- ☐ Baby soap and shampoo
- ☐ Baby bathtub
- ☐ Baby brush and comb
- ☐ Baby nail scissors or clippers

Toiletries and Medical Supplies for First Couple of Months

(See "Stocking Your Home First Aid Kit," page 635, for a more extensive list.)

- ☐ Mild laundry soap
- ☐ Petroleum jelly
- ☐ Rectal thermometer
- ☐ Antiseptic for cord care
- ☐ Nasal aspirator (an ear syringe may be used)
- ☐ Antibacterial ointment
- ☐ Cotton balls, cotton swabs
- ☐ Infant acetaminophen
- ☐ Vaporizer, type to be recommended by doctor
- ☐ Penlight, tongue depressors for checking mouth (sores, thrush, and so on)

Nursery Equipment and Furnishings

- ☐ Bassinet or cradle, or
- ☐ Crib and accessories, or
- ☐ Co-sleeper
- ☐ Changing table or padded work area
- ☐ Changing-table covers, two quilted mattress pads

☐ Rocking chair
☐ Storage chest for clothing

On-the-Go Accessories
☐ Baby sling for carrying baby
☐ Car seat

☐ Car-seat cover
☐ Car-seat head support
☐ Diaper bag

PACKING FOR BIRTH

Clothing for Mother
☐ Two old bathrobes (count on stains)
☐ Two nightgowns
☐ Loose-fitting clothes for going home
☐ Slippers or scuffs, washable
☐ Two pairs of warm socks
☐ Two nursing bras
☐ Nursing gown

Labor-Saving Devices
☐ Your favorite pillow
☐ Watch for timing contractions
☐ CD player with favorite music
☐ Massage lotion
☐ Rubber ball for back rubs
☐ Snacks, your favorite: lollipops, honey, dried and fresh fruit, juices, granola, sandwiches for father

Toiletries
☐ Soap, deodorant, shampoo, conditioner (avoid perfumes; may upset baby)
☐ Hairbrush, hairdryer
☐ Toothbrush, toothpaste

☐ Sanitary napkins (supplied by hospital)
☐ Cosmetics
☐ Glasses or contact lenses

Homecoming Clothes for Baby
☐ One undershirt
☐ Socks or bootees
☐ Receiving blanket
☐ One sacque or gown
☐ Cap
☐ Bunting and heavy blanket if cold weather
☐ Infant car seat
☐ Diapers for going home

Other Items
☐ Video and regular camera
☐ Insurance forms
☐ Hospital preadmittance forms
☐ Cell phone
☐ Address book
☐ Favorite book and magazines
☐ "Birthday" gift for sibling(s)
☐ This book

4

Getting the Right Start
with Your Newborn

Time seemed to crawl during your pregnancy. That elusive due date felt as if it would never come. Now the long-awaited moment is here, and everything happens so fast. Yesterday you were "still pregnant"; today you're a mother.

BABY'S FIRST MINUTES

In making the transition from womb to air breathing, baby experiences a lot of changes.

First Events

The first business at hand is to make sure baby has a safe and healthy entry into the world. Baby is born with his mouth and nose full of water (amniotic fluid). Your birth attendant suctions this fluid to make way for air. Baby gets his first "nose blow" within seconds after birth, sometimes even as his head emerges and the rest of his body is still inside. After suctioning the fluid from baby's breathing passages, your birth attendant cuts and clamps the cord, and baby begins life outside the womb. Most often these events can take

place with baby nestled on your abdomen, a soft cushion from which to be initiated into the rites of extra-uterine life.

First Touch

Birth is a hands-on affair. During the drama of birth, many mothers instinctively reach down and touch baby's head as it emerges from the birth canal, as if needing to get their hands on their baby during the delivery. (If the pushing stage is prolonged, the mother can be greatly encouraged if she can touch the small amount of her baby's head that is finally within reach. This helps her to organize her bearing down by showing her how to direct her efforts.) Some birth attendants encourage dad to touch baby's head or even to get his hands on the whole baby as she emerges from the birth canal, giving him a sense of taking part in the delivery.

I vividly remember the feelings I had at the birth of our sixth baby, Matthew. Because our birth attendant was late for the delivery, I had the privilege of "catching" our baby. (When I boast to friends that I delivered our baby, Martha is quick to correct me. *She* delivered Matthew; I caught. Why should dad get all the credit when mom did all the work? Martha is right.) I still remember the ecstasy I felt when my hands first held the head of my son. That was a very special relationship we had at the moment of birth; we still have a special relationship years later — any connection? That first touch Matthew may never remember, but I will never forget.

Since then, I've become a veteran baby catcher dad, as I also ushered babies number seven and eight (I was there for the birth of our adopted daughter as well) into the world. Many birth attendants are now offering fathers an opportunity to connect with their babies in this special way. This first touch isn't for all dads (or moms) — but if it is important to you, ask for it.

First Transition

As soon as the cord is clamped and cut, baby makes the most important switch of his or her life — the transition from womb breathing (via the placenta and the umbilical cord) to air breathing. Some babies click in immediately, or "pink up." Others need a few puffs of oxygen and/or gentle stimulation to initiate breathing.

First Meeting

After "all systems are go" — meaning baby is pink and breathing well — the birth attendant places baby on your abdomen (if he's not there already) skin to skin, tummy to tummy, his head nestling between your breasts, and covers him with a warm absorbent towel to get him dry and keep him warm. Encourage baby to nestle cheek to breast and lick or suck your nipple. If he

seems upset and continues to cry, realize he has just been through a very harrowing experience. Your warm hand firmly on his back can give him the feeling of being securely held. This safe, warm place, together with your rhythmic breathing, is just what he needs to calm his nerves from the stress of birth. Once he starts sucking at your breast, he will calm even more.

This first snuggle is not just sound psychology, it's good medicine. Newborns easily get cold. Draping your baby tummy to tummy, cheek to breast, allows a natural transfer of heat from mother to newborn. And sucking from your nipple stimulates the hormone oxytocin, which helps your uterus contract, minimizing postpartum bleeding.

This first meeting should be a private one. After the birth attendants are sure that mother and baby are well, and the theatrics of birth are over, request some family bonding time alone — just the three of you, mother, father, and baby (and siblings if allowed and desired). This is a special time of family intimacy that should not be interrupted by trivial routines.

First Impressions

Immediately after birth, babies usually appear distressed — pained grimace, wrinkled forehead, puffy eyes, tightly flexed limbs, and clenched fists. Within minutes after birth most newborns enter a state of quiet alertness. This is the prime state of receptivity in which a newborn can best relate with his or her new environment. Baby's eyes and body language reflect this state. When quietly alert, baby's eyes are wide open and searching for another set of eyes — give him yours. During the prime time of this premiere appearance, baby will look into your eyes, snuggle against your breasts, relax his fists and limbs, and quietly melt into the contours of your body. While in this intimate space, baby and mother share a mutual need: baby's need to be comforted and mother's need to be in touch with her baby. During this first interaction baby takes in the sound of your voice, your scent, the feel of your warm skin, and the sweet taste of his first food. As baby continues to suckle and you continue to soothe, you both feel right. Within an hour after birth, baby may drift contentedly into a deep sleep.

First Feelings

Imagine for a moment what your baby feels during this first meeting. By giving your baby a smooth transition from the inside womb to the outside womb of your skin, arms, and breasts, baby learns that *distress is followed by comfort;* that the world outside the womb is a warm and comfortable place. The connection continues, birth having changed only the way this connection is expressed.

The baby you now see is the baby you have been feeling all along, someone you have known and finally get to meet. We have noticed that in this first meeting mothers and fathers look at their newborn with a sort of wide-angle lens, getting an overall picture of the uniqueness of this little person. Then they gradually focus on their newborn's special characteristics. One first feeling we have noticed new parents express is that of immediately welcoming their newborn as a person, the newest member in the family. "She has your ears," mother may say to father. "She has her grandmother's nose," parents may exclaim.

BONDING — WHAT IT MEANS, HOW TO DO IT

Bonding — the term for the close emotional tie that develops between parents and baby at birth — was the buzzword of the 1980s. The concept of bonding was explored by Dr. Marshall H. Klaus and Dr. John H. Kennell in their classic book *Maternal-Infant Bonding.* These researchers speculated that for humans, just as for other types of animals, there is a "sensitive period" at birth when mothers and newborns are uniquely programmed to be in contact with each other and do good things to each other. By comparing mother-infant pairs who bonded immediately after birth with those who didn't, they concluded that the early-contact mother-infant pairs later developed a closer attachment.

When the concept hit the delivery room, it received mixed reviews. Parents and pediatricians enthusiastically welcomed the idea, mostly because it made sense. Behavior researchers were skeptical about whether the way a mother and baby spent the first hour together could have any lifelong effects.

We have carefully studied the concept of bonding. Based upon our review of bonding research and our own observations, here is what we believe is a balanced view of birth bonding.

Mother-Newborn Bonding

Bonding is really a continuation of the relationship that began during pregnancy, strengthened by the constant awareness of a growing life inside you. The physical and chemical changes that were occurring in your body reminded you of the presence of this person. Birth cements this bond and gives it reality. Now you can see, feel, and talk to the little person whom you knew only as the "bulge," or from the movements and the heartbeat you heard through medical instruments. Bonding allows you to transfer your life-giving love for the infant inside to caregiving love for the one outside. Inside, you gave your blood; outside, you give your milk, your eyes, your hands, your voice — your entire self.

Bonding brings mothers and newborns back together. Bonding studies provided the catalyst for family-oriented birthing policies in hospitals. It brought babies out of nurseries to room-in with their mothers. Bonding research reaffirmed the importance of the mother as the newborn's primary caregiver.

Bonding is not a now-or-never phenomenon. While there is little scientific basis for concluding that missing the initial bonding permanently weakens the parent-child relationship, we believe that bonding during this biologically sensitive period does give the parent-infant relationship a head start. Yet immediate bonding after birth is not like instant glue that cements a parent-child relationship forever.

What about the baby who for some reason, such as prematurity or cesarean birth, is temporarily separated from his mother after birth? Is the baby permanently affected by the loss of this early contact period? Catch-up bonding is certainly possible, especially in the resilient human species. The conception of bonding as an absolutely critical period or a now-or-never relationship is not true. From birth through infancy and childhood, there are many steps that lead to a strong mother-infant attachment. As soon as mothers and babies are reunited, creating a strong mother-infant connection by practicing the attachment style of parenting can compensate for the loss of this early opportunity for bonding. We have seen adopting parents who, upon first contact with their one-week-old newborn, release feelings as deep and as caring as those of biological parents in the birth room.

Father-Newborn Bonding

Most of the bonding research has focused on mother-infant bonding, with the father given only honorable mention. In recent years fathers, too, have been the subject of bonding research and have even merited a special term for the father-infant relationship at birth — "engrossment." We used to talk about father involvement; now it's father engrossment — meaning involvement to a higher degree. Engrossment is not only what the father does for the baby — holding and comforting — but what the baby does for the father. Bonding with baby right after birth brings out sensitivity in dad.

Fathers are often portrayed as well meaning but bumbling when caring for newborns. Fathers are sometimes considered secondhand nurturers, nurturing the mother as she nurtures the baby. That's only half the story. Fathers have their own unique way of relating to babies, and babies need this difference.

In fact, studies on father bonding show that fathers who are given the opportunity and are encouraged to take an active part in caring for their newborns can become just as nurturing as mothers. A father's nurturant responses may be a little less automatic and a little slower to unfold than a mother's, but fathers are capable of a strong bonding attachment to their infants during the newborn period.

Bonding After Cesarean Births

A cesarean section is a surgical procedure, but it is primarily a birth, the dignity of which needs to be respected. Bonding is not lost if a cesarean birth is necessary; it's just that the timing and the roles change a bit. Fathers have long been welcome at cesarean births, and it is a beautiful sight to see a father with his newborn during a surgical birth. Here are some ways to foster birth bonding following cesarean delivery.

For the mother. Epidural anesthesia, with which you are anesthetized from the level of the navel to the toes, is now routine for C-sections. Unlike general anesthesia, which puts you to sleep during the birth, an epidural anesthesia allows you to be awake and aware during the procedure, and you are able to enjoy bonding with your baby despite the operation. Expect the bonding time to be somewhat limited, since you may feel physically overwhelmed, have only one arm free to hold your baby (there will be an intravenous drip in your other arm), and your baby may be able to spend just a few minutes cheek to cheek and eye to eye with you. The important thing is that you connect with your baby immediately after birth, by either a visual or a touch connection. Though bonding is different after a surgical birth, an important connection is still made. (See the discussion of breastfeeding after a cesarean, page 184.)

For the father. You can sit at the head of the table holding your wife's hand during the operation. At the moment of birth, you are able to look over the sterile drape and see baby being lifted up and out. After being surgically removed from the uterus, baby is taken immediately to a nearby infant warmer, suctioned, given oxygen if necessary, and attended until all systems are go. As soon as the baby is stable (which usually takes a little longer than a vaginal birth) you or a birth attendant bring baby over to have some bonding time with mother. Then, while the operation is being completed and your wife is in the recovery room, go with your baby to the nursery and begin father-bonding time. Hold your baby in the nursery, rock your baby, talk and sing and stroke your baby — father bonding at its best. If your baby needs special care, you can still be there next to the isolette, and when the nursery staff gives the green light, you can get your hands on your baby and have your baby hear your voice. You'll find that your baby will respond to your voice because he's heard it all along in utero. I have noticed that fathers who get their hands on their babies and take an active part in their baby's care immediately after birth find it easier to get attached to their babies later.

As the former director of a university hospital newborn nursery, I have attended many cesarean births and personally escorted many fathers — some willing, some reluctant — from the operating room into the nursery, where I put them to work. Here's a story about Tim and what his cesarean-birthed baby did to him. I had met Tim and his wife, Mary, prenatally, and Mary shared with me that she had difficulty getting her husband involved in the pregnancy and feared that he was not going to be involved in the birth. She expected that he would probably be one of those dads who would become involved as soon as the child was old enough to throw a football. Tim thought this whole scene of delivering babies was strictly a woman's thing and that he would stay in the waiting room. As it turned out, Mary needed a cesarean, and I persuaded Tim to accompany her into the operating room and to be at her side during the delivery. After the baby was born and all her vital systems were stable, I wrapped baby in two warm blankets and orchestrated some bonding time among Mary, Tim, and baby Tiffany while the operation was completed. I then asked Tim to come with me to the nursery. It did not surprise me that his initial reluctance about getting involved in the birth was already melting. Tim was still in awe of all the theatrics surrounding the operation, but he willingly followed me.

While in the nursery, I said to Tim, "I need to attend another delivery. It's necessary that someone stay with your baby and stimulate her, because babies breathe better when someone is stroking them and talking to them." I encouraged Tim to get his hands on his baby, sing to her, rub her back, and just let himself be as loving and caring as he could. He looked around as though to be sure none of his cronies was watching and agreed to do these "motherly" things. I returned about a half hour later and saw big Tim standing there singing to and stroking his baby as the pair were really getting to know each other. I assured him that his initial investment was going to pay long-term dividends. The next day, when I made my hospital rounds and went in to talk with Mary, she exclaimed, "What on earth happened to my husband? I can't get our baby away from him. He's really hooked. He would breastfeed if he could. I never thought I'd see that big guy be so sensitive."

More Bonding Tips

Delay routine procedures. Oftentimes the attending nurse does routine procedures, gives the vitamin K shot, and instills eye ointment in baby's eyes immediately after birth and then presents baby to mother for bonding. Ask the nurse to delay these procedures for an hour or so, until your new baby has enjoyed the initial bonding period. The eye ointment temporarily blurs baby's vision or causes her eyes to stay closed. She needs a clear first impression of you, and you need to see those eyes.

Stay connected. Ask your birth attendant and nurses to put your baby on your abdomen and chest immediately after birth, or after cutting the cord and suctioning your baby, unless a medical complication requires temporary separation.

Let your baby breastfeed right after birth. Most babies are content simply to lick the nipple; others have a strong desire to suck at the breast immediately after birth. As stated previously, this nipple stimulation releases the hormone oxytocin, which increases the contractions of your uterus and lessens postpartum bleeding. Early sucking also stimulates the release of prolactin, the hormone that helps your mothering abilities click in right from the start.

Touch your baby. Besides enjoying the stimulation your baby receives from the skin-to-skin contact of tummy to tummy and cheek to breast, gently stroke your baby, caressing his whole body. We have noticed that mothers and fathers often caress their babies differently. A new mother usually strokes her baby's entire body with a gentle caress of her fingertips; the father, however, often places an entire hand on his baby's head, as if symbolizing his commitment to protect the life he has fathered. Besides being

enjoyable, stroking the skin is medically beneficial to the newborn. The skin, the largest
organ in the human body, is very rich with
nerve endings. At the time when baby is
making the transition to air breathing, and
the initial breathing patterns are very irregular, stroking stimulates the newborn to
breathe more rhythmically — the therapeutic
value of a parent's touch.

Gaze at your newborn. Your newborn can
see you best with an eye-to-eye distance of
eight to ten inches (twenty to twenty-five
centimeters) — amazingly, about the usual
nipple-to-eye distance during breastfeeding.
Place your baby in the *en face* position,
adjusting your head and your baby's head in
the same position so that your eyes meet.
Enjoy this visual connection during the brief
period of quiet alertness after birth, before
baby falls into a deep sleep. Staring into your
baby's eyes may trigger a rush of beautiful
mothering feelings.

Talk to your newborn. During the first
hours and days after birth, a natural baby-talk
dialogue will develop between mother and
infant. Voice-analysis studies have shown a
unique rhythm and comforting cadence to
mother's voice.

GETTING TO KNOW YOUR NEWBORN

Of course, bonding does not end at the delivery bed — it is just the beginning! Making
visual, tactile, olfactory, auditory, and sucking
connection with your baby right after the
birth may make you feel you don't want to

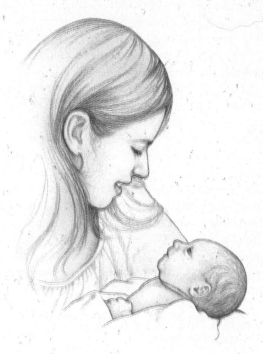

*Visual connection is an important part of the
bonding process; your newborn sees you best at
an eye-to-eye distance of around ten inches
(twenty-five centimeters).*

release this little person that you have
labored so hard to bring into the world —
and you don't have to. Your wombmate will
now become your roommate. We advise
healthy mothers and healthy babies to remain
together throughout their hospital stay.

Some babies make a stable transition from
womb to world without any complications;
others need a few hours in the nursery for
extra warmth, oxygen, suctioning, and other
special attention until their vital systems stabilize. Then they can return to the nursery of
mother's arms, "rooming-in."

Feelings after birth are unique to each
mother. Many mothers show the immediate
glow of motherhood and the "birth high"

excitement of a race finished and won. It's love at first sight, and they can't wait to get their hands on their baby and begin mothering within a millisecond after birth.

Others are relieved that the mammoth task of birth is over, that baby is normal. Now they are more interested in sleeping and recovering than bonding and mothering. As one mother said, following a lengthy and arduous labor, "Let me sleep for a few hours, take a shower, comb my hair, and then I'll start mothering." If these are your feelings, enjoy your rest — you've earned it. There is no need to succumb to pressure bonding when neither your body nor mind is willing or able. In this case, father bonds while mother rests.

ATTACHMENT-PROMOTING BEHAVIORS

Having your baby with you in your room is especially helpful for women who have difficulty jumping right into mothering. One day while making rounds I visited Jan, a new mother, only to find her sad. "What's wrong?" I inquired.

She confided, "All those gushy feelings I'm supposed to have about my baby — well, I don't! I'm nervous, tense, and don't know what to do."

I encouraged Jan. "Love at first sight doesn't happen to every couple, in courting or in parenting. For some mother-infant pairs it is a slow and gradual process. Don't worry, your baby will help you. But you have to set the conditions that allow the mother-infant care system to click in." And I went on to explain.

All babies are born with a group of special qualities called attachment-promoting behav-

iors — features and behaviors designed to alert the caregiver to the baby's presence and draw the caregiver, magnetlike, toward the baby. These features are the roundness of baby's eyes, cheeks, and body; the softness of the skin; the relative bigness of baby's eyes; the penetrating gaze; the incredible newborn scent; and, perhaps most important of all, baby's early language — the cries and precrying noises.

Here's how the early mother-infant communication system works. The opening sounds of the baby's cry activate a mother's emotions. This is physical as well as psychological. As discussed in Chapter 1, upon hearing her baby cry, a mother experiences an increased blood flow to her breasts, accompanied by the biological urge to pick up and nurse her baby. This is one of the strongest examples of how the biological signals of the baby trigger a biological response in the mother. There is no other signal in the world that sets off such intense responses in a mother as her baby's cry. At no other time in the child's life will language so forcefully stimulate the mother to act.

Picture what happens when babies and mothers are together. Baby begins to cry. Mother, because she is there and physically attuned to baby, immediately picks up and feeds her infant. Baby stops crying. When baby again awakens, squirms, grimaces, and then cries, mother responds in the same manner. The next time mother notices her baby's *precrying* cues. When baby awakens, squirms, and grimaces, mother picks up and feeds baby *before* he has to cry. She has learned to read her baby's signals and to respond appropriately. After rehearsing this dialogue many times during the hospital stay, mother and baby are working as a team. Baby learns to cue better; mother learns to respond better. As the attachment-promoting cries elicit a hormonal response in the mother, her milk-ejection reflex functions smoothly, and mother and infant are in biological harmony.

Now contrast this scene with the way an infant used to be cared for in the hospital nursery. Picture this newborn infant lying in a plastic box. He awakens, hungry, and cries along with twenty other hungry babies in plastic boxes who have by now all managed to awaken one another. A kind and caring nurse hears the cries and responds as soon as time permits. But she has no biological attachment to this baby, no inner programming tuned to that particular newborn, nor do her hormones change when the baby cries. The crying, hungry baby is taken to her mother in due time. The problem is that the baby's cry has two phases: The early sounds of the cry have an attachment-promoting quality, whereas the later sounds of the unattended cry are more disturbing to listen to and may actually promote avoidance.

The mother who has missed the opening scene in this biological drama because she was not present when her baby started to cry is nonetheless expected to give a nurturant response some minutes later. By the time the nursery baby is presented to the mother, the infant has either given up crying and gone back to sleep (withdrawal from pain) or greets the mother with even more intense and upsetting wails. The mother, who possesses a biological attachment to the baby, nevertheless hears only the cries that are more likely to elicit agitated concern rather than tenderness. Even though she has a comforting breast to offer the baby, she may be so tied up in knots that her milk won't flow, and the baby cries even harder. As she grows to doubt her ability to comfort her baby, the infant may wind up spending *more* time in the nursery, where, she feels, the "experts" can better care for him. This separation leads to more missed cues and breaks in the attachment between mother and baby, and they go home from the hospital without knowing each other.

Fortunately this scenario doesn't happen much anymore. Today baby awakens in his mother's room, his precry signals are promptly attended to, and he is put to the breast either before he needs to cry or at least before the initial attachment-promoting cry develops into a disturbing cry. Thus, both mother and baby profit from being together. Infants cry less, mothers exhibit more mature coping skills toward their baby's crying, and the infant-distress syndrome (fussiness, colic, incessant crying) is less common than when babies used to be in nurseries. We had a saying in the newborn unit: "Nursery babies cry *harder;* rooming-in babies cry *better.*"

A better term for "rooming-in" would have been "fitting in." By spending time together and rehearsing the cue-response dialogue, baby and mother learn to fit together well — and bring out the best in each other.

Martha notes: *I get behind the eyes of my newborn and realize that hunger is a new experience for him. He's never felt it before and doesn't know I will solve it for him quickly. A hungry baby becomes anxious, then frantic, quickly. I want to be there before this happens.*

BIRTHDAY "PICTURES"

Now come along with us as we take you through your first visual and tactile exam of your newborn.

Head. The asymmetrical watermelonlike shape of the head is caused by the movement of baby's skull bones, which shift to allow an easier passage through the birth canal. (The process is called molding.) As you run your hands over the top of your baby's head, you may feel ridges caused by the skull bones overlapping during the tight squeeze of labor. Molding is more noticeable in babies with larger heads and after long labors, giving evidence that baby labored, too. Molding is less noticeable in breech babies and, depending on whether or not labor occurred, may not be present at all in cesarean births. The molded head assumes a rounded shape within a few days.

Scalp. As your head caressing progresses, feel the relatively soft area (called a fontanel) in the center of your baby's head. Sometimes you can see and feel a pulse beneath the soft spot. You may feel a smaller soft spot in the center toward the back of baby's head. It's OK to touch and wash these soft spots. Actually, there is a tough membrane underneath. Enjoy this feel while you can; these soft spots gradually get smaller as your baby's skull bones grow together. Baby's scalp may range from bald to covered with a full crop of hair, matted and disheveled. Photo capture this first hairstyle quickly. As you feel baby's scalp, you may notice a "goose egg" — a soft swelling in one area due to the accumu-

Face: *flattened nose, pudgy cheeks; red patches on forehead and eyelids; neck obscured by fat folds*

Head and scalp: *elongated, lopsided; bumpy ridges; wrinkled skin, matted hair; soft spot where bones come together in center*

Skin: *white, cheesy covering, especially in creases; bluish hands and feet; fuzzy hair over shoulders and back*

Genitalia: *swollen vulva and scrotum*

Feet: *wrinkled skin; turned inward*

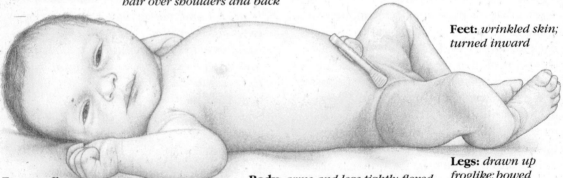

Eyes: *puffy, slitlike; opening occasionally; wandering movements*

Hands: *pudgy, wrinkled, bluish, tightly fisted*

Body: *arms and legs tightly flexed toward chest and abdomen; still, or random movements of limbs; rapid, irregular breathing, often with grunting noises during the first hour; springlike feel to muscles*

Legs: *drawn up froglike; bowed*

lation of fluid during birth. This is caused by tiny blood vessels beneath the scalp breaking during delivery. The lump may take several months to disappear and may feel very hard as the underlying blood calcifies. The overall contour of your baby's head and scalp changes quickly. Enjoy these fleeting features.

Eyes. Your first gaze into your baby's eyes may be a quick one. Notice the puffy eyelids and slitlike openings as baby squints to protect his sensitive eyes from bright lights. Appreciate your first quick glances at eye color, usually dark blue or gray at birth. Your newborn's eyes may wander a lot, squint, and, due to the pressure of labor, be temporarily bloodshot. Eyelids may droop for a few days or weeks, and baby may even open one eye at a time. Tears seldom appear for the first few weeks, but newborn eyes may occasionally have an easily wiped-out sticky film. While your baby's eyes may be closed most of the time, there will be intermittent periods of wide-eyed quiet alertness, during which baby's eyes enjoy connecting with another set of eyes — yours.

Face. Your baby's features may show the results of a tight squeeze: swollen blue eyelids, pudgy cheeks with bluish bruising and faint streaks of broken blood vessels, flattened nose, receding chin, and a bit of asymmetry. During the first day, baby takes off this birth mask and puts on a less puffy appearance, the facial bones spring back into position, and the facial features seem more in order. Photo capture this first face if you can. You will never see it again.

Skin. With your first caress you will notice your newborn's skin is covered with a white,

---

FIRST STATS

Approximately 95 percent of term newborns fit these statistics:

- They weigh between 5.5 and 9 pounds (2.5–4.1 kilograms), the average being 7.5 pounds (3.4 kilograms).
- They measure 18–21.5 inches long (46–55 centimeters), the average being 20 inches (51 centimeters).
- Their head circumference ranges from 12.8 to 14.8 inches (32.5–37.5 centimeters), the average being 13.8 inches (35 centimeters).

A newborn's breathing rate and heartbeat are twice as fast as an adult's.

---

cheesy, slippery material. Called vernix, this protected the skin during the time your preborn baby soaked in your amniotic fluid and acted as a lubricant during delivery. Since this coating has natural protective properties, let it soak in rather than rubbing it off. As you run your hand along baby's back, earlobes, cheeks, and shoulders, you will feel a fine fuzz of furry hair called lanugo. Enjoy the fleecy feel of this silky-soft early baby hair; it too will disappear. Newborn skin looks, feels, and fits differently from baby to baby. Some large term babies have smooth, well-fitting, thicker skin with a pink, ruddy complexion. Others, especially postmature and small-for-date babies, have loose-fitting, wrinkly skin. Some newborns have thinner skin with patches of blood vessels shining through, most noticeable on the bridge of the nose, the eyelids, and nape of the neck.

As if the blood in your newborns' immature circulation is deciding which way to go, newborn skin is various colors. Some areas may be a rosy red, others a pale pink. Because the final destination of mature circulation is the hands and feet, expect them to be cool and blue for the first few hours or days. When the baby is crying, her skin takes on a flushed appearance, and the patchy areas of extra blood vessels, especially in the middle of the forehead, intensify (see also the discussion of normal skin marks, page 107). For the first week or two baby's skin may be dry, flaky, and cracked, especially on hands and feet. No lotion is necessary.

Body. Most newborns have a pudgy appearance due to large fatty areas, called fat folds, along the back of the neck, the cheeks, the sides of the nose, and underneath the arms. The fat folds along the shoulders make it very hard to see baby's short neck. Because of the transfer of maternal hormones at birth, your baby's breasts may be swollen and even leak a few drops of milk. As you place your hand over baby's heart, the heartbeat is almost too fast to count. The plastic-clamped stump of the umbilical cord sits like a centerpiece in the middle of a rotund abdomen. The combination of the round abdomen and drawn-up legs nearly obscures the newborn's groin. The bowed legs and turned-in feet are pulled up beneath baby when he is lying on his tummy.

Hands. The hands are tightly fisted and pulled up toward the face as baby lies in a muscle-flexing position, and some newborns begin exploring their faces with their hands within the first few hours after birth. She may even scratch her delicate skin with paper-thin fingernails, which can be long. The skin of the hands is usually blue, wrinkled, and loose fitting, showing deep creases in the bracelet area of the wrists. Baby's clenched fists will unfold during states of quiet alertness and deep sleep.

Feet. Like the hands, the feet are blue and wrinkled. They are usually turned in, and the toes are frequently overlapping. The tiny toenails look ingrown but aren't.

Legs and arms. The legs are drawn up, froglike, and bowed inward in the squatting position baby assumed in the womb. As you play with your baby's limbs, you will notice that the arms and legs have a normal spring-back-to-the-body tightness, especially when baby is awake or upset, but they relax and unfold when she is in a deep sleep.

Genitalia. The vulva of female and the scrotal sac and testes of male newborns are swollen quite large due to the extra fluid accumulated at birth and the rush of hormones just before birth. The swelling in the vulva usually subsides within the first week, but the extra fluid in the scrotal sac may last for weeks or months. The foreskin of the penis is normally tight.

ROUTINE HOSPITAL PROCEDURES

To assess the general health of your baby and begin a bit of preventive medicine, the following procedures are done in all hospitals and even in some out-of-hospital births.

The Apgar Score

Immediately after birth your baby is given a "grade" — a reminder that your newborn is entering a quantitative world where humans are compared and scored from the moment of birth and throughout life. The Apgar score — devised by Dr. Virginia Apgar in 1952 — is a quick appraisal of the initial health of your baby. This score, determined first at one minute and then five minutes after birth, assesses your newborn's heart rate, breathing effort, skin color, muscle tone and activity, and response to stimulation.

Not a perfect ten. What does the Apgar score really mean? Is a 10 healthier than an 8? Not necessarily! The Apgar score was devised primarily for nursery personnel to determine which babies need more careful observation. A baby who has a 5 needs more intense observation than a baby who receives a 7 to 10. It is sort of a which-baby-to-worry-about score. A baby who receives an Apgar of 5 to 6 at one minute but increases to 7 to 10 at five minutes would be in the nonworry category. A baby who begins life with a one-minute Apgar of 5 and remains 5 at five minutes would need more careful observation, possibly in a transitional nursery, and then would be allowed to room-in with mother when the vital systems become stable.

There is seldom a perfect 10. Even though there are infants who are pink all over, breathe normally, have normal heart rates, show strong muscular movement, and cry lustily, most normal, healthy newborns do not achieve perfect scores. Because it takes a few minutes for a newborn's circulatory system to adjust to life outside of the womb, it is quite normal for a newborn to have blue hands and feet for the first few hours. Also, some babies

THE APGAR SCORE			
Signs Scored	**Points**		
	0	1	2
Heart rate	Absent	Below 100	Over 100
Breathing effort	Absent	Slow, weak, irregular	Strong, crying
Color	Blue, pale	Body and lips pink, hands and feet blue	Completely pink
Muscle tone, activity	Limp, weak movements	Arms and legs flexed	Strong movement
Response to stimulation (e.g., suctioning mouth and nose)	Absent	Grimace	Lusty cry, cough, protest

are naturally quiet immediately after birth. In fact, some of the healthiest newborns I have seen are in a state of quiet alertness at five minutes, but they would lose points on their Apgar for not "crying lustily."

Not an infant IQ test. The Apgar score should have a "For medical use only" label, but over the years this score has been given to parents who have perceived the number as a sort of infant IQ test — an unnecessary source of anxiety for parents of low-scoring babies. There is seldom a correlation between the Apgar score and the long-term development of babies. If your baby has pink lips and is breathing normally, chances are he or she is a healthy newborn.

Vitamin K

Newborns can be temporarily deficient in vitamin K. Immediately after birth an injection of vitamin K is given to your baby to promote normal blood clotting and lessen the risk of abnormal bleeding into vital tissues. You may request that the nurse delay this injection for a few hours until you and your baby have had bonding time.

Eye Ointment

To protect against germs that may have entered your baby's eyes during passage through the birth canal, an antibiotic ointment, erythromycin, is put into your baby's eyes. This ointment in no way harms your baby's eyes but may temporarily blur the vision. Because it is important for your baby to gaze into your eyes immediately after birth — one of the high points of bonding —

you may safely ask the nurse to delay administering this ointment until after bonding time.

Blood Tests

After birth a sample of your baby's umbilical cord blood is taken to the lab in case baby's blood type and Rh factor are needed later. After twelve to twenty-four hours, several drops of blood are taken from your baby's heel for screening tests for the following illnesses, listed in order of the diseases' frequency. (The newborn screening test is usually called the PKU test, but because hypothyroidism is the most common disease detected by newborn screening, this blood test should more accurately be called the thyroid test.)

Sickle cell disease. This condition can affect any ethnic group, but it is most common in people of African descent, occurring in about one in four hundred births. It also is not uncommon among people from India, Mediterranean nations, the Middle East, and Latin America. It is a disease that affects the red blood cells, causing them to change shape and not function properly. This results in anemia, as well as numerous other complications throughout the body. The newborn screening blood test will detect sickle cell disease, as well as various other red blood cell defects.

Hypothyroidism. An inadequate thyroid gland is the cause of hypothyroidism, a condition occurring in one out of every five thousand infants. If undetected and untreated, hypothyroidism may cause mental retardation. Treatment with thyroid hormone is more effective the earlier it is started.

Phenylketonuria (PKU). The early screening blood test also detects PKU, an extremely rare disease occurring in approximately one out of fifteen thousand infants. If left untreated, it can result in brain damage; if it is detected early and treated with a special diet, the child can develop normally.

Galactosemia. Among the diseases detected by this test, galactosemia is the rarest condition, occurring in one out of every sixty thousand infants. It is caused by an enzyme deficiency that allows harmful substances to build up in a baby's blood and damage vital tissues, resulting in death if not treated. Like PKU, this disease is treatable by a special diet.

Expanded newborn screening tests. The above-mentioned diseases are only a fraction of the genetic and metabolic disorders that can affect an infant. Some states now offer expanded testing that checks for dozens of such conditions. Commercial labs also do expanded testing for a fee. See page 36 for more information.

Newborn Hearing Screening Test

During the 1990s government-funded newborn hearing screening programs began in selected hospitals throughout the United States. Research showed that approximately one in 650 infants had some degree of hearing loss. Affected infants who received early learning interventional stimulation prior to six months of age scored significantly higher on developmental and academic tests during childhood than those infants with hearing loss who did not receive early intervention. The bottom line: Early detection results in early intervention, which leads to a higher functioning hearing-impaired child. More and more hospitals now perform free newborn

hearing tests prior to discharge. In the near future, every hospital will offer this.

Different methods are used to screen a newborn's hearing. In one, an earplug that emits a clicking sound is placed in baby's ear. Sensors in the earplug detect the inner ear's response to the sounds. Another method uses sensors attached to baby's scalp to measure brain wave activity in response to sounds. Both methods are painless and only take a few minutes. Some babies with normal hearing fail the initial test and the hospital may test the baby again the following day. If baby fails again, then a more detailed hearing evaluation is performed by a hearing specialist during the first few weeks of life.

Dr. Jim notes: Don't panic if your baby does not pass the first hearing test. Most initial failures go on to pass the next test with flying colors.

NEWBORN JAUNDICE

Browse through any postpartum ward, and you will notice that many of the babies have a yellow tinge to their skin and eyeballs. They have newborn jaundice, which, in most babies, is of no more concern than prickly heat. Most newborns develop some degree of jaundice, which is caused by the buildup in the blood of a yellow pigment called bilirubin and the deposit of this excess bilirubin in the skin. The bilirubin level is measured by obtaining a few drops of blood from your baby's heel.

Normal and Abnormal Jaundice

Newborns may develop two types of jaundice: normal (physiologic) and abnormal.

Babies are born with more red blood cells than they need. These excess cells, resembling tiny wafers packed with a yellow pigment called bilirubin, are broken down by the body's disposal system. During this process the yellow pigment is released. This happens every day in our bodies. We don't get yellow because our liver — the master filter — disposes of the excess bilirubin.

A newborn's immature liver can't handle the extra bilirubin, resulting in this yellow pigment's settling in the skin and reflecting a yellow color by the third or fourth day after birth. This is *normal jaundice.* As soon as your baby's bilirubin-disposal system matures and the excess blood cells diminish, the jaundice disappears — usually within a week or two, and *without any harm.*

Abnormal jaundice usually develops sooner, within the first twenty-four hours after birth. This type of jaundice is caused by too many red blood cells being broken down too fast. If too much bilirubin is released into the system (in medical terms, "if the bilirubin level is too high"), the excess bilirubin could cause brain damage (which, with modern prevention and treatment, *rarely occurs*). Even the abnormal type of jaundice almost never harms a term healthy baby. It is much more worrisome in premature or sick newborns.

This abnormal type of jaundice is usually caused by an *incompatibility* between mother's and baby's blood types. This means mother may have O-type blood and baby may have either A or B type. The mother may be Rh-negative and baby Rh-positive (to prevent an Rh problem in subsequent babies, mothers are given an injection of RhoGAM in the last month of pregnancy and immediately after birth). Some of mother's blood antibodies are circulating through baby's bloodstream, and if baby has a different blood type from mother, a sort of war develops between two opposing forces: baby's red blood cells and the foreign antibodies of mother's different blood type. As a result many red blood cells are damaged during the battle, bilirubin is released, and jaundice occurs quickly.

Your doctor will monitor the degree of jaundice by taking blood samples to determine bilirubin levels. If these levels are low, no harm, no worry. If these levels are too high and rapidly rising, your doctor may begin treatment by giving your baby more fluids to wash out the excess bilirubin and placing your baby under *phototherapy lamps,* which dissolve the extra yellow pigment in the skin, allowing it to be excreted in the urine, and reducing the bilirubin in the blood. Instead of placing the jaundiced baby under phototherapy lamps, your doctor may choose to use a more baby-friendly jaundice reducer called a bili-blanket. Baby is wrapped in a blanket containing jaundice-dissolving phototherapy lights. With a bili-blanket, you can hold and breastfeed your baby while she is receiving phototherapy instead of having her be separated from you in a Plexiglas isolette under phototherapy lamps. This new treatment often enables a jaundiced baby to be discharged earlier from the hospital.

If your baby develops jaundice — and most do — be sure your doctor explains to you, and you understand, what type of jaundice your baby has and whether you should worry. In my experience the anxiety level of the parents is always higher than the bilirubin level of the baby. In caring for newborn jaundice it is important that both the anxiety level in the parents and the bilirubin level in the baby be correctly diagnosed and treated.

Breastfeeding the Jaundiced Baby

Picture the following scenario. Baby has normal (physiologic) jaundice. He is healthy, term, and there is no identifiable reason in his blood for the jaundice. Baby is simply yellow. Upon seeing this "yellow flag," the doctor separates baby from mother and places him under phototherapy lamps. In addition to the fact that phototherapy causes baby to be sleepy and somewhat dehydrated, the separation makes baby disinterested in breastfeeding. Baby is then given supplemental bottles. Consequently, mother's milk supply diminishes at a vulnerable time, when frequent sucking and the continued presence of baby is needed to stimulate milk and at a time when more calories and fluid are needed to help excrete the bilirubin. (Studies have shown that breast milk is better than water or formula for helping babies get rid of jaundice, perhaps because of its laxative effect, producing more stools.)

This scenario should seldom happen. There is a general feeling in medical circles that breastfeeding babies get more jaundice. In my experience, newborns who are breastfed the way the feeding system was designed to work are no more yellow than their bottle-feeding friends. It is true, however, that scheduling breastfeeding and separating mother and baby do result in more breast-feeding babies becoming jaundiced because they wind up not getting enough calories due to the restricted feedings. This is appropriately termed *breastfeeding jaundice* (not breast-milk jaundice) — a preventable condition caused, not by your milk, but by the poor management of the breastfeeding. Here's what you can do to manage jaundice and get breastfeeding off to a good start.

• Follow the right-start suggestions for successful breastfeeding (page 127), specifically early frequent feedings and breastfeeding consultation. This will help reduce most causes of jaundice. A certain amount of fluids and calories, preferably from breast milk, are necessary to help the newborn clear the excess bilirubin out of his system.

• Consult your doctor and be sure you understand the type of jaundice. If baby is healthy and this is normal jaundice (which I call no-problem jaundice), don't worry; make milk. (Worry can cause you to make less milk.)

• Don't ignore a sleepy baby. Jaundice sometimes makes babies sleepy, and sleepy babies breastfeed less vigorously, thus aggravating the cycle of jaundice. (To circumvent this problem, see suggestions on switch feeding, page 142.)

• If your baby has the abnormal type of jaundice, requiring phototherapy and sometimes intravenous fluids to wash out the excess bilirubin, continue to breastfeed your baby unless the medical condition prevents it. (See "Breast-milk jaundice," below.)

Breast-milk jaundice. A rare type of jaundice, termed *breast-milk jaundice* (which is different from breastfeeding jaundice) accounts for less than 1 percent of significant jaundice in breastfeeding newborns. In this poorly understood condition breast milk may either increase the degree of jaundice or slow its normal resolution — for biochemical reasons that are still unclear. If your doctor suspects breast-milk jaundice, you may be asked to stop breastfeeding for twelve to twenty-four hours. If your baby's bilirubin level quickly drops by 20 percent, this is probably the right diagnosis. If so, most mothers can continue breastfeeding if the bilirubin isn't too high. If your doctor instructs you to delay breastfeeding for a few days, you will need to pump your breasts every three hours until you can resume breastfeeding.

It is rarely necessary to stop breastfeeding a jaundiced baby.

BABY'S FIRST CHECKUP

Within twenty-four hours after birth newborns get their first checkup. Ask to be present. You will learn about your baby's body and appreciate what your doctor looks for. Let's go head to toe through your baby's first exam.

Your doctor forms his or her first impression about the general health of your baby by just looking at her. Is she preterm, post-term, or done just right? Is she lying in the frog position, which indicates good muscle tone? Is she alert, active, pink, and healthy and breathing normally?

Next, your doctor examines baby's head to see if there are any abnormalities and may point out to you all the normal lumps and bumps on a newborn's head. Are the fontanels soft and flat? The head circumference is measured and compared with norms to be sure it is proportional to baby's length and weight.

By shining a light into baby's eyes, your doctor determines if there are any cataracts or internal eye problems. Are the eyes of normal size? Your doctor will reassure you that the few ruptured blood vessels in the whites of baby's eyes will clear up within a few weeks. (Sometimes a newborn's puffy eyelids prevent a thorough exam of the eyes, and your doctor may wait a few days.)

After making sure that the nasal passages are open wide enough to easily allow air through, your doctor checks the inside of baby's mouth. Is the front of the tongue attached too tightly to the floor of the mouth (called tongue-tie), which may prevent good latch-on during breastfeeding? (See "Tongue-Tie," page 137, for a full description.) Is the palate, the roof of baby's mouth, fully formed?

By shining a light into the ear canals your doctor can tell if they are correctly formed. The appearance of the outer ear varies greatly among babies. Some are pinned against the head; some fold over; some stick out. As the cartilage in your baby's ears develops, they will assume a more attractive shape. Bruised earlobes are normal.

Watch your doctor run his or her hands around baby's neck, checking for abnormal bumps, and over the collarbone, which sometimes breaks during a difficult delivery and seldom needs treatment. Your doctor then listens to baby's heart for any abnormal sounds and beats that may indicate structural problems and at the same time moves the stethoscope around baby's chest to be sure that air is properly entering and leaving the lungs.

The abdomen gets the next hands-on exam. Your doctor feels for the vital organs (liver, spleen, and kidneys) beneath the thin muscles of baby's abdomen and determines their size and if they are in the correct position; he also checks for abnormal growths in the abdomen.

The genitalia are then checked. Is the vaginal opening normal? An egg-white type of vaginal discharge, often blood-tinged, is normal. Are both testicles descended? Are there any hernias (protrusion of the intestines) beneath the skin of the groin?

The anus is checked to be sure that it is open and located properly. Your doctor may also check with you or the nurses if baby has passed any stools yet.

While looking at the groin area, your doctor will hold baby's thighs and move them around the hip joints. He or she is checking for *dislocatable hips* — a condition that is easy to diagnose and treat in the newborn period, but is more difficult to diagnose and treat later. While his hands are on the hips, notice your doctor placing a finger in the center of baby's groin, checking for the femoral pulse. The strength of the pulsation of these large arteries gives a clue that the vessel coming out of the heart is large enough.

Now on to the legs, which are normally bowed, and down to the feet, which normally curve in. However, if the front half of the foot is curved in too much in relation to the back half (called a clubfoot), it may need cast correction even in the newborn period. Toes are a familial curiosity. Webbed, oversize, and overlapping toes are common inherited traits. Your newborn's reflexes may also be checked, but by the time this head-to-toe exam is complete, the doctor has a general impression of your baby's neurological development.

Meanwhile back at the nurses' station, your baby's doctor reviews the birth events to see if any problem occurred that may require special attention. The mother's history and nurses' notes are looked at. The doctor also checks the mother's blood type to see if there is any potential incompatibility between mother's and baby's blood that may lead to an abnormal jaundice.

This concludes the usual newborn exam. Depending on special birth circumstances or physical findings, your doctor may perform other examinations or tests. While you are in the hospital your baby's doctor and your attending nursing personnel will help you get used to caring for you baby, especially feeding. In addition to the newborn exam, an important part of routine newborn care is what I call the discharge-from-the-hospital talk. Make a list of all your questions and concerns to ask your doctor before you leave the hospital. On the day you leave, your doctor will answer these questions, discuss your concerns, and go over what to expect when you get home. Also, be sure you know how to reach your doctor and when your first office appointment should be.

The first newborn checkup also has a special meaning to your doctor. He or she has made a new acquaintance; you have begun a lengthy friendship. It is the first in a long series of checkups as parents, doctor, and baby begin to grow together as a team.

5

Postpartum Family Adjustments

It's time to descend from the birthing highs and settle down to life with a new baby. During our prenatal counseling we try to prepare expectant couples for how physically and emotionally draining the early weeks may be. But their minds are so filled with images of perfect babyhood that our forewarnings of what life with a new baby is like seem to go right over their heads.

NESTING-IN

The opening weeks at home are a period we call *nesting-in* — a time to learn to fit together as a family. While life with a new baby may not be all rosy, here are some ways for feeling at home with your newborn.

Take maternity (and paternity) leave. What does most mothers in is not only attending to the incessant demands of the newborn but trying to do too many other things too soon. Consider what maternity and paternity leaves really mean — leave everything else to someone else and concentrate on your newborn. Baby will only be a new-

born for one month. Almost *anything* can wait four weeks.

Dress for the occasion. Don't take your nightgown off for two weeks; sit in your rocking chair and let yourself be pampered. As a busy mother of eight Martha has learned to dress for the occasion. Wearing her nightgown gives the rest of the family the message that mom is off call. Develop a language and mind-set — "Go ask daddy" — that directs the traffic of the other children from draining on mom. A phrase that works for Martha is "That is disturbing my peace." Teach siblings to respect the peace and quiet of the nest.

Get a doula. At no time in history have new mothers been expected to do so much for so many with so little help. Cultures around the world have always recognized the importance of mothers and babies nesting-in. In many places a mother is presented with a doula (from the Greek word for "one who ministers"), a servant who specializes in mothering the mother (*not* the baby), relieving her of household chores and interferences that drain her energy away from her baby. Tired mothers, perk up. The doulas are now in North America. Postpartum-care services are springing up all over the land. Try to find one in your community. These gems are well worth the price. If you are unable to hire a doula, husbands, relatives, and friends can become "servant for a day." If a friend asks, "What do you need?" reply, "Vacuuming and laundering" or, "Bring over dinner." (For doula services, see www.dona.org.)

ROLE ADJUSTMENTS

Bringing a new baby into the household means adjustments for everyone — not just mom but dad and siblings too. Here's what you can expect and some practical hints about ways to cope.

For Fathers Only

Fathers may have even more difficulty than mothers adjusting to life with a new baby. As protector of the nest, they have two jobs at home: sharing in the care of the newborn and caring for the mother. Many fathers are uncomfortable about getting their hands on tiny babies and equally uncomfortable caring for a postpartum mother whose normal hormonal changes may not make her the most fun person to live with for a while.

An understanding of what is occurring in the mother-infant relationship during the early weeks puts a higher value on dad's role. During the first few weeks a mother's feelings of attachment oscillate between oneness and separateness (bringing either confidence and euphoria or uncertainty and depression). Sometimes she feels in tune with her baby,

sometimes distant. As mother and baby practice their cue-response scene dozens of times each day, they grow into an attachment of mutual sensitivity, mother knowing baby and baby knowing mother. You will see this attachment unfold when your wife begins to exclaim, "I finally know what she needs" or, "I can read her." This is quality time for mother and baby. Dad creates an environment that allows this mother-infant attachment to mature. It's important for dad to understand this early mother-infant attachment (not be threatened by it) and support it. Here are some practical nest-keeping tips.

Keep the nest tidy. An upset nest yields an upset mother — and baby. In the postpartum period seeing one dirty dish unglues Martha, whereas normally she is unruffled by a whole sinkful. Take over the housekeeping yourself, or hire someone to do it. Stroll around the nest each day and take inventory of what needs to be done — and do it. TIDY is your memory word for the day: Take inventory daily — yourself.

Improve your serve. Stan, a professional tennis player, once asked me how he could help in the care of his newborn. I responded in the language of his trade, "Improve your serve." Pass out refreshments frequently during the day. Breastfeeding mothers need extra snacks and fluids. Serve breakfast in bed. Your wife's sleep has no doubt been disturbed, but you probably managed to stay asleep. Take a walk with your baby while you insist your wife indulge in a tub soak. Feel like a servant and waiter? You are.

Be sensitive. Many new mothers are unwilling to ask for help, perhaps for fear of shattering the supermom myth. Dads, be aware of your wife's needs. As one mother confided, "I'd have to hit my husband over the head before he'd realize I'm giving out."

Guard against intruders. While it is neither necessary nor healthy to become a postpartum recluse, socialize only when you want to. There will be times when you and your wife want to share the joys of a new baby with friends and be on the receiving end of new-parent strokes. Other times you will find crowds of well-wishers annoying. When you need to be alone, take the phone off the hook and put a "Do not disturb" sign on the door.

Take charge of the siblings. The other children are used to having mom all to themselves and may not be eager to share her with the new baby. If you are able to take a week or two (or more) of paternity leave, take over most of the sibling care. Trips to the playground and other out-of-the-house activities keep the nest quiet. Instruct the older children to pick up after themselves and tell them why a neat nest is important to mom. They are future mothers and fathers too. The postpartum period is a time when the little (and big) takers give to mom.

Be a gatekeeper against unhelpful advice. Love for her new baby and an overwhelming desire to be a good mother make your wife particularly vulnerable to any advice that implies she might not be doing the best for her baby. Guard your mate against well-meaning but intrusive visitors who may upset the harmony of the nest. Fend off purveyors of bad baby advice: "You probably don't have enough milk" or "You're spoiling that baby." Confusing advice plants doubts in the mind of even the most confident mother. If you sense outside advice upsetting your wife, protect her style of mothering. Put a stop to it, even if it's coming from your own mother.

Respect the nesting instinct. Avoid making major changes around the time of childbirth. This is not the time to move into a new house or to get a new job. If possible, make these changes long before the birthday. The nesting instinct is very strong in a new mother, and to upset the nest is to upset the mother.

Become a shareholder. Mothers do not have an exclusive patent on carrying babies. Fathers have an important role in the postpartum period. They form their own father-infant attachment and make their own contribution to the growth and development of their baby. It is not greater than mom's, nor less — it is different. Babies thrive on this difference.

Prove yourself. Dads, let me share with you some family secrets I've learned about new mothers. As a mother is developing an attachment to her baby, she experiences a reluctance to share the baby care with anyone else. As soon as baby cries, you stride over only to be outrun by your wife, sprinting toward her helpless infant. (See page 48 to read how a baby's cry affects mother.) If on rare occasion you win the race, be prepared for your wife to hover around waiting to rescue baby. Because baby seems to quiet more quickly in your wife's arms, you back off from becoming a baby comforter — and your wife lets you off the hook. Two problems arise from this: Father never gets a chance to develop his nurturing skills, and mother falls into the exhausting trap of "My baby needs me so much I can't do anything else." Dads, you first have to prove yourself as a baby comforter before your wife is comfortable releasing baby into your charge. Read about being a babywearing father on page 291, and other nurturing tips on pages 349–351 and 380–382.

Dads, don't miss out on baby. Mothers get plenty of bonding time with baby while breastfeeding and sleep sharing. Not so for fathers. New dads, want to form a close attachment to your baby like your wife has? Hold your baby as much as you can. Wear baby in a sling, especially during naps. This time with baby will give you a bond almost as close as the mother-baby bond. Don't concentrate so much on housework and the other kids that you miss out on your new baby.

For Mothers Only

If dad never gets his share of baby care, how can he learn nurturing skills? Want your husband to share those fussy moments and wakeful nights? Here's how to get it to happen.

Show and tell. Pick out the baby-care tasks you most need help with and tell your husband specifically what you need. Otherwise your husband may surmise that you want to do everything yourself. Rather than get teachy-preachy, do baby-care basics *together,* such as bathing baby, comforting, and changing diapers. Subtly (and sometimes not so subtly) point out to him techniques that work best for your baby.

Set up dad. Beginning with short solo walks around the block, periodically arrange for dad and baby to be home alone. When it's just baby and him, you may be surprised how dad measures up. To be fair, leave the breastfeeding baby with a full tummy, otherwise dad may really be stuck.

Delay the rescue. Your baby is crying, and dad picks her up. She's still crying. Dad bounces her and sings to her. She continues crying. By now you're a wreck. Your milk is leaking, and you have the overpowering urge to rescue crying baby from fumbling daddy. Rather than immediately hovering about, ready to say, "I'll take her," hold off a bit. Allow dad and baby some time to work it out. If the scene is obviously deteriorating, come to the rescue, but without casting doubt on his comforting abilities. A hungry baby, after all, needs to be fed. Part of his skill building as a cue reader is to know when to announce "Dinner is served" and hand baby over. Perhaps next time baby will settle better. And to be honest, there are times when baby isn't instantly comforted by you or your breast either.

Be patient. Baby care may not come as easily for some fathers, especially if they come from a family in which baby tending was exclusively left to females. Gradually encouraging dad's involvement and affirming his results will eventually get him hooked on infant care, at least as a pinch hitter if not as an equal shareholder.

Introducing a New Baby to Siblings

Children more than three years of age are usually excited by the birth of a new baby. They realize how much fun baby will be to play with. Children under three may not welcome a new baby with open arms, but here's how to foster an early friendship.

Make friends before birth. Get your older one acquainted with baby before birth. "Johnny, put your hand on the bulge — feel baby kick." This gives him an appreciation of a real baby inside. Talk to your preborn baby and let your child join the conversation. Soon he'll come up and begin talking to this little brother or sister, too. Take him along for pre-natal checkups, and let him hear the heart-beat. "Do you hear baby? . . . Soon he will be talking to you." Don't start talking about the baby with a younger child (say, under two and a half) until the last trimester or when he notices something about you is different. Giving notice too early will confuse him — he has no concept of months passing.

Pictures, pictures, pictures. Show pictures of how babies develop in the womb and use correct terms. Babies grow in mommy's *uterus* not in mommy's *tummy*. It helps to get a child in the mood for a baby-in-the-house atmosphere by reliving a page-by-page trip through his own baby book, commenting that what you'll be doing with your new baby you actually did with him. There are many good picture books — called sibling books — to prepare a young child for the arrival of a baby. Try *Baby on the Way* and *What Baby Needs* by William Sears and Martha Sears and Christie Watts Kelly (Little, Brown, 2001).

Prepare your child for your hospital stay. Your two-year-old is probably more interested in what's going to happen to him while you are gone than what's going to happen at the hospital. Present the thought of separation from you not as a loss, but as *something special* (a marketing phrase you will use many times). "Grandma is coming to our house and will bake cookies and bring you new toys. . . ." It is best to leave your two-year-old in his own home with someone he knows and enjoys.

Stay connected. While in the hospital, phone your child frequently and welcome lots of sibling visits. It's best not to bring home a stranger.

Play "big brother or big sister." Get into the mind of your child; his first thought is how the new baby will affect his life. The sooner he learns that having to share mommy with another child is not so bad after all, the more kindly he will take to the new baby. Make a game out of "mommy and daddy's little helper": changing diapers, loving, dressing, and bathing baby. The role of helper evolves to that of a teacher: "Show baby how to hold her rattle."

Help your child feel important, too. Siblings can get spin-off presents from the new baby. Rather than having him feel left out as everyone showers gifts on the new mother and baby, be sure your child reaps the bene-fits of the birth harvest. Wise gift-bearing friends will bring along an extra gift for the sibling. If they don't, keep a few of your own in reserve. And make sure he gets the mes-sage that he is still important to you, even though you have to spend so much intimate time with the new baby.

Give your child more of dad. During those early weeks when you are naturally preoccu-pied with your new baby, dad can take up the slack by doing special things with the older child. Where the child may feel she has lost some of mom, she gets more of dad.

Dr. Bob advises: Dads, spending extra time with your older children should be in addi-

tion to, not instead of, time spent with your new baby. Don't miss this fleeting time of early father-infant bonding.

Make double use of your time. Wearing your baby in a baby sling gives you two free hands to do fun things with your toddler while nurturing your baby. At the same time as you sit and breastfeed your baby in the sling, you can read a book or play with your older child. Babywearing also helps older children catch the spirit of having a new baby in the house. If your older children resent baby's being in mom's arms all the time, use your sling as much as possible and encourage them to "wear" a doll or even a pet in their own homemade slings. (See section on babywearing siblings, page 294.)

Getting the toddler involved in the care of your baby is like rewinding a tape of his own baby care. As you breastfeed, change, and care for your new baby, talk about what you are doing and how you did the same nurturing with your toddler when he was a baby. Reliving a bit of their own babyhood helps older children better understand family life with a new baby.

It is best not to try to convince the older one that he or she is a big boy or a big girl now, thinking that you can use ridicule to help the older one "grow up." One look at all the love and holding and time the baby gets is enough to convince any sibling that being little is best. It's normal for the sibling to regress in daily habits, toileting, eating, sleeping, and so on. Here's where more of dad will make up for less of mom. And it's helpful to point out that babies are cute but they sure can't do much, like go to the park to play, eat a popsicle, or ride a trike.

PREVENTING AND OVERCOMING POSTPARTUM DEPRESSION

You train for the big event for nine months. You finish the race and hold the prize. Hospital attendants cater to your every need at the push of a button. You're a star. You deserve the attention and the high feelings that go with it. After the incredible high of giving birth, most mothers experience baby blues, a temporary "down," about three days later. Hormonal shifts are partially responsible, as well as just the natural letdown your emotions go through after any mountaintop experience. This explains why you'll suddenly find yourself crying as you sit holding your newborn.

After a few weeks of parenting, things seem different. Baby's days and nights are mixed-up and so are yours; your milk may not be enough (or so somebody advises you). As soon as you crash on the couch for a much-needed catnap, baby calls. Your energy is going out faster than it's coming in. Add to this body fatigue, the healing of birth wounds (an episiotomy or a cesarean section), and possibly memories of a birth less fulfilling than you rehearsed, a baby who is not acting according to the books, and a husband who isn't either. Put all these daily scenes together, and by the end of two weeks you may have a case of more than just the baby blues.

More changes occur in the first month after birth than at any other time in a woman's life. It's no wonder that 50–75 percent of all mothers feel some degree of baby blues (the incidence would be 100 percent if males gave birth and fed babies). Besides simply feeling down, around 10–20 percent of mothers drift into postpartum depression, manifested by incapacitating anxiety, insomnia, fears, outbursts of crying, making mountains out of molehills, mental confusion, inertia, lack of interest in grooming and physical attractiveness, and a negative attitude toward husband — and sometimes baby.

The feelings of postpartum depression are your body's signals that you have exceeded your physical, mental, and emotional capabilities to adapt to all the recent changes and energy demands that have been put upon you. This does not imply a weakness on your part, only that you have exhausted your body's capacity to adjust to these changes. Besides the energy-draining events of birth and baby care, hormonal swings can contribute to postpartum depression. Even though after-birth blues and depression are common, there are ways to avoid or at least minimize these crippling feelings.

Respect the nesting-in period. Don't try to be all things to all people. Giving birth is your license to be pampered. You need time to settle in with your baby. You can't be gourmet cook (or even short-order cook), social hostess, housekeeper, and mother. You won't have the energy for all these, nor should you be expected to.

Stick to priorities. There will be days when you feel, "I'm getting nothing done." *You are doing the most important job in the world* — mothering a new human being. Especially if you have a high-need baby (we will meet this baby in Chapter 16, "Parenting the Fussy or Colicky Baby"), temporarily shelve all obligations that siphon off energy from yourself and your baby. The constant-baby-care stage does not last forever.

Get out — get moving. There is nothing in the new mother-baby contract that requires staying in the house. "Home" to a tiny baby is where you are. Wear your baby (see Chapter 14, "Babywearing") and take hours-long walks through parks, stopping periodically to let the peace of nature speak to you. Since inertia is part of depression, set aside a certain time of the day for outside living and stick to it.

Try group therapy. You are not alone in your depression. Nearly all new mothers have down days, some more than others. The traditional model for a mother and a baby has never been a mother alone in the home with a baby. It has always been mothers with babies sharing their joys and burdens together. Your childbirth class, friends and relatives, or a local support group such as La Leche League will help you get through this stage. You may also need to talk to a counselor who specializes in postpartum depression. More mothers are now aware of the value of counseling for this transition in their life. Many areas offer group counseling, in which women come together for support.

Martha notes: Shortly after the arrival of our eighth baby I felt overwhelmed with kids. I was not a pleasant person to be with. And — can you believe it? — I doubted my ability as a mother. I felt even more guilty when our fourteen-year-old daughter announced, "I'm never having any kids!" When I realized that my mood was getting the whole family down, I was determined to get help and get better. I don't want my daughters growing up thinking that being a mother is no fun.

Eat well. Depression causes lack of appetite, and inadequate nutrition feeds more depression. Some force-feeding of balanced nutrition must be in your daily menu (see page 149).

Practice good grooming. "I just don't have the energy to put a comb through my hair" is a common feeling in depression. Like poor nutrition, poor grooming contributes to the unattractive cycle of depression. If you look good, you're more apt to feel good. Invest in a simple, easy-care hairstyle to get you through the early months.

Treat yourself. You deserve a break today — and every day. Occasional trips to the hairdresser, a facial, a massage, an hour at the spa, along with daily showering and resting or a soak in the tub, is good medicine, and just what the doctor orders.

"But I don't have time; my baby needs me," you may argue. You *do* have the time and *your baby needs a healthy mother.*

Fixing a Poor Start

Susan, a first-time mother of a well-researched baby, had planned for the ideal birth and instant intimacy with her baby. But, through no one's fault, a medical complication required a surgical birth and mother-baby separation because baby was transferred to a newborn intensive care unit in another hospital for one week. When I saw Susan and her baby in my office for the two-week checkup, she did not have the spark that I recognized in her before birth. She was distant from her baby, perhaps angry, but didn't know whom to be angry with and was preoccupied more with mending her wounds, physical and emotional, than getting into motherhood to the depth she had envisioned. In fact, she con-

fided, "I feel like I'm holding someone else's baby." The start she had wanted was not the start she got.

Having a difficult birth experience is one of the main causes of postpartum depression. If this scene pushes a button in you, here's how to help yourself fix a poor start.

Take the first steps. First, the most important step in fixing a poor start is to realize that you had one and that grieving this loss is causing a distance between you and your baby. Next, hold a family council with your husband and reveal your feelings. Tell him specifically about the help you need — for example, with doing housework, with holding the baby, and so on. Let your husband know you want some time to bond. Temporarily shelve all in-home and outside activities that drain your energy away from time with your baby. Impress upon your husband that you require a time of nesting-in with your infant, and why. You need to go back to day one. Return to the mind-set you had on the day of birth and live these days over again now that you are able to focus on baby. You need to get connected, and that takes time and energy. You must do it now, because it will be harder to do it later.

Let baby be your therapist. Babies have a way of bringing out the best in a mother, provided she creates a baby-centered environment that allows this to happen. For a period of at least two weeks — longer if necessary — stay glued to your baby. If you are having trouble breastfeeding, seek help from a professional lactation consultant. Not only does baby need your milk, but you need the hormonal stimulation that breastfeeding provides. Breastfeeding gets your mothering juices flowing. If you are bottlefeeding, touch and groom your baby during the feeding as though you were breastfeeding.

Try a daily touch. To get more in touch with baby, give your newborn a daily massage (see page 95 for techniques). Let baby fall asleep skin to skin on your chest. As an added touch, *wear your baby* in a baby sling for many hours during the day. Take long walks together — as though spending time with someone you are in love with.

Think baby. Besides keeping physically attached, keep mentally close to your baby. While baby is napping or sleeping — better, if you and baby are napping or sleeping snuggled together — allow yourself the luxury of thinking motherly thoughts. All competing worries or preoccupations with business can be put on hold in favor of this important work that can only be done by you.

Journalize. Write your baby's birth story, emphasizing how it made you feel at the time and how you feel now. Write about both your feelings and the everday developmental changes you notice in your baby. It is easy to get so preoccupied with all the upsetting thoughts that you may forget the precious moments that you really do have with your baby. If you record these precious moments on paper, you won't feel robbed. Writing is therapeutic and can help you focus on the pleasant interactions you have with baby.

Large doses of baby touch, taken as directed, are the best medicine to heal a poor start. If this medicine is not working, seek professional help from a therapist knowledgeable in disorders of mother-infant attachment.

Tips for Dads

All these dealing-with-depression tips sound easy, but in reality your wife won't do them without a boost. Here's a prescription that's much quicker and cheaper than an hour with the doctor: "I've booked an hour at the spa for you and I'll drive you there. I'll pick you up at six P.M. and we'll stop by for pizza on the way home. Besides, I need an hour at the park with Junior."

When an hour with the doctor *is* advisable, recognize the red flags of serious depression that needs professional attention. If the symptoms mentioned earlier do not go

POSTPARTUM DEPRESSION IN FATHERS

While fathers do not experience the hormonal and physiologic changes that mothers do, a bit of letdown is common in new fathers. Fathers' postpartum-adjustment concerns are mainly caused by the increased responsibility of another mouth to feed, sudden changes in life-style, and changes that they had not anticipated in their relationship with their mate. The emotional, financial, and sexual adjustments that occur in the postpartum period usher in another season of marriage — a season in which more adjustments take place in a shorter period of time than in any other stage of married life. Just as the upsetting stages in baby's growth and development pass with time, the after-baby blues and depression in mothers and fathers also pass.

away after you and your wife have done what's suggested here, consult your doctor for advice. New approaches, including hormone therapy, are available now for treating postpartum depression. Just a word of caution — if the professionals recommend therapy that would result in mother-baby separation, get a second opinion. Separation, in our experience, only compounds the problem. For resources and referral for professional help, contact DAD — Depression After Delivery — at (800) 944-4773 or www.depressionafterdelivery.com.

NOW WE ARE THREE

No matter how much they have planned for a new baby, couples are taken by surprise at how this demanding little person challenges the husband-wife relationship. That's part of the parenting package! But being aware of the likely consequences can help you cope with this new season in your marriage.

For Fathers Only

Here are some normal feelings new fathers express: "I feel left out." "All she does is nurse." "She's too attached to our baby." "We haven't made love for weeks." "We need to get away — alone."

A Season of the Marriage

Both your feelings and your wife's attachment to baby are normal. It's natural to conclude that your wife is less interested in you. If you understand the changes that occur in the postpartum mother, it's easier to grasp why you feel this way and why your wife acts this way.

A woman has both sexual and mothering hormones. Before birth the sexual hormones are higher, and her desire to be a mate may have been greater than her desire to be a mother. After birth a hormonal reversal occurs. Her hormones to mother prevail over her hormones to mate. This shift from attachment to husband to attachment to baby is a sort of biological insurance policy that the young get mothered.

Besides these biological changes, another reason for your wife's apparent lack of sexual interest is she's just too tired. This new little person has big demands, and there's only so much of a woman's energy to go around. Most mothers feel so drained by the incessant demands of a new baby that all they want to do is sleep. Mothers describe these end-of-the-day feelings as: "I feel all touched out," "I feel all used up."

New mothers also realize their energy limitations and try to portion out their energy to meet needs and not wants. One tired mother told us, "My baby needs nurturing; my husband wants sex. I don't have enough energy for both." For several months after childbirth most wives do not have the energy for a high level of intimacy both as a mother and as a mate. It is normal to feel left out of the inner circle of mother-infant attachment and conclude that your wife has lost interest in you.

Dads, appreciate that a new mother is biologically programmed to nurture her baby. You are not being displaced by the baby, but some of your wife's energies previously directed toward you are temporarily redirected toward your baby. This is a time primarily to parent and secondarily to mate, and ideally a time to find opportunity and energy for both.

Dr. Bob notes: *Dads, if you're feeling left out of the mother-infant bond, jump on in and join your wife and baby in their new-found relationship. Staying on the sidelines will only increase the distance between you and your wife and baby.*

Sex After Childbirth

Be a supportive and sensitive husband and father during this early season of mother-infant attachment and the season to be sexual will return — and will be better. Here's how to spark the sexual fire after childbirth.

Go sensitively. Don't pressure. Pregnancy, birth, and postpartum adjustment leave the woman physically and emotionally drained. Let your wife's system recharge before making sexual overtures. For many men, sex equals intercourse. For women there is more of a mental component to sex. A woman's mind may not be ready for sex even when her body is; and her body isn't ready for intercourse until weeks after birth. Pressuring your wife to give too much too soon will not lead to satisfying sex. Sex motivated by desire is better than sex motivated by obligation.

Go slowly. "I don't care if the doctor said it's OK, he's not the one recovering from pregnancy and childbirth," said a tired mother to her impatient husband. The doctor's green light does not mean your sexual relationship will pick up, overnight, where it left off before pregnancy and childbirth.

Court and woo your wife all over again. New mothers do want to be sexually reunited with their mates, but in a progression similar to courtship. They want to be held, caressed, cared for, loved, and above all to feel that their mate is sensitive to their needs. Only then is intercourse likely to follow willingly.

A month after the birth of her baby, Joan was beginning to feel sexual again. Meanwhile, her husband, Larry, hovered like a sexually thwarted male ready to pounce. When the doctor-prescribed waiting period was over, Larry moved too quickly. Joan stopped him and said, "Please hold me for a while instead of making love right away." This couple needed a more gradual process of lovemaking for the sexual reunion to be fulfilling. If Larry had been making the right moves all month long (holding, courting, serving, and so on) he might have gotten a green or at least a yellow light instead of a red one.

The First Reunion

Sensitivity and gentleness are the keys to postpartum sex. Dads, respect the physical changes that are going on as your wife's body is returning to its prepregnant state. Fathers often describe their sexual reunion with their wives as "getting to know her body all over again." Here are some tips to help you and your wife to get sexually reacquainted.

Opening night. The bulge is now gone, and you will be able to snuggle close together again. Make the first night you plan to have intercourse after childbirth a special time of courtship and romance, complete with a candlelight dinner and flowers.

Comfortable positions. Postpartum women often experience vaginal discomfort during intercourse. Vaginal dryness is common in the months after birth because the hormones that usually prepare the vagina for intercourse by releasing a protective lubricant are at a lower level during lactation. Also, an incompletely healed episiotomy may contribute to vaginal pain. To ease the dryness, use a water-soluble lubricant (such as K-Y Jelly). Experiment with positions that do not put pressure on your wife's episiotomy — for example, the side-lying and woman-on-top positions. Ask her to guide your penetration in the most comfortable position, and move slowly to avoid pain.

Leaking milk. Milk leaking from breasts is a natural part of sex after childbirth and is a sign your wife's body is responding to your lovemaking. Be careful not to give your wife the message that this normal body function is distasteful. Also, avoid lovemaking positions that apply pressure to full breasts, as this is uncomfortable for the mother. Emptying the breasts by feeding baby prior to lovemaking alleviates much of the leaking and discomfort — and may prevent an untimely interruption.

More Keys to a Better Marriage Adjustment

Remember baby comes first. Respect the mother-infant bond. Dads, don't try to compete with baby — you'll likely lose. Remember that the mother-infant bond that forms after birth is stronger than any sexual urge. A father once confided to us, "I feel like I'm making love to a split personality." It is normal to feel that while your wife's body may be in your arms, her mind is with her baby. If baby and daddy both want mommy at the same time, guess who wins. Be prepared for this sexual scene in a home with a new baby: Baby is asleep (you hope), but as love-

making begins, baby awakens and within a millisecond mother's radar shifts from you to baby. How would you handle this? The wrong way: You could let loose with an angry "foiled again" reaction, giving your wife the message that baby has had enough of her and it's your turn. This selfishness is a guaranteed turnoff, and not-very-satisfying sex, if any, will follow.

Here's a better way. Since birth, perhaps even during pregnancy, you have given your wife the message that baby will be high priority. Now, in the middle of sex, you have a chance to prove yourself. Either get up and go comfort your baby and then return to your wife or say to her, "Go comfort baby first, and we'll make love later." Nothing will earn you more points (and better sex!) than giving your wife the sincere message that you understand why she feels that baby's needs come before yours. After comforting baby she will likely return to your side feeling even more loving and responsive because you have encouraged her to meet baby's needs first.

Share baby care. Dads, while you can't (and shouldn't) fight biology, you can fight fatigue. Your wife may be too tired to make love. Besides sharing baby care, take over or hire help for all the household chores that drain your wife's energy away from you and baby.

Part of maturing as a person is being able to give yourself to another person and to delay your gratification because someone else takes priority. That's just what becoming a father does. Baby takes; you give; you wait. These are real facts of a new father's life. Every time you feel you are suffering from an acute lack of sex, realize that sharing your wife with your baby and delaying your gratification is a temporary season of the marriage. There is sex after childbirth! It is a selfless kind of sex that matures a man into a husband and a father.

For Mothers Only

While you may feel your husband doesn't understand the changes in your body and hormones after pregnancy and childbirth, do you realize that your husband's urges *haven't* changed? His hormones are the same before and after birth.

Talk it out. Talk about sex — or a lack of it — after childbirth. Explain to your husband the hormonal changes described earlier that are occuring in you, why they occur, and how this is a normal season of the marriage. Be sure your husband knows *it's not his fault* that your sexual feelings are not what they were before childbirth.

Tell him you still need him. If your husband feels displaced by the baby, impress upon him that you still need him, but those needs may be temporarily different while baby is still a baby. Tell him exactly what you need, when, and how much. "I need to be held tonight" is a good start.

Keep your mind on what you're doing. Your husband can sense when you are physically connected to him but mentally connected to your baby. He does not expect you to be thinking primarily of him during breastfeeding; should you be thinking about your baby during lovemaking? If you have trouble releasing yourself physically and mentally from your baby to enjoy your husband, these are normal new-mother feelings that you need to work out.

Avoid the "But my baby needs me" syndrome. You do not have to make an either/or choice between your mothering and your marriage relationship. They can complement each other. Like many issues in parenting, these relationships are a question of balance as you learn to juggle new roles and new relationships to fit one another.

Here's a situation we frequently encounter in our counseling practice. Steve and Marcia, both professionals, married in their late twenties and had their first baby a few years later. Marcia had been very successful in her career and wanted to carry on this high level of success as a mother. She wanted to "do it right." She became deeply attached to her baby, day and night, and it seemed to be working — for her. Steve was a bit uncomfortable handling babies. He was more at home on the fast track of his career. Sensing Steve's uneasy feelings about baby care, Marcia was afraid to leave him alone with the infant and seldom allowed Steve to comfort him. As an added stress they were blessed with a baby who needed to be held most of the time. Even when Steve did hold his son, Marcia would hover around, ready to come to the rescue at the first whimper, so Steve never had a chance to develop comforting skills. Because he fumbled at fatherhood, Steve immersed himself in his work. He felt left out of the inner circle of mother-baby attachment. He got more strokes at work. Gradually he and Marcia drifted down different interest paths, Marcia into her mothering, Steve into his work. Marcia became more attached to her baby, Steve became more attached to his job, and they became less attached to each other.

One day Marcia came into our office for marriage counseling and began, "But I tried to be such a good mother, and my baby needed me. I thought Steve was a big boy and could take care of himself." We told Marcia, "What your baby needs is two parents." We counseled Marcia that she needed Steve if she was to avoid burning out. No mother can continue a high level of solo giving to a high-need baby without having someone give to her and share the parenting. Steve needed her attention and her help in building up his confidence to take care of the baby. They could take care of each other's needs as well as baby's. Fortunately, Marcia and Steve went on to mature as parents and as mates.

For Couples Only

During the three years preparing for and writing this book we had our seventh baby, Stephen, celebrated our twenty-fifth wedding anniversary, and adopted our eighth child, Lauren. Friends always ask us how we have any time for each other. Answer — we *make* time for each other. Early in our marriage we realized the danger of two high-output people getting so involved in their careers and in parenting that it would be easy to drift apart as a couple. We vowed never to let that happen. We realized that children have insatiable appetites in draining energy from their parents. We had to learn to save energy for ourselves, because indirectly this would make the whole family function better. *It's OK to say no to your kids.*

One custom we have stuck to — and our children have learned to respect it — is our weekly dinner for two, sometimes at home, sometimes out on a date. Our older children have grown accustomed to our weekly date and even remind us if we forget. Sometimes when we dine at home they make a game out of it and act as our waiters or perform a skit for our after-dinner entertainment. We have

continued this custom even when there is a newborn in the house, sometimes making it a dinner for three.

Moms and dads, working hard to become a couple is as important as working hard to become a parent. The most difficult times are the early months, but remember your baby is a baby a very short time. This high-maintenance stage soon passes. Yes, there is romance after birth.

SHAPING UP AFTER CHILDBIRTH

For months after giving birth, your body shows many telltale signs and feelings that you have grown and delivered a baby. The excess fat accumulated during pregnancy — normal reserve energy stores for you and your baby — may leave you with unwanted postpartum bulges. Pushed-out tummy muscles may weaken normal abdominal support for the back and contribute to backache.

Losing weight and toning muscles are an important concern of most new mothers. Patience and persistence are the keys here.

Losing Weight While Breastfeeding

It took nine months to put it on, expect nine months to take it off safely. Breastfeeding mothers require, theoretically, an average of 500–600 extra calories per day to provide adequate nutrition for themselves and their babies. These figures are averages. If you were underweight prior to or during your pregnancy, you may require more calories to prevent undernourishing yourself. If you were overweight, you may require fewer calories as the excess fat stores in your body are gradually used up. Several studies in the late 1980s showed that metabolic efficiency is enhanced during lactation, so that the theoretical recommended daily values (RDVs) for lactating women may be higher than what is actually needed. The key to weight loss during lactation is to find the level of calorie intake that works for you individually.

Here is our safe weight-loss program, which considers the nutritional health of both mother and baby if breastfeeding.

Set what you feel is an optimal number of calories for your health and well-being. We advise most breastfeeding mothers to eat at leat 2,000 *nutritious* calories a day, balanced among the basic food groups. With less than this amount most lactating women cannot supply enough calories for their health and well-being.

Set a safe and realistic goal. A gradual weight loss should be your goal; usually around two and a half pounds per month, slightly more if overweight, less if underweight, prepregnancy.

Exercise for one hour per day. By choosing an activity you enjoy — preferably one that you can do with your baby — you are more likely to stick with it. A very comfortable exercise for mother and baby is to put baby in a sling-type carrier and walk for at least one hour every day. Walking briskly for one hour while carrying baby burns off an average of 400 calories (see Chapter 14, "Babywearing"). This exercise plus one fewer chocolate-chip cookie or its daily equivalent in junk food burns off about a pound per week (a deficit of 500 calories a day, or 3,500 calories per week, results in a weekly one-pound weight loss). Exercising after feeding is more comfortable, since your breasts are less full and weighty. Wear a supportive bra during vigorous exercise, and use soft breast pads to prevent friction on your nipples.

Breastfeeding mothers in our practice have been surprised with the effects of strenuous exercise such as jogging and aerobics. Some women have reported a drop in their milk supply if they worked out more than two days per week. Exercises that work the upper arms, such as jumping rope, have been known to cause breast infections, and there have been reports of breast milk developing an unpleasant taste after too much vigorous exercise. So besides making mother more comfortable, breastfeeding before exercising also seems more desirable for baby. We advise each breastfeeding, exercising mother to stick to an activity that works for her. In our experience swimming is an ideal exercise.

Chart your progress. If you are losing weight according to your goal, feeling good, your baby is thriving, and your milk supply is not lagging, then you have selected your optimum level of calories. A breastfeeding mother at her "ideal weight" can usually eat 500 extra nutritious calories a day without abnormal weight gain. This figure depends upon your body type and whether or not you were overweight or underweight before lactation. If you are losing more than one pound a week you are probably eating too little, and we would advise consulting your doctor and a nutritionist. If you are still gaining weight while following this program, you are probably eating too much. In short, a consumption of 2,000 nutritious calories a day plus one hour a day of comfortable exercise will usually result in a weight loss between two and a half and four pounds per month, which is a safe range for most mothers and their breastfeeding babies.

Exercise to Get Back in Shape

Perhaps the best reason to exercise after childbirth is to feel good. A happier woman is likely to be a happier mother. In addition to the daily hour of comfortable exercise recommended above, there are a number of structured exercises you can do to help the muscles most directly affected by pregnancy and childbirth.

Don't hurry your body back into its prepregnant state. Some postpartum-exercise instructors recommend not doing any structured exercises for the first two weeks, except pelvic muscle exercises. They believe the abdominal muscles naturally shorten during the first two weeks, so that much "muscle work" is being accomplished even though you think you are doing nothing. Just being up and around and going through daily living activities is enough exercise initially.

When you are ready to begin structured postnatal exercises, here are a few that most women can safely handle. Begin gradually, working up to an average frequency of ten times, twice daily.

➤ **SPECIAL NOTE:** *Before beginning any exercise program, be sure to check with your doctor regarding when to begin and at what pace. You may have special circumstances (such as a cesarean birth) that require adding or omitting some exercises.*

POSTPARTUM POSTURE

Why: To correct the forward sag and swayback posture caused by the weight of your baby and uterine contents naturally pushing your abdomen forward during pregnancy.

How: Stand with your back against the wall and heels about four inches from the wall. Flatten the small of your back against the wall by pulling in your abdominal muscles and tucking in your buttock muscles. Raise your chest so that your upper back is flat against the wall. Now walk away and try to maintain this posture during the day.

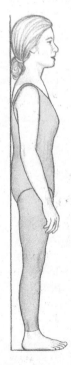

Postpartum posture.

PELVIC MUSCLE EXERCISES (KEGEL EXERCISES)

Why: To restore the tone of the vaginal muscles for intercourse and to prevent leaking of urine during coughing. (The muscles and tissues surrounding the vagina and urethra — which are called the pelvic-floor muscles — have been loosened by the hormonal changes of pregnancy and the stretching of delivery.)

How: You can do Kegels in almost any position. Begin by lying down on your back or front, whichever is more comfortable (face-down is the most comfortable position if you have had an episiotomy). Also, practice these pelvic exercises standing, squatting, and sitting cross-legged against a wall. The muscles you are exercising are the same as those used for control of urination and during intercourse. Tense your vaginal muscles and hold

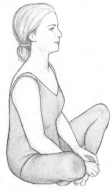

Pelvic muscle exercise (Kegel exercise): cross-legged position.

for around five seconds. Contract and release these muscles fifty times a day, or as often as you think about it.

PELVIC TILT

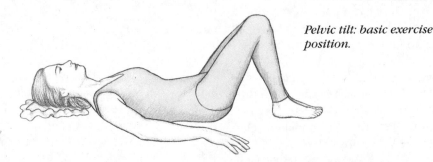

Pelvic tilt: basic exercise position.

Why: To strengthen abdominal and lower back muscles and to improve posture. (The pelvic tilt decreases the curve in the lower part of the spine and strengthens the lower back muscles that have been stressed and stretched by the forward-leaning position of your weighty abdomen.)

How: Lie on your back in the basic exercise position, bent knees together and feet flat.

(You may want to use a thin pillow under your head, but this isn't essential.) Slowly breathe in deeply, let your abdomen rise, then while exhaling pull your abdomen in tightly and push the small of your back flat against the floor. Hold for five seconds. Release and repeat ten to fifteen times.

ABDOMINAL CONTRACTIONS

Why: To strengthen the abdominal muscles.

How: This can be done standing or cross-legged, or in all-fours position. Take a deep breath, then exhale slowly while drawing in your abdominal muscles tightly, and hold these muscles tight for a few seconds after you have completely exhaled. (Be careful to keep your back straight; do not sag.) Do these several times daily.

HEAD LIFT

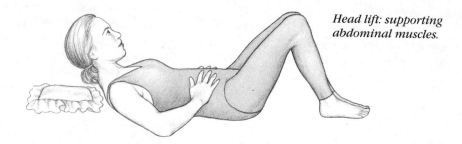

Head lift: supporting abdominal muscles.

Why: To strengthen abdominal muscles and stabilize the posture by flattening the back.

How: Lie on your back with your knees bent (the basic exercise position). You can do the head lift exercises along with the pelvic tilt. Place one or both hands on your tummy to remind you to keep your backbone flat to the floor and avoid overstressing abdominal muscles. (If you had a lot of separation of abdominal muscles during pregnancy and birth, support your abdominal muscles with both hands during the early weeks of abdominal muscle–strengthening exercises.) Take a deep breath and raise your head slowly while exhaling. Then lower your head slowly while inhaling. Raise your head a little higher each day. Keep your eyes toward the ceiling. This keeps your chin off your chest and avoids muscle strain from too much curl. As your abdominal muscle tone gradually improves over the next month or two, take your hands off your abdomen and raise your arms toward the ceiling. Progress from head lifts to lifting your shoulders off the floor and finally to a full sit-up.

KNEES TO CHEST

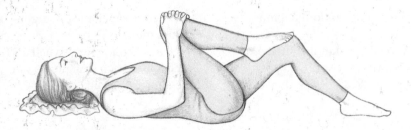

Why: To strengthen lower back and hip muscles.

How: Beginning with a back-lying pelvic tilt, slowly raise one knee to the chest, grab the knee with your hands, and pull gently toward your chest. Hold for five seconds, then release and relax leg. Do this ten times with each leg. Again raise one knee to your chest, and this time while holding it to your chest stretch the opposite leg out flat. Hold for a few seconds, then return to the starting position. Repeat this ten times with each leg. Finally, progress to flexing both knees to your chest: Slowly raise one knee to your chest, then the second. Pull both knees toward the chest with your hands. Hold for five seconds, then release and lower each leg slowly and separately. Repeat ten times.

LEG LIFTS

Why: To strengthen abdominal, lower back, and thigh muscles.

How: Lie on your back with knees bent. Flex one leg up toward your chest as in the knees-to-chest exercise and then extend it as far as you can overhead while keeping the opposite leg bent. Also, you can try raising and lowering one leg at a time while keeping it straight.

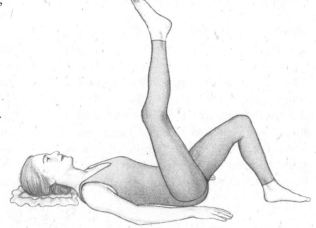

6

Caring for Your Baby's Bodily Needs

The high-maintenance stage of the first two years is often tedious, sometimes fun, but it's also a chance to get to know your baby. In this chapter you will find practical ways to take good care of your baby — and enjoy it.

DIAPERING YOUR BABY

During the early years your baby will spend a lot of time in diapers, and you will spend a lot of time changing them. Here's how to be kind to your baby's bottom and to your time.

Making Changing Time Quality Time

During life before toilet training, expect to change around five thousand diapers, an interaction surpassed only by the frequency of feeding your baby. Rather than being a mundane task to be handled with dispatch and distaste, diapering can be a satisfying time to interact with your baby. More happens during diapering than baby's going from wet to dry. Baby feels your touch, hears your voice, watches your face, and responds to your giggles (and you to your baby's). Before you even begin to change the diaper, connect with your baby. Focus on the child, not the job. Reserve some special facial expressions, jingles, and massage strokes just for diapering time so that baby looks forward to getting more than a clean diaper, and be sure to convey this diapering attitude to any substitute caregiver.

Look forward to diapering as a time to communicate to your baby that he or she is special. Avoid expressions of disgust with the sight or smell (here's where breastfed babies have an advantage — the odor is not unpleasant!). Your face is baby's mirror. Baby regards himself by what he sees on your face. We chatter to our babies about finding "treasures" and keep the tone of our voice excited and loving. Of course, not every diaper change will be a magical, happy, playful time. Sometimes you just want to get it over with so you can move on.

Choosing a Diaper and Diaper Cover

Whether you choose cloth or disposables is a matter of convenience, cost, and your concern for ecology. And, of course, your baby's skin should be a factor. Which type of diaper is kindest to your baby's skin? Many parents use both: 100 percent cotton cloth diapers for home use and disposables when on the go. The bottom line is to choose a diapering system that is user friendly for parents, skin friendly for your baby, and kind to our environment.

One day I was asked what I thought was the biggest recent breakthrough in child care. I responded, "The elimination of diaper pins." As a frequently stuck father of eight, I don't like diaper pins, and they don't like me. Cloth diaper covers with Velcro fasteners have eliminated stuck babies and parents. They're great! And because they breathe, cloth diaper coverings are kinder to baby's bottom than plastic pants, which aggravate diaper rashes.

Changing Diapers

Here is the basic approach to changing your baby's diapers. These steps may vary, depending on what kind of diapers you use.

Preparing Baby

Change baby in a warm room and on a safe and soft surface. Before starting, be sure you have all the necessary equipment within arm's reach. You will need:

- Clean diapers ready. There is nothing more frustrating than getting baby naked, then reaching for a new diaper and finding the bag or stack empty. For cloth diapers, fold the new one before you begin changing.

- Baby wipes. For newborn girls, use warm wet washcloths for the first few weeks, or rinse the baby wipes in warm water before using them. The cleansing ingredi-

ents in wipes can irritate the vagina during the first few weeks of life.

- Changing pad or towel to lay baby on.

- Diaper rash ointment. Most newborns get a rash as their sensitive skin adjusts to life in diapers. We suggest using a small amount of Original A & D Ointment (looks like Vaseline) to protect baby's skin during the early weeks. Use a white zinc oxide cream if a persistent rash develops. Eventually you may not need to use any ointment at all, except periodically during flare-ups.

- Change of clothes. Baby will inevitably leak onto his clothes, and it always seems to happen when you don't have a new outfit handy. Keep a few outfits near the changing table.

- Cotton balls or swabs and alcohol during the first weeks for umbilical cord care.

- Diaper covers. If using cloth diapers, always keep a stack of covers ready because baby will frequently leak.

- Diaper pins or clips (if using them). Warning: Keep them out of baby's reach.

It is best to have a changing table or a designated changing counter where all the items you need are conveniently arranged.

If you are having difficulty with diaper rashes, see "Dealing with Diaper Rashes," page 110.

Safe and Fun Diaper-Changing Tips

- Don't take both hands off baby; babies can fall off changing tables during diaper changing, especially as they approach four or five months and begin rolling over. While your back is turned or you are searching for a diaper, it takes your infant one second to roll off the counter or changing table. Use the safety strap on the changing table, but don't rely on it.

- Handle pins safely. Don't leave open pins within grabbing distance of your baby. Avoid putting diaper pins in your mouth, as baby may imitate this dangerous habit. For easy storage, stick pins in a bar of soap, which keeps the pin sliding smoothly into the cloth.

- We recommend that baby-sitters and other people not used to changing diapers use the floor. It is much safer.

- Change diapers frequently, especially if your baby is prone to diaper rash. It is difficult to tell when baby is wet if using superabsorbent disposable diapers. These should be changed just as often as you would change cloth diapers. With cloth diapers you don't have to count cost each time you change baby.

- Beware! Babies like to pee when naked. Have an extra cloth diaper or towel nearby in case baby decides to "spray" all over the place. Trust me, it will happen!

- A caution about baby wipes: Some babies' sensitive skin will not tolerate them. Try using an unscented brand or rinse the wipes with warm water prior to use.

- After baby is past the stool-a-feeding stage (usually by the end of the first month), change baby's diaper (if soiled or wet) just *before* a feeding. Baby can then drift into an after-feeding slumber without being interrupted by a diaper change.

- Be especially careful when baby has a painful rash — this is a very sensitive area.

ALL-IN-ONE DIAPERS

Diapering does not have to be the ordeal it once was. Gone are the days when the diapering ritual necessarily involved custom folding a rectangular piece of cloth, pinning it snug (without sticking baby or yourself), and snugly fitting a diaper cover over waving legs and a rolling bottom to ensure an elimination-tight system — only to have baby often repeat his performance before leaving the changing table. Now you can get a package deal that contains a cotton diaper, nylon cover, and Velcro or snap fasteners all in one easy-to-put-on diaper. A bit more expensive, but a real boon to busy parents. Ask your diaper service or infant clothing store about pinless diapers. While writing this book we cared for two babies in diapers. All-in-ones were our salvation, and I suspect the delight with easy diapering helped us enjoy this time spent with our babies.

Either soak baby's bottom clean in warm water in a shallow basin or tub or use a warm cloth compress to apply soothing heat, and pat the area clean with minimal rubbing. Generously apply a barrier cream, spreading it gently without rubbing.

Changing the Wiggly Baby

Dr. Jim notes: *Diapering wiggly babies often amounts to an unfinished wrestling match and a half-diapered baby. Parents often ask me, "Why won't my toddler let me* *change her diaper anymore? She kicks and screams, and it turns into a battle every time." Well, older infants and toddlers are supposed to act this way. They are naturally going to resist anything in which they are restrained.*

- Reserve special entertainment only for diaper changing. Sing a song that you have saved just for this event. When your baby hears this song, he is likely to calm down and listen.

- Dangle a special toy from your mouth (your third hand) to try to settle the squirmer; let him grab for it and play with it. Keep this toy only for diaper changing, and change the toy periodically.

- Place a mobile or similarly entertaining toy over the changing area to distract baby.

- Walk your fingers up and down baby's legs and abdomen during the change while singing a song. (Our babies have enjoyed this.)

- Have him "find" his belly button, eyes, nose, and so forth.

- Reserve special, funny facial expressions and contortions to hold your baby's interest during the diapering, getting him to focus on your face rather than the bottom cleaning.

- If baby is a real squirmer, use the floor, the safest place to change a diaper.

Be creative in your diaper-changing techniques, especially with a toddler. A strip of masking tape can entertain a toddler long enough to get the job done while the two of you discuss this sticky subject. (The tape comes out only at changing time.) Some toddlers like holding the wipe or the diaper for you. Keep a dialogue going so baby senses your focus is on her and your enjoyment of this special time. If you are negative about diaper changing, she will be, too.

CORD CARE

The nurse or birth attendant usually removes the plastic clamp from your baby's cord by twenty-four hours of age. In the first few days your baby's cord may be swollen and jelly-like. Over the next few days it begins to dry and shrivel up, usually falling off within two or three weeks. To prevent infection and enhance the drying of the cord, go around the base of the cord, getting into the crevice, with a cotton-tipped applicator dipped in alcohol, or whatever antiseptic solution your doctor recommends, at least three times a day or after most diaper changes. After the cord has completely fallen off, continue this cord hygiene for a few days more. It is normal to see a few drops of blood the day the cord falls off.

If your baby's cord has a puslike discharge and/or an increasingly offensive odor, visit your doctor, who may apply a silver-nitrate solution to help dry it out. A slight odor from the drying cord is normal, but a particularly putrid odor may be a sign that an infection is brewing and it's time to step up the use of the antiseptic solution. If the skin around the drying cord looks normal and is not inflamed, there is seldom any reason for concern. A sign of infection for which you should call your doctor is a red, hot, swollen, and tender area the size of a half-dollar around the base of the cord.

To avoid irritating the cord, do not cover the cord area with a diaper or plastic pants, and, if using disposable diapers, be especially careful to fold the irritating plastic away from the cord area. Whether or not it is safe to immerse baby in a bath until the cord falls off is controversial. Some physicians feel getting the cord wet increases the risk of infection; some do not. If there is pus draining at the base of the cord, it would be unwise to immerse baby in a bath for fear of contaminating the water and spreading infection. In this case sponge bathe baby until the cord falls off and the stump is well healed.

CARE OF THE CIRCUMCISION SITE

Your doctor will instruct you on caring for the circumcision site. Apply a protective lubricant over the site every time you change baby's diaper for about a week. The circumcised site will go through the typical healing process. Initially it is swollen, then a yellow scab appears. The swelling and the scab resolve by one week. Be sure your doctor informs you how to tell if the circumcision site becomes infected. Surprisingly, circumcision sites rarely become infected, but here are signs to call your doctor: The entire penis is red, warm, and swollen, and the surgical site is draining pus. A yellow, nondraining scab is normal during healing.

DISAPPEARING PENIS?

Oftentimes, during the first two years boys develop an increased accumulation of fat, called the pubic fat pad, around the base of the penis. This mound of growing fat may appear to bury the penis. (I have gotten phone calls from worried mothers exclaiming, "His penis is gone.") No, it is not gone. It resides comfortably buried beneath the mounds of fat. As your baby goes through the normal stretching and lengthening of his whole body, the mounds of baby fat melt away and the penis reappears. This curious relationship between fat and penis occurs in both circumcised and uncircumcised infants.

NAIL CARE

Some newborns enter the world with fingernails so long that they need to be cut right away to prevent them from scratching their faces. Expect your newborn's nails to grow very fast and don't be afraid to cut them. If you're timid about cutting your baby's fingernails, as many parents are, here's how to make it easier:

- Trim your baby's fingernails while baby is in a state of deep sleep, recognized by the *limp-limb sign:* Baby's limbs dangle limply at his side, and the hands are wide open.

- Use a miniature nail clipper designed especially for babies. They are much easier and safer than scissors or adult-sized clippers, and baby's paper-thin nails are so easy to cut anyway. If not using a nail clipper, use safety scissors with blunt ends in case baby startles during the cutting.

- To avoid snipping the fingertip skin as you clip the nail, depress the finger pad away from the nail as you cut. As a beginning nail cutter, have your spouse hold baby's hand while you manipulate the finger and the nail clipper. After a while you will be able to trim baby's nails by yourself.

- Drawing a drop of blood is part of learning nail trimming. Apply a bit of pressure and a dab of antibiotic ointment to the little nip.

- If you're squeamish about cutting tiny nails, cover them with cotton mittens to prevent scratches.

A baby's toenails do not grow as fast, and quite often the nails are surrounded with heaped-up skin, making trimming difficult. Don't worry that the toenails may grow into this skin. Ingrown toenails are rarely a problem in newborns.

BATHING BABY

Most babies are overwashed. In reality, newborns don't get very dirty. The toddler–mud puddle friendship has not yet begun.

When to give baby her first bath is a matter of some debate. It is still general practice to advise parents to sponge bathe baby until the cord falls off and the circumcision heals. Some physicians question the necessity of this advice, feeling that an immersion bath does not increase the risk of infection. Check with your doctor. Our own personal recommendation is to sponge bathe baby until the cord is no longer moist and the circumcision is well healed.

Sponge Bathing

Let's go step-by-step through baby's early bath.

Select a bathing area. Try the kitchen or bathroom counter next to the sink. The room should be warm and draft free. Take the phone off the hook so that you will not be tempted to leave baby unattended even for a moment.

Have your bath kit ready in the bathing area before you start. You will need:

- two washcloths
- a mild soap and baby shampoo
- cotton balls
- a hooded towel
- rubbing alcohol
- cotton-tip applicators
- diapers
- clean clothes

While some babies like to be bare, most don't, so remove all clothing except the diaper and swaddle baby in a towel. You can hold baby on your lap while sitting in a chair with your bath kit on an adjacent table, or stand up at the counter with baby lying on a pad of thick towel, or lay baby on a sponge pad in an empty baby bathtub.

Have your swaddled baby's head and face exposed. Begin washing his face with warm water, especially behind the ears, in the ear crevices, and in the neck creases. Unless baby's skin is sweaty, oily, or dirty, plain water is enough; otherwise use a mild soap, but not on the face.

Hold baby in the clutch hold (see illustration on page 132). Squeeze a bit of warm water on top of baby's head, apply a dab of baby shampoo, and gently massage the entire scalp. Use no special caution over the soft spot. It's really tough underneath. (If baby's scalp is flaky or crusty, see instructions for caring for cradle cap, page 109.) Rinse over the sink with running water. Blot dry with a towel hood. Meanwhile, baby is still swaddled in a towel, with only his head and face exposed, not getting cold. As you proceed with the rest of the body, cover the head with a towel hood.

Unswaddle baby, remove his diaper, and wash the rest of his body. Extend the arms and legs to wash the groin, knee, and elbow creases, where there are likely to be oily collections. Clean around the base of the cord with a cotton-tipped applicator dipped in rubbing alcohol.

Turn baby over on his tummy and clean the crevice just above his buttocks and around the diaper area. Or you can lift both feet up and clean the lower back and buttocks while baby is lying on his back. To keep baby from getting cold and upset, cover the rest of the body while cleaning the diaper area.

Clean the genitalia. Hold baby's legs outward like a frog's. For girls, spread the labia and, using a moistened cotton ball, gently wipe between the labia. When cleaning around the vagina always wipe from front to back. You may notice that secretions and diaper creams collect and cake between the vulva and the outer labia. This area requires the most cleansing. A normal egg-white vaginal discharge is common between the inner labia and vagina. It is not necessary to clean away this normal discharge. For boys, clean the creases beneath the scrotum and the skin

> ## KID GLOVES
>
> Here's a washing tip that we have used to make bathing baby safer and easier: Wear a pair of old white gloves and rub a little mild baby soap on the white gloves. You have an instant washcloth that automatically shapes itself to baby's body and reduces the slipperiness of bare hands on soapy skin.

of the groin and buttock and around the base of the penis. Clean the circumcision if necessary after it heals. Do not retract the foreskin if the penis is uncircumcised. (See page 110 for further suggestions on the care of the diaper area and preventing diaper rash.)

Quickly diaper baby and dress him in clean clothes before he has a chance to get cold and more upset.

Additional Bath Tips

- As you move from one area of the body to another, change the parts of the washcloth in order to keep clean cloth on cleaner parts of the body.

- *Pat the skin* with a washcloth and *blot dry* with a towel rather than vigorously scrubbing, which may irritate baby's sensitive skin.

- Spot cleaning works best for babies who do not like either a total sponge bath or an immersion bath. Clean the areas that get the most oily, sweaty, or dirty.

- Clean the eyes on an as-needed basis rather than during the regular bath. Babies often protest eye cleaning, which may set off a protest for the entire bath. Using cotton balls and warm tap water (always squeeze a few drops of the water from the cotton ball on the inside of your wrist to make sure it is not too hot), wash accumulated discharge out of the corners of baby's eyes.

• Cotton-tipped applicators are handy when cleaning little crevices in and behind the outer ear, but never try to clean inside the ear canal, for you may damage the canal or eardrum.

A Rub in the Tub

After the sponge-bath stage, the real fun begins. First, choose the right tub that's safe and easy to use. There are many types of baby tubs on the market, or you can simply use the kitchen sink, which makes great pictures for your baby book. The kitchen sink is easy to use because it is the right height. If using the kitchen sink, observe the following safety tips: Purchase an insert-type plastic or rubber tub that fits into your sink, or line the bottom of the sink with a folded towel or sponge mat to keep baby from slipping. There are even inflatable baby bathtubs. If you have a movable faucet, be sure to turn it away from baby.

Before the splash begins, make sure the water is comfortably warm but not too hot. Tie a towel around your own neck like a bib to keep yourself dry during the bath and in case baby needs to be picked up quickly and cuddled. Most newborns do not eagerly await their bath. Singing a few songs, making eye-to-eye contact, and gently massaging baby during the bath often relaxes the reluctant bather.

Questions About Bath Time

Here are some questions new parents commonly ask us about the bath-time routine.

How often should we bathe our baby?

Bathing is primarily playtime. Babies don't get dirty enough to *need* a daily bath. For busy parents this is good news. Once or twice a week is enough bathing, providing you clean your baby's diaper area sufficiently well each time there is a bowel movement. Daily spot cleaning is necessary in areas that get particularly sweaty, oily, or dirty, such as behind the ears, in the neck folds, in the creases of the groin, and in the diaper area.

Which soap and shampoo should I use when bathing our baby?

Baby's skin, especially a newborn's, is sensitive, and all soaps are mild irritants. The function of a soap is to suspend particles and oils on the skin surface so that they can be more easily removed from skin with water. Without soap, some oils, dirt, and surface secretions would simply stick to the skin and require vigorous rubbing with a cloth and water to remove them, which in itself would irritate the skin. Every baby's skin has an individual tolerance to different soaps. How much soap, how often, and which kind can be determined only by trial and error, but here are some general guidelines:

• Use soap only on areas that are caked with secretions, such as oil or sweat, that are not easily removed with plain water without much rubbing. Do not use soap on the face.

• When first using a soap, try a test rub on one small part of the body. If, over the next few hours, the skin reddens or dries or noticeably changes in any way relative to other areas, ban that soap and try another.

- Use a mild soap. Baby soaps are regular soaps with fewer additives such as anti-microbials, fragrances, or abrasives.

- Limit the soap's time on the skin to less than five minutes to avoid drying or irritating the skin. Wash it off as soon as possible and rinse the skin well.

- Above all, avoid vigorous scrubbing of any area of the skin with soap.

If your baby is prone to eczema or has allergic dermatitis, use a moisturizing soap such as unscented Sensitive Skin Dove.

Shampoos are similar to soaps, and over-use can irritate the scalp and rob the hair of natural oils. Shampooing once a week is enough for most babies. Use a mild baby shampoo; like baby soaps, baby shampoos contain fewer additives than other commercial shampoos. It is seldom necessary to massage shampoo deep into the scalp. If your baby's scalp is covered with the flaky, crusty, oily substance called cradle cap, after shampooing massage a vegetable oil into the crust to soften it, and remove it carefully with a very soft toothbrush.

Here is a final thought about soaps and shampoos that many mothers have expressed to me over the years. Sensitive mothers feel that too much soap and shampoo (and scented oils and powders) camouflage natural baby scents that mothers find irresistible. Also, it is better not to mask the mother's natural scent, which baby needs, and perfume is irritating to some babies.

Should I use powders and oils on our baby's skin?

Gone are the days when a baby was sprinkled with perfumed talcum after every bath. Powders and oils are unnecessary, since your baby's skin is naturally rich in body oil, and they may be irritating and even harmful. Moisturizers such as Soothe and Heal with Lansinoh may be used on patchy areas of dry skin; otherwise, they are unnecessary. Powders easily cake and build up in skin creases and can actually contribute to skin irritation and rashes. Powders, if inhaled, can irritate baby's nasal and air passages. Cornstarch is not recommended. It can serve as a medium for the growth of harmful fungi.

My baby screams every time I try to give her a bath. How can we both enjoy bath time more?

If your baby screams every time you try to put her into the water, it either means that she is hungry, the water is too hot or cold, or you have a baby who doesn't like to be alone in the water. Her security may be threatened. Here's how we have enjoyed bathing our babies. Take your baby into your bath with you. Get the water ready, slightly cooler than you usually have it, then undress yourself and undress your baby. Hold her close to you as you get into the water and then sit back and enjoy this warm skin-to-skin contact. If your baby still protests, sit in the tub first, showing that you are enjoying your bath. Then have someone else hand your baby to you while you are sitting in the bathtub. Mothers, don't be surprised if your baby wants to breastfeed at this time. It is the natural result of being close to your breast. In fact, if your baby still fusses upon entering the water in your arms, relax her by putting her to your breast first, slowly ease your way into the tub, then gradually let your arms lower baby into the water as she continues to suck. This is a special way to enjoy mothering and bathing your baby. As your baby gets older, bath toys such as the traditional rubber ducky may entice the reluctant bath taker. When bathing together in a tub, take special precautions to avoid slipping. While you are getting used to bathing with baby, it is safer to hand baby to another person or place her on a towel rather than holding baby as you get in and out of the tub.

Here's another Sears family trick for enticing the reluctant bather. This involves getting baby into the mind-set that a pleasant event will follow one that he or she may have mixed feelings about. After the bath you may have a special cuddle time. Or follow the bath with a soothing massage. Baby will develop an association with the bath as the wet stage to put up with in order to get the total body massage. (See the section on infant massage at the end of this chapter.)

Over the years we have bathed a lot of babies. There is no one right way to bathe baby, just one that works for you safely with a minimum of hassles. We have learned to regard bath time as more of a parenting ritual than a cleaning regimen; that way the pressure is off in case we miss a crevice. Enjoy bathing your baby and bathing with your baby as just another ritual for getting in touch with your infant.

KEEPING BABY COMFORTABLE

New parents also ask us about their baby's general comfort. Here are a few common questions.

How should I dress our one-month-old at night?

As a general rule, dress and cover your baby in as much or as little clothing as you would wear yourself, plus one more layer, such as a blanket of appropriate weight. Get used to feeling your baby's body temperature. Cold hands and feet indicate the need for more warmth; hot, sweaty head means a need for less clothing and/or a cooler sleeping environment. If your baby was premature or weighs under eight pounds and has little insulating body fat, dress him even more warmly. Cotton clothing is best because it absorbs body moisture and allows air to circulate freely. Your baby's clothing should be loose enough to allow free movement but well fitting enough to stay on the proper body parts. If your baby's sleepers do not contain feet, cover these cold little feet with cozy bootees. Avoid dangling strings or ties on your baby's sleepwear (and yours as well), since these could cause strangling. While blanket sleepers are great for babies who sleep alone, a baby who shares his parents' bed also shares their body warmth and can easily become overheated, which will cause him to be restless. In this situation even a thin polyester sleeper can be a problem, and cotton would be better. (See "Irritating Sleepwear," page 325.)

How warm should we keep our baby's nursery?

Regarding the temperature of your baby's room, the *consistency* is more important than how hot or cold it is. Premature or small babies under five and a half pounds have incompletely developed temperature-regulating systems at birth and need a reasonably consistent temperature to avoid cold stress. Term healthy babies over eight pounds usually have enough body fat, and their temperature-regulating systems are mature enough to feel comfortable in an environment in which an average adult would be comfortable. Since babies do not adjust to marked swings in room temperature in the first few weeks, a consistent room temperature around 68–70°F (20–21°C) is preferable.

Besides the temperature of baby's environment, humidity is important. Best is a consistent *relative humidity* around 50 percent. Dry air may lead to a stuffy nose, a common contributor to night waking. A warm-mist vaporizer in your baby's sleeping area helps maintain an adequate and consistent relative humidity, especially with central heating during the winter months. And the constant hum is an additional sleep inducer. As a rule, if the heat goes on, so should the humidity. When traveling with a baby during the winter, take along a vaporizer, especially if you are staying in motels or cabins with electric heat. Heating, particularly dry forced air or heat from electric baseboard heaters, is drying and not conducive to sleep. Unless it's very cold, turn off central heat at night. Here's a healthier alternative: An inexpensive warm-mist vaporizer (available at pharmacies and department stores) adequately heats and humidifies a fifteen-by-fifteen-foot room with normal ceiling height. (See page 666 for vaporizer tips.)

Is it better to put our newborn down to sleep on her stomach or her back?

Unless advised otherwise by your doctor, put your baby to sleep on her *back*. Most newborns do seem to sleep "better" on their stomachs than on their backs, accounting for the traditional advice of putting babies down to sleep on their tummies. But research has shown that sleeping "better" may not equate sleeping safer. New insights into infant sleep patterns have resulted in a reversal of the traditional tummy-sleeping position to back-sleeping, mainly because of the reduced risk of Sudden Infant Death Syndrome (SIDS) in infants who sleep on their backs. "Back to Sleep" campaigns have reduced the incidence of SIDS by 50 percent. Babies who sleep on their backs awaken more easily and sleep less deeply than tummy sleepers, and easier arousability from sleep seems to be a protective mechanism against SIDS. Be sure to check with your doctor to see if your baby has any medical condition that necessitates front-sleeping, such as small jaw bones or other oral structural abnormalities that may compromise the airways when she is sleeping on her back; a mucus-producing respiratory infection; or gastro-esophageal reflux (GERD). (For more information on safe sleeping, see page 641 for the possible relationship between baby's sleeping position and SIDS; crib safety, page 603; and safe ways to sleep with your baby, page 341.)

How soon can we take our baby outside?

Follow the guidelines mentioned in the preceding discussion about baby's clothing and room temperature. Consistency of temperature is still necessary in the first month. A newborn's immature temperature-regulating system may not tolerate exposure to extreme temperature swings. Traveling from a heated house to a heated car maintains this consistency. If your baby is term, healthy, and has enough body fat (usually with a weight of at least eight pounds), baby is mature enough to tolerate brief exposure to extremes of temperature (such as house to car and back). If your baby is premature or small and does not yet have a generous amount of body fat, avoid extreme temperature changes for at least a month. In climates where the inside and outside temperatures are similar, you and your baby can enjoy a walk outside within the first few days. Passersby love to stop and peer at a tiny baby. To avoid unnecessary exposure to germs, shun crowds, shopping malls, and handling by — or being within sneezing distance of — persons with colds. Going outside won't make baby sick. Being around sick people will.

PACIFIERS: IN OR OUT?

Every age has its props, but none is so controversial as this tiny plug. Some babies like them, grandmothers turn their heads, parents are unsure, and psychologists offer no comment. Babies have an intense need to suck, and some have more intense needs than others. Babies even suck their thumbs in the womb. Next to holding and feeding, sucking is the most time-tested comforter. Even preemies grow better when they can suck on pacifiers. These silicone "peacemakers" have their place, but they can also be abused.

When Pacifiers Are Out

In the early weeks of breastfeeding. When learning how to breastfeed, a baby should have only mother's nipple in his mouth. One thing a newborn has to "learn" is how to suck on mother's nipple the right way to get the most milk. A baby sucks on a pacifier differently than on mother's nipples. Some newborns, but not all, develop nipple confusion when given a pacifier or bottle nipple at the same time as they are learning to suck from mother. Pacifiers have a narrow

---

PACIFIERS VERSUS THUMB-SUCKING — WHICH IS BETTER?

We would vote for the thumb. It's easily found in the middle of the night, it doesn't fall on the floor, it tastes better, and baby can adjust the position to her own sucking needs. Pacifiers get lost, get dirty, and are always falling on the floor. Those of the pacifier set claim, however, that it is easier to "lose" the pacifier than the thumb; and *intense* thumb-sucking, if prolonged three to four years, may lead to orthodontic problems. Parents of tiny thumb-suckers, don't choose your child's orthodontist yet. Most babies suck their thumbs at some time. Most outgrow it, and if their sucking needs are appropriately met in early infancy, they seldom carry the thumb-sucking habit into childhood.

---

base, so baby doesn't have to open his lips wide. This often results in poor latch-on techniques, sore nipples, and a difficult start at breastfeeding. Many sensitive babies gag on every pacifier you might try. The texture, taste, and smell are rejected hands down. Other babies make the transition from rubber to flesh nipples without any confusion or complaint. Our advice: Avoid pacifiers until your newborn learns to latch on properly and you have a good milk supply. If your own nipples are wearing out, or at least the mom they are attached to is, use your finger (or, better yet, get dad or someone else to give you a break). The skin-to-skin element is still there, and your index finger (or dad's little finger) can be placed more properly farther back in baby's mouth to simulate sucking at the breast. Your fingernail should be trimmed short and the nail should be turned down toward the tongue so it won't poke baby's palate. Many of our babies have been soothed by the touch of my well-scrubbed pinkie.

As habitual substitutes for nurturing. Ideally, pacifiers are for the comfort of babies, not the convenience of parents (but I have yet to meet the ideal parent or the ideal baby). To insert the plug and leave baby in the plastic infant seat every time he cries is unhealthy reliance on an artificial comforter. This baby needs picking up and holding. Always relying on an alternative peacemaker lessens the buildup of baby's trust in the parents and denies the parents a chance to develop baby-comforting skills. *Pacifiers are meant to satisfy intense sucking needs, not to delay or replace nurturing.* A person should always be at the other end of a comforting tool. The breast (or the finger) has the built-in advantage of making sure you don't fall into the habit of just plugging up the source of the cries as a mechanical gesture. When baby cries, if you find yourself, by reflex, reaching for the pacifier instead of reaching for your baby, pull the plug — and lose it.

When Pacifiers Are In

If used sensibly and used for a baby who has intense sucking needs — in addition to, not as a substitute for, human nurturing — pacifiers are an acceptable aid. If you have one of these babies and experience times when the human pacifier wears out, use the rubber one, but don't abuse it. There will be times when being a baby is socially unacceptable, for example, during a sermon in church or in a quiet theater. If baby is finished feeding and won't accept finger sucking, a pacifier may keep the peace. Since pacifiers stimulate the flow of saliva, which is a natural digestive aid and intestinal lubricant, extra sucking on a pacifier may help babies with intestinal upsets, such as gastroesophageal reflux.

Pacifiers bother adults more than they harm babies. I confess that while examining a baby and needing an unobstructed view of baby's face, I wish *that thing* were not there. Besides, pacifiers obstruct those adorable smiles. But in defense of the much-maligned pacifier, I soon relax my unfair judgment of the rubber comforter as baby sucks contentedly during the entire exam.

Choosing and Using a Safe Pacifier

• Select a sturdy one-piece model that will not break into two pieces, allowing baby to choke on the bulb. Also, be sure it is dishwasher safe and easy to clean.

• Be sure the base of the pacifier has ventilation holes. Avoid large circular shields that may obstruct baby's nasal passages when baby draws in the pacifier during intense sucking.

• One size doesn't fit all. Choose a smaller, shorter, newborn-sized pacifier for the early months.

• Pacifiers come in a variety of nipple shapes. Some are symmetrically round, like a bottle nipple. Others are preshaped, supposedly to duplicate the elongated, flattened breast nipple during sucking. Preshaped nipples, however, may not always fit baby's mouth, especially if the pacifier turns during sucking or is inserted upside down. Some pacifier manufacturers claim orthodontic benefits, but these are questionable. Try various shapes and let baby's discerning mouth decide.

• Avoid attaching the pacifier to a string or ribbon around baby's neck or pinning the pacifier string onto baby's clothing. This is a setup for strangulation. "But it's always falling on the floor," you plead. Answer: Keep one hand on baby and the other hand on the pacifier. (Or pin the pacifier ring directly onto baby's clothing.) *Perhaps babies are not meant to be left unattended with anything in their mouths. Good safety and good nurturing go together.*

• Do not make your own pacifier out of a cotton-stuffed bottle nipple. Baby may suck the cotton through the hole.

• Resist the temptation to sweeten the offering by dipping the pacifier in honey or syrup. If baby does not yet have teeth, he is too young for honey or syrup. If he has teeth, he is too old for the decay-producing sweets — and probably the pacifier, too. If he has to be enticed to suck by sweetening, he would probably benefit from some other form of comforting — having a change of scene, going out in the fresh air, playing, cuddling with you, rocking to sleep, being worn more, and so on.

Our advice about pacifiers: In the early weeks only the real nipple belongs in a baby's mouth. If you have a baby who really needs a pacifier, then use it, don't abuse it, and quickly try to lose it.

SHORTEN SWADDLING TIME

Once upon a time, wrapping babies burrito-style in a blanket was advised to help them settle easier. New insights, however, have shown that swaddling babies too often and for too long may harm their hip development. In order for the ball-and-socket structures of the hip joint to develop properly, babies need to have freely swinging motion of their legs and lie or sleep with their legs outward in a frog position. Leaving their legs unbound is especially crucial in the first few months, when the hip joint is rapidly developing. Swaddling your baby for a few hours every few days won't harm her hip development, but avoid letting her sleep tightly swaddled for long periods of time, such as through the night.

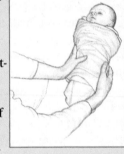

THE RIGHT TOUCH: THE ART OF INFANT MASSAGE

It's one of life's simple pleasures (massage has long been enjoyed by adults), and research is showing that babies grow better and act better when they are on the receiving end of the right touch. Infant massage is a skin-to-skin connection that helps parents and baby better read each other's body language — without saying a word.

Why Massage?

Besides the fact that it is just plain fun to touch your baby, infant massage helps babies grow and develop better. Other cultures highly value touch to help babies grow. In some Eastern societies a mother is expected to give her baby a daily massage. One of the most exciting areas of research is the connection between touch and growth. Touched babies thrive and here's why.

Touch stimulates growth-promoting substances. Health care providers have long known that babies who are touched a lot grow better, and now there is research to back up this observation. There seems to be a biological connection between stroking, massaging, and grooming infants and their growth. Touch stimulates growth-promoting hormones and increases the enzymes that make the cells of the vital organs more responsive to the growth-promoting effects of these hormones. For example, premature infants in a "grower nursery," where they can gain needed weight, showed 47 percent more weight gain when they received extra touch.

Animal researchers have recognized the connection between a mother animal's licking her offspring and how well her babies grow. When newborn pups were deprived of their mothers' frequent licking (equivalent to infant massage), the level of growth hormone decreased, and the pups stopped growing. Even injecting growth hormone into the untouched pups would not cause them to grow. Only when the mother animal's touching and licking were restarted did the pups resume their growth.

Researchers have found that human babies, too, when deprived of touch showed decreased growth hormone and developed a condition called psychosocial dwarfism; even more amazingly they also did not grow when given injections of growth hormone. Only when given human touch did these infants grow. This finding implies that touch causes something beneficial to occur at the cellular level that makes the cells respond to growth hormone. Yes, there is something magical about a parent's touch.

Touch promotes brain growth. Not only is touch good for the body, it's good for the mind. Studies show that newborns receiving extra touch display enhanced neurological development. Why this smart connection? Researchers believe that touch promotes the growth of myelin, the insulating material around nerves that makes nerve impulses travel faster.

Touch improves digestion. Babies receiving extra touch show enhanced secretion of digestive hormones. Researchers believe that this is another reason that touched infants grow better. It seems that touch makes the babies' digestive system more efficient. Babies with colic caused by the irritable colon syndrome may have less trouble in the colon when massaged frequently.

Touch improves behavior. Research shows babies receiving extra touch become better organized. They sleep better at night, fuss less during the day, and relate better to caregivers' interactions. Touch settles babies. Massage can be a wonderful tool for helping baby go to sleep at night.

Touch promotes baby's self-esteem. Being on the receiving end of loving hands helps babies develop a feel for their body parts by learning which areas of the body are most sensitive and which need relaxing. Being touched gives value to a person, like an adult feeling "touched" by the remarks of a friend.

Touch helps parents. A daily massage helps you to get in touch with your whole baby, to read her body language, and to learn her cues. Giving your baby the right touch is just one more step up the ladder of learning about your baby. Infant massage is especially valuable for the parent and infant who had a slow start — for example, when separated by a medical complication. Massage helps parent and baby reconnect. For the slow-start mother who doesn't feel naturally "motherly" toward her newborn, massage is the extra spark to ignite the fire. Likewise for the slow-to-warm-up baby, massage helps break down the barrier so that the uncuddly baby gets to like being handled — and the parents get used to handling their baby.

Several employed mothers in our practice use an evening infant massage as a tool to help them reconnect with their baby after being away for the day. This special touch enables them to tune in to baby and tune out their work as they reenter home life.

For dads who are novices at caring for babies, massage is a hands-on course in baby handling. Also, it's important for baby to get used to dad's touch as well as mom's. Babies thrive on different strokes.

Special touches for special babies. Handicapped infants — and their parents — particularly benefit from infant massage. Studies show that massage helps motor-impaired infants better communicate their needs to the parents — a process called social cueing. Massage puts you in touch with your infant's body signals.

Learning the Right Touch

Massage is a touch you do *with* your baby, not to your baby. It's an interaction, not a task. You learn which strokes your baby enjoys and, as if dancing, go with the flow of your baby's body language. While it is nearly impossible to rub your baby the wrong way, here's how to learn the right touch for your baby.

Get Ready

Choose a warm, quiet, draft-free place. Our favorite is in front of a floor-to-ceiling window with the rays of sunlight warming baby. Do this ritual wherever you and baby are comfortable: on the floor, a padded table, grass, beach, or bed. Put on soothing music (see discussion of soothing sounds, page 324). Infant-massage instructors are a good reference source for music to massage by.

Choose a time when you are not in a hurry, not likely to be interrupted, and baby is most in need of relaxing. Some parents like to start the day off with a morning massage. Some prefer a before-nap massage. Babies with evening colic are best massaged toward late afternoon or early evening before the "happy hour" of colic begins. Sometimes a late-afternoon massage can prompt the colicky infant to forget his evening blast.

Choose the right massage oil. Infant-massage instructors and their selective infant clientele prefer fruit or vegetable oil ("edible oils"), vitamin E enriched and unscented. Look for "cold pressed" on the label, which means the oil has been extracted only by the use of pressure, not by heat or chemical solvents, which change the characteristics of the oil. Avoid oils made from a petroleum base. Massage oils that have stood the test of time are coconut, almond, apricot, safflower, and avocado oils. Watch for a possible skin allergy rash to occur within an hour, especially to nut oils.

Get Set

Position yourself and baby so you're both comfortable. Sit on the floor with your back against the couch or wall, or kneel alongside your bed. In the early months babies like to lie in the natural cradle formed in your lap when you sit cross-legged; or just stretch your legs straight out in front of you. Place baby on a diaper-covered lambskin or a dryer-warmed towel draped over your legs as a pillow. When baby grows out of your leg cradle, stretch out your legs alongside baby. Be sure to keep a spare diaper handy for the unexpected sprays.

Veteran infant-massage instructors stress the importance of respecting baby's desire for a massage. They advise, before laying on hands, asking baby's permission — "Would you like a massage?" Babies become attentive to a *setting event,* a group of events that signal a familiar event will follow. When baby sees you rubbing oil into your hands and hears you pronouncing the cue word "massage," watch for his face to light up approvingly. If baby is upset, it's best to postpone the massage and just hold him awhile or use one of the comforting techniques in Chapter 16, "Parenting the Fussy or Colicky Baby." Remember, massage is something you do *with* your baby; if he's not "with" you, wait till a better time. If he becomes upset during the massage at any point, stop and just hold him. Massage is not meant to be like a Band-Aid that you apply to a baby who is hurting but rather is a process that equips baby (and you, too) to be better able to handle life's stresses.

If baby is wiggling or appears stiff and tense, open the ritual with a *touch-relaxation technique:* Engage baby in eye-to-eye contact

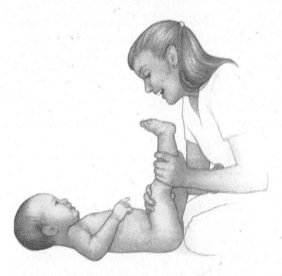

Regular massage sessions can help you and your baby stay "in touch."

before you start. Grasp baby's wiggly or tense legs and bicycle them while speaking softly, "Relax, relax . . . " This opener sets baby up to associate the touch-relaxation motions and sounds with the pleasant ritual to follow. This is baby's opening cue that the play is about to begin. And relax yourself. A tense baby doesn't relax to the touch of tense hands. Read and feel the response of your baby rather than making massage a mechanical exercise.

Go!

Begin with the legs, the easiest part to work with and the easiest for baby to accept. Hold the foot with one hand and "milk" the leg from ankle to thigh with the other. Then, hold the thigh with both hands, as if holding a baseball bat, and using a gentle twisting and squeezing motion, move your hands from thigh to foot. Finally, roll the leg between your hands from knee to ankle. As you move down the leg to the foot, do a series of thumb presses with your hand encircling the ankle and foot. For the finishing touch, lightly stroke the legs from thigh to feet before you move on to the trunk.

To massage the abdomen slide your whole palm and fingers in a hand-over-hand circular motion, working from the rib cage downward. Next, slide both hands around the abdomen in clockwise circular movements. To relax a tense, bloated abdomen try the "I Love U" stroke (see page 403). Finally, using fingertip pressure, try "walking" over the abdomen.

For the chest, slide both hands along the rib cage from center to sides and back again, like flattening the pages in a book.

The arms and hands are done in the same fashion as the legs and the feet, beginning, however, with a "pit stop" (massaging the lymph nodes in the armpit).

The face has special strokes all its own — whole-handed smoothing; lightly pressing, pushing, and circling with the thumbs; and finally combing from forehead over cheeks with light fingertip strokes.

Last, do the back, everyone's favorite. With the pads of your fingers, lightly rub small circles all over the back. Then gently comb with the fingertips from back over buttocks and legs to ankles.

There are many other creative touches that you and your baby will work out together as you learn the art of infant massage. You might also take a look at the book *Infant Massage: A Handbook for Loving Parents* by Vimila Schneider McClure (Bantam Books, 2000), complete with photographs illustrating the strokes. Remember, as in all aspects of parenting, *read your baby* along with the book. You can also purchase videotapes to learn the technique or obtain the services of a certified infant-massage instructor who can

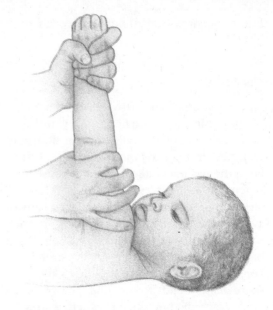

teach you personally. For more information or to contact a local instructor, consult the International Association of Infant Massage, U.S. Chapter, at www.IAIM-US.com; e-mail IAIM4US@aol.com; (805) 644-8524; fax (805) 644-7699.

Giving your baby a massage is like reading a long poem. If both of you are in the mood to hear the whole poem, you start at the beginning and go line by line in an orderly sequence (baby knows what to expect). If time is short or the setting not conducive to poetic retreat, you can jump in anywhere with a few favorite lines that you have memorized. For example, if you have had the whole massage earlier in the day, then at bedtime it is possible to savor the beauty of the whole by doing only the arm or the back massage to send your little one off to dreamland. Since he has learned to associate this with relaxing, you have a wonderful finishing touch to your bedtime routine, and one that can be administered by father.

7

Common Concerns in the Early Weeks

So much happens so fast as your baby adjusts to life outside the womb and you adjust to life with this little person. Knowing what to expect and understanding why babies do what they do will help you ease more comfortably into parenting.

EARLY NEWBORN CHANGES

Big changes occur in your newborn. Part of getting to know your child is cherishing these fleeting changes.

Breathing Patterns and Sounds

Watch your newborn breathe. Notice the irregular patterns. Baby takes many short breaths of varying lengths, an occasional deep sigh, and even has a worrisome ten-to-fifteen-second period when she doesn't appear to breathe; then baby breathes deeply (and so do you), and the cycle continues. Called *periodic breathing,* this irregular pattern is normal for the first few weeks. Breathing becomes more regular by the end of the first month. The younger or more pre-mature the baby, the more irregular the breathing.

First "cold." Because the nasal passages are small in the newborn, even a slight amount of clogging can cause noisy, uncomfortable breathing. You may think that this is your baby's first cold. But, although very loud and noisy, these early sniffles are usually not caused by an infection. Babies' nasal passages are easily congested with lint from blankets or clothing, dust, milk residue, or environmental irritants such as cigarette smoke, perfumes, hair sprays, and aerosols. A stuffy nose may cause baby a lot of difficulty breathing because newborns are obligate nose breathers, meaning they need to breathe through their noses rather than their mouths. A newborn with a stuffy nose does not switch easily to breathing with her mouth but rather struggles to get more air through her nose. One of the reasons that newborns sneeze a lot is to clear their nasal passages. It is unlikely to be her first cold. She is trying to clear her nose.

Gagging and choking. Your baby's lungs were filled with fluid while in the womb. Most of this fluid was squeezed out of the lungs during passage through the birth canal or was suctioned by the doctor or nurse after birth. Your baby may cough up some remaining mucus, which momentarily sticks in the back of the throat. Baby gags, then swallows the excess mucus and is all right. Placing baby on her side prevents this mucus from pooling in the back of the throat.

Noisy breathing. In addition to being uneven breathers, newborns are noisy breathers. Toward the end of the first month you may hear a gurgling sound in baby's throat and feel a rattling in her chest. Your baby seems generally well and happy — she is just noisy. This is not a cold, since it is seldom caused by an infection. Near the end of the first month or during the second month of age, babies begin to produce a lot of saliva, often more than they can comfortably swallow. Some of the saliva pools in the back of the throat. Air passing through it produces gurgling noises. When you place your hand on baby's back or chest, the rattle you hear and feel is not really coming from the chest but from the vibrations produced by air passing through saliva in the back of the throat. These normal sounds subside when baby learns to swallow the saliva at the same rate she produces it.

You may notice that baby seems quieter in her sleep. This is because saliva production lessens when babies fall asleep. Your baby will not choke on these secretions and will eventually learn to swallow the excess saliva. No medicines are necessary.

Normal noises. Newborns are anything but silent, even when they are asleep. Most noises are caused by too much air passing too fast through small passages. Here are our favorite precious sounds: *gurgles* caused by

---

CLEARING LITTLE NOSES

Here's how you can help your newborn breathe more easily.

- When your newborn is awake, place her on her stomach with her head turned to one side. This position allows the tongue and any saliva in the throat to come forward, making more room for air to pass.
- Keep your baby's sleeping environment as fuzz free and dust free as possible. Remove dust collectors such as feather pillows, fuzzy animals, and the dozens of furry gifts that surround most newborns. (There is no need to defuzz baby's sleeping environment if her nose is not congested.)
- Keep baby away from nasal irritants: cigarette smoke, paint and gasoline fumes, aerosols, perfumes, and hair sprays. Do not allow smoking in the same house as baby. This is one of the most common irritants to baby's sensitive nasal passages.
- Hose the little nose. Use saline nasal spray or drops to loosen the nasal secretions and stimulate baby to sneeze the secretions from the back of the nose toward the front, where you can gently remove them with a bulb syringe, called a nasal aspirator, available at your drugstore. (See page 665 for how to make and use nose-clearing solutions.)

---

air passing through pooled saliva in the back of the mouth; if accompanied by nasal congestion they are a combination of a snort and a gurgle we call *snurgles.* A burping sound may pass through mucus in the mouth or nose and become a *blurp* or, if accompanied by bubbles, a *burble.* Normal breathing may take on a *purring* quality when air and saliva compete for the same space. During sleep the already narrow breathing passages relax and become even narrower, causing each breath to take on either a musical, grunting, or sighing quality. And don't forget those delightful birdlike chirps and squeaks. Enjoy these sounds, for they won't last long.

Hiccups. All babies hiccup, in the womb and outside. Hiccups frequently occur after burping. We don't know the cause, and they don't bother baby. Feeding during hiccups usually settles the spell.

Baby's Elimination Patterns

Changes in your baby's stools. Expect your newborn's stools to progress from black to green to brown to yellow. The first few days baby's stools contain a black, tarlike, sticky substance called meconium, which is composed of amniotic-fluid debris from the newborn's intestines. Your newborn should have a meconium stool within the first twenty-four hours. If not, notify your doctor. Near the end of the first week your baby's stools will become less sticky and turn greenish brown. Between one and two weeks later they assume a yellowish-brown color and more regular consistency.

Breastfed versus bottlefed. The stools of breastfed and formula-fed infants are different. If you are breastfeeding, after a week or two, as your baby gets more of the fatty hindmilk, expect his stools to become yellow, seedy, and mustardlike in consistency. (See page 117 for a discussion of what's in mother's milk.) Because breast milk has a natural laxative effect, the stools of breastfed babies are more frequent, softer, more yellow, and have a not unpleasant buttermilk-like odor. The stools of the formula-fed infant tend to be less frequent, firmer, darker, greenish, and have an unpleasant odor. While the stools of the newborn baby are usually mustard yellow, an occasional green stool is of no significance if your baby seems generally well.

How frequent. How many stools a day varies greatly among newborns. As mentioned previously, breastfed infants usually have more stools than formula-fed infants. Some babies have a loose stool after or during every breastfeeding. And mothers often hear the gurgly sounds of the soft stool a few minutes into the feeding. An occasional watery gush (called an explosive stool) is usual and not to be confused with diarrhea. (If worried, read about diarrhea and signs of dehydration, page 686.) A newborn who is getting enough breast milk usually has two to five bowel movements a day, but it can also be normal to have one or two a day. Occasionally baby may even go two to three days without a bowel movement as a normal bowel pattern, but usually not until one or two months of age. Infrequent stooling in a breastfed baby less than two months old may mean the baby is not getting enough milk.

Blood in the stool. Occasionally babies have a hard stool, or a sudden explosive stool, that causes a tiny tear in the rectum, called a *rectal fissure.* If you notice a few spots of bright red blood on baby's diapers or streaks of blood in the stools, a fissure is probably the cause.

RX FOR INCONSOLABLE CRYING

Sometimes a baby who is generally not colicky and was previously well suddenly shows an outburst of unexplained, inconsolable crying. Before racing to the phone to summon your doctor, go through the following checklist.

☐ Does baby have an emergency medical problem? Two concerning signs are (1) persistent vomiting and (2) pale all over. If neither of these signs is present and baby does not look sick, it is not necessary to call your doctor immediately before going through the next steps.

☐ Is baby hurting? Undress baby completely and observe the following:

- Are any of baby's limbs not moving normally? Do you notice any unusual lumps or swelling? These observations are important to detect any injury from a recent fall; consult your doctor if a problem is noted.
- Is there swelling in the groin? This could indicate intestinal obstruction from a hernia, which requires medical attention.
- Is baby's abdomen tense and bloated, with more swelling on one side than on the other; or tense or tender when you try to massage it? These signs plus sudden onset of colicky behavior could indicate an intestinal obstruction, but this emergency medical problem is usually associated with persistent vomiting and a pale, generally ill-appearing baby. Be sure to feel baby's abdomen between outbursts because crying babies often swallow air and have tense-feeling abdomens.
- Does baby have a scalded-skin type of diaper rash? This can be very painful. (See treatment of diaper rash, page 110.)
- Is there a thick yellow discharge from the nose? This is often a sign of ear infection. (See treatment tips, page 680.)
- Has baby been straining to pass a stool? This suggests constipation; try a glycerine suppository. (See page 405.)
- Does baby have swollen gums with profuse drooling? He may be experiencing teething pain. (See pages 325 and 496.)
- Does baby have a hair wrapped around a finger or toe? Carefully remove it.

If your parent exam does not suggest any of the above problems or trigger an alarm that you need to seek immediate medical attention, proceed to the next step.

☐ Have you introduced any new foods that could upset baby? If breastfeeding, have you eaten any gas-producing foods within the past few hours? (See page 152.) If bottlefeeding, have you recently changed formulas? Have you introduced baby to a new solid food? (See page 271 on food allergies; see also page 385 for deflating gassy babies.)

☐ Is your baby just upset? If your parent detective work does not suggest any medical, physical, or allergic cause of baby's crying, try the following soothing techniques:

- putting baby in a sling and taking a walk
- nursing while carrying baby
- infant massage, especially the abdomen (see pages 95 and 403)

If none of these suggestions yield either cause or consolation, consult your baby's doctor. (For more soothing tips and for detailed insights into the cause and comfort of hurting babies, see pages 378–388.)

These heal easily by lubricating baby's rectum with over-the-counter pediatric glycerin suppositories (cut in half lengthwise).

Wet diaper changes. In the first week baby's urine is very unconcentrated, like water. After a few weeks the urine may assume a more concentrated yellow-amber color. During the first week your newborn may normally have two to three wet diapers a day. Thereafter expect your baby to wet at least six to eight cloth diapers (four to five disposables) a day.

What about reddish urine? Within the first week it is common to see a few orange or reddish spots on the diaper that may alarm you, since they resemble blood. These red spots are caused by urates, normal substances in the urine of the newborn that form an orange-to-red color on the diaper.

The Newborn's Body

Weight changes. Newborns usually lose around 6–10 ounces (170–280 grams), or about 5–8 percent of their birth weight, during the first week. Babies are born with extra fluid and fat to tide them over until their mother's milk can supply sufficient fluid and nutrition. How much weight a newborn loses depends on the following factors.

Large babies with a lot of extra fluid tend to lose the most weight; babies who are fed frequently on cue and room-in with their mothers tend to lose the least weight. How quickly your milk appears also influences your newborn's weight loss. If you room-in with your baby and breastfeed every two hours, your high-calorie hindmilk will appear sooner, and baby will lose less weight. Babies who are separated from their mothers a lot during the first week or who are fed on a three- to four-hour schedule, tend to lose the most weight. Remember to record your baby's weight upon discharge from the hospital. This is an important reference for measuring weight gain at your baby's first checkup.

Normal lumps. When you run your hand over baby's head you may feel lots of bumps and ridges, especially on top of the head, on the back of the head, and behind the ears. Babies' skull bones consist of many small bones that are unconnected to allow for brain growth and also for molding to the birth canal. During the second year baby's head will feel much smoother.

Another normal lump is a hard bump in the center of baby's chest, just above the tummy. This is the end of the breastbone, and in some babies it sticks out for a few months. Around the second or third month you will find several pea-sized lumps beneath the skin on the back of the head and along the neck. These are normal lymph glands.

Swollen scrotum. The testicles begin inside the abdominal cavity and, usually before birth, push through the groin tissue forming a scrotal sac. (Occasionally, one or both testes do not descend into the scrotum by birth time but may come down later. If the testes remain undescended by one year of age, they can be brought down by hormonal or surgical treatment.) The opening in the abdominal wall through which the testes migrated usually closes. Sometimes this passageway remains open, allowing fluid to accumulate around the testis. Called a hydrocele, this swelling seldom bothers baby and usually subsides by the first birthday. During your son's checkup the doctor may shine a penlight on the scrotum, illuminating the water around the testicle to confirm the diagnosis.

CROOKED FEET

A newborn's legs and feet reflect the scrunched-up position of "no standing room" in the womb. The legs are normally very bowed, and the feet turn in. Since the bones were curved that way for many months inside, expect several months of free kicking before the legs and feet straighten. You can help the straightening process by not letting baby sleep in the fetal position — with feet and legs curled beneath (see page 550). For the persistent fetal sleeper, sewing the pajama feet together prevents sleeping in this tucked-in position.

When not to worry. Pick up those precious feet and look at the soles. It's normal for the front of the foot to be curved in a bit. Now hold the heel of baby's foot with one hand and gently stretch the front of the foot to the straight position. If the foot straightens easily with gentle stretching, this is normal curvature that will self-correct within a few months. To help these little feet straighten, do these stretches with each diaper change and minimize sleeping in the fetal position, as mentioned above.

When treatment may be needed. If the front of the foot is curved inward and you see and feel the following features, your doctor may suggest treatment:

- The front half of the foot is very curved in relation to the back.
- You are unable to straighten the foot with gentle pressure.
- There is a deep crease in the sole where the front of the foot begins to curve inward.

If your baby's foot or feet (usually it's both) have these features at birth and show no signs of self-correcting over the following month or two, your doctor may send baby to an orthopedic specialist for a simple and painless treatment called *serial casting*. Plaster casts resembling little white boots are placed over your baby's feet. The doctor changes these casts every two weeks, each time straightening the foot a bit, over the course of two or three months. After the cast treatment your doctor may prescribe special shoes for a few more months to keep baby's feet straight.

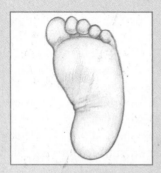

Crooked foot.

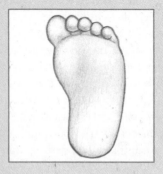

Normal foot.

Occasionally a loop of intestines may poke through this opening into the scrotum. This is called an *inguinal hernia*. Unlike a hydrocele, which is round and soft, a hernia feels more firm and oblong, about the size of a thumb. A hernia swelling comes and goes, usually disappearing back into the abdomen when baby is asleep or relaxed and bulging out again during crying. Mention this swelling to the doctor on baby's next checkup. The hernia will need to be repaired by a minor surgical procedure, usually without an overnight stay in the hospital.

Rarely, the loop of intestines gets stuck in the scrotum, prompting immediate surgical release to prevent damage to the intestines. Call your doctor right away if the swelling suddenly gets larger, harder, darker, tender, or baby is vomiting and suffering colicky pain.

Lump in the labia. The labia are equivalent to the scrotal sac in males. Sometimes an ovary can migrate into the labia and feels like a movable marble beneath the skin. Mention this to your doctor, who will arrange to have the ovary repositioned in the abdominal cavity by a minor surgical procedure.

Baby's swollen breasts. Because of a surge of breast-enlarging hormones at birth, your baby's breasts may become swollen, firm, and lumpy within a week after birth. And these baby breasts may even produce a few drops of milk. These are normal physiologic changes in both girl and boy babies. The swelling should subside within a few months.

Closing vagina. Commonly during the first year or two you may notice that the slitlike opening in your daughter's vagina begins to close. Mention this to your doctor during your baby's regular checkup. Called labial adhesions, this condition occurs because the sides of the vaginal opening are so close to each other that they begin growing together. This does not cause baby any discomfort or harm. Oftentimes these adhesions open by themselves. But if the adhesions are becoming thicker or obstructing the whole orifice enough to block the flow of urine, your doctor may gently open the adhesion. You can prevent them from growing back together again by daily gently spreading the labia apart. If they continually grow back, the doctor may prescribe an estrogen cream to be applied around the edges to prevent further adhesion. Around two years of age, as your daughter begins producing her own estrogen in this tissue, the labial adhesions will subside.

Protruding navel. Babies are born with an opening in the abdominal wall through which the umbilical-cord vessels connect with the placenta. When the cord is cut, the stump shrivels up. Sometimes the newly formed navel bulges out — other times it stays flat or inverts. Whether it's an "outie" or an "innie" depends on the individual way a stump heals, not the way it's cut. Most outies flatten with time.

Two large bands of muscles grow down the center of baby's abdomen and encircle the navel. Sometimes there is an opening between these muscles, and when baby cries or strains the navel protrudes. The intestines poke through beneath the skin, and you feel a squishy bulge of intestines in the protruding navel. This is called an *umbilical hernia*. It may be the size of a golf ball or a fingertip. As the muscles grow, the opening in and around the navel seals, and the hernia disappears. Umbilical hernias are particularly common in African American babies. They do not hurt baby. Above all, don't tape over the hernia. This doesn't speed the closure and can lead to irritation. Nearly all heal with only the treatment of time, usually by the second birthday.

Quivers and shakes. Baby's immature nervous system causes frequent muscle twitches: quivering chin, shaking arms and legs, and grinlike lip twitches. These normal movements, especially noticeable while baby is drifting off to sleep, subside by three months.

Creaking joints. When you move baby's joints you may hear crackles or "joint noises." These are normal, caused by loose ligaments and loose bones.

SPITTING UP

The spots of dried milk on your clothing are telltale signs that you are the parent of a spitter. Most babies regurgitate, or spit up, their milk or formula several times a day during the early months. This is more of a laundry problem than a medical problem and seldom bothers baby. Dress for the occasion. If you are blessed with a baby who shares a bit of each meal with your clothing, wear prints and avoid dark-colored clothing. Keep a cloth diaper handy as a burp cloth.

Not much lost. When baby spits up, you may feel she has lost the whole meal of the milk your body worked so hard to produce or wasted the expensive formula you bought. But you are likely to vastly overestimate the volume of regurgitated milk. Pour a tablespoon of milk or formula on the countertop and watch the huge puddle it makes. Now, does that amount match the spot on your dress? Most spit-up measures only a teaspoonful.

Why babies spit up. Babies spit up because they are just being babies. They gulp milk and air, and the air settles beneath the milk in the stomach. When baby's stomach contracts, like an air gun the stomach shoots some milk back up the esophagus, and you have sour, curdled milk on your shoulder. Some ravenous eaters gulp too much milk too fast, and the overloaded tummy sends some back. Jostling babies after eating may also trigger regurgitation.

Settling the spitter. Here are some suggestions that may help your spitter:

- Slow the feedings. Respect that tiny babies have tiny tummies. If you are formula feeding, give your baby smaller-volume, more frequent feedings.

- Burp baby during and after the feedings. Formula-fed spitters should be burped after every three ounces (ninety milliliters) of milk, and breastfed spitters should be burped when switching sides or during a pause in baby's sucking if baby lingers on one side. (See "Burping Baby," page 213.)

- Feed upright and keep baby upright twenty to thirty minutes after feeding. If you do not have time simply to sit and hold your baby upright, wear your baby in the upright position in a baby sling as you go about your work. Gravity is the spitter's best friend.

- Avoid jostling or bouncing baby for at least a half hour after a feed.

- If bottlefeeding, be sure the nipple hole is neither too large nor too small. (See pages 210 and 213 for how to judge the right nipple-hole size.)

When to expect the last spat. Most spitting up subsides around six to seven months when baby sits upright and gravity holds down the milk. (See discussion of gastroesophageal reflux, pages 388–397.)

Blood in spit-up. Don't panic at baby's first bleed. If you breastfeed, most often this is your blood, not baby's. It usually comes from cracked nipples during breastfeeding and subsides when your nipples heal. Occasionally baby may retch or spit up forcefully and tear a tiny blood vessel at the end of the esophagus. This also heals quickly. If neither of these causes seems likely and the bleeding continues, notify your doctor.

SPITTING UP: WHEN TO WORRY

Spitting up becomes a problem and needs medical attention if any of the following occur:

- Baby is losing weight or not gaining weight sufficiently.
- The vomiting increases in frequency and volume and becomes projectile (the spit-up flies across your lap and onto the floor).
- The vomitus is consistently green (bile stained).
- Painful colicky behaviors accompany the vomiting. (See the discussion of gastroesophageal reflux, pages 388–397.)
- Baby gags and coughs during every feeding.

EYES

Discharging Eyes

Most newborns' eyes begin tearing by three weeks of age. These tears should drain into the nose through tiny tear ducts at the inside corners of the eye. During the first few weeks or months you may notice a yellow, sticky discharge from one or both eyes. This is usually caused by a blocked tear duct. At birth, the nasal end of these ducts is sometimes covered by a thin membrane that usually breaks open shortly after birth, allowing proper drainage of tears. Often this membrane does not fully open, causing the tear ducts to remain plugged and tears to accumulate in one or both eyes. Fluid that does not drain properly becomes infected. If this happens, the discharge from your baby's eyes will be persistently yellow, indicating infection in the region of the blocked tear ducts.

Here's how to unclog your baby's tear duct. Gently massage the tear duct that is located beneath the tiny "bump" in the nasal corner of each eye. Massage in a downward and inward direction (toward the nose) about six times. Do this tear-duct massage as often as you think of it — for example, before each diaper change (after washing your fingers). Massaging the tear duct applies pressure on the fluid backed up within the ducts and eventually pops open the membrane and clears the ducts.

If you still notice persistent tearing or yellow drainage from one or both eyes, during your well-baby checkup ask your doctor to instruct you in how to massage the tear ducts. If the yellow drainage persists, your doctor may prescribe antibiotic ointment or drops to treat this infection. Mothers often report that squirting a few drops of their breast milk (which is loaded with germ-fighting substances) will clear up the eye discharge.

Blockages may recur intermittently, but tear ducts usually remain open by six months. Occasionally this conservative treatment does not work, and between nine months and one year it becomes necessary for an eye doctor to open these tear ducts by inserting a tiny wire probe into them. This is usually a short, minor office procedure but may require out-patient surgery under general anesthesia if done after one year. Discharge from the eyes in the first few months is almost always caused by blocked tear ducts; in the older infant and child, discharging eyes may be caused by an eye infection called conjunctivitis or, more commonly, may be part of an infection in the ears and sinuses. (See conjunctivitis, page 708.)

Red Streaks in Eyes

Shortly after baby's birth you may notice a red streak in the whites of one or both of baby's eyes. Don't worry! These are called *conjunctival hemorrhages* and are caused by blood vessels broken during the squeeze of delivery. These do not harm baby's eyes and disappear within a few weeks.

BABY'S MOUTH

You look inside your baby's mouth and see white cheesy patches on the inside lips or cheeks or on the tongue or the roof of the mouth. These spots weren't there before, and new spots bother new mothers. You can't wait to share your newly found spots with the doctor, who is only a phone call away.

Thrush

Hold the phone — it's only thrush, a yeast infection inside baby's mouth. Yeast is a fungus that normally resides in warm, moist areas of the skin, such as the mouth, vagina, and diaper area, and thrives on milk. Yeast infections commonly flare up following antibiotic therapy, since antibiotics also kill the good bacteria that normally keep the yeast germs under control.

Unless it is left untreated, thrush seldom bothers babies, though it may itch and cause an irritable soreness in the mouth. It is more a nuisance than a medical problem, although some babies with thrush may become quite cranky during feeding. Milk deposits on the tongue and membranes of the mouth may be confused with thrush, but milk can be easily wiped off; thrush cannot. When you try to wipe the thrush off the tongue or mucous membranes, it may leave a superficially eroded area, and sometimes even tiny points of bleeding.

Most likely your newborn did not "catch" thrush from another baby. Rather, it is probably due to an overgrowth of baby's own yeast organisms, which normally reside in the mouth and skin, usually living there harmoniously without anyone's knowing they're there. In fact, baby was probably first introduced to yeast during passage through your birth canal.

Treatment. Notify your doctor (no emergency call necessary), who will prescribe an antifungal medication. Using your fingertips or the applicator that comes with the medicine, paint the thrush medicine on the patches of thrush and the rest of the mucous membranes of your baby's mouth and tongue four times a day for ten days. Here's a simple home remedy to use in addition to the medicine for thrush: Spread a fingertipful of acidophilus powder (available in capsules in the refrigerated section of a nutrition store) on the thrush twice a day for a week.

Yeast residents may often be resistant to eviction from the mouth. Several courses of treatment may be needed. If baby is using rubber nipples, teething toys, or pacifiers, boil them for twenty minutes once daily. Oral thrush may be accompanied by a fungal diaper rash. (See suggestions for treatment of diaper rash later in this chapter.)

Sharing thrush. Your baby's first bit of sharing may be to transfer his oral thrush to your nipples during breastfeeding. Signs of nipple thrush: Your nipples are sore; they are slightly reddened or pinkish; the skin is slightly puffy, dry, and flaky. Your nipples may feel itchy and burn, and you may experience a deep shooting pain, which radiates inward from the nipple after feeding. The same treatment as for your baby's oral thrush, a prescription antifungal cream medication, will chase the yeast from your nipples. If the fungus infection on your nipples is severe, your doctor may prescribe an oral antifungal medication. Mother can take acidophilus capsules as directed to help clear up this nuisance.

Lip Blisters

During the first month blisters or calluses may develop on your baby's upper lip. Called sucking pads, these develop in response to baby's vigorous sucking and subside toward the end of the first year. They are normal and do not bother baby, so leave them alone. You may also notice a few tiny white cysts on baby's palate or gums. Dubbed "pearls," these usually resolve within a few months.

NEWBORN SKIN MARKS AND RASHES

Run your hand over your baby's skin. So soft, so smooth, but not perfect. You feel dry patches, flaky areas, areas that are rough and wrinkled, and some areas where the skin doesn't seem to fit, such as around the chin, neck, wrist, and heels. But don't worry, your baby will grow into it. Let's run your hands and eyes, head to toe, over the variety of skin changes in most newborns.

Normal Baby Marks

When you look at your baby's skin, it doesn't look perfect either. There are spots and specks, blotches and bruises, streaks and stains — a coat of many hues that your newborn wears. But newborn skin has a remarkable quality — the ability to change — sometimes before your eyes.

Stork bites. Most newborns have areas where lots of blood vessels bunch up and show through their thin skin. These smooth reddish-pink marks are most prominent on the eyelids, the nape of the neck, and in the middle of the forehead. They are not, in correct skin talk, rashes. These are called *nevi* or, in parent terms, birthmarks. Grandmothers dubbed them stork bites. But the mythical stork did not bite your baby. These skin curiosities stem from bunches of overgrown blood vessels showing through the newborn's thin skin. As the excess blood vessels shrink and your baby's skin thickens, they nearly always disappear or fade by the first birthday. Some nevi, especially on the nape of the neck, persist but are obscured by hair. Sometimes these distinguishing marks fade but reappear when baby strains or cries, prompting parents to exclaim, "His forehead lights are on."

Strawberries. While stork bites appear at birth and fade with time, other birthmarks appear a week or two later and grow with time. Most begin as a raised red circle and gradually enlarge to coin size during the first year. Between one and three years they begin to shrivel up. You will know when the growth has reached its peak when you see the center turn gray.

Called *strawberry hemangiomas* — they look and feel like a strawberry — these birthmarks come from blood vessels that went astray and kept growing. Most babies have at least one. And, like a bunch of strawberries, they come in various sizes and shapes, ranging from freckle size to as large as a golf ball.

While cosmetically unattractive, most of these strawberry hemangiomas are best left alone to self-destruct. Sometimes they are a nuisance by location. Such a growth on the eyelid, for example, may interfere with lid opening and strain baby's developing vision. Others reside in areas such as the arms and legs where they bleed when struck. Rarely do they persist as a cosmetic nuisance. In these situations, disfiguring or annoying hemangiomas can be shrunk and removed by injections and laser treatment.

Moles. Called *pigmented nevi,* these brown-to-black moles range from freckle size to large, hairy patches. The moles usually remain the same, so they appear relatively smaller as your baby grows. They are benign and need neither worry nor treatment. When you start using sunscreen (see page 735), be sure to cover the moles with it. Very large pigmented hairy nevi should be removed because of their potential for becoming malignant.

Mongolian spots. Never a year goes by that I don't get an embarrassing call from someone accusing a parent of child abuse because of black-and-blue marks on baby's bottom. These bruiselike spots, common in African American, Latino, Asian, Indian, and Native American babies, are prominent on the lower back and buttocks and sometimes also on the shoulders and legs. These "spank" marks fade in time, but most never completely disappear.

Café-au-lait spots. These are flat, brown birthmarks, resembling tiny puddles of coffee and cream. Most remain the same size, becoming relatively smaller as baby grows.

Baby's First Spots

Milia. In the early weeks you may see and feel tiny whiteheads sprinkled over your baby's face, especially the nose. Caused by secretions plugging the skin pores, these milia are normal and disappear within a few months without any treatment.

Toxic erythema. Don't be frightened by its alarming name. The dotlike spots appear as yellowish-white pimples surrounded with a red blotchy ring. They look like bites. These normal spots appear during the first week most commonly on your baby's abdomen, and disappear without treatment by two weeks.

Prickly heat. A reddish pimply rash, prickly heat appears on excessively moist areas of the skin, such as between the neck folds, behind the ears, in the groin, or in areas where clothing fits tightly. Run your fingers gently over the rash, and you will know why parents call this rash prickly. It has a coarse, sandpaperlike feel. I suspect prickly heat can bother a baby. To take the heat and the prickles out of the rash, dress your baby in light-weight, loose-fitting cotton clothing and gently wash the skin with plain cool water or a solution of baking soda (one teaspoon to a cup of water). Remember to dab, wash, and blot dry; do not scrub and rub sensitive newborn skin.

Newborn acne. Around the third or fourth week be prepared for the picture-perfect baby face to show its first complexion problem.

In a situation similar to the hormonal stages of puberty, the increased hormones at birth may cause the overproduction of a waxy, oily substance called sebum in the oil glands of the skin, most noticeably in the face and scalp. Plugging of these glands leads to inflammation and the formation of pimples. Parents call it baby acne. The medical term is *seborrheic dermatitis.*

Like teenage acne, the red, pimply, oily rash covers much of baby's face, and the previously soft, smooth cheeks feel sandpaper rough. Hold the camera; this first puberty is short-lived (in fact, veteran baby-face watchers plan first photos or christenings before or after the acne period). Newborn acne usually peaks around the third week and clears within a month or six weeks.

Newborn acne bothers parents more than baby. Cut baby's fingernails short to prevent scratching. Gentle washing with water and a mild soap will remove the excess and sometimes irritating oil. If the acne pimples get infected (red area around the pimples or honeylike oozing), your doctor may prescribe an antibacterial cream. Most newborn acne disappears completely without any special care of the skin.

If the condition appears early (that is, in the second week) and/or worsens quickly, spreading past the face into the hair and down onto the neck and even the shoulders, you may be observing one of the first signs of allergy to a nutrient in baby's formula or in your breast milk. This happened with our seventh baby, Stephen, and the acne retreated dramatically when cow's milk products were eliminated from Martha's diet.

Cradle cap. In another form of seborrheic dermatitis, you will notice and feel a crusty, oily, plaquelike rash on baby's scalp, especially over the soft spot. In a mild case of cradle cap the flaky, dry skin on the scalp resembles dandruff. This seldom needs any more treatment than gentle washing and increased humidity. Wash the scalp with a mild shampoo no more often than once a week. Too-vigorous and too-frequent hair washing will only dry out the scalp and make the cradle cap worse.

Here's how to treat a more severe case of cradle cap:

- Massage cold-pressed vegetable oil into the crusty areas to soften them. Give the oil fifteen minutes or so to soak in.

- Using a very soft toothbrush, gently remove the scales.

- Wash off the excess oil with a mild baby shampoo.

If the cradle cap is persistent, severe, and itchy, try an over-the-counter (OTC) mild tar shampoo twice a week until it clears up. (See "Rx for Healthy Baby Skin," page 113.)

You may also notice a crusty, oily rash behind your baby's ears and in the skin folds of the neck. This seborrheic dermatitis is usually cleared with gentle washing with warm water, but sometimes hydrocortisone cream may help. Skin enjoys humidity. This is why most rashes worsen during the winter months, when central heating dries the air. A vaporizer or humidifier in your baby's sleeping room will moisturize dry skin.

DIAPER RASH: PREVENTION AND TREATMENT

Take a close look at your newborn's blemish-free bottom. Its complexion may never be so clear for the next year. When you begin diapering, a rash is soon to come. Diapers and skin just don't go together without friction. To protect the surroundings from baby's excrement, diapers were invented — and baby's skin rebels at losing its freedom to enjoy fresh air and sunshine.

Where does diaper rash come from? Start with ultrasensitive skin, add the chemicals of urine and stools, occlude the area with a big "bandage," and rub it all together. Presto! You have diaper rash. Keep this mixture together long enough, and bacteria and fungi begin to

---

HEALING CRACKED SKIN

Many newborns, especially if post-mature, have dry flaky skin, most noticeably on the hands and feet. Baby's natural skin oils suffice; no lotion is necessary. If cracks develop in the creases around the wrists and ankles, apply a moisturizing cream such as Soothe and Heal with Lansinoh or an infant massage oil, such as coconut, almond, safflower, apricot, or avocado oil.

---

grow into the weakened skin, and you have more diaper rash.

Excessive moisture on sensitive skin is the main culprit in diaper rash. Too much moisture removes the skin's natural oils, and wet skin is more easily damaged by friction. Once the skin has been irritated by excessive moisture, it is no longer a good natural barrier. Infants have a lot of fat folds around the groin. These moist folds of skin rubbing together is the reason a rash is most often seen in the creases of the groin. Just as the skin gets used to the wetness, solid foods present different chemical irritants, and the rash changes — the bottom's reflection of something changing at the other end.

Dealing with Diaper Rash

Don't take diaper rash too personally. "But I change him as soon as he wets," mothers often say, apologizing for their baby's persistent rash. Babies of even the most attentive diaper changers get rashes. But here are ways to lessen it.

Change frequently. Studies have shown that infants who are changed at least eight times a day have fewer cases of diaper rash.

Try different types of diapers. While each brand claims victory over diaper rash, experiment with both cloth and different brands of disposable diapers to see which one causes the least diaper rash.

Rinse irritants from diapers. If washing your own diapers, to remove soap residues and alkaline irritants add one-half cup of vinegar to the rinse cycle. You can also request this treatment from your diaper service.

Rinse or wipe well. During each change rinse baby's bottom, especially if the diaper is soaked or you smell ammonia. Experiment with what gets along well with your baby's bottom. Sensitive skin does best with plain water; some bottoms need a mild soap. Some sensitive bottoms rebel at the chemicals in disposable baby wipes, especially those that contain alcohol; some bottoms accept them without a rash. Try different wipes until you find the one that works.

Pat gently. *Blot* dry with a soft towel or a clean cotton diaper. Avoid excessive towel rubbing or scrubbing with a strong soap on irritated skin. One of our babies had such sensitive skin that even towel blotting reddened the skin. We used a hair dryer (lowest setting, twelve inches away) to blow-dry her bottom.

Air-condition baby's bottom. Allow the diaper area to breath by applying disposable diapers loosely. Avoid tight-fitting diapers and occlusive elastic pants that retain moisture; reserve these pants for occasions when a leaky diaper would be socially unacceptable.

Keep bottoms up. While baby is sleeping, expose his bare bottom to the air and occasionally to a ten-minute ray of sunlight near a *closed* window. Place naked baby on a folded cloth diaper with a rubberized pad underneath to protect bedding and blankets. In warm weather and after the newborn period let baby nap outside with his bare bottom exposed to fresh air.

Remove friction. To reduce friction, try a larger-size diaper. Fold the plastic liner of disposable diapers outward so that only the soft area of the diaper touches baby's skin. A "border" rash around baby's belt line reveals friction as the culprit. Besides this diaper-to-skin friction, the fat folds around baby's groin rub together during cycling of the legs or during toddler walking. Apply a lubricant such as Original A & D Ointment or a zinc-oxide cream to reduce chafing along the groin creases.

Barrier Creams

For most rashless bottoms, creams and ointments are not needed, as they may prevent the skin from breathing naturally. But if your baby's bottom is prone to rashes — "As soon as I get the rash cleared up, it starts again" — barrier creams may be a good ounce of prevention. At the first sign of a reddened, irritated bottom, *generously* apply a barrier cream containing zinc oxide. Barrier compounds protect the underlying skin from irritants and friction rubs. Cornstarch, one of the oldest protective compounds, can be used in groin creases to prevent friction rubs, but in our experience cornstarch cakes and is more of a nuisance than a help.

Dietary Changes

When conditions change at one end, expect changes at the other. Changing the diet — including formula changes and beginning solids — teething, or taking medicines all result in a change in the chemistry of stools and urine, producing a rash. (Incidentally, studies have shown that breastfeeding babies have less severe diaper rashes.) As soon as these "mouth end" conditions change, apply barrier creams before the rash begins, especially if your baby is prone to diaper rash.

If baby is taking antibiotics, give a daily teaspoon or break open a capsule of acidophilus or *Lactobacillus bifidus* powder to lessen the antibiotic-produced diarrhea and resulting rash. (See "Probiotics," page 691.) If the rash doesn't improve quickly, try an antifungal cream (see below).

How to Be a Diaper Rash Detective

"Diaper rash" is really an umbrella term for a number of skin rashes in the diaper area. Here are tips for identifying and treating some specific types of diaper rash.

Allergy ring. A red ring around baby's anus reflects a dietary irritant as the culprit, similar to a rash around baby's mouth when beginning a new food. Excess citrus fruit and juices and wheat are the main irritants. Discontinue the food to see if the red ring goes away. You may even need to drop the food from your diet if you are breastfeeding. (See

page 267 for a thorough discussion of food allergies.)

Contact dermatitis. A red, flat, scald-type rash, contact dermatitis appears over the area of rubbing by the diapers, usually around the belt line and upper thighs. A telltale sign of this type of rash is the sparing of the creases where the skin is not in intimate contact with diapers. Causes of the rash include a chemical irritant in the diaper itself or in the detergent, or the chemical irritants that form after urine and stools remain in the diaper for a period of time. Chafing of synthetic material on sensitive skin is another possible cause, as are the chemical changes in the stools during diarrheic illness or antibiotic treatment.

To treat, soak baby's bottom in warm water for five minutes; after soaking, if you detect a whiff of ammonia on baby's diaper area, soak longer. Leave your baby diaperless as much as is practical. Experiment with different diapers and apply an over-the-counter 1 percent hydrocortisone cream twice daily for a few days in addition to your usual cream.

YOUR OWN DIAPER RASH RX

Try this "prescription" to treat your baby's diaper rash:

- zinc cream with each diaper change
- antifungal cream (Lotrimin)
- 1 percent hydrocortisone cream (do not use for more than three days without consulting your doctor)

Apply *each* twice daily at different times. (All three are available in over-the-counter preparations.)

Intertrigo. In appearance, intertrigo is just the opposite of contact dermatitis. It occurs where the skin folds rub together, such as in the groin. This is caused by the "tropical climate" heat and moisture retention in the creases, resulting in irritation of the skin. When urine touches the irritated areas of the intertrigo, it may burn the skin, causing baby to cry. To treat, apply Original A & D Ointment to the irritated skin with each diaper change.

Seborrheic dermatitis. The margins of seborrheic dermatitis are sharply demarcated, and the condition looks like a big red patch over the groin, genitalia, and lower abdomen. This is one of the most sore-looking diaper rashes — more raised, rough, thick, and greasy than any of the others. Besides the preceding preventive measures, this type of rash is usually treated with an OTC ½ percent or 1 percent cortisone cream or, if severe, a prescription cream. A word of caution: Do not use cortisone cream on the diaper area longer than prescribed by your doctor, as overuse may damage the skin. (See also "Treating Eczema," page 703.)

Yeast rash (candida). If your baby's diaper rash persists despite all of the preventive measures and over-the-counter creams already mentioned, suspect yeast, and try an over-the-counter or prescription antifungal cream. A yeast rash is a reddish-pink, raised, patchy rash with sharp borders, primarily over the genitalia but with satellite spots sprinkled around the main area of rash and often appearing as tiny pustules. Yeast infection may occur on top of any of the preceding diaper rashes if they last more than a few days. Sometimes for

RX FOR HEALTHY BABY SKIN

Healthy baby skin depends not only on what the skin touches and is exposed to (what I call the outside job), but also on what feeds the skin — the inside job! Besides being kind to baby's sensitive skin by not using irritating clothing and not exposing baby to the damaging rays of the sun, feed baby's skin the right nutrients and you will continue to see and feel that adorable baby skin for a long time.

Hydrate baby's skin. Like fertile soil, babies need lots of fluids to keep skin from drying out. Formula-fed babies should drink one bottle of water every day. Breastfed babies do not need extra water.

Oil baby's skin. Next, healthy skin needs to be rich in healthy oils. The best oils for healthy skin are omega-3 fatty acids. Besides breast milk the best food source of omega 3's is cold-water fish, such as deep ocean salmon. Flax oil and, to a lesser extent, canola oil, are also rich sources of skin-healthy omega-3 oils. In our pediatric practice, I have seen dramatic results in my little patients with dry, scaly skin when I prescribe extra omega 3's for the breastfeeding mother's diet or one teaspoon of flax oil added daily to a bottle of formula for infants. For toddlers I prescribe one tablespoon of flax oil added daily to a fruit-and-yogurt smoothie. (For more skin health tips, see "Treating Eczema," page 703.)

persistent yeast rashes it is necessary to give an antifungal medication orally, as in treating thrush.

Impetigo. Caused by a bacteria (usually streptococci or staphylococci), impetigo appears as coin-sized blisters that ooze a honey-colored crust. These are spotted around the diaper area, primarily around the buttocks. This type of diaper rash needs a prescription antibiotic cream and sometimes oral antibiotics.

Diaper rash is a fact of civilized, bottom-covering baby life. Like all the nuisance stages of infancy, it too will pass.

II

Infant Feeding and Nutrition

Baby feeding is a learned art with a pinch of science and a touch of patience. Becoming your child's own nutritionist takes knowledge of good nutrition, awareness of infant development, and skill in creative marketing. Both the food choices and the eating patterns you instill into your toddler will help shape his young taste for lifelong healthy eating habits. Reading the feeding cues of your baby, introducing solid foods wisely, and encouraging self-feeding all lead to an important principle of infant nourishment — creating a healthy feeding attitude. To a baby, feeding is not only a developmental skill but a social event. There's a person at both ends of the feeding, whether it be by breast, bottle, or spoon. During the first year you will spend more time feeding your baby than in any other interaction. Here's how to make the most of it.

8

Breastfeeding: Why and How

Breastfeeding is a *life-style* — and a way of feeding. In the early weeks, you will have days when you are ready to toss in the nursing bras and reach for a bottle. But when you realize how breastfeeding benefits mother, baby, and family, you will strive to conquer the problems and master the art of providing the oldest and choicest in infant nourishment. Breast milk does good things for baby. Breastfeeding does good things for mother. Martha has breastfed all eight of our children and was breastfeeding our new baby as we wrote this book. We wish to share the self-help techniques we have learned in our eighteen years of personal breastfeeding experience, our thirty-year professional experience in counseling breastfeeding families, and our work as codirectors of a breastfeeding center. Breastfeeding matters!

WHY BREAST IS BEST

Mother's milk is special. No two mothers make the same milk; no two babies need the same milk. Your milk is custom-made to meet the needs of your baby. Every milk has what is called *biologic specificity* — meaning every species of mammal formulates a milk that is unique for the young of that species, ensuring their growth and enhancing their survival. Mother seals, for instance, make a high-fat milk because baby seals need high body fat to survive in cold water. What is a human baby's survival organ? The brain. And human milk contains special nutrients that promote brain growth.

Components of Mother's Milk

Let's pick out the main ingredients from the oldest living recipe and see how each is tailor-made to fit *your* baby.

Fats

The most changeable ingredients of breast milk, fats vary according to the caloric needs of your growing baby. The fat content of your milk changes during a feeding, at various times during the day, and as your infant grows, adjusting like a self-formulating fuel to the energy needs of your baby. At the start of a feeding your *foremilk* is low in fat, like skim milk. As the feeding progresses the fat steadily increases until your baby gets the

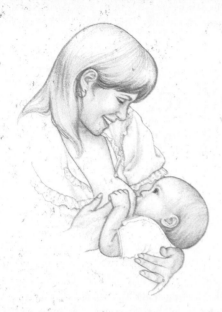

Because breastfeeding is an exercise in baby reading, it helps you get to know your baby.

"cream," the higher-fat *hindmilk*. This milk contains a built-in *satiety factor* that gives your infant a feeling of contented fullness, and baby stops eating. Watch breastfeeding babies at the end of a feeding. Notice how they radiate an "I feel good" look.

Suppose your baby is just thirsty. She will suck for only a few minutes and be satisfied with the lower-fat foremilk. Throughout the day babies enjoy an occasional two-minute feeding — little pick-me-up periods of emotional refueling. When truly hungry, your baby will suck longer and more vigorously, eventually being rewarded with the more-filling, higher-calorie hindmilk. As their rate of growth decelerates, older babies need fewer calories per unit of body weight. You guessed it! The fat content of human milk lessens as baby grows, automatically changing from "whole milk" to "low fat" during the last half of the first year.

Then come those frequent growth spurts, when every few weeks baby seems to feed continuously for a few days — called frequency days or marathon feeding — to get more energy for more growth. As intervals between feeds shorten, the fat content increases to accommodate the increased energy needs of a rapidly growing infant.

The moral of this fat story is that breastfeeding infants are not just passive players in the feeding game. They take an active part in shaping the food and the feeding to satisfy their individual needs.

Smarter fats. Human milk contains brain-boosting fats, namely DHA (docosahexaenoic acid) and ARA (arachidonic acid), omega-3 fatty acids vital for the growth and development of nerve tissue. DHA is needed to form myelin, the insulating sheath around each nerve that helps electrical nerve impulses travel faster and get to where they should go. Studies have shown that DHA concentrations are highest in the brains of babies who are breastfed and highest of all in those who are breastfed the longest. Recently, manufacturers in the United States have begun to include DHA and ARA in infant formula. It is likely, however, that DHA is only one of hundreds of yet to be identified ingredients in human milk that work together to give breastfed babies an edge in brain development.

Better fats, less waste. Not only does breast milk contain better fat than cow's milk or infant formula, less of it gets wasted. Human milk contains an enzyme, *lipase* — a substance that helps digest fat so that more gets into the baby and less in the stools. Formulas do not contain any enzymes, because they are destroyed by the heating process. The malodorous stools of the formula-fed infant

"MOTHER'S MILK: FOOD FOR SMARTER KIDS"

This was the headline in the February 2, 1992, issue of *USA Today.* While numerous studies have shown that breastfeeding boosts development, this has been attributed more to nurturing than to the type of milk itself. But this study suggests that it's *mother's milk* rather than (or in addition to) the process of breastfeeding that gives the developmental advantage. Researchers in England divided three hundred premature infants into two groups: those who received their mother's milk and those who didn't. Prematures who got their mother's milk during the first four to five weeks of life averaged 8.3 points higher on IQ tests at age seven and a half to eight years. And the research suggested a dose-response relationship: The more mother's milk they got, the better the children scored.

The difference could not be explained by increased nurturing, since the babies were fed breast milk by tube. At least eleven more scientific studies (some tracking children for as long as eighteen years) have come to the same conclusion: The longer babies are breastfed, the greater their intellectual advantage. Why breast milk builds better brains is not fully known, but researchers attribute it to the effects of the hormones and growth factors not found in formula as well as the special fats that contribute to the structural development of the nervous system. There are around four hundred nutrients in breast milk that are not present in formula. To give your baby a good intellectual start, breast milk is the best milk for growing brains. Breastfeeding does make a difference!

give a clue that the intestines are unhappy with having to process the types of fats in formula. The intestines — the body's food judge — reject some of the fat of formula or cow's milk and allow this excess to pass into the stools, giving them an unpleasant odor — which makes for unpleasant diaper changes.

Cholesterol: good or bad for baby? The next important component of the fat family is cholesterol. Is this vital fat really the nutritional gremlin it is portrayed as? Not in babies. Like other fats, cholesterol promotes brain growth, and it provides basic components of hormones, vitamin D, and intestinal bile. Cholesterol is high in human milk, scant in cow's milk, and nearly absent in formulas. Recent studies show that during the first year exclusively breastfed infants have higher

blood cholesterol than formula-fed babies. Higher blood cholesterol at the stage of most rapid brain growth — what a smart idea! Nutritionists are uncertain about the possible short-term effects of low-cholesterol milk on the infant's brain versus the long-term effects on the heart. For our children we chose to go with the oldest successful nutritional design — human milk for human babies.

Powerful Proteins

If the fat facts are not heavy enough to convince you your milk is special, listen to the protein story. Proteins are the building blocks of growth. (For more about proteins, see page 241.) Quality protein is most important during your baby's first year because your baby grows faster during this period than at any other time. Your milk contains proteins specifically designed for infant growth. These powerful growth-promoting substances cannot be manufactured or bought. Each of these special factors does good things for your baby.

Milk (cow's, formula, and human) contains two main proteins: whey and casein. Whey is a gentle protein, easy to digest and very friendly to human intestines. Casein, the curd protein of milk, is lumpy and less easy to digest by human intestines. Your milk contains mostly whey. Cow's milk and some formulas contain mostly casein. Your baby's intestines recognize breast milk proteins as the right stuff. They digest these nutrients easily, absorb them quickly, and do not reject them as foreign foods. The intestines do not so eagerly welcome the foreign proteins in formula or cow's milk because they must work harder to digest the lumpier curd. The intestines are the body's nutritional gatekeeper, letting into the blood the right proteins and keeping out of the blood proteins that may harm the body — called allergenic proteins, or allergens. In the early months your baby's intestines are more porous; the "gate" in the intestinal lining is open, allowing foreign proteins to get through. Around six months the intestines mature and the gate begins to close, selecting some proteins and rejecting others — an intriguing process called *closure*. Giving your baby only your milk until the intestines mature is the safest way to keep potentially allergenic proteins out of baby's blood.

Besides whey, your milk contains other select proteins not naturally found in milks made by cows or companies. Let's meet this elite group. *Taurine,* the brain protein, is believed to enhance the development of the brain and nervous system. *Lactoferrin* is another protein unique to human milk, acting like a ferryboat transporting valuable iron from your milk into your baby's blood. This special protein also polices the right kind of bacteria that reside in your baby's intestines. Throughout your baby's lower intestines reside good and bad bacteria. The friendly, useful bacteria, in return for a place to live, do good things for your baby, such as make vitamins. The harmful bacteria, if not kept in check, can overwhelm the intestines, causing diarrheal illnesses. Besides suppressing the harmful bacteria in your baby's intestines, lactoferrin keeps candida (a yeast organism that produces toxins) in check. Another group of natural antibiotics in your milk is called *lysozymes,* special proteins that help ward off harmful bacteria.

Nucleotides are another type of helpful protein in human milk. These valuable proteins help tissues grow stronger, similar to the way strength-enhancing elements are added to structural steel. Nucleotides help the lining of your baby's intestines develop better by boosting the growth of intestinal *villi* — the tiny fingerlike projections that process and absorb food. These substances in your milk also help promote the bacteria that belong in your baby's intestines and eliminate those that don't — a process called maintaining the normal *ecology of the gut*.

How Sweet It Is!

Try the taste test. Sample formulas and breast milk, and you will instantly know why babies prefer the real thing. Breast milk tastes fresh. Formula has a canned taste. Human milk contains more lactose (sugar) than the milk of any other mammal — 20–30 percent more than cow's milk. Formulas add corn syrup or lactose to make up the difference. So why should your baby have this better sugar? Answer: Baby's brain needs it! Nutritionists believe that one of the products of lactose, galactose, is a vital nutrient to developing brain tissue. To lend support that lactose is important for central nervous system development, researchers have shown that among all mammals the higher the lactose content of the milk, the larger the brain of that species. Lactose also enhances calcium absorption, which is vital to developing bones. Not only does lactose help growing brains and growing bones, your baby's intestines need this natural sweet. Lactose promotes the growth of a useful intestinal bacteria, *Lactobacillus bifidus*.

Vitamins, Minerals, and Iron

No one can make these nutrients as well as you can. These nutrients are unique because of their high *bioavailability* — meaning most of what is in the milk gets used by the body. What gives a food high marks is not how much of a particular nutrient it contains, but what percentage is absorbed through the intestines into the bloodstream. What you see on the formula labels is not what babies get into their blood. The vitamins, minerals, and iron in your milk have high bioavailability. Most of these high-efficiency nutrients in your milk get into your baby's tissues. There is very little waste. Not so with company-made or cow-made milk. These have low efficiency, low bioavailability. With breast milk iron, for example, 50–75 percent gets into the baby's blood and tissues. Less wasted iron is left unabsorbed in the intestines. Not so with the "other brand." Only 10 percent of cow's milk iron and as little as 4 percent in iron-fortified

formulas gets into the blood. Not terribly efficient.

Spare the leftovers. Besides the low efficiency of commercial nutrients, the excess nutrients that are not absorbed overtax the baby's waste-disposal system, for which baby pays a metabolic price. Excess unabsorbed nutrients upset the ecology of the gut, encouraging the growth of harmful bacteria. We do not yet know all the possible long-term effects of these excesses.

Changing as baby grows. Another tribute to the efficiency of your milk is how the amounts of these nutrients change as your baby grows. The vitamin and mineral content of colostrum (your first milk), transitional milk (first-week milk), and mature milk is formulated just right for your baby's rapidly changing needs. There is no such commercial food as colostrum or transitional formula.

Facilitators. To further upgrade nutrient bioavailability, human milk contains *facilitators* — substances that help their fellow nutrients work better. The higher vitamin C in human milk, for example, increases absorption of iron. In an intriguing experiment researchers added equal amounts of iron and zinc to samples of human milk, cow's milk, and formulas and fed them to human volunteers. More of these nutrients in the human-milk sample than in the other milks got into the bloodstream. Indeed, breast milk is a unique recipe.

Protection Factors in Breast Milk

To nourish and protect is the nutritional goal of every mother. You have learned how breast milk so perfectly nourishes babies;

now you will see how this rich nutrient further protects them.

White blood cells. Each drop of your milk is alive with millions of tiny white blood cells that circulate throughout your baby's intestines ingesting and destroying harmful bacteria. So valuable are the nutritional and disease-fighting properties of breast milk that in ancient times it was known as white blood. Like a vigilant mother, these protective cells are most plentiful in the early weeks of life, when your newborn's own defense system is weakest. As your baby's immune system matures, the concentration of white blood cells in your milk gradually decreases, yet they are still present in your milk at least six months postpartum.

Besides gobbling up infection, these precious cells, like blood, store and transport priceless elements such as enzymes, growth factors, and infection-fighting proteins — other partners in good health, which we will now examine.

Immunoglobulins. In addition to living white cells, your milk also contains immunoglobulins — infection-fighting proteins that circulate, like natural antibiotics, throughout the body and destroy germs. In the first six months of life, baby's immune system is immature, or deficient in protective antibodies. Your infant makes some antibodies shortly after birth, but these do not reach adequate protective levels until nine to twelve months of age. Enter mother. To defend your baby against germs, you as mother make up for baby's insufficient immunity in many ways. One is by giving your baby your blood antibodies across the placenta. But these blood immunoglobulins are used up by nine months. As your blood antibodies in your baby go down, your milk immunoglobulins go up;

your milk completes the job of your blood, protecting your baby until his or her own defense system matures — a process that is well on its way by the end of the first year. Your breasts function after birth as your placenta did before birth — to nourish and protect.

Milk immunization. Colostrum, the first milk you produce, is the highest in white blood cells and infection-fighting proteins at the most opportune time, when your newborn's defenses are lowest. Another perfect match. Consider colostrum your baby's first immunization.

To appreciate milk immunization, let's follow an important member of the immunoglobulin team, IgA, through your baby's intestines. In the early months a baby's immature intestines are like a sieve, allowing foreign substances (allergenic proteins) to pass into the infant's blood, potentially causing allergies. The IgA in breast milk provides a protective coating, sealing these leaks in the intestinal lining and preventing the passage of unwelcome germs and allergens.

Defense system continually updated. Your milk is a custom-made infection repellent, fighting off germs in your baby's environment. The germs around you are continuously changing, but your body has a protective system that selectively recognizes friendly and harmful germs. This system is immature in babies. When a new germ enters mother's body, she produces antibodies to that germ. This new army of infection fighters then enters her baby, via her milk. Baby is now also protected. This dynamic process of milk immunization constantly adapts to provide the mother-infant pair with the best defense system.

►*IMMUNIZE YOUR BABY EVERY DAY!* *BREASTFEED. (Advised by the International Lactation Consultant Association)*

New Discoveries

Several times a year I pick up a medical journal and read about a new element discovered in breast milk. Because the exact makeup of these substances is often unknown, researchers call them factors. We have discussed the satiety factor and the brain-building factors. A new member of the factor team is epidermal growth factor (EGF), so named because it promotes growth of important cells. The epidermal cells lining your baby's intestines do a very important job in processing food. The EGF acts like a tonic to enhance the growth of important cells like these throughout your baby's body. Your milk also contains many of your hormones — vital substances that help important organs work better.

We have only skimmed the surface in pointing out the unique qualities and components of human milk. There are many other valuable nutrients in human milk that are not in formula, but because we do not yet know their significance, we often discount their importance. As new technologies allow us to study these special nutrients, we will cherish breast milk even more as baby's best nutritional start. Science is only now beginning to discover what mothers have long known — something good happens to babies and mothers when they breastfeed.

Best for Mother

Not only is your milk best for baby, but breastfeeding is also best for you. There will be those marathon days when baby wants to "breastfeed all the time"; you will feel drained of milk, of energy, and of patience. As a patient of mine once said, "I feel like breastfeeding is one big give-a-thon." Breastfeeding is not all giving, giving, giving. The return on your time and effort is immeasurable, both while you are breastfeeding and in years to come.

One of the main benefits of breastfeeding — and a theme of this book — is the concept of mutual giving: You give to baby; baby gives to you. When your baby sucks, you give baby your milk. Baby's sucking stimulates nerves in your nipple to send a message to your pituitary gland — the master control panel in your brain — to secrete the hormone prolactin. One of the mothering hormones, this magical substance travels throughout the highways of mother's body telling her which turn to take and stimulating her motherly feelings.

Breastfeeding Gets You Back in Shape

Sucking stimulates the release of the hormone oxytocin, which contracts your uterus to (nearly) its prepregnant size. Mother shapes the baby — baby shapes the mother. And breastfeeding does not cause your breasts to lose their shape. Pregnancy is what brings on the breast changes.

Relax, Relax!

Breastfeeding relaxes mother and baby. Watch a breastfeeding pair. Notice how the mother mellows, and the baby drifts peacefully to sleep as if given a natural tranquilizer. In fact, this happens. Your milk contains a natural sleep-inducing protein that, in addition to the aforementioned satiety factor, puts baby into a restful slumber. The hormones induced by sucking tranquilize mother. This natural calming is especially helpful for the baby (and mother) who has difficulty getting to sleep. This aspect of breastfeeding is a beautiful example of mutual giving when we let it happen naturally.

The relaxing effect of breastfeeding is particularly helpful to mothers with busy lifestyles. Tanya, a dual-career mother and part-time breastfeeder, declared, "When I come home after a busy day at work, I breastfeed my baby and it helps me unwind!"

Other Fringe Benefits

Breastfeeding contributes to mother's health. Women who breastfeed have a lower incidence of breast cancer — an important consideration if you have a strong family history of cancer. Breastfed babies tend to be healthier, saving money in medical bills. Breastfeeding is less expensive, and it's better milk — truly one of nature's best food bargains. And, for family planners, breastfeeding is a natural child spacer.

Breastfeeding Is Good Discipline

Breastfeeding is an exercise in baby reading. In studying the long-term effects of breastfeeding on babies in my practice one feature stands out — these children are well disciplined. Very simply, my basic recipe for discipline contains two ingredients: *Know your child and help your child feel right.* Breastfeeding serves both these components. A responsive mother knows her baby. The mother-infant interaction of the breastfeeding pair is repeated at least a thousand times in the first three months, leading mother to a deep perception of her baby's behavior. During breastfeeding more than milk flows into the baby. A baby who is on the receiving end of nature's best nurturing learns *trust,* and the right feeling that goes with it. The mutual

sensitivity that both members of the breastfeeding pair have for each other helps both behave better.

PREPARING FOR BREASTFEEDING

Just as preparing for the birth of your baby increases your chances of having a good birth experience, preparing yourself for breastfeeding helps you better enjoy feeding your baby.

If you feel uncomfortable handling your breasts, consult a breastfeeding friend or a lactation consultant about the art of breast massage. This technique increases your comfort in handling your breasts and is useful later on when you're learning to express your milk manually.

Notice the changes in your body. The hormones of pregnancy naturally prepare your breasts for feeding. In fact, breast changes may have been one of the first changes you noticed in your body at the beginning of your pregnancy. Breasts are bigger in early pregnancy as the amount of milk-making tissue in them increases, and they may feel tender at times. In the last months of pregnancy, breasts may secrete small amounts of colostrum, the yellow sticky substance that is your baby's first nourishment. This is a time to appreciate the wonderful ways that a woman's body not only grows a baby but prepares to care for that baby after birth.

Should you prepare your nipples? Years ago women were advised to toughen their nipples during pregnancy to prepare for breastfeeding. They were told to rub their

BREASTFEEDING HEALTH BENEFITS FOR MOTHER AND BABY

Breastfeeding does lots of good things for baby, mother, and family. Here is a system-by-system overview of the most important health benefits of breastfeeding.

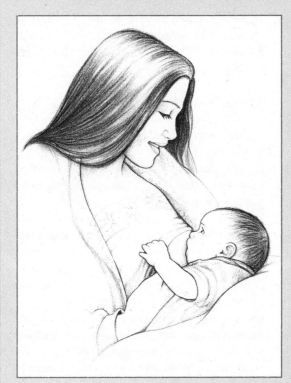

Breastfed babies enjoy:
- brighter brains
- better vision
- fewer ear infections
- better dental alignment
- healthier hearts
- fewer respiratory infections
- improved digestion
- fewer intestinal infections
- less constipation
- leaner bodies
- less diabetes
- healthier skin
- increased immunity
- healthier growth

Breastfeeding mothers enjoy:
- relaxation
- less depression
- natural child spacing
- less osteoporosis
- less breast, uterine, and ovarian cancer
- faster postpartum weight loss

nipples with a rough towel, leave their bra flaps down to expose the nipples to air, and if they had flat or inverted nipples, to do nipple exercises to make their nipples more erect. Doesn't that sound like a lot of work — and not too pleasant either? Fortunately, recent studies by lactation specialists have found that prenatal nipple preparation is neither necessary nor helpful. In fact, paying so much attention to nipples prenatally may even set women up to fail at breastfeeding by creating unnecessary anxiety whether their natural nipple shape will be adequate. Nowadays, those in the know about breastfeeding remind mothers that babies feed from *breasts*, not nipples, and that being careful about how baby latches onto the breast will prevent nipple soreness.

Instead of worrying about your nipples, let them prepare themselves. The glands around your nipples and areolas (the dark portion of your breast surrounding the nipple) secrete a natural lubricating substance. Avoid using soap on your nipples, because soap will remove these natural oils and leave the skin dry and more likely to crack. If you are concerned about flat or inverted nipples, contact a lactation consultant to assist you in the first days after birth as you teach your baby to latch on and suck properly.

Prepare your mind as well as your body. Linda, a mother in our practice, confided: "Intellectually I thought I was prepared for breastfeeding, but emotionally I was not." She knew that breast milk is best for her baby, but she did not realize the level of commitment it would take during those first few weeks when "all baby wants to do is suck." Then she went on to say, "If only someone had told me that after the first few weeks, breastfeeding would be less draining and more fulfilling."

Join your local La Leche League or other breastfeeding-support group. Successful breastfeeding is not automatic for many first-time mothers who have no models or family support. La Leche League International (LLLI) is a volunteer organization of women members and group leaders who have practical breastfeeding experience and special training in counseling new mothers. Since the extended family is not usually available to most new parents, a support group such as La Leche League often becomes the extended family for the new mother. In the last trimester of your pregnancy attend a series of La Leche League meetings, which cover right-start techniques, the effects of breastfeeding on the family, and practical tips on making breastfeeding a more enjoyable experience. Besides being informative, these meetings help you get acquainted with other new mothers and will be a valuable support resource after your baby is born. Watch those mothers so effortlessly tend to their babies'

needs, as if mother and baby have been rehearsing this breastfeeding scene for years — and some have. You can usually find your local La Leche League through your doctor's office, or check with your hospital, childbirth class, or local library. You can also call or write LLLI headquarters for the name and number of your local leader. (See "Breastfeeding," in "Resources," page 745.)

Take a breastfeeding class. Breastfeeding classes instruct you on right-start techniques and put you in touch with a lactation specialist who may later be your personal breastfeeding consultant. Hospitals and birthing centers usually offer breastfeeding classes as part of the childbirth class.

Choose health care providers who know about breastfeeding. When choosing your baby's doctor, impress upon him or her that breastfeeding is a high priority in your overall parenting style. Choose a doctor who gives more than just lip service to breastfeeding. During the early months of your baby's medical care, you'll be interacting with your doctor more about feeding questions and problems than any other concern. You want this person to whom you are entrusting the care of your baby to be *knowledgeable and supportive* in giving your baby the best nutritional start. La Leche League has a medical associates program to help you locate just such a doctor.

Talk with supportive friends. Seek out those who encourage your feeding choices rather than sabotage your choice of parenting styles. Nothing divides friends like differences of opinion on child rearing. The defeating cliché "It must be your *milk*" is used for every conceivable problem: colic, constipation, diarrhea, night waking, and so on. This is a damaging and inappropriate remark. Love for your baby makes you particularly vulnerable to any suggestion that your milk is bad, therefore you are a bad mother. In fact, you are likely to get the most critical advice from mothers who have never breastfed. Surround yourself with supportive friends who inspire confidence and affirm your choices.

Learn proper positioning and latch-on techniques. In addition to your breastfeeding class, contact a certified lactation consultant (see page 31) before birth. Within twenty-four to forty-eight hours after your baby is born, ask the lactation consultant to give you a hands-on demonstration of correct positioning and latch-on techniques, as described in the following section.

RIGHT-START TECHNIQUES

Early in our medical practice and our parenting career we naively felt that breastfeeding was such a natural process that if you put a lactating mother and hungry baby in the same room the pair would automatically get together, milk would flow, and baby would grow. Actually most new mothers and babies need to be taught the right skills — correct *positioning* and *latch-on techniques.* Our desire is not only to encourage you to breastfeed, but, more important, we want you to enjoy this relationship.

First Feedings

You can put your baby to your breast just minutes after birth. Unless a medical condition (breathing difficulties, for example) prevents it, right after birth your baby can be draped over your chest, tummy to tummy, cheek to breast, skin to skin (with modifications for a cesarean birth), and covered with a warm towel. Then just relax and enjoy each other. Don't force or rush things. This is not a time to practice everything you learned in the class. It's a time to *introduce* baby to the breast. A whole meal is not needed. Most babies take a few licks, a few sucks, pause, and then resume a few more gentle licks and sucks. Sucking in frequent bursts and pauses is the usual pattern for the first few hours and sometimes even the first few days.

Within a few minutes after birth most babies enter a state of quiet alertness — the optimal behavioral state for interaction with you. When baby is quiet and alert her eyes are open wide, attentive, and looking for another set of eyes — and for the breast. In fact, immediately after birth some newborn babies, when draped over mother's abdomen, make crawling motions toward the breast and often find their target with minimal assistance. When baby is in this state of quiet alertness, massage her lips with your nipple, stimulating her to open her mouth and seek the breast (the rooting reflex). She may latch on and suck or she may just enjoy the skin-to-skin contact.

This first interaction is important for several reasons. The first milk you produce, colostrum, is the best food — the sooner baby starts the better. Sucking is good for helping the newly delivered baby to ease the tension that has built up from the stress of labor and birth. Sucking is a familiar and comforting function from the womb, so it helps baby adjust to the new environment. When you see your baby begin to open her eyes, look around, and put her fist in her mouth, it's time to offer her your breast.

Frequent feedings get the mothering hormones flowing and the mother–baby care system going.

Positioning and Latch-on Skills

We cannot overemphasize the importance of proper positioning and latch-on. Most of the breastfeeding problems we see in our practice and breastfeeding center (sore nipples, insufficient milk, mothers not enjoying breastfeeding) are due to not using these basic right-start techniques.

Position Yourself Correctly

Get comfortable before beginning to breastfeed. Milk flows better from a relaxed mother. Sitting up in bed or in a rocking chair or an armchair is the easiest position for breastfeeding. Pillows are essential for your comfort and for baby's positioning. Place one behind your back, one on your lap, and another under the arm that will support your baby. You can also buy a nursing pillow. If sitting in a chair, use a footstool — this raises your lap so you don't have to strain your back and arm muscles to get baby closer to your breast (see illustration on page 146). To best prepare your mind and body, think baby, and think mothering.

Position Baby Correctly

Start with your baby only lightly dressed (or even undressed) to promote skin-to-skin contact. Undressing babies who seem too sleepy to feed keeps them from falling asleep and helps them suck better. Then position her as follows:

1. Nestle baby in your arm so that her neck rests in the bend of your elbow, her back along your forearm, and her buttocks in your hand.
2. Turn baby's entire body on its side so she is facing you tummy to tummy. Her head and neck should be straight, not arched backward or turned sideways, in relation to the rest of her body. Baby should not have to turn her head or strain her neck to reach your nipple. (Try turning your head to one side and swallowing a sip of water. Then try it again with your head extended far back, then flexed toward your chest. It doesn't feel nearly as comfortable as when you hold your head naturally straight ahead.)
3. Raise baby to the level of your breasts by putting her on a pillow on your lap and by using a footstool. Let the pillow on your lap support your arm and baby's weight. Trying to hold your infant up with your arm will strain your back and arm muscles. If baby rests too low on your lap, she will pull down on your breast, causing unnecessary stretching and friction. Bring baby up and in toward you rather than your leaning forward toward her.
4. Get baby's interfering arms and hands out of the way. As you turn baby on her side tummy to tummy, tuck her lower arm into the soft pocket between her body and your midriff. If her upper arm keeps interfering, you can hold it down with the thumb of your hand that is holding her.
5. As you are positioning baby's arms, wrap her around you, tummy to tummy. This basic position is called the *cradle hold*. If your baby is premature or has trouble latching on, try the *clutch hold* (see page 132).

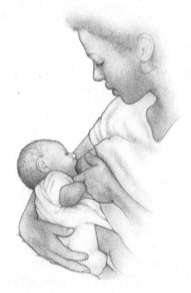

Cradle hold, showing correct head and body alignment for breastfeeding.

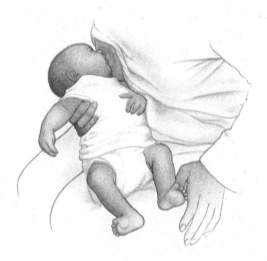

Incorrect position for breastfeeding: Don't let baby's body dangle away from yours.

Present Your Breast

With your free hand, manually express a few drops of colostrum or milk to moisten your nipple. Cup your breast, supporting the weight of your breast with palm and fingers underneath and thumb on top. Keep your hand back toward your chest wall so your fingers stay clear of the areola, away from baby's latch-on site. If you are very large breasted, use a rolled-up hand towel under your breast to help support its weight so that it doesn't drag down on baby's lower jaw and tire her out.

Encourage Proper Latch-on — The Most Important Step

Using your milk-moistened nipple as a teaser, gently massage baby's lips with your nipple, encouraging her to open her mouth wide, as if yawning. Babies' mouths open very wide and then quickly close, like little birds' beaks. The moment your baby opens her mouth wide (keep patiently teasing until she really opens wide), direct your nipple into the center of her mouth and with a rapid movement pull her in very close to you with your arm.

Many new mothers are a bit timid, expecting baby to do the latching on, and they do not pull their babies in closely enough or quickly enough to get baby's open mouth to latch on correctly. Don't lean forward, pushing your breast toward your baby; you *pull her close to your breast* by moving your arm. Otherwise you will wind up sitting hunched over, and you'll have a tired, sore back at the end of the feeding. If you move your arm too slowly or you hesitate until she's closed up a bit, she will probably slurp just the nipple

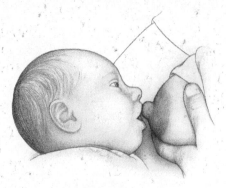

Teasing baby's mouth open wide.

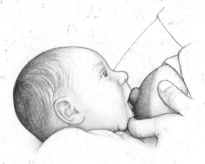

Helping baby open mouth wide enough for proper latch-on: depressing lower jaw and everting lips.

into her mouth, stopping short of the correct position for your nipple, which should be far back in baby's mouth.

Make sure baby sucks the areola. Your baby's gums should bypass the base of the nipple and take in at least a one-inch radius of the areola as you latch her on. After just one or two feedings "on the nipple," your nipples will be sore. Another reason it is so important that baby compress the areola is that the milk sinuses (the reservoirs for milk) are located beneath the areola (see the diagram on page 170). If these sinuses are not compressed, your baby will not get enough milk. *Babies should suck areolas, not nipples.*

Open wide! An important part of proper latch-on is getting baby to open her mouth wide enough. Many babies tighten or purse their lips, especially the lower one. Help your baby open her mouth wider by using the index finger of the hand supporting your breast to press firmly down on your baby's chin as you pull her on. You may need someone else to do this for you at first. If your nipple gives you the message that your baby is tight mouthing you, causing a pinching feel-

ing, temporarily remove the hand supporting your breast and use your index finger to evert (turn out) her lips. If baby does not cooperate, break the suction by gently wedging your finger between the gums, and start again. Even if you have to start over several times until you and baby get it right, hang in there. This is good practice, and it helps baby learn the right moves. Consider this your first opportunity to discipline (which means teach and guide), and take a deep breath and try again.

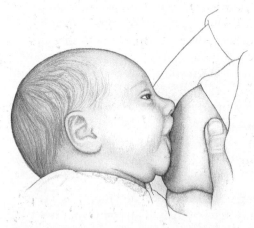

Proper latch-on. Notice baby's lips correctly everted.

In teaching breastfeeding techniques to nurses and interns, we made latch-on rounds in the maternity ward. After simply pressing down on baby's chin and everting the tight, inwardly turned lower lip, mothers would exclaim, "It doesn't hurt anymore; it feels right." The students dubbed this teaching session "Sears's lower-lip rounds."

Make adjustments for baby's breathing. As you get baby to open her mouth wide and evert her lips, pull your baby so close that the tip of her nose touches your breast. Don't be afraid of blocking her nose, since she can breathe quite well from the sides of her nose even if the tip is compressed. If baby's nose does seem to be blocked, pull baby's bottom closer to you, changing the angle of baby's position slightly, or if necessary use your thumb to press gently on your breast to uncover her nose.

Support your breast. After you have your baby correctly latched on, *hold your breast throughout the feeding* so the weight of your breast does not tire your newborn's mouth.

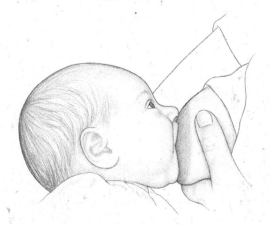

Incorrect latch-on. Notice baby's lower lip is tucked in.

As baby gets older and stronger, this supporting step will be less necessary, and you will have a free hand during most of the feeding. To avoid trauma to your nipples, do not pull your nipple from baby's mouth without first breaking the suction by inserting your finger into the corner of her mouth, wedging it between her gums.

Two Types of Sucking

After a few weeks you will notice that your baby exhibits two types of sucking: comfort and nutritional. Comfort sucking, the weaker suck, is most prevalent when baby is not hungry but simply needs comforting. With this type of sucking baby usually gets the less-filling foremilk. Nutritional sucking is more vigorous. The muscles of her face work so hard that even her ears wiggle during intense nutritional sucking. This type of productive sucking soon rewards your baby with the higher-calorie and more-filling hindmilk.

Alternative Breastfeeding Positions

In the first week it's wise to teach baby more than one latch-on position. Two other helpful breastfeeding positions are the side lying position and the clutch hold. These positions are useful in the early days of recovery from a cesarean birth.

Side-lying position. Think of this as the cradle hold, but with baby and mother lying on their sides facing each other. Place two pillows under your head, a pillow behind your back, another under your top leg, and a fifth pillow tucked behind your baby. Five pillows sounds like a lot, but you need to be comfortable. Place your baby on her side facing you and nestled in your arm, and slide your baby up or down to get her mouth to line up with

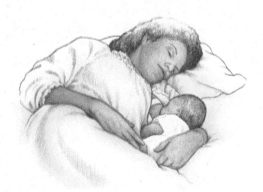

Side-lying position.

your nipple. Use the same latch-on techniques as previously described.

Clutch hold. Try this hold with babies with latch-on problems and those who squirm and arch their backs, detaching themselves from the breast. It's also useful for small, hypotonic (floppy), or premature babies. Sitting up in bed or in a comfortable armchair, set a pillow at your side (let's say your left side) or wedge it between you and the arm of the chair and place baby on the pillow. Position your baby in close along your left side and cup the back

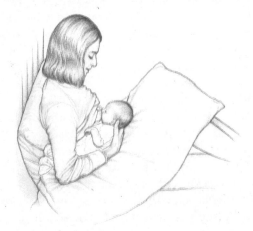

Clutch hold, sitting in bed. Notice how pillows help prop baby and mother to comfortable positions.

LATCH-ON AT A GLANCE

Here's a quick review of how to get your baby latched onto the breast:

- Get comfortable with pillows behind your back and under your elbow.
- Support baby at breast level on a pillow pulled in close, tummy to tummy with you.
- Massage baby's lips with your milk-moistened nipple to tease her mouth open wide.
- When baby's mouth opens wide, aim your nipple at the center of her mouth, and quickly pull her in close as she takes the areola into her mouth.

Once baby is latched on, check the following:

- Baby has one inch of areola in her mouth, all the way around.
- Baby's lips are turned outward. If not, pull down on baby's lower jaw.
- Baby's entire jaw moves as she sucks.
- You can hear baby swallowing milk.
- There is no pinching sensation or pain.

If baby is not latched on correctly, insert a finger to gently release the suction, take her off the breast, and try again.

of her neck in your left hand. Direct her legs upward so that they are resting against the pillows supporting your back. Be sure that baby is not pushing with her feet against the back of the chair or pillow, causing her to arch her back. If this happens, position baby bent at her hips with her legs and buttocks against the back pillow. Follow the same latch-on steps, cupping your left breast in your right hand, and pull baby in close to you. Once baby is sucking well, wedge a pillow up against her back to help hold her close.

Babies with lazy latch-on and weak sucking. Some babies initially need more support at the breast because of low muscle tone, prematurity, or weak sucking. Try these helpers:

- Position yourself comfortably, with pillows behind your back and under your elbow on the side you will be using to feed the baby. Use additional pillows on your lap to bring baby up to the level of your nipple.

- Hold baby on his side, tummy to tummy in the cradle hold (see pages 128–129).

- Support the breast with your hand in a U-shape, thumb and fingers one and one-half to two inches behind the areola. Press in and back slightly to make an areola "sandwich" for your baby.

- Tilt baby's head slightly backward and touch his lower lip with your nipple. As he opens his mouth wide, bring him onto the breast, "landing" the breast on his lower jaw and tongue first and then "rolling" the rest of the breast into his mouth. This will help him to get a big mouthful of breast and get his lower jaw far back on the areola for efficient feeding.

- Depending on the size of your breasts and your baby's strength and maturity, you may have to support the breast through the entire feeding. Watch that baby doesn't slip down to the end of the nipple as you do this.

- Seek hands-on help from a lactation consultant who is knowledgeable about "suck training" techniques.

COMMON POSITIONING AND LATCH-ON MISTAKES

- Letting baby's body turn and dangle instead of snuggling tummy to tummy.
- Not patiently waiting for baby's mouth to open wide enough as you are tickling her mouth with your nipple.
- Allowing the lips to be tightly pursed inward instead of loosely turned outward.
- Allowing baby to apply pressure on the nipple instead of the areolar tissue.
- Being too passive or reluctant to teach baby proper latch-on.

We encourage the first-time breastfeeding mother to seek the services of a lactation specialist within the first several days after birth in order to get a right start with proper positioning and latch-on before incorrect habits develop. As a result, breastfeeding problems dramatically decrease, and we find that mothers and babies better enjoy their breastfeeding relationship.

HOW YOUR BREASTS MAKE MILK

Understanding how your breasts produce milk helps you appreciate the womanly art of breastfeeding and realize why proper positioning and latch-on techniques are so important. You will notice that your breasts enlarge during your pregnancy, which is nature's message that your breasts will nourish your baby after birth just as your enlarged uterus nourished your baby before birth. Breast enlargement occurs primarily from the growth of milk-producing glands. It is the number of milk-producing glands and how they function that determine the mother's milk-producing abilities, not the size of her breasts. Differences in breast size are caused more by the presence of non-milk-producing fat tissue than by glands. Small-breasted mothers do not produce less milk than do large-breasted mothers.

Inside your breast the lactation system resembles a tree (see the illustration on page 170). Milk is produced in the glandular tissue, which is like the leaves of the tree; milk travels from these milk cells through the milk ducts (branches and trunk) into the milk sinuses (roots of the tree), which are the reservoirs where milk is stored. Located beneath the areola, these sinuses release milk through approximately fifteen to twenty openings in your nipple. To drain the milk sinuses effectively, your baby's mouth must be positioned over these reservoirs so that her tongue can compress the sinuses where the milk is pooled. If baby sucks only on your nipple, she will get little milk, unnecessarily traumatize your nipple, and not gain weight well.

Here's how this magnificent milk-producing system works. Your baby's sucking stimulates special nerve sensors in your nipple to send messages to the pituitary gland in your brain to secrete the hormone prolactin, which stimulates the glands in your breasts to produce milk. The first milk your baby receives at each feeding, the foremilk, is thin, like skim milk. As your baby continues sucking, the nerve sensors in your nipple stimulate the pituitary gland to secrete another hormone, oxytocin.

This hormone flows into your breasts and causes the elastic tissue around each of the many individual milk glands to contract like a rubber band, squeezing a large supply of milk and extra fat from the milk glands into the ducts and sinuses. This later milk, or hindmilk, is much higher in fat and slightly higher in protein and, for this reason, is more filling to baby and has greater nutritional value. Hindmilk is the growth milk.

Milk-Ejection Reflex

As the hindmilk is ejected from the milk glands into the milk sinuses, most mothers have a tingling sensation in their breasts. Because of the "letting down" of the creamier milk, this sudden outpouring of hindmilk used to be called the *let-down reflex.*

Instead of "let-down reflex," we prefer the more accurate term "milk-ejection reflex," because of an embarrassing incident that occurred in my first year of medical practice nearly thirty years ago. One day while making hospital rounds, I entered the room of a new mother breastfeeding her baby and asked if she had any problems. She answered, "Yes, I haven't yet experienced any letdown." Having no idea what she was really talking about, I assumed she was referring to depression, so I began counseling her about postpartum depression. It was only later, after asking my wife about the term "letdown," that I learned my patient was referring to her breasts and not her mind. At that point I realized that in all those years of medical training I had been taught nothing about how the breasts make milk, perhaps because it was not considered very scientific. Later when I became a teacher of young doctors, I resolved that this unpardonable lack of knowledge about such a beautifully human function would not be passed on to the next generation of physicians. Because I still find the older term "let-down reflex" somewhat depressing, we will use the term "milk-ejection reflex" (MER).

A good MER is the key to good milk. Different mothers feel different sensations when experiencing a milk-ejection reflex. Usually a mother feels a sensation of fullness or tingling occurring thirty to sixty seconds or more after her baby starts sucking. This feeling may occur several times during a feeding and may be felt at different times and varying intensities from mother to mother. First-time mothers usually experience the MER by the second or third week after beginning breastfeeding. Some mothers never feel it, but recognize it by the leaking that occurs during the MER. Because your milk production is tied to your emotions, when you feel well your MER is more likely to work well. Fatigue, fear, tension, and pain are the usual emotional enemies suppressing milk ejection. In this case your infant receives mostly foremilk, which is less satisfying and less nutritious. Because of the emotional link between hormones and milk production, an upset mother leads to upset milk production.

Supply and Demand

Milk production works on the principle of supply and demand. The more your infant sucks correctly, the more milk you produce, until you have both negotiated the proper balance. In fact, frequent sucking contributes more to milk production than how long your baby feeds.

Proper latch-on and sucking help your supply meet baby's need. Stimulated by the touch of your nipple to her lips and the scent and taste of your milk, your baby grasps the areola of your breast with her lips, and her sucking draws the nipple and the areola far back into her mouth. Because your breast tissue is very elastic, your infant's tongue "milks" the areola in a rhythmic motion, elongating your nipple and areola so that milk is delivered toward the rear of the tongue, far back into her mouth.

Babies suck milk differently through a rubber nipple. The rubber nipple stays the same length during feeding, so the bottle-feeding baby's tongue motion and suck-swallow actions are very different from a breastfeeding baby's. Also, if the baby sucks incorrectly on a rubber nipple, he still gets rewarded with milk. Sucking on the breast in the same way as from an artificial nipple is likely to produce sore nipples and a reduced milk supply. This nipple confusion is why breastfeeding experts frown on giving bottles to babies during the early weeks when they are still learning to suck properly.

COMMON BREASTFEEDING QUESTIONS AND PROBLEMS

The following questions represent only a few of the situations a breastfeeding mother is likely to encounter or wonder about. Many more suggestions can be found in later chapters.

Starting Out

When will my milk come in?

Your true milk appears between the second and fifth day after your baby's birth, depending on whether this is your first baby, what the fatigue level of your birthing experience was, how well your baby learns to latch on to your breasts, and how frequently and effectively your baby sucks. Until your true milk appears, baby is getting colostrum, the premilk that is very rich in protein, immune factors, and other ingredients that are beneficial to your newly born baby. For about a week you have transitional milk, a gradual changing from mostly colostrum to mostly milk. By ten to fourteen days after birth your milk has become mature milk. The following situations encourage your milk to be produced sooner and more comfortably:

• experiencing an uncomplicated birth
• encouraging early, frequent feedings
• learning correct, comfortable latch-on
• avoiding supplemental bottles unless medically necessary
• consulting with a lactation specialist
• having a supportive husband, friends, and health care professionals

How often and how long should I feed my baby?

"Watch your baby and not the clock" is the advice of breastfeeding veterans. Breastfeeding is not a mathematical exercise; as one breastfeeding mother put it, "I don't count the number of feedings any more than I count the number of kisses." In the early weeks of breastfeeding, baby sucks in varying intensities and durations (sometimes for long periods — even as long as an hour). Baby often falls asleep during a feeding and wakes up in a half hour and wants to feed again. Remember, it is the *frequency* of breastfeeding more than the duration that stimulates your milk-producing hormones.

There is no such thing as an "empty breast." You don't have to wait for your breasts to "fill up" again after a feeding.

There is always some milk there for baby. In fact, waiting a long time between feedings may be counterproductive. Lactation researchers have noticed that as the time between feedings increases, the fat level in the milk goes down. Frequent feedings give your baby the high-fat, high-calorie milk he needs to grow. Lactation science also reports that babies are remarkably adept at regulating how much milk their mothers make. Some women's breasts have lower storage capacities than others. (This is not necessarily related to breast size.) Researchers have found that babies of mothers with lower milk-storage capacity simply nurse more often to make up for the lower volume at each feeding.

Your nipples will not get sore from breastfeeding too frequently, as long as you have correct positioning and latch-on. Ignore the advice: "Begin with three minutes on each side and gradually increase by one minute each feeding until your baby is feeding ten minutes on each side. After ten minutes that is enough." Babies did not write these restrictive rules nor did experienced breastfeeding mothers. Often it may take two minutes of sucking for a new mother's MER to activate. Mellow newborns may take a longer time to get a full meal, whereas ravenous feeders can finish off a breast within ten minutes. After months of breastfeeding, when mother and baby are in harmony with each other, many babies can get all the milk they need within the first ten minutes, but most babies still linger at the breast for more sucking. Remember, sore nipples are caused by improper latch-on and suck, not by how long baby sucks. Even three minutes of incorrect sucking or latch-on makes nipples sore.

Realistically, expect your baby to breastfeed an average of every two hours around the clock for the first month to six weeks. Then gradually the frequency of feedings diminishes. In the early weeks when you and your baby are establishing appropriate milk-supply levels, let your baby breastfeed as frequently and as long as he wishes and your life-style permits. Once your milk supply is established and you and your baby have reached a mutually satisfying routine, when frequent and unrestricted breastfeeding is still preferable, your baby may accept forms of comforting other than frequent breastfeeding. (See related section on scheduling the breastfed baby, page 167.)

Sore Nipples

What if my nipples are getting sore?

At the first sign of nipple soreness, scrutinize your technique of positioning and latch-on to be sure that you are not letting your baby apply pressure directly on your nipple rather than on your areola. Be particularly certain that your baby is opening her mouth wide enough and everting both lips, especially the lower. It is often hard for the mother herself to see if baby's lower lip is everted. Ask an

TONGUE-TIE

Tongue-tie means that the membrane (called the frenulum) that attaches the tongue to the floor of the mouth is shorter than usual. If the tongue-tie is interfering with breastfeeding, the frenulum can be easily clipped to release the tongue, enabling baby to suck more efficiently. Signs that your baby's tongue is tight enough to warrant clipping are:

- Baby's tongue tip does not protrude past the lower gum.
- When baby cries, opens her mouth wide, or tries to suck, a dent forms in the tip of the tongue, resembling the dip in the top of a heart shape.
- Latch-on is painful to mother. Nipples are very sore, cracked, or bleeding.
- Baby needs to feed longer, more frequently, tires easily, and often bites or chews the nipple.

After the tongue has been clipped, mother almost immediately notices that latch-on is more comfortable and baby is able to nurse more effectively. Sometimes the tongue can look tight, but if baby has a good latch-on, is getting milk efficiently, and the nipples are not sore during the feeding, there is no need to clip the frenulum.

Clipping the frenulum is a quick and painless procedure that can be done in your doctor's office. In the early weeks, the frenulum is so thin that it's easy to painlessly clip, and it usually yields only a few drops of blood, or none at all. While baby's mouth is open (either normally open or when crying), the doctor holds the tip of the tongue with a piece of gauze (sometimes if the mouth is open wide enough, holding the tongue is not necessary) and uses scissors to clip the frenulum back to where it joins the base of the tongue. The longer tongue-tie is left unclipped, the more muscular the tether can become and the more extensive and difficult is the clipping procedure.

Over the years of counseling breastfeeding mothers, I have become more of a frenulum clipper. It is not worth enduring painful latch-on and an unsuccessful breastfeeding experience while waiting for baby's tongue to naturally loosen up as she grows.

experienced breastfeeding mother to observe your latch-on, and try the technique described earlier to evert his lower lip. If you immediately sense less nipple soreness, then a tight latch-on is the problem. Also, change the way baby is angled and put baby to the least-sore breast first.

Nipple care. Be sure the surface of your nipples is free of wetness when not "in use." Use fresh breast pads, without plastic liners, to be sure no moisture is in contact with your tender skin. (See page 161 for more about breast pads.) Before putting your bra flap up, gently blot the wetness off with a soft cloth. It used to be recommended that you air dry your nipples, expose your nipples to sun, or even use a hair dryer to speed drying. For some women, *quick* drying can actually make delicate nipple tissue crack more by disturbing the moisture balance needed for skin softness and elasticity.

Transitional tenderness. Many women experience a transitional period of tenderness as the skin of the nipple acclimatizes itself to the sucking. If you experience this tenderness, check your latch-on techniques. Also, massage your nipples after feeding to promote circulation to the tissues. The best massage medium is colostrum or breast milk. Additionally, the little bumps on the areola around your nipples are glands that secrete a cleansing and lubricating oil to protect the nipples and keep them clean. Therefore, avoid using soap on your nipples, since it removes these natural oils and encourages dryness and cracking.

First aid for nipples. Women with a predisposition to dry skin can develop dry, cracked nipples even when practicing correct positioning and latch-on. Do not use oils or creams that need to be washed off before breastfeeding, even if the hospital offers you one. Try Lansinoh, a pure, hypoallergenic, pesticide-free lanolin, if cracking and fissuring develop and breast milk alone as a massage medium is not helping. Lansinoh promotes healing by encouraging normal tissue moisture, and it does not have to be washed off before baby breastfeeds.

If your nipples become more sore, cracked, or fissured in spite of these remedies, you need hands-on help from a lactation consultant. She will work with your technique and/or your baby's suck and will help you manage the feeding of your baby until the problem is solved.

My baby feeds constantly, my nipples are wearing out, and I'm wearing out. Can I give him a pacifier?

Many babies love to suck for comfort, not only for nourishment; and there is no better pacifier than a mother suckling an upset baby peacefully off to sleep. Realistically, however, the human pacifier may need a rest. We discourage the use of artificial pacifiers in the early weeks while baby is learning correct sucking patterns at your breast. After his sucking patterns mature and nipple confusion is no longer a concern, a pacifier may be a real lifesaver for a tired mother, and a soothing comforter for an insatiable sucker. (See more on pacifiers, page 90.)

Is Baby Getting Enough?

How do I know my baby is getting enough milk?

After the first month or two you will know intuitively that your baby is getting enough milk. She will feel and look heavier. In the

BREASTFED BABIES ARE LEANER

A 1992 study from the University of California at Davis compared the growth patterns of normal, healthy breastfed and formula-fed infants. Dubbed the DARLING study (Davis Area Research on Lactation, Infant Nutrition, and Growth), the investigation found that the two groups showed similar weight gain during the first three months, but that the weight-for-length scores were higher for formula-fed infants between four and eighteen months, suggesting that breastfed babies were leaner. The breastfed infants averaged 1½ pounds (680 grams) less weight gain during the first twelve months.

What might this mean to new parents? This study suggests that growth chart norms — which don't differentiate between breastfed and formula-fed babies — may themselves be "overweight." Let *your baby* set the standard, not the charts. If your infant is gaining weight at a reasonable rate and appears healthy and content, he's probably doing just fine. (Growth charts are discussed in more detail on page 446.)

• Your baby's stool changes give you another clue to how much milk she is getting. In the first week your baby's stools should normally go from sticky black to green to brown; as soon as your rich, creamy hindmilk appears, stools become more yellow. Once your baby's stool becomes like yellow, seedy mustard, this is a sign that your newborn is getting enough of the higher-calorie hindmilk. In the first month or two a baby who is getting enough high-fat milk will usually have at least two or three yellow, seedy stools a day. Because breast milk has a natural laxative effect, some breastfed babies may even have a stool during or following each feeding.

• Your breasts may feel full before feedings, less full after feedings, and leak between feedings — all signs of sufficient milk production and delivery. After a few months leaking usually subsides, even though you have sufficient milk. Your baby's sucking styles and level of contentment are other guides to sufficient milk. If you feel your baby sucking vigorously, hear her swallowing, feel your milk-ejection reflex, and witness your baby drift contentedly off to sleep, chances are she is getting enough milk.

How much weight should my baby gain during the first month?

Your baby's weight gain is another indicator of sufficient milk. After the initial weight loss during the first week (usually 5–8 percent of your baby's weight, or between 6 and 10 ounces/170–280 grams), babies getting sufficient nutrition gain an average of 4–7 ounces (115–200 grams) a week for the first few weeks, thereafter an average of 1–2 pounds (450–900 grams) per month for the first six months, and one pound per month from six

first few weeks, however, it is not as easy to tell, especially if you are a first-time mother. Here are some signs baby is getting enough milk in the first few weeks.

• A baby who is getting a sufficient volume of milk will usually have at least six to eight wet cloth diapers (four to six disposable diapers) per day after the initial three days of start-up time. Enough wet diapers tell you that your baby is safe from dehydration.

months to one year. Babies usually lengthen about an inch (2.5 centimeters) a month during the first six months. Weight and height gains depend somewhat on baby's body type (see page 248).

New mothers are zealous weight watchers. While it is not true that good weight gain is an index of good mothering, I feel that a baby's weight gain may be some tangible reward for mothers for all those days and nights of breastfeeding, especially since breasts don't have ounce-measurement lines she can refer to.

My ten-day-old baby has plenty of wet diapers, but he has not yet regained his birth weight. Should I be concerned?

Your baby is probably getting big enough volumes of milk, but his slow weight gain suggests that he may not be getting enough calories to grow. If his eyes and mouth appear moist and he is wetting six to eight cloth diapers or four to six disposables each day, he is not dehydrated. He is getting the fluid he needs from your milk, but he may not be getting enough fat. He may look scrawny. When you pinch a piece of skin on an undernourished baby, it is loose and wrinkled because there is not much fat underneath. A baby who is not getting enough calories cries to be fed often but fusses because he is never satisfied. Breastfed babies who are growing and gaining well will have two to three goodsize stools every day. Some will soil their diapers at each feeding. What goes in one end quickly comes out the other. The baby who is not gaining weight may have infrequent stools — fewer than one per day, and that one is little more than a stain in the diaper.

The problem here is that your baby is not getting enough of the high-fat hindmilk. The thin, watery foremilk provides enough fluid for him, but it doesn't have the extra calories needed for growth. Your baby is getting "skim milk" when he needs whole milk. This doesn't mean there's a problem with your milk-making ability, but you do need to improve the delivery system. The high-fat milk is released later in the feeding, after your milk-ejection reflex has been triggered, sending the "cream" down into the ducts. If you automatically switch sides after five minutes or ten minutes on one breast, your baby may get only foremilk on both sides. Encourage your baby to nurse longer on each side until the milk becomes more creamy and helps him feel good and full. A good guideline for babies who nurse actively is "finish the first breast first." Let baby decide when to switch, rather than following the clock or a schedule.

If your baby tends to fall asleep after only a few minutes of nursing, you need to encourage him to nurse longer and more vigorously. When he starts to drift off, take him off the breast, wake him up by burping him gently, and then latch him on again. You may have to repeat this process several times until baby has nursed actively for at least ten to fifteen minutes. Longer, more vigorous nursing stimulates more milk-ejection reflexes and puts more meat on baby's bones. Many of the tips on increasing your milk supply, below, will help you get more of your high-fat hindmilk into your baby, especially double-feeding and massaging your breasts during feedings.

Dr. Bill notes: There are babies who are normally slow weight-gainers. They are often "banana" body-type (long, lanky) babies who put more of their calories into height than weight, or normal petite babies from petite parents. Unlike the failure-to-thrive infants, these babies produce the normal number of stools, and their skin does not have a loose, wrinkly appearance.

Does my breastfed baby need extra water and vitamins?

Breastfed babies do not need extra water, as formula-fed babies do. Your breast milk is very high in water, while formula is more concentrated. We discourage extra water, not because of the water itself, but because of the possibility of nipple confusion and breast-feeding disharmony if babies are given water in a bottle in the newborn period.

A healthy term baby who is getting enough breast milk does not need vitamin supplements, unless recommended by your doctor for your baby's special nutritional needs. When baby is around nine months of age, your health care provider may recommend a multivitamin with iron if baby's blood count or diet is low in iron.

Increasing Your Milk Supply

Our three-week-old baby doesn't seem to be gaining as much weight as she should, and I don't feel I have enough milk. How can I increase my milk supply?

Most delays in milk production are the result of one or several of the following: improper positioning and latch-on, interference in the harmony between mother and baby, a tired mother in a busy nest, or scheduled feedings. Go through the following steps.

Weigh baby more frequently. Consult your doctor and arrange to bring your baby into the office for a weight check twice a week.

Seek assistance. Consult a lactation specialist to review your positioning and latch-on techniques and to evaluate your baby's suck.

Get support. Contact breastfeeding and mothering organizations such as your local La Leche League.

Avoid negative advisers. "Are you sure she's getting enough milk?" "I couldn't breast-feed either. . . ." You don't need discouragement when you are trying to build up your confidence as a new mother. Surround yourself with supportive people. Breastfeeding is a confidence game.

Check your nest. Is your nest too busy? Temporarily shelve all commitments that drain your energy from breastfeeding your baby.

Take your baby to bed. Feed nestled close to each other. Nap nursing and night nursing are powerful stimulators of milk production, since the milk-producing hormones are best secreted while you are asleep.

Undress your baby during feeding. If she is small (under 8 pounds/3.6 kilograms), you need to keep baby warm by placing a blanket around her, but still allowing tummy-to-tummy contact. Skin-to-skin contact helps awaken sleepy babies and stimulates less enthusiastic feeders.

Increase the frequency of feeding. Give *at least* one feeding every two hours, and wake your baby during the day if she sleeps more than three hours. If you have a sleepy baby, let her sleep nestled against your breasts. This skin-to-skin contact stimulates milk flow.

BUILDING YOUR MILK BANK

Your breastfeeding is going great. Your supply meets baby's demand, and the thought of ever giving your baby canned milk is foreign to you. But the best-laid plans of breastfeeding mothers sometimes go astray. A circumstance beyond your control, such as a sudden hospitalization, may cause an abrupt, unplanned break in your breastfeeding. Be prepared for this rainy day. Open an "account" in your freezer. Stockpile at least a few days' worth of this white gold. It's a wise investment in your baby's nutritional future (see "Expressing Milk," page 168, for details on collecting and storing breast milk).

Think baby, think milk. While you are feeding, stroke and cuddle your baby, using a lot of skin-to-skin contact, a custom called grooming. These maternal behaviors stimulate your milk-producing hormones.

Sleep when your baby sleeps. This requires delaying or delegating the many seemingly pressing household chores. If you are blessed with a baby who feeds frequently, you may think, "I don't get anything done." But you are getting something done. You are doing the most important job in the world — mothering a human being.

Nurse longer. Don't limit the length of baby's feedings to a certain number of minutes per side. Give baby the chance to finish the first breast before switching to the second. He needs to get the high-fat hindmilk on the first side. This low-volume, high-calorie milk helps babies grow and rewards them for their sucking. If you switch breasts after only a few minutes, baby will get only the watery foremilk from both sides. This fills baby's tummy but may not give him enough calories to put on weight. Longer nursing stimulates more milk-ejection reflexes and brings more fat down to baby.

Try switch feeding. In the traditional method of breastfeeding, you encourage your baby to suck as she wishes at one breast (usually around ten minutes) and to complete her feedings on the second breast, reversing the process on the next feeding. Switch feeding, also called the *burp-and-switch technique,* operates as follows: Let your baby suck at the first breast until the intensity of her suck and swallow diminishes and her eyes start to close (usually three to five minutes). Don't watch the clock, but watch your baby for these signs that she is losing interest in continuing to suck on that breast. As soon as these signs appear, remove her from the breast, burp her well, and switch to the next breast until her sucking diminishes again; stop, burp her a second time and repeat the entire process back to the first breast and then to the other again. This burp-and-switch technique encourages a creamier, high-calorie hindmilk to be released because the milk-ejection reflex is stimulated each time you switch. This technique is particularly effective for the sleepy baby, the "nipper-napper," who does not feed enthusiastically. The frequent switching keeps her awake, and the burping makes more room in the tiny stomach for more milk.

Try double feeding. This technique operates on the same principle as switch feeding, increasing the fat content of your milk and giving baby a greater volume of hindmilk.

After you feed your baby and she seems content, burp her and carry her around in an upright position for ten to twenty minutes. Then offer her the breast again. With less air in her tummy, there will be room for more milk, and the milk that is there and ready for her in your breasts will be high in fat. You'll be topping her off with more of what she needs to grow. The longer you wait between feedings, the lower the fat content of your foremilk.

Wear your baby. Carry baby in sling as often as you can between feedings. The close proximity of baby to your breast not only stimulates more milk production but also reminds baby to feed. When she roots toward your breast, breastfeed her in the sling. Some babies feed better on the move. (See page 296 for suggestions on breastfeeding while wearing baby.)

Massage your breasts before and during feedings. Gentle breast massage before a feeding can help stimulate your milk-ejection reflex, so that the milk is ready and flowing when baby latches on. Compressing the breast during feedings helps move the milk down toward the nipple, mimicking a milk-ejection reflex. You can use this technique to encourage baby to nurse longer. When his sucking slows or he seems to be losing interest, use the hand that is supporting the breast to massage milk down toward the nipple. You will notice baby start to swallow and suck more actively as the milk flows into the breast's sinuses and out the nipple. Work your hand around the breast so that all the ducts get this extra stimulation.

Attempt to relax during breastfeeding. The milk-ejection reflex can be inhibited if you are physically and emotionally tense. Use the relaxation techniques you learned in childbirth class, use pillows, have someone rub your back, visualize flowing streams, play soothing tapes, feel confident in yourself. (See page 145 for more suggestions on how to relax during breastfeeding.)

Try herbal teas. Natural remedies to increase milk production are based more on folklore than on real evidence. In our practice and during our own breastfeeding we have found fenugreek tea helps milk production. Here's the Sears recipe: Steep one teaspoon of fenugreek seeds in a cup of boiling-hot water for about five minutes, or until the water is mildly colored and scented (the tea has a sweet maplelike flavor). Martha has found a few cups of this tea to be very helpful during times when her milk supply seems to be lagging. Some mothers report better success with Mother's Milk tea, which contains some fenugreek, and other teas reported in herbal literature to help with milk supply. Whether these teas really help physically or psychologically is irrelevant. So try them — relax and enjoy.

Engorgement

What happens if I have too much milk and become engorged?

Engorgement, a pronounced filling and swelling of your breasts that causes them to become very hard and painful, is your body's signal that the supply-and-demand mechanism is out of balance. Engorgement is a problem for both mother and baby. For mother, it can be very painful, and, if left untreated, can progress into a debilitating breast infection.

This condition is also uncomfortable for baby. If your breasts are engorged, the nipple angle flattens, preventing baby from properly latching on. When this happens, your baby sucks your nipple but cannot get enough of the areolar tissue into her mouth to compress the milk sinuses. As a result, the baby stimulates more milk to enter the breast but is unable to empty it, further aggravating engorgement and setting up a vicious circle. As the breast tissue swells, the milk cannot flow freely. Baby gets less milk and needs to feed more frequently; mother gets more engorged, and the breastfeeding pair is in trouble. You can prevent engorgement by following the right-start tips for breastfeeding; feeding on cue rather than on schedule and using correct positioning and latch-on techniques.

If engorgement occurs while you are still in the hospital, use an electric breast pump to release some of the extra milk in order to soften the areola, so that baby can latch on and more effectively empty your breasts. Usually, in the first week, your breasts slowly and steadily build up milk, and baby should drain your breasts at the same rate as the milk is produced. Some fullness is common as your milk increases during the first week, but it should subside with proper positioning and latch-on, frequent feeding, and lots of rest. Sometimes milk increases suddenly around the third or fourth day, causing mothers to exclaim, "I awakened with these two painful boulders on my chest." Use a breast pump, preferably electric, immediately to relieve this engorgement before it progresses. In the past, warm compresses were recommended, but now that engorgement is better understood, we realize that heat can actually do more harm by increasing tissue swelling. You will need to apply cold compresses or packs of crushed ice (use a thin cloth between your skin and the ice pack to prevent frostbite) until the swelling subsides enough for the milk to flow. This cool therapy will also relieve the heat and pain in your breasts.

You can keep fullness from developing into engorgement once you are home by standing in a warm shower, soaking your breasts in warm water in a basin, or applying warm compresses for ten minutes before expressing or feeding. This helps trigger your milk-ejection reflex so baby will get milk flowing sooner and empty your breasts better. If your areola is too full for your baby to latch on correctly, then express some milk before feeding to soften your areola enough so that your baby can grasp the areola and not only your nipple.

If fullness progresses to engorgement, do not sit patiently and wait for engorgement to subside. Use continuous ice packs between feedings to alleviate your pain and reduce swelling, and if possible rent an electric breast pump until you can reach a lactation consultant for help with your breastfeeding technique. If your baby is nursing well, pump only enough milk to relieve the fullness and soften the areola so that baby can latch on. If your newborn is not yet nursing effectively at the breast, you will need to pump every two to three hours to keep the milk flowing and to stimulate a good milk supply. Acetaminophen and a well-fitting bra that is not too tight for support are helpful, and rest is a must.

Above all, don't stop breastfeeding! *The breasts must be drained.* Unrelieved engorgement often leads to a breast infection called mastitis. The symptoms resemble the flu: fatigue, fever, chills, and aches. Your breasts may be generally engorged or you may feel a localized swollen, tender, red, warm area. To treat, apply moist heat (warm towel or jet of warm water in shower) to the sore area for ten minutes at least four times daily, take acetaminophen for fever and pain and a doctor-prescribed antibiotic (both safe while breastfeeding), and rest. Unless you are advised not to by your lactation consultant, it is helpful to continue breastfeeding. The breast must be emptied (either by baby or by pumping) for the infection to heal. (For information on taking probiotics with antibiotics, see page 691.)

If you have enjoyed uncomplicated breastfeeding and suddenly you are becoming engorged, take inventory of your feeding techniques, or take this as a signal that your nest or your schedule is too busy. Listen to your body; it is trying to tell you something.

Needs to Relax

I'm a tense person. How can I better relax during breastfeeding?

The hormone prolactin has a calming effect, yet emotional stress or physical stress (exhaustion, pain, illness) can actually interfere with the milk-releasing hormone, oxytocin, inhibiting the MER. Then if your milk doesn't flow, baby comes unglued. Babies are quick to pick up on mother's tension, so relaxation is a valuable skill to cultivate. Try the following tips.

Think baby. Before beginning to breastfeed, set the tone for the time ahead by focusing on the activity at hand — put aside conflicting concerns and think baby. Imagine yourself breastfeeding; imagine the movements and facial expressions of your baby that you enjoy most. Massage your baby. Stroke and cuddle your baby using a lot of skin-to-skin contact. All these images and activities get the relaxing hormones flowing, helping you to unwind before beginning to feed.

Minimize distractions. Prior to feeding eat a healthful snack and drink some water or juice. A hot shower, warm bath, or brief nap before feeding time is good relaxation therapy. Try the relaxation techniques and breathing exercises you learned during childbirth class. Play relaxing music prior to and during breastfeeding. Visualize a fountain flowing from your breasts. Ask someone to stand behind your chair and massage your neck, shoulders, and upper back. As you accomplish latch-on, with all your pillows in place, take a deep abdominal breath and exhale slowly, just as you learned for childbirth, letting all the tension flow away from your neck, back, and arms.

Feed in a warm bath. Water therapy helps if you are extremely tense. Sit in a warm bath with the water level just below your breasts. Breastfeed baby (who is also half-immersed in warm water) as you recline in the tub. A safety tip: Don't try to step into a filled tub while holding a baby. You may slip. Place baby on a towel next to the tub until you are comfortably settled, or have someone else hand your baby to you after you are reclining in the tub.

Prepare a breastfeeding station. This idea has helped Martha relax while feeding our babies amid all the activities of a busy family. This station is an area in your home especially set up as a nest for mother and baby, containing your favorite chair (preferably an armchair or a rocking chair with arms at a comfortable height to support your arms while holding baby), plenty of pillows, a footstool, soothing music, a relaxing book, nutritious nibbles such as fruit bits or trail mix, and juice or water. If you don't take the phone off the hook, a cordless phone or a long extension wire is a real help. You will be spending a lot of time in this nest, so make it inviting and functional. Anticipate your needs for the hour or so you may be spending there — for instance, extra diapering supplies and baby clothes, a burping cloth, a waste can. If you have a toddler and/or preschooler, include snacks for him and some favorite activities you save just for feeding time. You may need to have one feeding station located where you can keep him contained in a safe area. It's hard to relax if you have to worry about what he's getting into. Some toddlers tolerate new baby feeding time better if you

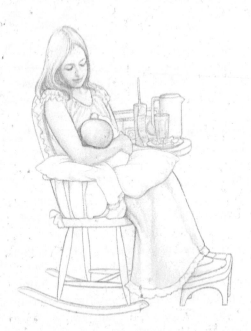

A breastfeeding station, a designated area set up with what you need for comfort and efficiency, can help make breastfeeding more relaxed and enjoyable.

actually set up your station on the floor. This gives the message that you are accessible. Breastfeeding itself is a self-relaxing cycle. The more you breastfeed, the more relaxing hormones you produce, which help you breastfeed better.

Make Time for Toddler

We have a two-year-old and I'm nursing a new baby. Every time I sit down to nurse he wants to play. Any suggestions?

Consider your toddler's viewpoint. Baby is getting all the attention, the milk, and the cuddling that *he* used to have. Here's how we have learned to juggle the needs of two children at the same time. Feed your baby in a baby sling. This frees one or both hands to play with your toddler. Sit on the floor and throw a ball, stack blocks, or read a book with your toddler while baby is comfortably feeding in the sling. Next, expand the feeding-station idea to include items for your toddler, a basket of reserved toys, favorite books, a tape player, and activities such as blocks. Sit down on the floor with your back against the couch and as you feed your baby, play with your toddler. Your toddler will view the feeding station as a special place for him, too. Regard the feeding station, toys, or activities as only for breastfeeding time so that your toddler learns that feeding time for baby is also a special playtime for him. Eventually your toddler will realize, "Mom does special things with me that she doesn't do at any other time." By sitting on the floor and feeding your baby, you avoid the scene of your toddler trying to climb up on your lap to be where the action is. Extending feeding time to include toddler activity also helps you relax. You don't have to wonder what mischief your toddler is getting into in the other room. Also include your toddler in the nap-nursing scene. While you nap nurse your baby, invite your toddler to snuggle up next to you — for a family nap.

If Baby Bites

Our seven-month-old bites during feeding, and I find this annoying. What can I do?

Your natural inclination is to pull your baby away from the breast and scream, "No!" You can hardly blame the mother for a violent reaction, especially if it is a hard bite, but some babies are so bothered by a harsh reaction to their biting that they actually stop breastfeeding for a few days — called a breastfeeding strike. Affectionate nibbling, those annoying nips from a baby who is experimenting with her teeth, will lessen.

Instead of the yank-and-yell response, when you sense baby's teeth coming down to bite, draw her way in close to your breast, and she will automatically let go in order to open her mouth more and uncover her nose to breathe. Don't try to disengage yourself from the clenched teeth. Your baby will lessen her bite as she realizes that she can't both bite and breathe. After several times of this counterinstinctive trick of pulling your baby in close to you when she bites, your baby will realize that biting triggers an uncomfortable position, and she will adjust it. It's OK to say no, because baby needs to learn that some undesirable action occurs when she bites, but don't frighten her.

Keep a log of what triggers the biting and when she bites. Biting can be baby's way of telling you she's finished eating. If she chomps at the end of a feeding, interrupt the feeding before she has a chance to bite. Teething can also create the urge to chomp. Keep some teething toys in the freezer, such as a frozen banana or a cold washcloth, and let her chomp on these before or at the end of a feeding. These techniques plus saying, "Ouch, that hurts Mama!" will help teach your baby breastfeeding manners and preserve your breasts. (For additional tips, see the discussion of the chomper, page 179.)

Breastfeeding As Birth Control

I have heard that breastfeeding can be a natural contraceptive. How reliable is this method of birth control?

Breastfeeding can be very effective as a natural method of birth control. Here's why. The milk-making hormone, prolactin, suppresses the release of the fertility hormones that cause eggs to develop and prepare the womb to nourish those eggs. When prolactin levels are high, women do not ovulate or menstruate. What keeps prolactin levels high? Frequent breastfeeding — feeding according to baby's cues. Long stretches of time without nursing allow prolactin levels to fall and fertility hormones to take over. The key to using breastfeeding as a natural contraceptive is to keep prolactin levels high with frequent feeding, both day and night. Breastfeeding can provide reliable birth control, *as long as you follow the rules.*

Researchers have developed guidelines for mothers who wish to rely on breastfeeding for birth control. These rules are the basis of the lactational amenorrhea method of family planning, or LAM for short. According to LAM, a mother can rely on breastfeeding for protection from pregnancy if she can answer no to the following three questions:

- Have your menses returned?
- Are you supplementing regularly, or allowing long periods without breastfeeding, either during the day (more than three hours) or at night (more than six hours)?
- Is your baby more than six months old?

Studies have shown that mothers who follow the LAM guidelines have a less than 2 percent chance of becoming pregnant in the first six months after birth. This compares favorably with the protection from pregnancy offered by artificial methods of birth control. Many mothers enjoy longer periods of infertility and no menses, as long as their babies continue to nurse frequently and rely on the breast for most of their nourishment. Studies have shown that the following practices can prolong the period in which you are unable to conceive:

- Encourage unrestricted breastfeeding without regard to daytime or nighttime scheduling.
- Sleep with your baby and allow unrestricted night feeding.
- Delay supplemental bottles or pacifiers. All of baby's sucking should be at the breast.
- Delay solid foods. When introduced they should add to baby's nutrition, not substitute for breastfeeding.

Mothers who follow these rules enjoy an average of 14.5 months of amenorrhea and infertility. Every mother and baby pair, however, is different, and periods will return sooner for some mothers and later for others. Some women may not ovulate during their first few cycles. Approximately 5 percent of women ovulate (and thus are fertile) before ever having a period; the longer you've gone without having a period, the more likely this is to happen.

9

The Breastfeeding Mother: Choices, Challenges

By now we hope you realize breastfeeding does make a difference — for mother and baby. But there are medical, social, and economic situations that may challenge this way of nurturing. Here are some ideas for making breastfeeding easier in a variety of circumstances.

EATING RIGHT DURING BREASTFEEDING

Just as your body provided the nutrients your baby needed to grow during your pregnancy, your milk delivers the nutrients baby needs to develop outside the womb during the first year of life. Your body uses nutrients more efficiently while you are lactating so that there is enough for both baby and you. It also relies on fat stores left over from pregnancy for energy to make milk. But you are still "eating for two." You need between 300 and 500 extra *nutritious* calories a day to make milk for your baby.

Your eating plan for breastfeeding should include the nutritious foods you normally eat, but more of them. If you eat foods that are good for you, you will have more energy and feel better as you recover from birth and weather the stress of new motherhood. Avoiding the empty calories of high-fat, high-sugar foods will also help you regain your prepregnancy weight and figure. Candies, desserts, soda pop, and packaged snack foods offer little nutritional value. Instead, eat nutrient-dense foods that provide a lot of nutrition for each calorie. For balanced nourishment, include nutrient-rich foods from the five basic food groups:

- whole grain bread, cereal, rice, and pasta group (six to eleven servings daily)
- vegetable group (three to five servings daily)
- fruit group (two to four servings daily)
- fish, meat, poultry, dry beans, eggs, and nuts group (two to three servings daily)
- milk, yogurt, and cheese group (two to three servings daily)

Each day consume foods from each of these groups, portioned for balanced nutrition into the three basic calorie groups:

- *Carbohydrates* should supply 50–55 percent of your total daily calories, and the

149

major portion of this energy source should be in the form of healthy sugars, which give a steady release of energy, chiefly pasta, grains, and fruit. (See the discussion of healthy sugars, page 240.)

- Healthy *fats* should make up around 30 percent of your total daily calories. (For a list of foods that contain healthy fats, see page 239.)
- *Proteins* should make up 15–20 percent of your daily calories. (For a list of protein-rich foods, see page 242.)

Calcium Is Good Bone Food

You need a lot of calcium during pregnancy and lactation. To nourish rapidly growing bones, calcium is important to baby. Don't let the fear of depleting your own calcium reserves scare you from breastfeeding. Recent studies show that breastfeeding may actually protect mother's bones against osteoporosis. The calcium that is taken from mother's bones during lactation is returned during and after weaning, resulting in greater bone density than before pregnancy.

SMART FATS FOR BABY, HEALTHY FATS FOR MOM

Dr. Bill advises: *Low-fat diets are not healthy for infants. Instead, feed baby a* ***right-fat*** *diet.*

Not all fats are created equal, and not all fats are bad. Babies need fat to build brain and nerve tissue, and 50 percent of the calories in your milk come from fat. The fats you eat affect the amount of the different kinds of fat — good and bad — that appear in your milk.

For example, you can boost the levels of good fats in your milk by eating more fatty fish, such as salmon, which contains omega-3 fatty acids. (See "Go Fishing!," page 243.) Omega-3 fatty acids include the "smart fat" DHA, which builds better baby brains. Flax oil, canola oil, and soybean oil give your body the raw materials it needs to manufacture DHA for your milk. Most standard prenatal and multivitamins do not contain omega 3's. Compared with mothers in cultures that eat a lot of sea-food, American mothers tend to have lower levels of omega-3 fats in their milk.

Bad fats include hydrogenated fats. These are fats that are chemically altered to stay solid at room temperature so that they will have a longer shelf life. You will find hydrogenated fats in many processed foods if you take time to read the labels. The problem with hydrogenated fats is that they contain trans fatty acids, or trans fats, a type of fat that is created during the hydrogenation process. Trans fats may raise cholesterol levels and interfere with immune functions. Compared with mothers in cultures that eat less packaged foods, most American mothers have higher levels of trans fatty acids in their milk, probably because of the hydrogenated fats in their diet. This may not be the best thing for their infants. For your own health and that of your baby, become more aware of the hydrogenated fats in the foods you eat. Then cut back or eliminate them entirely from your family's diet.

You don't have to drink milk to make milk; cows don't! If you don't like milk or are allergic to or intolerant of it, you can get all of the bone-building mineral you need from the following calcium-rich nondairy foods: sardines, soybeans, broccoli, beans, salmon, tofu, watercress, kale, collards, okra, dried beans, greens, raisins, dried figs, and carrot juice. Since dairy products are still one of the best sources of calcium, cheese and yogurt are good sources if you dislike milk but are not intolerant of or allergic to it.

Iron — The Blood-Building Element

Sufficient iron intake is vital to the postpartum mother. Several iron-rich foods are fish, poultry, prune juice, and iron-fortified cereals (see page 246 for more iron-rich foods). To improve the absorption of iron from food, eat or drink vitamin C–rich foods (for example, fruit and vegetable juices) along with it — combinations like meatballs and tomato sauce, iron-fortified cereals and orange juice. As an added nutritional perk, breastfeeding has an iron-preserving effect by suppressing your menstrual flow.

Extra Vitamins?

Because of the extra nutritional needs of mother and baby, continue your prenatal vitamin supplements during breastfeeding, unless your doctor advises otherwise. (Occasionally, we have found that some brands of prenatal vitamins cause colicky symptoms in the baby, which disappear when switching to another brand.) To boost your vitamin D naturally, treat yourself to short, frequent doses of sunlight.

LACTADE

To the smoothie recipe on page 257 add 1 serving of soy lecithin and 1 serving of soy protein. Studies suggest that lecithin can improve milk duct drainage, and extra soy protein can increase the volume of a mother's milk.

Extra Fluids

A breastfeeding mother's best noncalorie drink is water. Enjoy a glass of water or juice just before breastfeeding. Most mothers drink at least eight glasses of fluids a day. As a volume guide, drink as your thirst urges. Prepare something to drink *before* you sit down to breastfeed. If you wait to drink after feeding, you may not drink sufficient liquid. While extra fluids are prescribed as the universal elixir for nearly all breastfeeding ills, don't flood yourself. Excess fluids may actually hinder milk production. Shun caffeine-containing coffee, teas, and colas, and alcoholic beverages, as these may have a diuretic effect, causing you to lose valuable minerals and fluids.

Environmental Pollutants

Pesticides and other contaminants are an increasing concern. To minimize these harmful substances entering your milk, avoid fish from waters known to be contaminated, peel and thoroughly wash fresh fruits and vegetables, and cut away the fatty portions of meat, poultry, and fish, since chemicals tend to concentrate in fat. (See page 276 for more pesticide-prevention tips.)

UPSETTING FOODS IN BREAST MILK

Mother-infant dining partners can enjoy a bountiful menu. But some babies are sensitive to certain foods in mother's diet. Upsetting foods can enter your milk and upset baby as early as two hours after you eat them. A clue to food sensitivities as a cause of fussy, colicky behavior is a pattern called twenty-four-hour colic — a definite episode of hurting that occurs within twenty-four hours after the breastfeeding mother eats a suspect food but that does not recur until the next time she eats the same food. Watch for these offenders:

Dairy products. Potentially allergenic proteins in dairy products may enter the breast milk and produce colicky symptoms in baby. (This is discussed in detail in "The Colic–Cow's Milk Connection," page 397.)

Caffeine-containing foods. Soft drinks, chocolate, coffee, tea, and certain cold remedies all contain caffeine. While some babies may be more caffeine sensitive than others, usually a mother must consume a large amount of these products to bother her baby.

Grains and nuts. The most allergenic of these are wheat, corn, and peanuts.

Spicy foods. Your milk may have a distinctive taste after you eat spicy or garlicky foods. Salads, pizzas, and a binge at your local ethnic restaurant introduce baby to these foods.

Occasionally they may evoke a gastric protest from your baby, causing him to refuse to feed or to be colicky.

Gassy foods. Broccoli, onions, brussels sprouts, green peppers, cauliflower, cabbage — these vegetables in the raw state may bother babies, but they are less likely to be offensive when cooked. We find it difficult to explain scientifically how these foods bother babies, but our personal breastfeeding experience validates what veteran breastfeeding mothers have known for a long time — gassy foods make gassy babies.

Tracking Down Foods That Bother Baby

This simple three-step technique for identifying foods in your breast milk that may be upsetting your child is virtually identical to the approach to take in identifying food allergies that may arise after baby is no longer consuming breast milk exclusively. (See page 270 for details.)

Step one: Make a fuss-food chart. From the preceding food possibilities, select and list the foods in your diet that are most suspect. Cow's milk is the most common culprit. Across from these list your baby's upsets, usually fussiness, crying and colicky episodes, bloating, severe constipation or diarrhea, a very gassy baby, unexplained night waking, or a red ring around baby's anus.

Step two: Eliminate foods. One by one, starting with cow's milk (or all at once if necessary), eliminate the most suspect foods from your diet for ten to fourteen days.

ALMOND MILK RECIPE

If your breastfeeding baby does not tolerate cow's milk in your diet, here's an alternative. (Note: Almond milk should not be given to babies in place of standard infant formulas.) Almond milk or a prepared mix can be purchased in a nutrition store, or you can make your own.

½ cup blanched raw almonds
2 cups water (more as needed)
Salt, honey, maple syrup, vanilla
    or almond extract (optional)

Place the blanched raw almonds in a blender. Add 1 cup of the water and blend until smooth — about five minutes in a high-speed blender. Add the remaining cup of water to thin the milk to the desired consistency, using more water as needed. Chill before using for best flavor. You may wish to flavor the milk by adding a few grains of salt, a bit of honey or maple syrup, or a touch of vanilla or almond extract. Almond milk can be used as a beverage, on cereal, or in baking and cooking.

Observe your baby to see if the symptoms of upset diminish or disappear. If they do not, try eliminating a different fuss food. If they do disappear, go on to step three.

Step three: Challenge the result. If some or all of the troublesome symptoms subside, challenge this result by reintroducing the suspicious food. If baby's symptoms reappear within twenty-four hours, temporarily scratch this food off your menu. Though mothers are often wise detectives, the reintroduction challenge keeps you more objective. Love for your baby and hurting when your baby hurts make you vulnerable to quickly labeling a certain food as the culprit of baby's problems, which may unnecessarily deprive you and your baby of a valuable source of nutrients. Even if you do pin the problems on a particular food, most babies are only temporarily intolerant of certain foods, allowing you to eventually include your favorite foods again.

Other Fuss-Food Hints

Don't overdose on any one food. While some babies are exquisitely sensitive to drops or crumbs of an offending nutrient, others are bothered only if mother eats or drinks large quantities. Wheat products and citrus foods are examples of this: Too much may bother baby, but a small amount may be tolerated.

If you find yourself eating fewer foods, yet baby is fussing more, consult a lactation consultant to be sure your breastfeeding technique is not the problem, a nutritionist to be sure you are consuming a balanced diet, and, most important, your baby's doctor for non-food-related causes of your baby's problem. See our *Fussy Baby Book* (Little, Brown, 1996) for tips on eliminating fuss foods and on comforting and coping with unhappy babies. For food lovers, let's dangle a final carrot. Don't let fear of food restrictions discourage breastfeeding. Often these intolerant babies also have serious problems with some or all formulas. For most breastfeeding pairs, what mother eats does not upset baby.

MEDICINES FOR TWO: TAKING MEDICINES SAFELY WHILE BREASTFEEDING

At some time during lactation, most mothers will need medicines to deal with an illness. Besides wondering how the drug will behave in your own body, you now have another body to consider. Most drugs taken by the mother enter her milk, but usually only around 1 percent of the dose appears in the milk. Here's how to safely take medicines while breastfeeding.

General Considerations

Before taking any medication during breast-feeding, consider the following:

- Will the medicine harm your baby?
- Will the medicine diminish milk production?
- Are there safer but equally effective alternative treatments?
- Are there ways to juggle medicine taking and breastfeeding to lessen how much of the drug gets into your baby?

You should be aware that advice for a mother about a medication is sometimes based more on legal considerations than on scientific knowledge. A physician who does not know if a drug is safe may tell the mother not to breast-feed. Pharmaceutical companies also legally protect themselves (with package inserts and in the drug reference book *Physicians' Desk Reference*) by advising a mother not to breast-feed while taking a certain drug. This precautionary advice is usually less expensive than researching how much of the medicine enters

breast milk and its effect on the baby. As a result of erroneous advice given about a harmless medication, babies are often weaned prematurely, abruptly, and unnecessarily.

Juggling Medicine Taking and Breastfeeding

If you need to take a medicine, here's how to reduce the amount that gets into your baby.

Ask yourself if you really need the medicine. If you have a cold, can you achieve the

RESOURCES

The information in this section is based upon thorough research and up-to-date sources. Because new information on the safety of a particular drug may be discovered after this writing, we advise checking with your doctor before taking any medication while breastfeeding.

American Academy of Pediatrics, Committee on Drugs. "Transfer of Drugs and Other Chemicals into Human Milk." *Pediatrics* 93 (1994): 137–150.

Briggs, Gerald G., Roger K. Freeman, and Sumner J. Yaffe. *Drugs in Pregnancy and Lactation: A Reference Guide to Fetal and Neonatal Risk* (William and Wilkins, 1998).

Hale, Thomas. *Medications and Mothers' Milk*, 10th ed. Amarillo, Texas: Pharmasoft, 2002. (See Dr. Hale's website, http://neonatal.ttuhsc.edu/lact/.

Drug Information Service at the University of California, San Diego, (900) 288–8273. The service charges $3 for first minute and $2 for each additional minute.

same benefit by steam, extra fluids, and a tincture of time? Can you get by with a *single-ingredient* rather than a multiple-ingredient cold medicine?

Find out if you can delay your treatment. If you need a diagnostic procedure (for example, X-ray studies with a radioactive material) or elective surgery, can you wait until baby is a few weeks or months older? The drug may affect exclusively breastfed newborns more than an older infant who has alternative sources of nutrition and whose more-mature systems are better able to handle the drug.

Choose a medicine that passes poorly into your milk. Let your doctor know how important breastfeeding is to you and your baby and that you don't want to stop unless medically necessary. Your doctor can choose a medicine (such as an antibiotic) that passes poorly into your milk. Also, your doctor can choose an alternative route of administration so that more of the medicine gets directly to the site of the problem and less gets into your bloodstream. For example, instead of pills try locally applied creams for skin infections, inhalant medications for asthma or bronchitis, and decongestants sprayed into the nose instead of taken orally. Because they clear more quickly from your milk, short-acting medicines (taken three to four times a day) are generally regarded as safer during breastfeeding than long-acting drugs (taken once or twice a day).

Juggle feeding and medicine times. Ask your doctor when the time of peak concentration is. (This is when the medicine reaches the highest level in your blood — usually the same time that it's highest in your milk.) Most drugs reach their peak concentration one to three hours after you take the medicine and are nearly cleared from the milk after six hours. If there is doubt about the safety of a drug, try these tactics:

1. If possible, before beginning the medicine, pump and store a few feedings' worth of milk. (See "Expressing Milk," page 168, for details on collecting and storing breast milk.)
2. Breastfeed just before taking the medicine.
3. Take the medicine just prior to baby's longest sleep period, usually after the last feeding at night.
4. If baby requires a feeding within the next three to six hours, use the "safe" milk from your storage supply, or use formula.
5. Pump and dump. Because most drugs leave the breast milk as quickly as they enter it, some authorities feel that waiting six hours is just as effective as pumping and discarding the milk, but pumping may help prevent engorgement. In addition, some fat-soluble drugs are stored in the fat of breast milk, so it may be helpful to pump and discard a feeding's worth of milk up to three or four hours after taking the medication.

This timing of the sequence is a general guide and may vary according to the type of medication and the feeding pattern of your baby. (Some radioactive medications may take twenty-four hours to clear your system, for example.) *Check with your doctor on the best juggling schedule.*

If the safety of a drug you must take is questionable, but medically your baby must breastfeed (for example, baby is allergic to formula), besides observing the preceding juggling tips, consult your doctor about monitoring the amount of drug that enters your milk or baby's blood.

Most Common Medications

The following guidelines will help you when dealing with some of the most frequently used drugs.

Pain and fever relievers. Acetaminophen is the safest analgesic to use during breastfeeding; only 0.1–0.2 percent of the maternal dose enters the milk. Several doses of narcotic analgesics (Demerol, codeine, and morphine) after delivery or surgery may cause baby to be temporarily sleepy, but not enough to discourage breastfeeding. Prolonged use of narcotic pain relievers may not be safe during breastfeeding.

Cold, cough, and allergy remedies. These nonprescription medicines are safe to take while breastfeeding, but observe the following precautions: Try single-ingredient medications (either decongestant or antihistamine, for example) before using combinations; short-acting medicines are usually safer than long-acting ones. Before bedtime, cough syrup containing codeine is all right; dextromethorphan (DM) is preferable. It is best to take these remedies after breastfeeding and before bedtime, and to limit them to one or two days at a time. Watch baby for hyperirritability following your taking decongestant medications or for excessive sleepiness after an antihistamine, and adjust the medicines accordingly. Nasal sprays (cromolyn, steroids, decongestants) are safer than oral medications while breastfeeding.

Antibiotics. Nearly all antibiotics are safe to take while breastfeeding, especially if taken for the usual one- to two-week course for common infections. Even though only a trace amount of the most commonly used antibiotics (penicillins and cephalosporins) enter the milk, baby may be allergic to the antibiotic (allergy-type rash) or develop oral thrush or diarrhea from a prolonged effect of the antibiotic on the intestines. Sulfa antibiotics should be used with caution during the newborn period. Your doctor may take special precautions with the prolonged use of any antibiotic such as tetracycline, with some high-dose intravenous antibiotics, or with special antibiotics like Flagyl.

Caffeine and chocolate. No, you don't have to give up your coffee, tea, soft drinks, or chocolate candy during breastfeeding. Studies show that only 0.5–1 percent of the maternal dose of caffeine or chocolate enters the breast milk. The occasional baby may become irritable, showing a hypersensitivity to caffeine or the theobromine in chocolate.

Oral contraceptives. Most authorities believe the low-dose progestin-only pill (the "minipill") is safe while breastfeeding. And for mothers who exclusively breastfeed, the minipill is as protective as the older progestin-estrogen combination, which decreases the quality and quantity of milk and is not safe. Studies have shown the progestin-only pill does not alter the quantity or quality of breast milk or interfere with infant growth, and some studies show that this type of pill may even enhance milk production. An occasional mother, however, may report a decreasing milk supply even with the minipill. Although an eight-year follow-up of breastfed infants of mothers taking a fifty-microgram progestin pill showed no harmful development or effects, the primary concern is the possible long-term effects when these babies begin to procreate. Like the progestin-only pill, levonorgestrel implants are generally regarded as safe, but their long-term effects are also unknown. Because longer-term effects of oral contraceptives on breastfed infants are being studied, consult your gynecologist for the latest information on the safety of oral contraceptives while breastfeeding. (See the discussion of breastfeeding and birth control, page 147.)

Antidepressants and other psychiatric medications. These drugs are in the *use-with-caution* category. Most of these drugs appear in breast milk in greater or lesser amounts, and there is little information available about long-term effects on infants. However, a mother who is suffering from serious postpartum depression may benefit from medication, and treating the mother's depression will indirectly benefit the baby.

The most commonly used antidepressants are collectively known as SSRI's (selective serotonin reuptake inhibitors). They boost the brain's levels of serotonin, a mood-elevating neurochemical. Zoloft (sertraline) seems to be the safest SSRI to use while breastfeeding. Studies of infants whose mothers are taking Zoloft have found either insignificant amounts of the drug in the infant's blood, or the drug has been undetectable. Paxil (paroxetine) is the next best choice, and Prozac (fluoxetine) is also considered compatible with breastfeeding.

In addition to medication, consider professional counseling and peer support. Getting help at home, regular exercise, and the relaxing effects of breastfeeding can also help mothers weather a mild depression. Life-style changes are important, even if you are also taking medication.

Other psychiatric medications that are sometimes prescribed for mothers include antidepressants from the tricyclic category. Your doctor can choose one of these that is safe to take while breastfeeding. An occasional dose of Valium (diazepam) is considered safe while breastfeeding, but prolonged use is not advisable. Lithium, used to treat bipolar disorder, is in the yellow-light category (that is, use it with caution) for mothers who are breastfeeding. If treatment with lithium is necessary for mother and premature weaning is undesirable, the levels of lithium in the baby's blood should be closely monitored, approximately every two to four weeks.

Herbs and vitamin supplements. Herbs and dietary supplements are drugs. Use the same caution about taking these as you would about taking any over-the-counter medication. Prenatal vitamins are fine to take while breastfeeding, but megadoses of vitamins may not be a good idea while breastfeeding. Herbal teas promoted as galactagogues (substances that increase your milk supply) are harmless and may work, though there are no scientific studies that confirm this. Herbs to be avoided or used with caution during lactation include comfrey, sassafras, ginseng, and licorice.

Alcohol. New research is questioning the wisdom of traditional breastfeeding folklore that wine is good for relaxing the breastfeeding mother and beer is good for increasing milk supply. Studies suggest two major concerns when a mother drinks alcohol while breastfeeding. First, alcohol enters breast milk very rapidly and in concentrations nearly equal to that in the maternal blood. Second, the tiny infant may have a limited ability to detoxify the alcohol from his or her system. Alcohol has also been shown to inhibit the milk-ejection reflex, and the higher the dose the greater the effect. Studies in animals show that alcohol reduces milk production. A study in humans has shown that infants take less milk from the breast in feedings following their mother's consumption of alcohol. It's possible that alcohol alters the flavor of human milk, making it less appealing to babies. In another study, the infants of breastfeeding mothers who regularly consumed two or more alcoholic drinks daily scored slightly lower on tests of motor development at one year. For these reasons mothers would be wise to limit their alcohol consumption during breastfeeding or eliminate alcohol altogether. The occasional glass of wine with a special dinner should not be a problem. Sip it slowly with food, and, if possible, wait an hour or two before breastfeeding your baby.

Smoking. Nicotine passes into a mother's milk, into the baby, and causes colicky symptoms. Secondhand smoke irritates a baby's nasal and respiratory passages, causing frequent colds, runny noses, and difficulty breathing. Studies show that mothers who smoke have a delayed milk-ejection reflex and a decreased milk supply, and they tend to wean earlier than nonsmoking women. Mothers who smoke also have lower prolactin levels.

Clearly, there are plenty of reasons to quit smoking before you become a parent and even more reasons not to smoke around your

baby. (See page 620, "Smoking and Babies Don't Mix.") If you smoke, we encourage you to seek help if quitting is difficult for you. If you cannot quit, do not smoke around your baby and do not smoke while breastfeeding. If you must smoke, have one cigarette immediately after feeding your baby, allowing the nicotine to clear from your body before the next feeding.

Recreational drugs. Research on the effects of some recreational drugs on the breastfeeding infant is inconclusive at this writing. The problem chemical in marijuana, THC, appears in the breast milk of users, and marijuana has been found to lower the levels of prolactin in the mother. Animal studies have shown structural changes in brain cells of breastfeeding infants after their mothers were exposed to marijuana. These experimental hazards, in addition to the possibility that marijuana may lower a mother's attentiveness to her baby, dictate, by common sense, that mothers avoid marijuana if breastfeeding.

Cocaine, a more dangerous and powerful drug, enters the milk of the breastfeeding mother and agitates the baby's nervous system, causing irritability, sleeplessness, and colicky symptoms. This drug, as well as depressing and addicting drugs such as heroin, should obviously be completely avoided.

BREASTFEEDING HELPERS

There once was a time when a baby, a breast, and an experienced grandmother were all that was needed to breastfeed successfully. As families drifted apart and breastfeeding declined, the supply of knowledgeable breast-

GREEN LIGHT: GO AHEAD!

Common Medications and Ingredients That Are Safe While Breastfeeding
The safety of the following medications is established for short-term use only. Consult a physician before taking prescription drugs or if using an over-the-counter medication for more than two weeks.

acetaminophen	aspartame	Kaopectate
acyclovir	asthma medicines	laxatives
anesthetics, local (e.g., for	(cromolyn, inhalant	muscle relaxants
dental work)	bronchodilators)	naproxen
antacids	barium	pinworm medications
antibiotics (cephalosporin,	chloroquine (antimalarial)	propranolol
erythromycin, penicillin,	cortisone	propylthiouracil
sulfa,* tetracycline,†	decongestants	silicone from implants
trimethoprim)	digitalis	thyroid medications
anticoagulants	diuretics	vaccines
anticonvulsants	ibuprofen	vitamins
antihistamines	insulin	

Use caution in the newborn period.
†Avoid taking tetracycline for longer than 3 weeks.

YELLOW LIGHT: USE CAUTION!

Drugs That Are Compatible with Breastfeeding but Need Careful Monitoring by a Physician
Whether these drugs and medications are safe to take while breastfeeding depends on many factors: the dosage, age of infant, duration of therapy, and timing of dosage and breastfeeding. Consult a physician knowledgeable about drugs during breastfeeding if you need to take any of the following medications long-term.

alcohol	indomethacin	oral contraceptives
antidepressants	isoniazid	(progestin-only)
aspirin	lithium†	Paxil
codeine	metoclopramide	phenobarbital
Demerol	metronidazole	Prozac
ergots	(Flagyl)	Valium
general anesthetics*	morphine	Zoloft

It is safe to breastfeed six to twelve hours after most general anesthetics.
†Some authorities consider lithium absolutely contraindicated while breastfeeding; others believe lithium can be used cautiously, as long as blood lithium concentration in the baby is monitored.

(continued)

RED LIGHT: STOP!

Drugs That Must Not Be Used While Breastfeeding

amphetamines	cyclosporine	methotrexate
antimetabolite drugs	heroin	Mysoline
(anticancer drugs)	lindane	Parlodel
cocaine	marijuana	PCP

---

feeding helpers dwindled. If problems arose, well, there was always someone eager to give the baby a bottle. Commitment runs high among today's breastfeeding mothers, and because more women are now breastfeeding in a variety of medical situations and lifestyles, a variety of ingenious aids and resources are now available to make breastfeeding easier and more enjoyable. (See "Breastfeeding," in Resources, page 745.)

What to Wear

Your breastfeeding wardrobe should include the following:

- bras for breastfeeding (at least three)
- breast pads
- clothes in which you can breastfeed discreetly
- a baby sling

Selecting the Right Bra

Special bras for nursing are designed with a flap on the cup that is opened for feedings. Here's how to choose and use the right bra:

- Before birth, purchase one or two bras that are one numerical size and one cup size larger than what you're wearing while pregnant, to allow for breast enlargement when your milk appears.

- When your milk is established and your breasts reach postengorgement size (usually around the second week), purchase three bras (one to wear, one in the laundry, one on standby).

- Be sure your bras fit comfortably enough in the cups to accommodate the change in breast size as your breasts fill before a feeding; tight-fitting bras encourage breast infections.

- Select a bra that fastens and unfastens easily with one hand, so that you don't have to put the baby down when you open or close the cup. Look for a style that opens via a self-closing slit along the inner edges of the cups. Avoid bras that have a row of hooks down the front, which give no support to either breast when open. Bras with a hook at the top of each cup offer more support and easier access, letting you uncover one breast at a time.

- When the flap is down, the cup of the bra should support the entire lower half of the breast in its natural position.

- Choose a 100 percent cotton bra cup. Avoid synthetic fabrics and plastic liners that are not absorbent and do not allow the skin to breathe.

- Avoid bras with underwires, since these wires may compress the breast, leading to plugged ducts.

Breast Pads

Disposable or washable cotton cloth pads can be worn inside the bra to absorb leaking milk. Here are a few tips for using these breast pads:

- Avoid synthetic fabrics and plastic-lined pads, which prevent air circulation, retain moisture, and encourage bacterial growth.

- Make your own breast pads by placing a folded all-cotton handkerchief in each cup of your bra, or cut out four-inch circles from cotton diapers.

- Change pads promptly after leaking, and if the pad sticks to your nipple, moisten with warm water before peeling it off. Leaking is usually a problem only in the early weeks of breastfeeding.

Breastfeeding Fashions

After the birth of our first baby I went clothes shopping with Martha. When I protested that she was taking too long, Martha explained, "For the first time in my life I have to consider the needs of another person." Then there was a first-time mother in my office in her one-piece dress, frantically trying to disrobe to comfort her screaming baby. Somewhere between a pile of clothing and a half-stripped mother nestled a breastfeeding baby. We both laughed, and the mother acknowledged, "Next time I'll dress for the occasion."

Consider the following when selecting a wardrobe for breastfeeding:

- Patterned fabric won't reveal milk that might leak through; avoid solid colors and clinging materials.

- For discreet feeding, a patterned, loose sweater-type top that can be lifted from the waist is best. Your baby will cover your bare midriff during breastfeeding.

- Blouses especially designed for breastfeeding women have slits hidden with pleats over the breasts.

- Front-buttoned blouses allow easy access; remember to unbutton the blouse from the bottom up, using the unbuttoned flap of the blouse to cover baby for modest feeding.

- To accent the limited designs available, drape an attractive shawl or scarf over your shoulder and use it to cover baby for discreet feeding.

- In cold climates, even a little bit of bare midriff can be a chilling experience. A letter in La Leche's bimonthly magazine *New Beginnings* has this solution for cold climates: Wear an old T-shirt with the top front cut away, tucked in at the waist under your loose top. The T-shirt completely covers mother from icy northern air when baby needs your nice warm breast.

- Off-the-rack one-piece dresses are impossible for convenient and discreet breastfeeding. Look for dresses designed especially for nursing mothers in maternity shops or look on-line by searching for "breastfeeding fashions."

- Two-piece outfits and warm-up suits are practical, as are pullover sweaters. The top should be loose and easily lifted from the waist.

- Don't try to squeeze into your pre-pregnancy clothes too soon. Tight tops rub against your nipples, are uncomfortable, and can trigger an untimely milk-ejection reflex.

A suggestion for new mothers sensitive about breastfeeding in public: Choose your breastfeeding wardrobe carefully and practice breastfeeding in front of the mirror. It's all a matter of tucking your baby's face inside your clothing rather than bringing your breasts out.

Use a Baby Sling

Breastfeeding mothers for centuries have fabricated sling-type carriers as an extension of their native dress, wearing their baby in this sling very near mother's breast. A baby sling is an indispensable item, making life easier and breastfeeding more enjoyable for mother and baby. The sling-type carrier is much more practical for the breastfeeding pair than either a front or hip carrier or a backpack. It allows baby to breastfeed discreetly in public and can be used in a variety of feeding positions. Don't leave home without it. We recommend the Original Babysling, an infant carrier that has been designed with the breastfeeding mother and infant in mind. (See Chapter 14, "Babywearing," to learn how to breastfeed in a sling. To obtain the Original Babysling, visit www.AskDrSears.com or www.nojo.com or call (800) 421–0526.)

Using creative apparel with the breastfeeding baby in mind, Martha has been able to carry on a busy life-style while breastfeeding our babies. Four times she has breastfed a baby on national television. The babies were calm, and she was calm. Because she was dressed for the occasion no one on the set or in the audience was astonished at having a breastfeeding pair on camera.

Alternatives to Supplemental Bottles

For breastfeeding an adopted baby (see page 190), a premature baby (see page 184), or in any circumstance in which the newborn is unable to get enough nutrition from mother alone, we advise using cups, breastfeeding supplementers, or syringes in lieu of supplemental bottles during the first few weeks when baby needs to learn to suck properly from mother's breast.

Cup Feeding. Cup feeding is a safe, low-tech method for supplementing a breastfed baby while avoiding the use of artificial nipples. Cup feeding has been used with newborns and even with premature infants. When a medical situation temporarily delays breast-feeding, or if baby must be supplemented during the first few days of life while learning to nurse effectively, cup feeding is an easy alternative to bottles. It may also work for the older baby who refuses bottles offered by dad or a substitute caregiver.

Use a small cup that holds just one or two ounces of human milk or formula. (Flexible plastic cups designed especially for feeding babies are available from lactation consultants and La Leche League International.) Fill the cup at least half full. Support baby upright on your lap, with a cloth diaper, towel, or bib under her chin to catch any drips. Swaddle her in a receiving blanket if her hands get in the way. Hold the cup to baby's lips and tilt it so that the liquid touches her lips. Allow baby to lap and swallow the milk. Don't pour it into her mouth. Let baby set the pace. Refill the cup as needed or fill two or three before you start the feeding. (For more on cup feeding, see page 234.)

Breastfeeding Supplementers

A supplementer consists of a plastic container to hold breast milk or formula, connected to a feeding tube to deliver it. The supplementer is suspended by a cord around mother's neck and rests between her breasts. Tiny flexible tubings extend from the supplementer and rest over mother's nipple. (Some supplementer systems, such as the Medela Supplemental Nutrition System, or SNS, have two tubings, one for each breast). While sucking at mother's breast baby draws the breast

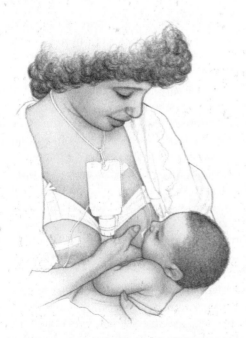

Use of a supplementer such as the Medela SNS (Supplemental Nutrition System) makes it possible to breastfeed in circumstances in which baby cannot get enough nutrition from mother alone.

milk or formula from the supplementer through the tubing. Any milk present in the breast also comes to baby through mother's nipple.

Supplementers have the advantage of teaching baby to suck only from mother's breast, so as not to confuse him by presenting a variety of artificial nipples. As an added benefit, mother gets hormonal stimulation as baby sucks at her breast. A supplementer should be obtained through a lactation consultant, who can supervise progress of the baby.

Martha notes: *In the early weeks of fumbling with plastic tubing I had a love-hate relationship with my supplementer. I needed it and Lauren needed it, but I still missed the naturalness of breastfeeding without gadgets. But after four weeks, life with the supplementer became easier, as I realized that this plastic breast was a tool that let me have, as closely as possible, a breastfeeding relationship with our adopted daughter.*

Syringes

Syringes are helpful to supplement a breastfeeding newborn. In our breastfeeding center we use a periodontal syringe, which has a long, curved tip from which supplemental milk (either breast milk or formula) is syringed into the baby's mouth during breastfeeding or during finger feeding if baby has trouble at the breast.

The *syringe-and-finger-feeding method* is especially helpful for fathers to supplement the primarily breastfed infant. Let baby suck on one and a half inches of your index finger (most fathers and women with large fingers use the pinkie finger) and slide the tip of the syringe inside the corner of baby's mouth alongside your finger, squirting in the

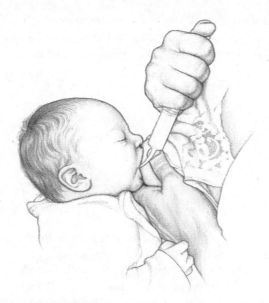

Syringe feeding.

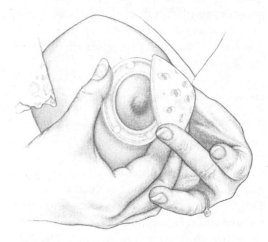

A breast shield, perforated to allow air circulation.

supplemental milk as your baby sucks. You can use a supplementer in similar fashion, placing the tubing along the tip of your finger, so that when baby sucks he also gets milk or formula from the tubing. Once again, supervision from a lactation consultant is strongly recommended.

Breast and Nipple Care

Here are some items you should know about in caring for your breasts, especially your nipples. (For nipple creams and moisturizers, see page 138.)

Breast Shields

Also called breast shells or milk cups, breast shields are two-part plastic cups that fit over mother's nipple and areola and are held in

place by her bra. The pressure of the shell on the breast encourages the nipple to protrude through a hole in the inner part of the cup. Meanwhile, the outer part of the cup protects the nipple from contact with the bra fabric.

Lactation experts used to recommend that mothers with flat or inverted nipples wear breast shells prenatally and postnatally between feedings to encourage the nipples to stand out. However, research on breast shells has not shown that they are helpful. Most specialists believe that a baby who knows how to latch on properly can shape any kind of nipple to deliver milk.

Breast shields can be used to protect sensitive sore nipples from rubbing against clothing. The pressure from the shields encourages leaking, so milk may collect in the shells between feedings. You should discard this milk, since germs can multiply rapidly in the warm environment inside your bra.

Nipple Shields

Rubber or silicone shields that fit over mother's nipple and the areola during feedings are sometimes recommended to protect sore or cracked nipples while they heal. It is wiser to prevent and correct improper positioning and latch-on than to rely on the use of nipple shields. Babies learn to latch on to the shield rather than the breast, and it can be very difficult to persuade them to take the breast without the shield. Breasts do not receive as much stimulation through a nipple shield, and this can compromise mother's milk supply. We do not recommend the use of nipple shields, except in situations where a baby cannot latch onto the breast in any other way — for example, a tiny preemie whose mother has large nipples, or for a few days if mother's cracked nipples are not healing with the standard treatment.

Footstools

A footstool makes life easier for the mother by lifting her lap to the correct and most comfortable height for breastfeeding. The nursing stool is especially designed for the breastfeeding mother and eliminates stress on a mother's back, legs, shoulders, and arms. (See illustration on page 146.)

Nursing Pillows

Pillows designed especially for the breastfeeding mother provide firm support for the baby in her lap and raise baby to breast height. They fit around mom's middle, and some also offer extra support for mom's lower back. Nursing pillows are especially handy for mothers who are juggling twins at the breast and for mothers of babies who need extra support because they are premature or have low muscle tone.

GETTING IT TOGETHER: WORKING AND BREASTFEEDING

Are working and breastfeeding compatible? Yes! It boils down to commitment — how serious you are about giving your baby the best nutritional start. I was a Harvard intern when our first baby, Jim, was born. We couldn't live on an intern's meager salary, so a few weeks after Jim's birth Martha returned to part-time work as a nurse. Driven by an intuitive desire to give Jim her milk, yet facing the financial realities of life, Martha found a way. Doctor and nurse would shuttle their precious baby between workplaces, home, and substitute caregivers. We juggled. We chose to. Some folks would say this wasn't ideal parenting, but at the time we could not achieve the ideal. We did the best we could under less-than-perfect circumstances. Here are some ideas for blending breastfeeding and working.

Basically, you have three challenges to consider: how to feed baby while mother is gone, how to keep up mother's milk supply when she's away from baby, and how to minimize the amount of time mother and baby spend away from each other. Many mothers choose to pump their breasts every two to four hours during the time that they are away from their babies. This helps to maintain their milk supply, and the expressed milk can be stored and later given to baby while mother is away at work. When mother and baby are together — nights, weekends,

BENEFITS OF CONTINUING TO BREASTFEED WHILE WORKING

Once you realize the benefits of extended breastfeeding for baby, mother, and family, you will find a way to do it.

- **Mothers miss fewer workdays.** Because breastfed babies are healthier, mother (or father) will need to stay home less often with a sick baby.
- **Breastfeeding saves money.** Even considering the cost of a high-grade breast pump, breastfeeding is cheaper than buying formula. Also, because breastfed babies are healthier, you will need to spend less on medical care.
- **Breastfeeding helps you feel connected.** Pumping and storing your milk helps you feel connected to your baby even while you are apart. This is a special relationship that no other caregiver will have with your baby.
- **It's the modern thing to do.** Years ago breastfeeding while working was considered unusual. Now most mothers do it, and workplaces are becoming more breastfeeding friendly.

(For more information on expressing milk, and on getting a breastfed baby to take a bottle, see below.)

We have seen mothers come up with the most creative plans for minimizing their time away from their babies while working. They find ways to enjoy longer maternity leaves, work from home, commute with their babies, or even bring baby to work. Here are some possibilities to keep in mind as you plan your working and breastfeeding lifestyle.

Plan Ahead — But Not Too Much

Over the past ten years I have become increasingly concerned about new mothers dwelling on "the day I have to go back to work." They are so concerned with all of the what-ifs: "What if he won't take a bottle?" "What if he won't settle for the babysitter?" "Should I get him used to the bottle and start leaving him right away so he won't get spoiled?" Mothers confide that their preoccupation with leaving baby dilutes their attachment to their newborn. This subconscious detachment does not seem right, to me or to my patients. Mothers should have the joy of being absorbed into mothering, at least for a few weeks! Focus on your baby for the first few weeks; it will do both of you good. (For a fuller description of this principle, see "Shortening the Distance," page 417.)

Work and Wear

Mothers the world over blend their mothering and working, and we are attempting to popularize this wonderful custom in the Western world. If you have the kind of job that allows you to take your baby with you,

holidays — mother encourages baby to nurse often, so that they can continue to enjoy their breastfeeding relationship. As baby gets older and starts to eat a variety of foods, mother may pump less at work but continues to breastfeed her baby when they are together.

get a sling-type carrier and wear your baby to work. Many mothers in our practice do this. (See pages 298 and 417 for tips on working and wearing.)

Your Schedule, Baby's Schedule

Enjoy a happy departure and a happy reunion. Breastfeed your baby at the caregiver's before leaving for work and as soon as you return. Instruct your caregiver not to feed your baby within an hour before you leave work. An eager baby and a full mother make for a happy reunion. It depends on your work hours, but you can usually get in an early morning feeding at home, one at the caregiver's, a late-afternoon feeding after work, a couple of evening feedings, and a before-bed feeding. An alternative if you live close to your workplace is for your caregiver to bring baby to you for a feeding once or twice during the day or for you to return to the baby during your lunch break. With work-based day care, some mothers are able to totally breastfeed their baby during lunch and coffee breaks. Return to full-time breastfeeding on weekends, holidays, and days off, as periodic full breastfeeding days are necessary to keep up your milk production. Your breasts will be fuller than usual on Monday if you have been full-time breastfeeding over the weekend.

Expect baby to wake up and want to breastfeed more often at night after you return to work. Experienced mothers who have successfully managed breastfeeding while working accept this nighttime attachment as a natural part of working and mothering. They simply take their baby to bed and enjoy nighttime breastfeeding. Fairly quickly, mother and baby learn to sleep while breast-feeding. Nestling together and breastfeeding at night give baby and mother the touch time they both miss during the day and help compensate for the time apart. Many mothers who have achieved nighttime harmony with their baby report they sleep better, possibly due to the relaxing effects of breastfeeding helping mothers unwind from a busy day. As an added family benefit, this nighttime arrangement gives daytime working *fathers* extra touch time with baby, too. (For additional information, see Chapter 17, "Working and Parenting.")

Store Up a Milk Supply

Some babies either refuse to take formula or are allergic to all the commercial formulas and only thrive on your breast milk. To avoid being caught empty-handed, you will need to express and stockpile a supply of your milk before returning to work. (See the section "Expressing Milk," below.)

Introducing the Bottle

Present the bottle around two weeks before going back to work. After baby has had his first bottle, he doesn't need one every day. Two bottles a week should be enough practice to prevent a cold turkey experience for baby. Encourage dad or your substitute caregiver to offer your baby the bottle. Baby may be more willing to experiment if he is not desperately hungry — try when he is happy and alert. It is usual for babies to be rather selective in their eating behavior and refuse to accept a bottle from mother. This is not in their nutritional mind-set. The box on page 169 offers additional details on bottlefeeding.

EXPRESSING MILK

At some time in your breastfeeding career you will almost certainly encounter medical or life-style circumstances for which you need to express milk. Whether by hand, by pump, or a combination of both, the methods of expressing milk are a matter of personal choice. Experiment with the following techniques, modifying them in ways that work for you.

How to Hand Express Your Milk

The advantages of using a manual technique rather than a mechanical pump include the following:

- Some mothers find pumps uncomfortable or ineffective.
- Mothers often feel put off by the gadgetry and prefer the natural approach.
- Skin-to-skin stimulation can actually produce the milk-ejection reflex better.
- Your hands are "handy" — convenient, portable, always available, and free!

Martha notes: The techniques for manual expression of breast milk can be very individual. I learned how to do it in 1975 when our third baby was born. When he was one month old I was back at work several afternoons a week, and I wanted to leave breast milk for him. I found that I could express between six and eight ounces [180–240 milliliters] of milk in about twenty minutes during a midafternoon break. I learned to do this first at home, so my trial-and-error practice was more relaxed. A week or two before going back to work, I started to build up a supply by expressing just an ounce or two in the morning when my breasts were the fullest. So I had several four-ounce bottles in the freezer — a little stockpile to give me some leeway in learning how the routine would work away from home.

Here's how I did it at work. I locked the washroom door to ensure privacy, washed my hands, then got relaxed and comfortable. A big drink of water helped me "prime the pump," so to speak, and I thought of my little Peter as he was at my breast just a few hours earlier, feeding just before I left him. Before I actually began to express milk, I massaged my breasts (both at once), which helped to relax me even more and sometimes even activated the MER (milk-ejection reflex) so that the milk began dripping. I had a clean plastic bottle as my only tool, and I simply directed my nipple into the opening. This was rather awkward, but it worked fine after I got the hang of it.

I started with the fullest, drippiest breast and learned how to press with my forearm against the other nipple to stop the leaking (no sense wasting any of this liquid gold!). Holding the collecting bottle with one hand, I held my breast with the other. I started with the hand on the same side as that breast and then switched hands later on to get different angles so as to empty all the sinuses around the "clock" (that is, the thumb and fingers at twelve and six o'clock and then at ten and four, then switched to the other hand for two and eight). As the MER activated, the milk would often spray out on its own. When the spraying stopped, I went back to the firm rhythmic movements and continued until the flow of milk was just dribbling. Then I changed to another position with that hand and released more milk, then proceeded to

BOTTLEFEEDING THE BREASTFED BABY

When part-time breastfeeding is necessary or desired, expect the mostly breastfed baby to be less than enthusiastic about the new container and its contents. Try these suggestions on your little connoisseur. (Additional bottlefeeding suggestions are on page 213. See also "Combo Feeding: Breast and Bottle," page 211.)

- If baby is a confirmed breastfeeder, enlist an experienced bottlefeeder such as grandmother or another bottlefeeding mother. A breastfeeding mother normally feels a bit awkward in offering her baby a bottle, and the baby may smell his mother's milk and sense her ambivalence. After baby has learned to accept the bottle from an experienced feeder, father is next in line to bottlefeed his baby.

- Don't confuse your little gourmet. Some babies accept a bottle while being held in the breastfeeding position; others reject the bottle if given in the situation or position that reminds them of breastfeeding. If baby is baffled by the cradle hold, expecting the bosom to mean more than a cushion, try holding baby at a less suggestive angle, sitting in places different from the ones used during breastfeeding, or putting baby in a sling carrier and walking around while offering the bottle.

- Use nipples that resemble the real thing. Choose a nipple that has a wide, areolalike reservoir beyond the tip. Avoid nipples that offer only a nubbin to latch on to. The slow-flow nipple that baby really has to suck on is less likely to be rejected than the quick-gush type that overwhelms the eager feeder, causing choking. (See nipple suggestions, page 210.)

- Encourage baby to latch on to the artificial nipple using the same techniques employed with his favorite nipples: mouth wide open, lips everted, and gum pressure at least an inch beyond the tip of the nipple. (See the illustration on page 130.) If baby learns lazy latch-on habits on the rubber sub, making daily transitions to your nipples may be a confusing and painful experience.

- To further entice the discerning feeder, warm the bottle nipple in warm water, making it more supple, like the breast. Try changing the temperature of the nipple for the changing needs of the baby. A chilled nipple may be more inviting to a baby who is teething.

- Instruct the caregiver to interact with your baby during bottlefeeding much the way you do when breastfeeding. Advise the caregiver to undress baby and wear a short-sleeved blouse to promote skin-to-skin contact. Maintaining eye contact during the feeding is important; feeding is not only giving milk but enjoying social interaction.

- Show your caregiver how to let baby suck on her finger between feedings. This helps satisfy baby's sucking needs and will warm baby up to a substitute caregiver.

- Avoid bottle propping. It is unsafe to leave baby unattended in a crib or infant seat to take his own bottle.

Manually Expressing Breast Milk: The Marmet Technique

HOW THE BREAST WORKS

The milk is produced in milk producing cells (alveoli). A portion of the milk continuously comes down the ducts and collects in the milk reservoirs. When the milk-producing cells are stimulated, they expel additional milk into the duct system (milk ejection reflex).

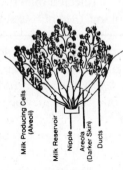

Milk Producing Cells (Alveoli)

Milk Reservoir

Nipple

Areola (Darker Skin)

Ducts

EXPRESSING THE MILK

Draining the Milk Reservoirs

1. **POSITION** the thumb and first two fingers about 1" to 1½" behind the nipple.
   - Use this measurement, which is not necessarily the outer edge of the areola, as a guide. The areola varies in size from one woman to another.
   - Place the thumb pad above the nipple and the finger pads below the nipple forming the letter "C" with the hand, as shown.
   - Note that the fingers are positioned so that the milk reservoirs lie beneath them.
   - Avoid cupping the breast.

2. **PUSH** straight into the chest wall.
   - Avoid spreading the fingers apart.
   - For large breasts, first lift and then push into the chest wall.

3. **ROLL** thumb and fingers forward as if making thumb and fingerprints at the same time.
   - The rolling motion of the thumb and fingers compresses and empties the milk reservoirs without hurting sensitive breast tissue.
   - Note the moving position of the thumbnail and fingernails in the illustration.

4. **REPEAT RHYTHMICALLY** to drain the reservoirs.
   - Position, push, roll; position, push, roll . . .

5. **ROTATE** the thumb and finger position to milk the other reservoirs. Use both hands on each breast. These pictures show hand positions on the right breast.

Push into Chest Wall

Roll

Finish Roll

Right Hand   Left Hand

AVOID THESE MOTIONS

Avoid squeezing the breast. This can cause bruising.

Avoid pulling out the nipple and breast. This can cause tissue damage.

Avoid sliding on the breast. This can cause skin burns.

Squeeze

Pull

Slide

ASSISTING THE MILK EJECTION REFLEX

Stimulating The Flow Of Milk

1. **MASSAGE** the milk producing cells and ducts.
   - Start at the top of the breast. Press firmly into the chest wall. Move fingers in a circular motion on one spot on the skin.
   - After a few seconds move the fingers to the next area on the breast.
   - Spiral around the breast toward the areola using this massage.
   - The motion is similar to that used in a breast examination.

MASSAGE

2. **STROKE** the breast area from the top of the breast to the nipple with a light tickle-like stroke.
   - Continue this stroking motion from the chest wall to the nipple around the whole breast.
   - This will help with relaxation and will help stimulate the milk ejection reflex.

STROKE

3. **SHAKE** the breast while leaning forward so that gravity will help the milk eject.

SHAKE

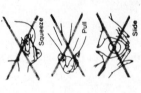

change hands and went to yet another hand position on the areola "clock." The Marmet technique (see page 170) of manual expression is the one I use now with my babies and teach as a lactation consultant.

Choosing and Using a Breast Pump

Breast pumps are convenient and often necessary for expressing milk to relieve engorgement, to preserve a mother's milk supply when baby cannot nurse, and to collect milk when mother and baby are separated because of the mother's employment. Here are some general considerations for choosing the right breast pump for you, as well as some ideas for more efficient and comfortable pumping:

- Unless you must frequently pump in an area that does not have an electrical outlet, consider a high-quality electric pump. These are best at mimicking a baby's natural sucking pattern. You can pump both breasts at once, which saves time. Some electric pumps can also be used as manual pumps.

- If you are pumping to keep up your milk supply because your baby is premature or ill and is not nursing, use a hospital-grade electric pump. These are the most effective pumps and the most convenient to use, which really makes a difference if you are pumping six to ten times a day. Studies have shown that pumping both breasts at the same time with a hospital-grade electric pump produces higher prolactin levels than pumping with a manual or battery-operated pump. Maintaining your milk supply for the day when your baby can

breastfeed is an important job. It takes good tools to do it well.

- Cost varies widely. Hand pumps are the least expensive, and hospital-grade electric pumps (usually rented) are the most expensive. Some insurance companies reimburse the cost of renting an electric pump, provided you submit a doctor's prescription (with *baby's* name on it, not yours).

- If your nipples become sore during pumping, massage an emollient, such as Lansinoh, on your nipples prior to pumping.

- Before pumping, look at a picture and think motherly thoughts of your baby. In some mothers, just *anticipating* breastfeeding or pumping may stimulate the milk-producing hormones to flow.

- There are many breast pumps for different occasions and life-styles. The list of breast pumps on pages 174–175 is a useful guide, but because breast-pump technology is rapidly improving to meet the varying demands of today's mothers, we recommend contacting your lactation consultant for the most up-to-date information on selecting the right breast pump and accessories for you.

What It's Like When You Begin Collecting Milk at Work

When you begin pumping your milk, don't be discouraged if you initially obtain only a small amount. With practice most mothers are able to pump at least several ounces within ten to fifteen minutes. It is normal for you to experience high-production and low-production

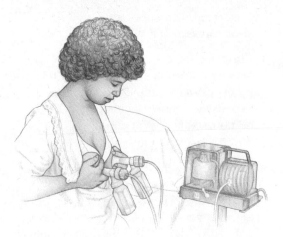

Large electric breast pump with double-pumping system.

days. Don't expect your relationship with the mechanical pump to be love at first sight. It will take time to warm up to the metal and plastic when you'd rather be holding your soft baby. While pumping your milk, think baby and look at a picture of your baby. This stimulates your milk-producing hormones and activates your milk-ejection reflex, which gets your milk flowing. Pump as much milk as you can at least every three hours and store it in a refrigerator or use a portable cooler (see page 176). If you are unable to take time off during your regular schedule to pump your milk, collect your milk during coffee breaks, lunch breaks, or more frequent bathroom breaks. Choosing an electric pump that uses a double (both breasts at once) pumping system should cut your pumping time in half.

At first your breasts may leak milk, perhaps when you think about your baby or during usual feeding times. To deal with this tug from your hormones, nonchalantly fold your arms across your chest, applying pressure directly to your nipples for a minute or two.

Also during the first week after going from full-time to part-time breastfeeding, expect your breasts to fill up periodically at feeding times as a reminder to pump. After the first two weeks your body will naturally make biological adjustments to adapt to this change in routine.

▶ *NEWS FLASH! A 2002 law in the state of California requires employers to provide a private location (not the bathroom!) for mothers to express their milk. Score state points for preventive medicine.*

Storing and Transporting This Liquid Gold

Stockpiling a supply of nature's most valuable nutrient is an investment in the future nutrition and health of your baby, especially as a reserve when you return to work, during a major illness, or in any other situation that may temporarily separate mother and baby. Here's how to take care of this valuable product.

Storing Expressed Milk

Reusable items involved in the collection and storage of breast milk need to be cleaned and sterilized. Rinse all milk containers, bottles, and accessories with cool water, then wash them well with soap and hot water. A dishwasher with a water temperature of at least 180°F/82°C adequately sterilizes these items. (For an alternative approach, follow the directions given on page 212. Follow manufacturer's directions for sterilizing breast-pump parts.)

To safely store the milk, follow these suggestions:

- Wash your hands well before collecting your milk.

- Use hard plastic or glass containers.

- If you find disposable plastic storage bags the easiest to store and transport, be sure to double bag in case the outside bag tears.

- Use four- to six-ounce containers, a few of them filled with only two ounces (one ounce equals approximately thirty milliliters). This makes thawing easier and wastes less.

- Freezer bags sold through the La Leche League catalog are especially designed for freezing and storing breast milk (self-sealing and presterilized).

- Leave space in the container at the top of the milk, allowing for expansion as it freezes.

- Date each serving, placing the oldest in front, and note anything that you've recently ingested that is not routine — for example, any unusual food, medication, even aspirin.

- You can add to milk that is already frozen, but be sure to *chill* the new milk first in the refrigerator, as adding warm milk can defrost the top layer of the frozen milk.

- Breast milk may be safely kept unrefrigerated in a *clean container* for six to ten hours. However, we advise refrigerating milk as soon as possible after it is expressed.

- Breast milk may be stored in a refrigerator for up to *eight days* before use, after which it should be frozen. Fresh breast milk is better for baby than frozen, so if

> ## A VALUABLE BREASTFEEDING AND WORKING WEBSITE
>
> For more information on pumps, products, and practical tips on breastfeeding and working, see www. breastfeedingandworking.net.

you know you will be using it within a few days, store it in the refrigerator.

- Milk can be stored in:
  - the freezer section of a one-door refrigerator for two weeks
  - the freezer of a two-door refrigerator/freezer for three to four months
  - a deep freeze at constant 0°F (–18°C) for six months or longer

Using Stored Milk

Freshly expressed breast milk may be given to baby within several hours without any special storage. Milk that has been stored, however, requires special care.

- To defrost milk, place the container of frozen milk upright in a bowl of warm water.

- As you warm the milk, turn the container around and around to mix the separated cream and milk, and swirl the bottle of milk again before feeding. Don't heat beyond body temperature, as heat destroys enzymes and immune properties.

- If you do not use all of the milk in the container, you can refrigerate the remaining milk and use it again within the same day. Don't refreeze thawed milk.

A USER'S GUIDE TO BREAST PUMPS

Type of Pump	How It Works	Useful When . . .
Bulb-type hand pump (also called "bicycle-horn" pump)	Squeezing the bulb causes suction, drawing milk into the pump.	
Hand pump	Various mechanical means are used to create suction.	. . . mother wants to pump milk for occasional separations from her baby and pumps no more than once a day.
Low-cost electric or battery-operated pump Medela MiniElectric Medela DoubleEase	A small motor creates suction. Used with batteries or an electrical outlet.	. . . mother wants to pump milk for occasional separations from her baby and wants the convenience of an electric pump.
Portable electric pump Ameda Purely Yours Medela Pump In Style Medela Lactina Select Ameda Nurture III Whittlestone Breast Expresser	A motor creates a suction/release cycle. Some can be used with batteries as well as with an electrical outlet.	. . . mother is pumping during daily separations from her baby or to maintain a milk supply when baby cannot nurse at the breast.
Full-size automatic piston pump (hospital-grade pump) Medela Classic Ameda Elite	A high-quality motor creates suction/release cycles for efficient pumping.	. . . mother is pumping during daily separations from her baby or to maintain a milk supply when baby cannot nurse at the breast.

PRACTICAL POINTERS FOR PUMPING

- Buy or rent your pump from a lactation consultant who can instruct you in how to use it and can answer your questions about pumping. If you're not sure about how to assemble and use the pump, or if you are not able to pump much milk, talk to your lactation consultant. There may be a problem with the pump that is easily solved, or you may need to use a better pump.
- Don't select a pump based on cost alone. Good pumps are expensive, but if you are pumping several times a day at work or pumping at home to maintain a milk supply for a baby in the hospital, the ease and convenience of a better-quality pump are well worth the money. Renting a pump is cheaper than buying formula.
- Pump parts do wear out. If you are not able to pump as much milk as you once did, the problem may be the pump, not you. Talk to your lactation consultant or contact the pump manufacturer. Note that all but the hospital-grade pumps are made to be single-user products. A used pump may not work as well as a new one.
- Follow a set routine. As often as possible, pump in the same place, in the same chair, with the same "get ready, relax, and pump" routine. This conditions your milk-ejection reflex and you'll be able to pump more milk.
- Use breast massage before and during pumping to help you relax and bring more milk down to the nipple. (See "Assisting the Milk Ejection Reflex," page 170.)
- Take some slow, deep breaths and let go of the day's worries. Visualize flowing water, fountains of milk — whatever helps to get your milk moving down into the pump. Picture yourself nursing your baby in a quiet, comfortable place.
- Use a portable stereo with headphones to enjoy your favorite music or background sounds from nature.
- Pumping should not make your nipples sore. Be careful that the nipple doesn't rub against the side of the breast shield when the pump is operating. Adjust the suction level if your nipples are hurting.
- Pumping calls for clothing that makes it easy to get at your breasts. Dresses and blouses designed for discreet breastfeeding also make pumping more convenient. Some of the companies that make and market nursing fashions specialize in sophisticated clothes for breastfeeding working moms.
- Network with other breastfeeding mothers at your workplace. Perhaps you can pump at the same time and enjoy each other's company. If you are the only breastfeeding mother at your workplace, you may have to educate co-workers about breastfeeding and why you are pumping. Be patient and tolerant of others' opinions, while remaining confident that you are doing what's best for your baby and yourself.

through a growth spurt, which occurs typically around three weeks, six weeks, three months, and six months, with smaller spurts in between. Your baby is obeying the law of supply and demand: The more he sucks, the more milk you produce, and the better he grows. Also, your baby may be going through a high-need period in which he needs a day or two of frequent feeding and holding as he becomes adjusted to life outside the womb. Here are some survival tips:

• During high-need days, temporarily shelve all outside commitments that may drain your energy. Your baby is a baby only a very short time, and no one's life is going to be affected if the housework doesn't get done on time. In our experience, mothers become burned out, not so much because of the demands of their baby, but because of too many other family expectations and commitments and because they are not being nurtured themselves.

• Be sure your baby is getting mostly milk at each feeding and not a lot of air, otherwise as soon as she burps up the air she will be hungry again. Burp her well as you pass from one breast to the other and after feeding. (See burping suggestions, page 213.)

• Attempt to get more of your hindmilk into your baby to satisfy her longer. Allow baby to finish the first breast before switching her to the other side. Try double feeding and other techniques discussed earlier for improving your milk supply.

• Wear your baby in a baby sling. Babywearing not only makes breastfeeding easier and more accessible, but it may be that your high-need baby wants the comfort of your closeness and not always the breastfeeding.

• Periodically offer your baby your finger as a pacifier. This satisfies her need to suck when she is not hungry. Call in the reserves, letting your husband or a trusted caregiver comfort your baby.

• Avoid the filler-food fallacy. You may be advised to give your baby a supplemental bottle or cereal with the implication that you don't have enough milk. This is rarely necessary; but if your baby is truly hungry, it may be necessary in order to satisfy baby *if all the other measures are not working.* Most of the time your baby is simply signaling that she needs to suck more in order for you to increase your level of milk to meet her level of need. If your doctor is advising a supplement, you need to be aware that this could lead to a gradual cessation of breastfeeding as you and baby come to depend more and more on the bottles. Supplementation can be done in such a way that it does not have to jeopardize your breastfeeding relationship. This would be an important time to obtain the services of a lactation consultant. She can help you get your baby's weight gain back on track and maximize your milk supply.

• Sleep when your baby sleeps and don't be tempted to "finally get something done." You need to recharge your own system to cope with these high-need periods. Nap nursing and night nursing are very effective for a persistently hungry baby and tired mother.

Mr. Suck-a-Little, Look-a-Little

Sometime between two and six months of age, expect your baby to suck a minute, pull away, suck another minute, and pull away again. The development of your baby's visual acuity accounts for this common breastfeeding nuisance. By this age baby is able to see things clearly across the room, notice passersby, and is so distracted by all the goings-on in his interesting environment that he stops eating to look. Sometimes baby will be so into his meal, yet interested in someone who walks by, that he may suddenly turn his head and seem to take a bit of your breast with him. You'll laugh only once at this antic. Your nipple can stretch just so far.

Experienced mothers have handled this with the strategy of sheltered feedings. Several times a day take your baby into a dark, quiet, uninteresting room (such as the bedroom with drapes drawn) and get him down to the business of eating. Lie down in a quiet dark room and nap nurse, drawing baby's attention to you as his close nap partner. Covering baby with a shawl or placing him in a sling during feeding also shelters Mr. Suck-a-Little, Look-a-Little. This is a passing nuisance that creative feeding techniques and a bit of humor will solve. Your baby will soon discover that he can eat and look at the same time.

The Nipper-Napper

While many babies feed at least twenty minutes every three hours, the nipper-napper likes to eat and sleep continually. He sucks a few minutes, sleeps awhile, sucks again for a few minutes, and then drifts back into sleep. This temporary nuisance occurs in the early weeks when some babies prefer sleeping to eating — and prefer small packages of each. If your baby is gaining enough weight and you have the time to luxuriate, put your feet up, turn on soothing music, and enjoy these prolonged feedings. This stage soon passes. If your sleepy baby is not gaining enough weight, try switch feeding (see page 142) to keep her alert long enough to fill her tummy at the breast.

The Gourmet

This baby prolongs the meals as if savoring every drop and touch of breastfeeding. He relishes not only the taste of the milk, but the whole ambience of a gourmet meal at a fine restaurant. Enjoying every minute of this fine cuisine, baby licks, sucks, fondles, nestles, and goes to great lengths to draw out the feeding time. As another ploy to stall the end of the meal, he will turn away as if finally finished, only to smack his lips, stretch a bit, and reposition himself for another course. If you have the time and baby has the desire, cherish every lingering meal, as breastfeeding is a phase of life with your baby that passes all too quickly.

The Yanker

This close relative of Mr. Suck-a-Little, Look-a-Little frequently pulls his head away while feeding, but occasionally forgets to let go. Ouch! To save your nipples, use the clutch hold (see page 297) to secure the back of baby's neck in your hand. Feed baby in the cradle hold in the sling (see page 297) to steady his head. Finally, be ready to insert your index finger into baby's mouth to break the suction just as baby begins to pull away.

The Chomper

A baby with this nursing nuisance is often dubbed "Jaws." You are comfortably into a feeding, beginning to nod off into the sea of tranquillity, when suddenly Chomps clamps down, and your tender nipples become a human teething ring. This uncomfortable nuisance occurs when baby is around five to six months old as he begins to experience pre-teething gum pain. If baby gets an attack of sore gums while feeding, he may regard your breasts as a source of teething comfort as well as milk. Letting your baby gum your finger or a frozen teething ring before and after feeding will usually pacify Chomps. Also, as you feel the gums gripping, put your finger between gums and nipple or use your index finger to depress baby's lower jaw — a reminder to respect the breast that feeds him. (If he evolves into the biter, see page 147.)

The Intruder

You have been feeding your infant all day long, chasing a busy toddler around the house, and carpooling children. By the end of the evening you have had it with kids, and you and your husband are comfortably nestled together in bed. The lights are out, lovemaking begins. Suddenly from outer space comes the familiar cry for milk. Your pulse goes up, your milk lets down. Your husband feels foiled again. A breastfeeding mother's radar system is so finely tuned, that baby's "need noises" traverse thick walls and closed doors. These intrusions will soon pass. Their *is* sex after birth, and certainly after baby has been resettled. All good things are worth waiting for.

The Twiddler

Between six and nine months babies love to use their top hand to pinch your breast, which can be annoying, or play with your face, which can be amusing. One antic you want to discourage immediately is the twid-

dling of your other nipple. It often starts with just touching or holding, as though baby wants to be sure it will be there when needed. It may seem very sweet, but the escalated version we call twiddling can be very irritating.

The Gymnast

Just as you and your baby are quietly nestled into a comfortable position, baby starts kicking his upper leg, as though keeping time with his sucking rhythm. Babies try all sorts of contortions while feeding, even flipping around nearly 180 degrees without letting go. Here's how to corral the gymnast: Contain both the young and the older baby in a baby sling to prevent him from flinging his head back to explore his environment and taking your breast with him. Try the "toddler tuck," wedging your baby's legs between your arm and body while baby is in the cradle hold. Also, babies don't like the feeling of dangling or falling while feeding; hooking his top leg over your arm gives him a feeling of security. Containing your baby during breastfeeding is baby's first lesson in mealtime manners. As motor skills mushroom, babies like to try out their body during situations in which they seem most relaxed, like during feeding. They may even *try* a somersault without missing a suck.

The Snacker

The snacker likes to eat on the run. When your toddler becomes too busy to enjoy prolonged gourmet meals, expect two-minute feedings several times a day. Toddlers often go through periods during which they want to suck as often as they did as a tiny baby. Your toddler gets into these fast-food habits due to the need for frequent pick-me-ups, a sort of pit stop for emotional refueling as the busy baby races around the house exploring new adventures, but routinely needs to return to a familiar home base.

The Pouncer

A cousin to the snacker, the pouncer is a frequent nuisance to mothers of breastfeeding toddlers. You are sitting on the couch treating yourself to a well-deserved rest, and you open your favorite book. Suddenly your toddler descends and pounces; he's maneuvering across your lap and under your blouse like it's old home week. Picture this scene from his point of view. You are sitting in his favorite place to feed, which triggers in baby's mind a replay of his favorite memories nestled comfortably in mother's arms at this very same place — sort of déjà vu. Here's how one mother, wishing to wean, tamed her pouncer. "As soon as he made advances I became a moving target, remembering not to sit in places that reminded him of feeding."

Other Breastfeeding Behaviors

Over time, your baby is likely to exhibit several of the "personality traits" described above. Similarly, don't be surprised if you encounter one or more of the following behavior patterns at one time or another during the course of breastfeeding.

Breastfeeding Strike

Some babies abruptly refuse to breastfeed for several days, then with coaxing resume their previous breastfeeding routine. Humorously called a breastfeeding strike, this behavior is usually caused by physical upsets, such as teething, illness, or hospitalization, and emotional upsets, such as a recent move, illness in the mother, family discord, or the busy-nest syndrome (too many visitors, too many outside responsibilities, holiday stress, and so on). Our first baby, Jim, refused to breastfeed after a trip to the emergency room for stitches following a fall at eight months of age. Being young parents, we interpreted this as his time to wean. After all, he was eight months old, taking solids, and drinking well from a cup, and in those days nearly all babies were weaned by eight months. We made no attempts to encourage him back to the breast. Now we know that Jim was on a breastfeeding strike.

Here's how to negotiate with a striker. First, spot this as a temporary loss of interest and not a sign that your baby is ready to wean. Rarely do babies under nine months of age want to wean from the breast. Try to pinpoint the possible physical or emotional upset that triggered the strike. Then woo your striking baby back to your breast. Pretend you are just beginning to breastfeed your baby as a newborn. Get reacquainted. Temporarily shelve all obligations that take you away from baby. Explain the breastfeeding strike to your husband and other family members, telling them why you need to focus intently on your baby over the next few days. Take the phone off the hook, relax at a comfortable feeding station (see page 145 for how to prepare one), soak in a tub together, and turn on soothing music and just hold your baby skin to skin most of the day. Wear your infant in a carrier as much as possible to keep baby close to your breast. Nap nursing and night nursing are proven ways to woo baby back to the breast; babies who resist the breast when awake often suck when falling asleep, or even in their sleep. Snuggle up with your baby at night. Sometimes re-creating the ambience of breastfeeding reminds baby of what he is missing. If baby continues to withdraw from the breast, don't force-feed. Let your baby fall asleep, skin to skin, with his head nesting on your breast. Remember, "nursing" means comforting, not just feeding. Sometimes babies need to go through a few days of holding or comfort feeding before they resume breastfeeding.

A breastfeeding strike may be a message that baby wants to renegotiate the mother-infant contract. Try to relive the feeding environment that you and baby enjoyed before the strike: your baby's favorite feeding position, rocking chair, location in the house, or cuddle position in bed. With creative mother-infant attachment, most strikes are over within a few days. But we have known babies who refused to breastfeed for nearly a week and then gradually resumed. These mothers persevered, made themselves super-available, pumped to maintain milk supply, offered this milk to baby in a cup, and followed their intuition that baby was not ready to wean. In this case, support from a mother who has gone through this helps — call La Leche League. If after all these negotiations baby does not resume breastfeeding, be reassured that this truly is baby's idea, and your infant is, in fact, ready to move on to the next level — weaning. There is no room for regrets; appreciate that your baby is ripe ahead of schedule.

Band-Aid Breastfeeding

To a baby, breastfeeding is a source of nourishment and comfort. Expect your toddler, even after you thought he had weaned, to run to you and climb into your arms to be nursed following a fall, a scrape, or a cut. So vivid in your baby's mind is the memory of breastfeeding that he automatically clicks in to the mind-set of breastfeeding as a quick fix to repair the leaks in his "fragile" body.

The One-Sided Baby

If baby prefers one breast over the other, or will feed only on her favorite, don't worry. Some babies quickly learn which breast works better and stay with the easier side. And babies usually grow well from the nourishment of only one breast. Twins do. You may feel a bit lopsided for a few months, but your body is never going to be the same after birth anyway.

Rather Fight Than Switch

Finally, to make life even more challenging for the breastfeeding family, there is the baby who refuses to take a bottle. You worry if you return to work, you worry when you go out. Yet the little food critic waits for his favorite meal and waitress to return, and rejects schemes to sell second-class service. Some babies also refuse to take a bottle (even with breast milk in it) from the breastfeeding mother. It's like walking into your favorite restaurant, sitting at your favorite table, hearing familiar music, being served by the waitress of your choice, and being presented the wrong menu. For babies who are hooked on breastfeeding, any alternative cuisine may not be in their program. You can feel flattered that your baby is so discerning!

We frequently tackled this problem on our live call-in radio program, "Ask About Your Baby." One day a father called and offered his advice on substitute bottlefeeding. "I'm a policeman, and I enjoy our baby while my wife's at work. I take my shirt off and let her nuzzle against my fuzzy chest. Then I hold the bottle under my arm like I am used to holding my flashlight while I walk the beat. I hold the baby very much like my wife does at the breast while baby drinks from the bottle between my upper arm and chest. We both seem to get a kick out of this innovation." Chalk up one for father's intuition.

If you've already tried the suggestions for bottlefeeding the breastfed baby given on page 169 and baby still refuses to accept a bottle, relax; there are other strategies in your feeding repertoire. Try cup feeding your baby using a small, flexible plastic cup. (See page 234 for instructions.) If baby likes sipping milk, try a trainer cup with a drinking rim on the top instead of a nipple. Avoid cups with spouts.

Fortunately, all of these nursing nuisances have one thing in common — they soon pass. Then comes more growth and development, and you are blessed with a new set of challenges. But babies are like that.

BREASTFEEDING SPECIAL BABIES IN SPECIAL CIRCUMSTANCES

Breastfeeding is even more important for babies with special needs and their parents. Breastfeeding gives you a higher level of maternal hormones, which increase your intuition and perseverance to meet the needs of your special baby. Because of its physical, psychological, and medical benefits, breast-feeding is even more important for these babies. Over our many years in medical practice we have witnessed a phenomenon for which we have coined the term "need-level concept." A baby has special needs. Parents develop a style of caring for their baby and in so doing elevate their level of intuition and sensitivity toward their baby to match the level of baby's needs. Let's discuss the most common situations in which babies with

SEXUAL FEELINGS WHILE BREASTFEEDING

The same hormones that make milk and make women feel motherly (prolactin and oxytocin) are also a normal part of female sexuality. They promote feelings of relaxation and pleasure and help mother bond to her baby. Breastfeeding is supposed to be pleasurable. The human race would not have survived if breastfeeding were not enjoyable.

Some women become alarmed at the intensity of the feelings that are generated when a baby sucks at the breast. Especially once the baby is older, women worry whether these feelings are normal. They are! La Leche League International advises: "Women do experience physical sensations during breastfeeding. Depending on the time and context, these feelings will be interpreted differently — as physical arousal, as an overall sense of well-being, or as warm and loving feelings towards the child. All are a natural part of a woman's experiences and her relationship with her child."

special needs in unique situations bring out a special kind of parenting.

The Cesarean-Birthed Baby

Following a surgical birth a breastfeeding mother has a double job: healing herself and nurturing her baby. Here's how to do both:

- Ask the lactation consultant in the maternity unit to show you the side-lying position and the clutch hold for breastfeeding. These positions keep baby's weight off your incision. (See pages 131–133 for a description of these positions.)

- If you would rather sit up to nurse your baby, sit in a straight-backed armchair rather than in your hospital bed. This is easier on your abdominal muscles. Use pillows along your side to bring baby up to breast height and to protect your incision.

- Be sure that dad observes how the professionals help you position yourself and your baby for comfort and for correct breastfeeding technique so that he can take over this role when you go home. Ask them to instruct dad on holding baby's lower jaw down and everting baby's lip outward, since it may be uncomfortable for you to bend over to see how baby is latching on.

- Take whatever pain medications you need to be comfortable. Pain suppresses milk production and interferes with your milk-ejection reflex. The usual medications used for post-op pain are safe, since very little goes into your milk.

- If post-operative complications prevent breastfeeding for a day or two, father or a nurse can give baby formula, but preferably not by bottle. Cup feeding or finger feeding with a syringe or a supplementer (see pages 162–164 for an explanation of these techniques) is better than using a bottle, which may lead to nipple confusion.

- Breastfeed your baby frequently, night and day. Studies have shown that it may take longer for a mother's milk to come in after a cesarean birth. Frequent feeding will build up your milk supply more quickly. If baby is not breastfeeding yet, you need to begin pumping your breasts as soon as possible so that your baby can benefit from your colostrum produced during this time, and so you will have an ample milk supply when baby does start breastfeeding.

- Baby should room-in with you as soon as possible. Because of post-operative sedation this is usually discouraged for cesarean mothers. We still advise rooming-in if someone can stay with you to help care for the baby.

Be patient. It takes more time, support, and perseverance to achieve a successful breastfeeding relationship following an operation. Some of the energy that would otherwise go toward breastfeeding is shared with healing your own body. Breastfeeding harmony will come, though not as easily or quickly. (See related section on bonding with the cesarean baby, page 45.)

The Premature Baby

These special babies have special needs for extra nutrition and comfort. Here is where the breastfeeding mother shines. The recent advances of newborn intensive care have increased the chances of taking home a healthy baby, but the same technology that is saving more babies has, by its very definition, displaced the mother. But you *are* an indispensable part of the medical team.

Sue and her baby, Jonathan, were a mother and a premature baby I cared for in the hospital. During most of the day, she lived at the side of her baby's incubator. As a participating witness in Jonathan's progress, Sue exclaimed, "It's like he's in an outside womb, and I have the opportunity of seeing him grow."

Supermilk!

A premature baby has an even greater need for mother's milk. Premature babies need more proteins and calories for catch-up growth. Researchers have discovered that the milk of mothers who deliver preterm babies is higher in proteins and calories — a vivid testimony to how the milk of a species changes to ensure the survival of the young of that species. Supermilk for early babies — how exciting!

While the nutritional benefits of breastfeeding are important for premature babies, the immunological benefits are even more critical. Breast milk protects these babies against bacteria and viruses that their own immune systems cannot cope with. In addition, human milk is the perfect first feeding for immature gastrointestinal tracts. Human milk offers protection against necrotizing enterocolitis, a life-threatening bowel disease that affects premature babies. Your baby's neonatologist may order that baby's diet of human milk be fortified or supplemented with a commercial product. This is because in order to grow as they did in the womb, very young preemies may need larger amounts of some nutrients than mother's milk can provide. But this does not mean that mother's milk should not be used also. Human milk provides premature babies with important health and developmental benefits unavailable in commercial formulas and fortifiers.

It used to be the policy in most newborn intensive care units not to let premature babies breastfeed until after baby was able to tolerate bottlefeedings. Research has shown that premature babies actually do better with breastfeeding than bottlefeeding, and that the ability to breastfeed precedes the ability to bottlefeed. Researchers found that a breastfeeding baby sucks and swallows in a burst-and-pause rhythm that uses less energy than the less rhythmic bottlefeeding. They found that breastfeeding babies actually grew better and had fewer stop-breathing episodes and tired less during breastfeeding than with bottlefeeding. Not only is breast milk superior for premature babies, so is the way it is delivered.

What Mother Can Do

To understand your important role in the care of your premature infant, let's go through the usual case of the premature baby whose breathing is stable but who is in the intensive care unit for "growing." Here are some care-by-mother steps to consider.

Practice kangaroo care. One way that a breastfeeding mother can join the medical team is through an innovation called *kangaroo care* — an affectionate nickname derived from the method's similarity to the kangaroo pouch and the easy self-feeding of the premature baby kangaroo. Research by Dr. Gene Cranston Anderson at Case Western Reserve in Cleveland has shown that preemies receiving kangaroo care gain weight faster, have fewer stop-breathing episodes, and experience a shorter hospital stay.

Using a baby sling, mother wears her diaper-clad baby skin to skin on or between her breasts. The combination of mother's warm body, warm blankets, and mother's clothing keeps the premature baby toasty. Many premature babies initially react to this comfortable environment by falling asleep and sleeping more peacefully than in their high-tech cribs. When baby awakens, the closeness to mother's breasts stimulates baby to feed as his little stomach requires — a system called self-regulatory feeding. Live at the side of your baby's incubator and sit in a rocking chair with baby wrapped skin to skin at your breasts. Unless your baby must be attached to medical instruments, walk around while wearing your baby. Even more than rocking in the chair, the rhythm of walking helps baby breathe more regularly because, presumably, this is a pattern he had been used to in your womb. (See discussion of the vestibular system, page 302.) Kangaroo-cared-for babies cry less. Because it wastes oxygen and energy, excessive crying can keep premature babies from growing optimally. Breast-feeding, kangaroo care, holding and rocking, and wearing your baby lessen crying and speed growth.

Besides being good for babies, there is something in kangaroo care for mothers, too. The closeness of baby nestling on the breasts triggers the mothering and milk-producing hormones. Mothers who are invited to participate in kangaroo care are more inclined to breastfeed, produce more milk, and breastfeed longer. They develop a deeper attachment to their infants, feel more confident about their mothering skills, and feel a valuable part of the newborn intensive care team.

Newborn specialists believe that one main reason kangaroo care helps premature babies thrive is that mother acts as a breathing pacemaker for her premature infant. Preterm babies have frequent stop-breathing episodes, called apnea, which contribute to these babies' slow growth and even slower departure from the hospital. You probably never thought of yourself as a breathing machine, but picture this: Baby is snuggled comfortably against your chest, his ear over your heart. You have a rhythm in your breathing and your heart rate, and your baby senses it. The rhythm of your breathing, your heartbeat, your voice, which baby was accustomed to hearing in utero, and even the warm air flowing from your nose onto baby's scalp at each breath are translated into breathing stimuli for your baby, as if reminding the forgetful premature to breathe. Attached babies catch the rhythm of their parents.

Pump your milk. Rent an electric breast pump and start pumping your milk as soon as possible after birth. Store this milk and begin giving your baby your milk as soon as baby is medically able to take it by whatever method works best.

Ask for help. Seek assistance from a lactation consultant who will show you special techniques to help your premature baby latch on correctly and suck efficiently.

Avoid the bottle. Ask the nursing staff to feed your baby with a cup, syringe, or a finger-feeding system (see page 163) instead of with bottles and artificial nipples. Another alternative is to continue tube feeding while your baby learns to nurse at the breast. Some premature babies do not experience nipple confusion and eagerly advance from bottle to breast. Others are prone to nipple confusion, so avoid the bottle stage unless medically necessary. When you take your baby home from the hospital, you may need to continue to offer supplements for a week or two.

Ease baby on. Instead of pulling your baby in very close with a rapid movement (see page 129), as you would to latch a term baby onto your breast, it's better to *ease* the breasts into the premature baby's mouth. Use the *compress-and-stuff* technique. With your hand shaped like a C (thumb on top and fingers beneath the breast), cup your breast well behind the areola. Compress the breast, tease baby's mouth open wide, and gradually ease the "areola sandwich" into baby's mouth.

Forget the clock. The concept of schedule has little meaning for term babies and none for prematures. Expect your baby to suck weakly, feed slowly, tire quickly, and fall asleep frequently during the feedings. (They do this with bottlefeeding, too.) Preterm babies tire more easily, need more calories for catch-up growth, and have small tummies. This is why they need small, frequent feedings. Premature babies have more bizarre sleep-and-wake cycles, so that every mother-baby pair must work out a feeding pattern that gets the most milk into the baby without tiring him out.

The Ill or Hospitalized Baby

Breastfeeding is good medicine. Besides helping preemies thrive, the breastfeeding mother is a valuable part of the medical team if her baby is ill, particularly if he is hospitalized. When one of my patients is in the hospital, it has always been my practice to encourage care by parents. I have noticed that babies get better more quickly, and parents feel involved as part of the team. The more involved they are, the better they understand the nature of the illness and the methods of treatment.

Breastfeeding is particularly valuable to infants who are hospitalized for breathing problems such as croup or bronchitis. In these conditions, the more upset baby is, the more the breathing is upset. Relaxing baby also helps relax the breathing. Let me share with you the story of one-year-old Tony and his breastfeeding mother, Cindy. Early one morning Tony awakened barking like a seal and having difficulty breathing. I hospitalized Tony for treatment of croup, but his condition worsened. Tony was in a vicious cycle — the more difficulty he had breathing, the more anxious he got, which further aggravated his breathing. I told Cindy that unless Tony relaxed, his condition would deteriorate, and we would have to do a tracheostomy (surgically open his windpipe below the inflamed vocal cords so that he could breathe more air). Without taking a breath Cindy volunteered, "I'll relax him," and she did! Through the opening in Tony's oxygen tent came Cindy's breast, along with soothing words of encouragement and a

---

NO MORE, PLEASE. I'M TIRED!

It is important not to jostle and tire premature babies, and others with medical problems, by becoming too enthusiastic and vigorous with feedings, lest babies burn more energy than they take in during feeding and consequently grow too slowly. Watch for cues (flutter-type sucking and drifting off to sleep) that baby has had enough. Ease baby off your breast, but be ready to feed again in a couple of hours, or even sooner.

familiar touch from someone who cared enough to give her child the very best. Tony listened, looked, and sucked. Immediately he relaxed and breathed better. I relaxed, mother relaxed, and so did the surgeon, waiting with his lifesaving instruments. Tony got the ultimate pacifier.

During an illness babies often regress to a more primitive and familiar pattern of self-comforting, such as thumb-sucking and curling up like a fetus. Being breastfed while sick lessens the anxiety of being in the hospital by helping the infant latch on to a comfortable and pleasurable pattern that he has learned to love and trust.

Breastfeeding is also valuable for the infant who has a diarrheal illness from inflamed intestines (called gastroenteritis). These infants may not tolerate commercially prepared formula, but they generally can tolerate breast milk. In our practice we have seen many infants with gastroenteritis continue to breastfeed without aggravating the diarrhea or getting dehydrated; whereas their formula-feeding friends with the same illness often wind up in the hospital with dehydration and need intravenous feedings. Chalk up another bonus for mother's milk. And the very act of sucking is very comforting to a baby who doesn't understand why she feels so crummy.

Breastfeeding Helps Hearts

Babies who are born with heart defects (called congenital heart disease, or CHD) have one of two problems: They may have too much blood flowing to their lungs, causing overload on the heart and resulting in heart failure. Or they may not have enough blood flowing to their lungs, resulting in cyanosis (blueness); a baby with this condi-

tion is termed a "blue baby." In both of these conditions babies with CHD tire easily during feedings and grow more slowly. Years ago, breastfeeding a baby with CHD was discouraged because it was erroneously thought that breastfeeding would tire these babies out. As we discussed for premature babies, research has shown the opposite. These babies may actually use less energy and breathe more efficiently during breastfeeding than bottle-feeding. Breast milk contains less salt than formula, so it is better for babies who are prone to heart failure. The same suggestions recommended for feeding premature babies apply to feeding babies with CHD: small, frequent feedings, often with a supplementer system, and large doses of patience.

Babies with Down Syndrome

Our seventh child, Stephen, has Down syndrome. As a lactation consultant, nurse, and mother, and as a pediatrician and father, Martha and I both wanted to give Stephen the best start. We went through a checklist of the most common medical problems we could expect in Stephen. While certainly no panacea, breast milk could help each one of these problems:

- Babies with Down syndrome are prone to colds, especially ear infections; breast milk provides extra immunity.

- Babies with Down syndrome are prone to intestinal infections; breast milk promotes the growth of friendly bacteria in the intestinal tract, a factor that lessens infections.

- Babies with Down syndrome are prone to constipation; breast milk has a laxative effect.

- Babies with Down syndrome are prone to heart problems; breast milk is lower in salt and is more physiologic.

- Babies with Down syndrome may have a weak suck; breastfeeding has an energy-sparing rhythm.

- Babies with Down syndrome have delayed mental and motor development; breast milk is good brain food, and breastfeeding optimizes oral-facial development and socialization.

There is a lot we don't know about babies with Down syndrome; there are a lot of valuable nutrients in breast milk yet to be discovered. We had a special baby who needed special parenting. After Stephen's birth, as we held each other and cried together, we vowed that he would have it — beginning with breastfeeding.

Typically, babies with Down syndrome have a hypotonic (low tone, weak) suck requiring lots of support, training, and patience until mother and baby get the hang of it. Not until he was two weeks old did Stephen open his eyes and become more receptive to breastfeeding. Until then Martha did what she could to get him latched on. This was a very scary time for us, as we feared he might never breastfeed well. Martha had to initiate most of the feedings. All our other babies were demand feeders. But if we had waited for Stephen to "demand," he would never have gained weight. He was what we call a happy-to-starve baby.

For the next two weeks she pumped several times a day and syringe and finger fed Stephen one ounce before each breastfeeding to "suck train" him. It was amazing to see how well he was making up for lost time — some days gaining two ounces.

Though most babies with Down syndrome have a more difficult breastfeeding start and need to be taught to breastfeed, they do eventually learn these skills. The profound benefits make the extra work worthwhile. Be sure to contact a lactation consultant who has experience working with babies with Down syndrome.

All of the tips for attachment parenting have magnified benefits for babies with special needs. We found that constant contact through sharing sleep, breastfeeding, and babywearing gave us the boost we needed for bonding with Stephen. We joined a support group that helped us get *excited* about our baby. As he began to gain weight and breastfeed, we found that we could stop worrying about him and begin enjoying him. Martha still remembers the day she discovered that he responded to high-pitched baby talk from her — worry had kept her from relating to him in a normal way. It felt so good to see the many ways he was similar to our other babies rather than focus on how he was different. Now we cannot imagine life without Stephen. Our world is a better place because of Stephen. He has taught us how to value every person, no matter what his or her handicap might be.

The Baby with Cleft Lip or Palate

Babies with a cleft lip or palate pose a special challenge to the breastfeeding mother, but the benefits of breastfeeding are worth the investment. The location and severity of the cleft will determine whether baby can learn to breastfeed effectively and which positions and techniques you should use. Mothers of babies with a cleft lip or palate should obtain professional help from a lactation consultant by the second day after birth. Choose a lactation consultant who has some experience helping babies with clefts breastfeed.

A baby with a cleft lip may or may not have difficulty forming a seal on the breast. If baby does have trouble, mother's soft breast tissue will fill in some of the space at the cleft, and mother's thumb can close off the rest of the gap, allowing baby to suck normally. Clefts are repaired in stages in the early months. Some surgeons feel that breastfeeding immediately after the surgery does not interfere with healing; others may insist that you pump your milk and feed it to your baby with a special device until the repair has healed.

A baby with a small cleft of the soft palate may be able to nurse with few problems, but a baby with a more extensive cleft may not be able to breastfeed at all. Because of the opening in the palate, a baby with a cleft palate cannot use suction to keep the breast in his mouth, and with part of the hard palate missing, it is difficult for baby to milk the breast with pressure from his tongue. Milk may run into baby's nose and ears. A lactation consultant can help you evaluate the problems your baby has with breastfeeding and suggest solutions. Even if your baby is unable to breastfeed, you can still pump milk and feed it to him in other ways.

The Adopted Baby

Where there's a will, there's a way. Yes, you can breastfeed your adopted baby; it takes high doses of commitment, a few special tools, and professional breastfeeding help. Martha was breastfeeding our adopted baby, Lauren, when we were writing the first edition of this book. We have counseled many adopting mothers who have successfully breastfed their babies, using a technique called *induced lactation*. These are the steps to go through:

- Seek advice and support from mothers who have successfully breastfed their adoptive babies. You can locate adoptive breastfeeding mothers through your lactation consultant or La Leche League, or ask your pediatrician for names of adoptive mothers in his or her practice who have breastfed their babies.

- Consult a lactation consultant as soon as you know you are getting a baby. The ideal situation is to know before the baby is born. A month's preparation is best, but not absolutely necessary.

- Here are the tools you need: Rent an electric breast pump, preferably one with a double pumping system, and simulate sucking at the breast by pumping your breasts as often as you would feed a newborn, around every two to three hours. Your lactation consultant will show you how to use the pump and work out a schedule. You will also need a breastfeeding supplementer, which is described on page 163. (An adopting mother in our practice was so thrilled at breastfeeding her baby and used the supplementer so much she had it bronzed.) You may begin to produce drops of clear or opaque fluid and then actually get small amounts of milk even before you have your baby, especially if you have previously or recently breastfed. Lactation is a very individual system, dependent on each individual's levels of milk-producing hormones. (It does *not* depend on your reproductive hormones.)

- Choose a pediatrician who is experienced in counseling adoptive breastfeeding mothers.

- Make arrangements if possible to be present at delivery so baby can begin bonding with you. In this way your baby knows right away to whom he or she belongs. You, baby's mother, will be the first one to feed your baby. (See page 430 for making hospital arrangements.)

- While baby is in the hospital try to be present for as many feedings as you can. With the help of your lactation specialist, begin feeding baby formula at your breast with a supplementer. If you're not able to be present for all the feedings (and few mothers are), instruct the nurses to use the finger-and-syringe method of feeding or to use the SNS for finger feeding (see page 163). Try to avoid bottlefeeding in the early days and weeks while baby is learning to feed at your breast. This method of feeding takes no longer than bottlefeeding.

- Remember, it is the *frequency* of sucking that stimulates milk. The frequent sucking at your breasts induces your own milk-producing systems to click in. Most mothers will begin producing some milk within three to four weeks. (In addition to pumping and using a supplementer, wear your baby a lot, sleep with your baby, and massage your baby. All these ways of just being close to your infant also increases your milk supply.)

- Do not focus on how soon you will produce milk or how much. Even after your milk appears do not establish milk supply expectations; the quantity of milk produced is not the ultimate goal. The close bonding that breastfeeding helps you achieve is the main benefit of breastfeeding your adopted baby.

Breastfeeding is ideal for the adoptive baby, and it does good things for mothers, too. The sucking at your breast stimulates the flow of your mothering hormones, giving you an added boost to become attached to your baby. In breastfeeding the adopted baby, you give the best start to baby; baby gives the best start to mother.

Twins (Even Triplets)

Twice the investment, twice the return. Here's how to both survive and thrive while breastfeeding your twins.

Get the right help early on. In the latter weeks of pregnancy, consult other mothers who have breastfed twins. Your local La Leche League or Mothers of Twins affiliate (see pages 126 and 431 for more information) can help you find some. Prenatally, attend La Leche League meetings to become acquainted with support persons that you are really going to need. Arrange for a lactation specialist experienced in helping mothers breastfeed multiples to help you within a day or two postpartum and teach you right-start techniques.

Get the right start. As an extra challenge to breastfeeding, many twins are premature and tend to be sleepy, not sucking well for a week or two. With the help of your lactation specialist, learn the right positioning and latch-on techniques immediately, before your babies develop poor sucking habits, your nipples get sore, and you don't produce sufficient milk. Proper positioning and latch-on techniques are important enough for single babies; double that for twins.

Breastfeed the babies separately, then together. In the first week or so most mothers find it easier to feed one baby at a time, giving undivided attention to teaching each baby proper latch-on. Once both babies have learned to latch on correctly, you may find simultaneous feeding easier, especially if both babies have similar feeding needs and temperaments. To give each one some individual attention, try mostly simultaneous feedings and give individual feedings once or twice a day, especially when one twin is hungry and the other is asleep. Simultaneous feeding works best if babies are on a similar sleep schedule. As an added boost, research has shown that mothers who breastfeed twins simultaneously have higher elevations of the mothering hormone prolactin than those who nurse one baby at a time.

Many twins have similar birth weights and nutritional needs, but oftentimes one wombmate robs the other of placental nutrition, so that one twin shows obvious signs of having been nutritionally shortchanged. This baby is likely to need more-frequent feedings for catch-up growth. Sometimes one twin is a high-need baby, the other easy; and one may simply be hungrier than the other. Let the hungrier and more frequent feeder set the pattern. As you are about to feed the hungrier baby, periodically wake the less demanding baby for feeding to ensure that you get at least some simultaneous feedings during the day. Otherwise you may find that you are *always* (literally) feeding one or the other.

Holding patterns for twins. Experiment with all these positions to find which combination works best for you and your babies.

- Unless sitting in bed, use a footstool to elevate your lap to better contain both babies. The double clutch hold allows you to control the babies' head movements in case one or both tend to throw their heads back during breastfeeding (see page 132 for a description of the clutch hold). When breastfeeding in this position, be sure to support yourself and the babies with lots of pillows, or purchase a specially designed nursing pillow (available from La Leche League).

- For the *cross-cradle position,* put one baby in the cradle hold, then put the other baby to the other breast in the cradle hold — they'll have their heads apart and their legs and feet crisscrossing. Again, use lots of pillows for support.

- In the *parallel position,* one baby is in the cradle hold and one is in the clutch hold so that their bodies are lying in the same direction. The cradled baby is on your arm (on a pillow) and the clutched baby is on a pillow, the back of his neck held by your hand.

Dad as the second mother. Father should be involved in the breastfeeding relationship with any baby. With twins it's an absolute must. In parenting twins the mother-father roles are not so well defined. It is true that only mom can make milk, but dad can do everything else. Fatigue is what does most breastfeeding mothers in. Mothers we have counseled who have successfully breastfed twins have mastered the art of becoming armchair household executives directing traffic and delegating responsibilities to any friend or family member they can draft. Father can give supplemental feedings, bring babies to the "executive" for feeding (espe-

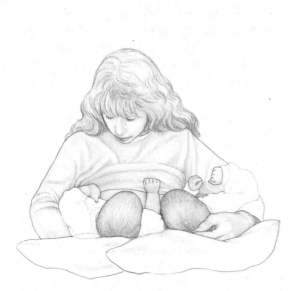

Breastfeeding twins: the double clutch hold.

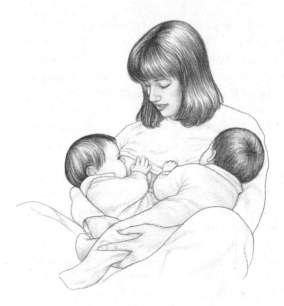

Breastfeeding twins: the cross-cradle position.

cially at night), and do or delegate household chores. One father of twins in our practice proudly described their shared parenting: "Our babies have two mothers; she is the milk mother, and I'm the hairy mother." Breastfeeding twins: double the commitment, double the sense of humor. (For more about parenting twins, see Chapter 18.)

Breastfeeding While Pregnant

Yes, you can! Mothers are often cautioned not to breastfeed during pregnancy. Here's the reason. Breastfeeding stimulates the release of the hormone oxytocin into your bloodstream. *In theory* this hormone could stimulate uterine contractions, possibly inducing a miscarriage. We have interviewed experts knowledgeable about the hormonal system during pregnancy and have received the following go-ahead: The uterus is not receptive to hormonal stimulation by oxytocin until around twenty-four weeks of gestation. And with a healthy uterus and cervix, this oxytocin is not sufficient to bring on labor unless your pregnancy is term and your cervix is ripe. Many mothers breastfed during part or throughout all of their pregnancy without doing any harm to themselves or their preborn baby. If, however, you have a history of frequent miscarriages or experience unusual uterine contractions during breastfeeding, or if your doctor advises against breastfeeding because of your individual obstetrical situation, it is wise to stop. If you are at risk for preterm labor, any and all stimulation of your nipples (even showering your nipples) and orgasm must be avoided beginning at around twenty weeks of gestation, when the oxytocin receptors in the uterus activate.

If your doctor gives you the green light, here's what to expect. You may experience nipple tenderness, making breastfeeding rather uncomfortable. You can negotiate with an older toddler, or enlist father's help to carry around and distract a younger one, to get the frequency and number of minutes of breastfeeding to a level you can tolerate. Some of the ideas in the following section on weaning will be helpful. In the final trimester or earlier, expect your milk to develop a different taste, and in the middle trimester expect your supply to diminish.

Some mothers begin to resent breastfeeding one while carrying another, as though not only your breasts but also your mind is telling you it's time to wean. Like so many things in parenting, if it isn't working, change it. This is usually the time at which a toddler will naturally wean, although a few hardy souls (very giving mother, very high-need toddler) continue through the pregnancy.

Martha notes: One day during my pregnancy with Erin, our high-need daughter, Hayden, announced, "I don't like the milk anymore. I'll wait until after baby is born when it will be good again, then I'll nurse." When Erin was breastfeeding through my pregnancy with Matthew, I quizzed her one day: "Why do you want to nurse? There's no milk, is there?" Her reply was "I don't care" — with a big grin on her face. Obviously there was something there she wanted that couldn't be measured in ounces or drops.

WEANING: WHEN AND HOW

All good things come to a timely end. While timely weaning is the ideal, we realize that the ideal is not achievable for many families. Nevertheless we feel obligated to present the ideal and then offer alternatives that make allowances for life-styles. We have taken many pages to portray one of parenting's most beautiful relationships, breastfeeding. Now here's how to guide it to a graceful finish.

What Does "Weaning" Really Mean?

"Weaning" is not a negative term. Weaning does not mean a loss or detachment from a relationship, but rather a *passage* from one relationship to another. Our first three infants were weaned before their time. We were young and uninformed parents. We misread our babies' cues, lacked confidence in our own intuitions, and yielded to the norms of the neighborhood. We were able to give our later babies their rightful heritage. In the process of our discoveries, we researched the real definition and history of weaning, and here's what we found.

In ancient writings the word "wean" meant "to ripen" — like fruit nourished to readiness, its time to leave the vine. When a child was weaned it was a festive occasion, and not because of what you may think — "Now I can finally get away from this kid. . . ." Weaning was a joyous occasion because a weaned child was valued as a fulfilled child; a child was so filled with the basic tools of the earlier stages of development that she graduated to take on the next stage of development more independently. A child who is weaned before his time enters the next state of development more anxiously and is consequently less prepared for its challenges and less ready for its independence.

An insightful description of weaning is found in the writings of King David: "I have stilled and quieted my soul; like a weaned child with its mother, like a weaned child is my soul within me." The psalmist David equates his feeling of peace and tranquillity with the feeling of fulfillment that a weaned child has with his mother. In ancient times, and in many cultures today, a baby is breast-fed for two or three *years.* Our Western culture is accustomed to thinking of breast-feeding in terms of months. We wish to challenge this mind-set.

When to Wean

We have a sign in our office, "Early weaning not recommended for babies." If you view parenting as a long-term investment, why sell your options short? Timely weaning occurs when the sucking need dissipates — sometime between nine months and three and a half years. Medically speaking, nutritionists and physicians advise breastfeeding at least until your child's first birthday, and there is nothing sacred about one year. Many babies given the opportunity choose to breastfeed much longer. Nutritionists and physicians advise at least one year because by that time most infants have outgrown most of their food allergies and will thrive on alternative nourishment. Weaning is a personal decision. Basically, when one or both members of the mother-infant pair are *ready,* it's time to wean.

Weaning Before Baby's First Birthday

Does weaning under a year mean you have failed Parenting 101? No! There may be life-style choices, circumstances beyond your control, and medical situations that require premature weaning. Also, the occasional baby *will* be filled and ready to wean before a year, though not as a rule.

Breastfeeding After the First Year

If you breastfeed longer than a year, you may wonder if you are spoiling your child, being possessive, or making him too dependent. Spoiling is what happens when you leave something (or some person) alone on the shelf — it spoils. As any breastfeeding veteran will attest, a breastfeeding baby is anything but left alone. Possessiveness means keeping a child from doing what he needs to do because of some need *you* have. Then comes the myth of overdependency. Be prepared for well-meaning advisers to shake your confidence a bit by exclaiming, "What! You're still breastfeeding?" This statement shows a lack of appreciation of a toddler as a little person with big needs. Both experience and research have shown that extended breastfeeding does not foster dependency. The opposite is true. As we stated in Chapter 1, securely attached babies (those who are not weaned before their time) eventually grow to be more independent, separate more easily from their mothers, move into new relationships with more security and stability, and are, in fact, easier to discipline.

If breastfeeding in terms of years sounds strange to you, ask yourself this: Who gets horrified at the sight of a two-year-old still having a bottle? The need to suck can be an extended need for many babies, breastfed or bottlefed. A need that is filled goes away. A need that is not filled may surface later to cause trouble.

How to Wean

The American Heritage Dictionary defines "wean": "To withhold mother's milk . . . and substitute other nourishment." There are two phases in weaning — withholding and substituting. As you *gradually* withhold your milk, substitute solid foods, alternative milks, and other forms of emotional nourishment. Here's how.

HOW LONG TO BREASTFEED — OPINIONS FROM THE EXPERTS

It used to be that few physicians openly advocated extended nursing, and the mothers who breastfed babies past a year or two years (or longer) kept mum about their child's continuing to nurse. Long-term breastfeeding may not yet be universally accepted, but it is getting more backing from health professionals and other scientists. The American Academy of Pediatrics stated in 1997 that breastfeeding should continue "for *at least twelve months,* and thereafter for as long as mutually desired." The World Health Organization, which concerns itself with public health issues in developing nations as well as in the developed world, recommends breastfeeding for *at least two years.* Perhaps these statements from respected organizations will usher in an era when more babies will get to breastfeed longer and more mothers will learn how much easier it is to mother a toddler when that toddler is still nursing.

Wean from Person to Person, Not from Person to Thing

Don't rely on a fluffy teddy bear or plastic toys to bribe your baby from the breast. Babies are not like that. As baby begins to wean from comfort at mother's breast, you begin to substitute other forms of emotional nourishment. Also, another person, ideally the father, takes on a more significant role in comforting.

Wean Gradually

Avoid weaning by desertion — leaving baby to go on a getaway vacation. Sudden detachment from mother's breast and from the whole mother all at once may be a combined stress that is too much for baby to handle. The key to healthy weaning is that it must be *gradual.* Some mothers purposefully start skipping the least favored feeding, for instance the midmorning time when mom and baby would really rather go to the park or read a book or have a snack. Other mothers find they are doing this without actually planning it. It just happens. After a while they make another adjustment, then another, either intentionally or just as life unfolds, so that months (and months) later they find they are down to just one or two feedings, usually nap time and bedtime. (In Chapter 15, "Nighttime Parenting," we discuss how to wean at sleep times.)

The time-honored weaning method of "don't offer, don't refuse" seems to work the best for most mothers and babies. Weaning means *releasing,* not rejecting. Minimize situations that encourage breastfeeding (for example, sitting down in the familiar, inviting rocking chair), but be open during needful periods of the day. It is quite normal, as babies are naturally weaning into other relationships, for them to use mother as their home base for nutritional and emotional refueling. Be prepared to back up a step or two if you see negative behavior (tantrums, anger, sadness) cropping up, telling you that you are going too fast. During illness the frequency of breastfeeding will pick up, becoming an important comforting tool, as well as supplying needed disease-specific antibodies.

Be Prepared for "Regressions"

Between eighteen months and two years baby may have occasional spurts of marathon breastfeeding, as if it were newborn time again. Here's why: As your budding explorer comes across new situations, it is necessary for him to check into home base frequently for a brief boost, reassuring himself that it is OK to resume exploring unknown territory. Breastfeeding, like a familiar friend in a strange crowd, helps the child to progress from the known to the unknown, from dependence to independence. A problem can develop here if mother is too busy to accommodate these brief but frequent pit stops. Baby may then insist on lengthy hour-long feedings, as though once he gets you to where he needs you, he knows he better hang on for dear life.

It's OK to Say No

In day-to-day dealings with their toddlers some mothers feel trapped by a breastfeeding contract without an escape clause. They think "don't offer, don't refuse" means they can never say no. There are many creative ways to say no that will not be regarded as "Mama is hardening her heart" but rather as "Mama wants to help me find a way to be content."

Develop Creative Alternatives

If you are comfortable letting your child take the lead in weaning, realize she may be two or three (or older if you have a family history of allergies) before she decides to wean. Although this is not part of our culture, there are definite benefits to those children who need a prolonged weaning process. On the other hand, if you feel it is time to wean (a clue is that you chronically resent continued breastfeeding), you *can* take the initiative. There is a unique book we recommend that thoroughly explores the benefits of longer-term breastfeeding and includes two chapters

on nudging the weaning process along a bit: *Mothering Your Nursing Toddler,* by Norma Jane Bumgarner (La Leche League, 2000).

If your child resists weaning, picture what is going on in her mind. In what we call our *deep groove theory* of child development, we believe the developing memory is like a big, blank phonograph record; experience cuts grooves in this record. The breastfeeding groove is probably one of the deepest your child will ever cut, and this is why she returns to it frequently until alternative grooves are etched into her memory record. Your goal is to encourage these alternative grooves at a pace that is neither too fast for your child nor too slow for you. One key is to keep your child busy. Nothing triggers the desire to breastfeed like boredom. Next, minimize scenes that remind her of breastfeeding. Many mothers relate, "As soon as I sit down in the rocking chair, she pounces." Expect nap nursing and night nursing to be the last to go. Many toddlers retain a desire to be breastfed to sleep well into the second or third year. When one (or both) of you is ready to drop breastfeeding as the ultimate sleep inducer, you will have to come up with something equally convincing. You should already have a bedtime routine, or nap routine, which includes quieting activities. Reading bedtime stories (over and over), a sling ride through the house saying night-night to everything and everybody, or a back rub accompanied by a lullaby can be the finishing touch to the standard fare of healthful snack, bath, and pajamas. (See also the suggestions on page 359.)

Plenty of exercise earlier in the day sets your little one up for the sandman. Wind-down, mood-setting tools can be thrown in: Turn off stimulating TV programs, turn on relaxing music, dim the lights, or draw the drapes. A variation of the bedtime story is to sit together and watch a classic, low-key video such as *Winnie the Pooh*. The favorite in our house is to tell a story from when we were children (or make one up using the current favorite fictional hero) and weave in a lot of lulling repetition and counting. The main feature of all these routines is that dad or anyone other than mother can do the honors. And remember, if your toddler has not had much time with dad, he will resist sleep just because of father hunger. So dads, don't try to shortchange this necessary contact time.

Finally, weaning is easier if you gradually develop creative alternatives to breastfeeding when your baby needs comforting. If you automatically offer the breast as a solution to every cry and setback in your baby's life (because it works so well), it will be more difficult for your baby to settle for anything else as he gets older, and it will be more difficult for you to get out of the rut, so to speak, of your limited comforting resources. Stories, toys, games, songs, outings, projects, may be just the reserves you need. Consider weaning as *broadening* your relationship with your baby, not losing it. As with all parenting styles there is a balance. Some mothers are overly attached to their babies, so that their total relationship revolves around breastfeeding. Consequently it is the only form of relating that their babies know. If you begin to feel that you are resenting so much breastfeeding, it's time to slow it down and consider other ways of relating to your child. As you develop more playful interactions as alternatives to breastfeeding, your child will gradually learn to be content with them and actually prefer them as a substitute.

Our Experience — Our Recommendations

Life is a series of weanings for a child: weaning from your womb, weaning from your breast, from your bed, and from your home to school. The pace at which children go from oneness to separateness should be respected in all of these weaning milestones. To hurry children through any of these relationships before their time increases the risks of what we call *diseases of premature weaning:* anger, aggression, habitual tantrumlike behavior, anxious attachment to caregivers, and less ability to form deeper and more intimate relationships. We have studied the long-term effects on thousands of children who had timely weanings and have observed that these children

- are more independent
- gravitate to *people* more than things
- are easier to discipline
- experience less anger
- radiate trust

LONG-TERM BENEFITS OF BREASTFEEDING

Breastfeeding, like all the other Baby B's of attachment parenting, is a wise long-term investment. For an account of our experience in attachment-parenting kids, as well as the latest scientific studies on the long-term effects of attachment parenting, see our books *The Successful Child: What Parents Can Do to Help Kids Turn Out Well* (Little, Brown, 2002) and *The Attachment Parenting Book* (Little, Brown, 2001).

Ideally, try to give your baby the best physical, emotional, and mental start — a gradual and timely weaning. In the normal process of oneness to separateness, it is not the mother who weans the baby, but the baby who weans from the mother. In our many years as baby watchers, studying the long-term effects of long-term breast-feeding, the most secure, independent, and happy children we have seen are those who have not been weaned before their time.

10

Bottlefeeding with Safety and Love

While human milk is certainly best for human babies, there may be a medical reason for needing to feed your baby formula. Or perhaps your life-style requires you to both breast- and bottlefeed your baby, dubbed "combo feeding." If you regard feeding as a time to interact with your baby, not just deliver food, and if you understand the subtle differences among formulas, together with your baby's doctor you can, using the following information, make the right choice of the right formula and style of feeding for your baby.

FORMULA FACTS

The more you know about how infant formulas are made and marketed, the better equipped you will be to make an informed choice.

How formulas are made. Using human milk as the nutritional gold standard, formula manufacturers follow a basic recipe that combines proteins, fats, carbohydrates, vitamins, minerals, and water in similar proportions to those found in human milk. The basic nutritional building blocks of proteins, fats, and carbohydrates are taken from cow's milk, soybeans, or other vegetable (corn syrup or sugar cane) sources. Commercially made vitamins, minerals, and other nutrients are then added to the milk-based or soy-based formula.

How formulas are marketed. Once upon a time parents relied *only* on their baby's doctor to choose the right formula. It was generally felt that advertising infant formulas directly to the consumer was unethical. Both the American Academy of Pediatrics and the World Health Organization have strongly discouraged marketing formulas directly to parents and bypassing the baby's health care provider. Unfortunately, this nutritional code of ethics is not followed by all formula companies.

How formulas are regulated. Don't be confused by the parade of formula cans on the supermarket shelves. You'll notice that the amounts of all the nutrients in each brand are about the same. That's because by law they have to be. The Infant Formula Act mandates that the FDA tightly regulate infant formula manufacturers so that all formulas contain all the nutrients that babies need. In fact, the FDA so tightly regulates infant formulas that all formulas are nutritionally equivalent. A formula manufacturer cannot make any nutritional changes in their formula without FDA approval.

How formulas differ. Although the nutritional content of infant formulas is tightly regulated, formulas differ in three ways: packaging, digestibility, and cost.

Packaging: Commercial formulas are packaged in three forms:

- powdered formula, with directions for how much water to add
- liquid concentrate, to be mixed half-and-half with water
- ready-to-feed liquid, to be put directly into the bottle

Your choice of packaging is mainly a question of time and economics. Powdered formulas are the least expensive but the most time-consuming to prepare; ready-to-feed formulas are the most expensive but the easiest to use, especially while traveling or when you are too busy to prepare formula.

Digestibility: With different food sources and processing methods, formulas can be more or less allergenic and easier or harder to digest. While all formula makers claim superiority when it comes to intestinal tolerance, your baby's individual digestive system will be the final judge.

Cost: Because the FDA so tightly regulates formula composition, parents don't need to worry that a less expensive formula is nutritionally inferior to a pricier one. Formulas from the "big four" (Enfamil, Similac, Carnation, and store brands) are nutritionally equivalent, though they may differ in cost. If your baby needs a special hypoallergenic formula, expect to pay considerably more.

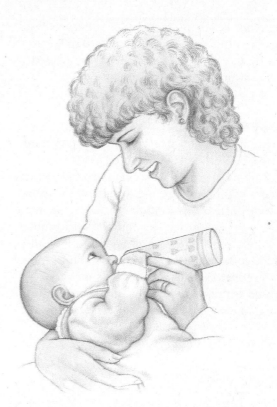

The bottlefeeding interaction.

Types of Formula

Reading the labels on formula cans may leave you feeling like you need a Ph.D. in biochemistry to make an intelligent choice. There are three basic categories of infant formulas: *milk-based* formulas (also known as *standard* infant formulas), *soy-based* formulas, and *hypoallergenic* formulas.

Milk-Based Formulas. These formulas use cow's milk as the food source of the protein and sugar (lactose). Cow's milk–based formulas enjoy a much longer history of experience and research and are well tolerated by most infants. Unless recommended otherwise by your baby's doctor, use a standard milk-based formula. Around 70 percent of formula-fed American babies consume this type of formula.

Soy-Based Formulas. As an alternative for infants who are allergic to or cannot tolerate milk-based formulas, soy formulas use soybeans as their protein source. Around 25 percent of formula-fed American babies consume some form of soy formula because it is touted to be less allergenic than milk-based formulas. However, we share the opinion of the Committee on Nutrition of the American Academy of Pediatrics that soy formulas should not be used as the starter formula for most infants for the following reasons:

- 30–50 percent of infants who are allergic to cow's milk protein are also allergic to soy protein.

- Where there is a family history of allergies, formula-feeding parents are sometimes advised to begin feeding their baby a soy formula in hopes of preventing later allergies. Research does not support this practice. Starting a newborn on a soy formula does not decrease the later incidence of allergy. Nor does the use of soy formula lower the risk of infant colic. For these reasons, the American Academy of Pediatrics' Committee on Nutrition recommends against the use of soy-protein formulas in the routine management of colic or routinely in potentially allergic infants. Instead of soy, hypoallergenic formulas (see below) are recommended.

- Giving an infant soy at a young age, when the intestines are more permeable to allergens, may predispose the child to soy allergies later on, even as an adult. He may

then find himself unable to tolerate many foods, since soy is present in a wide range of foods, often as a hidden filler.

- The wisdom of using lactose-free formulas, as most soy formula labels now boast, is questionable. Lactose is the sugar in human milk, as it is in the milk of all other mammals. Why tamper with nature's oldest nutritional experiment? Lactose enhances calcium absorption and helps colonize babies' intestines with favorable bacteria. The substitute sugar in some soy formulas is corn syrup, itself a potential allergen.

- Most soy formulas contain more minerals than the infant needs — adding extra work for little kidneys and possibly shaping tiny tastes to prefer salty foods.

- The bioavailability of the added iron and zinc in soy formulas may be less than in other formulas.

- The Committee on Nutrition of the American Academy of Pediatrics recommends that soy formula be reserved for *term* infants only and that it not be used for preterm or small-for-date infants.

At present, soy formula is used for:

- infants who are lactose deficient, a digestive problem which is uncommon in babies, or who have a rare disease in which they cannot metabolize lactose

- some infants who are intolerant of cow's milk–based formula

If you believe your baby is allergic to cow's milk formulas, always consult your physician before switching to a soy formula.

Hypoallergenic Formulas. The terms "hypoallergenic" and "hydrolyzed protein" on the formula label mean that the potentially allergenic protein has been pre-digested, that is, broken up into tinier proteins that are theoretically less allergenic. Infants who are allergic to protein in milk-based formulas may better tolerate these formulas — but at a price. The *proven* hypoallergenic formulas (Nutramigen, Pregestimil, Alimentum, and Neocate) are more expensive. Another disadvantage in some of these formulas is the absence of lactose as a carbohydrate source and the substitution of corn syrup and modified cornstarch. A third problem is their unpalatable taste.

Choosing a Formula

You're staring at the dazzling array of formula choices on the supermarket shelves, understandably confused by which formula to choose. Here's how to make the right choice for your baby:

- Consult your baby's doctor before selecting a formula for your baby. If you have a formula preference based upon experience with a previous formula-fed baby, share it with your doctor.

- Begin your baby on a *milk-based* formula unless advised otherwise by your doctor. If your doctor gives you a choice of several formulas, purchase a small amount of each or ask for a sample of each. Try each formula to see which one is best tolerated and most eagerly accepted by your baby.

- If one of your children was allergic to milk-based formula, don't assume subsequent children are also allergic to it. Try a milk-based formula first.

- Use an iron-fortified formula unless your doctor advises otherwise. Formulas that are labeled "low iron" contain insufficient iron, and in my opinion there is no reason to use them. Iron-fortified formulas contain the amount of iron recommended by the American Academy of Pediatrics and other organizations. Because the iron in formula is not absorbed as much as the iron in breast milk, expect your formula-fed infant's stools to be greenish (since iron is green). In this case, green stools are of no significance. Some parents feel that iron-fortified formulas upset their baby more than formulas without iron, but controlled studies comparing formulas with and without added iron showed no difference in gastrointestinal upsets.

- Choose a DHA- and ARA (or AA)-enriched formula. Beginning in February 2002, docosahexaenoic acid (DHA) and arachidonic acid (ARA), the brain-building fats that are found in breast milk, were added to some infant formulas made in the United States. These fats, which are so important for optimal development of the central nervous system, have for many years been added to infant formulas in over sixty other countries. Multiple studies have shown that infants fed a DHA- and ARA-enriched infant formula enjoyed increased visual and central nervous system development compared with infants fed a formula without these added fats. Since many researchers attribute the intellectual advantage that breastfeeding babies enjoy to the fact that breast milk contains lots of these omega-3 fats, it stands to reason that formula-fed infants should receive DHA- and ARA-enriched formula. Look for "DHA/ARA-enriched," or a similar notice, on the label.

COMPARISON BETWEEN HUMAN MILK AND FORMULA

	Human Milk
Fat: Provides calories for growth; needed for brain development	• High in cholesterol (used for building nerve tissue) • Contains the brain-building omega-3 fatty acids DHA and ARA • Easily digested because human milk contains the enzyme lipase • Level changes during feeding in response to baby's sucking; level declines as baby gets older
Protein: Provides amino acids for tissue growth; other proteins have special functions	• Contains mainly whey protein, which is easy to digest • Nonallergenic; babies aren't allergic to human milk protein • Some proteins help baby fight infection; see "Immune Factors," below • Contains the ideal balance of types of amino acids for brain growth, tissue development, and body building • Contains sleep-inducing proteins
Carbohydrates: Needed for brain development; sweet flavor that infants love	• Rich in lactose • High levels of lactose promote the growth of lactobacillus bifidus in the infant gut, responsible for better-smelling stools and resistance to gastrointestinal infections
Vitamins and Minerals: Needed for growth and physiologic processes	• High levels of bioavailability, especially for zinc, calcium, and iron • 50–75 percent of the iron in human milk is used by baby • The right balance of different vitamins and minerals ensures that all are well absorbed

Infant Formula	Comment
• No cholesterol; contains vegetable fat • Some brands now include DHA and ARA • No lipase; fat not completely absorbed — fat ends up in baby's stools • Fat level remains constant during feeding, doesn't adjust to infant's changing needs	A growing body of evidence shows that longer periods of breastfeeding may protect against high blood pressure and high cholesterol in later childhood and adulthood. High cholesterol levels in human milk may prepare infants to handle cholesterol better after weaning. The better intellectual skills observed in breastfed infants may be attributed to DHA and other fatty acids in human milk, which contribute to brain development.
• Many contain mostly casein protein, which forms a rubbery curd in baby's tummy • Protein comes from cow's milk and may cause allergies; soy formulas may also cause allergies • Offers no special immune protection • Higher levels of protein are hard on baby's kidneys • Amino acid profile, which is different from human milk's, may affect tissue development • Does not contain as many sleep-inducing proteins	Formula has more protein than human milk, but more is not always a good thing.
• Because cow's milk does not contain as much lactose as human milk, lactose and corn syrup are added to infant formula • Less gut-friendly	Animal species with bigger brains have more lactose in their milk.
• Extra amounts of vitamins and minerals are added to formula to compensate for poor absorption • Iron-fortified formula contains higher levels of iron, but only 5–10 percent is absorbed by baby • The complexities of how vitamins and minerals in human milk work together are not	Vitamin and mineral levels in infant formula are based on those in human milk, with an added margin of safety. Infant formula may contain more of many vitamins and minerals, but they may not be as available to baby as they are in human milk. Too much of one nutrient may make it harder for baby to use another nutrient. *(continued)*

COMPARISON BETWEEN HUMAN MILK AND FORMULA *(continued)*

	Human Milk
Immune Factors: Protect baby from infection until his own immune system matures	• Living white blood cells in human milk destroy bacteria in baby's intestines • Immunoglobulins protect baby against specific germs in the environment; other immunoglobulins line baby's digestive tract and prevent foreign proteins from getting through and causing allergies • Lactoferrin, lysozyme, and other specialized proteins prevent bacteria and viruses from multiplying in baby's gut
Enzymes and Hormones	• Contains digestive enzymes which help baby use the nutrients in human milk • Contains many hormones that may contribute to infant growth and development
Effects of Breastfeeding on Mother	• Lowers risk of breast and ovarian cancer • Lactation hormones aid in relaxation, help mother bond with baby • Easier weight loss • Exclusive breastfeeding provides protection from pregnancy for several months • Saves money • Healthier baby is easier to care for

Infant Formula	Comment
completely understood; infant formula may not contain the right balance of these nutrients.	
• No live cells in infant formula • Immunoglobulins come from cows — not the kind humans need; most are destroyed in processing • Minimal amounts of specialized proteins (or none at all) in formula	Mother manufactures antibodies to the germs to which she and baby are exposed. Baby gets these through mother's milk. Baby is protected by mother's more mature immune system.
• Enzymes from cow's milk are destroyed in heat processing • Hormones from cow's milk are destroyed in heat processing	Science is just beginning to investigate the role of the many enzymes, hormones, and growth factors in human milk. Working together in complex ways, these substances may account for differences in the health and development of breastfed and formula-fed babies.
• Risk of breast and ovarian cancer not lowered • Caregivers other than mother can feed baby, though time must be spent preparing formulas, cleaning bottles, etc. • Fertility returns sooner • Costs $1,200 a year or more • Formula-fed babies visit the doctor more often in the first year	When mothers are struggling with breastfeeding in the first days after birth, it may seem simpler to switch to formula. Yet the benefits of breastfeeding for both mother and baby are long-lasting. Even if it is difficult at the beginning, the rewards will come. Human milk for human babies — it makes sense!

Switching Formulas

During the early months you may join the formula parade, experimenting with different formulas before choosing the one that baby enjoys the most and that is least upsetting. Sometimes it's a matter of taste. Sometimes it's a matter of preparation: Your baby may show a preference for the liquid or powdered form of the same formula. Here are the signs that your baby may be allergic to or intolerant of a particular formula:

- bouts of crying after feeding
- vomiting immediately after nearly every feeding
- persistent diarrhea or constipation
- colic with a distended, tense, painful abdomen after feeding
- generally irritable behavior and/or frequent night waking
- a red, rough sandpaperlike rash, especially on the face and/or around the anus
- frequent colds and/or ear infections

If your child persistently has one or more of these features, change the formula in consultation with your doctor.

HOW MUCH? HOW OFTEN?

How much formula your baby takes depends upon your baby's weight and rate of growth, metabolism, body type, and appetite. The following guidelines on feeding volumes are meant to satisfy your infant's basic nutritional requirements. Your baby's individual desire may change from day to day and sometimes may be more or less than the average recommended volumes.

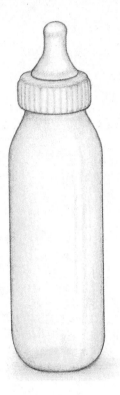

Rule of thumb for formula feeding: 2–2½ ounces per pound per day (125–150 milliliters per kilogram per day)

You may use the following rule of thumb for how much formula to feed your infant from birth to six months of age: *Two to two-and-a-half ounces of formula per pound per day (125–150 milliliters per kilogram per day).* If your baby weighs ten pounds, for example, he may take twenty to twenty-five ounces per day. Don't expect your baby to drink this much immediately after birth. Many newborns need and take only an ounce or two (30–60 milliliters) at each feeding for the first week. Use the following as a general guide:

- newborns: 1–2 ounces at each feeding
- one to two months: 3–4 ounces per feeding

- two to six months: 4–6 ounces per feeding
- six months to a year: up to 8 ounces per feeding

Small, more frequent feedings work better than larger ones spaced farther apart. Your baby's tummy is about the size of his fist. Take a full bottle and place it next to your baby's fist and you'll see why tiny tummies often spit the formula back up when they're given too much at one time.

Sometimes baby is thirsty and not hungry. Offer a bottle of water if you think baby may be thirsty. Because formulas are more heavily concentrated than breast milk, we advise parents to give their baby at least *4 to 8 ounces of water a day* (breastfed babies do not need extra water).

Scheduling the Bottlefeeding Baby

Formula-fed babies are easier to schedule than breastfed babies. Because formula is digested more slowly (the protein curds are tougher) the interval between feedings is usually longer for bottlefed babies.

There are two types of infant feeding practices: *demand feeding* (we prefer the term "cue feeding"), in which baby is fed every time his little tummy desires, and *scheduled feeding,* when baby is fed at certain fixed times during the day, usually every three hours, and when awakening during the night. Cue feeding is for infant satisfaction; scheduling is for your convenience. (We prefer the term "feeding routine" rather than the more rigid-sounding "feeding schedule.") Your overall infant-care routines, especially feeding, are challenging negotiations between baby's needs and yours. Tiny babies have tiny tummies. Most babies do best on smaller, more-frequent feedings. Giving your baby a bottle every three hours (rather than every four hours) is most in keeping with a balance between baby's satisfaction and parents' lifestyle. Most bottlefeeding parents arrive at a compromise, or semidemand type of schedule, giving baby one or two feedings at specified times each day, interspersed with cue feedings.

During the first few weeks, awaken your baby for feeding if he sleeps longer than four hours during the day. Allowing baby to sleep longer than four hours between feedings during the day may result in the exhausting day-sleeper-and-night-feeder routine. Try to arrange for the longer stretches of sleep to occur at night. More frequent feedings during the day and bottles at 7:00 P.M. and 10:00 P.M. generally seem to be the most comfortable feeding routine for most parents. This allows parents some free time in the later evening; and giving baby a bottle before you retire will often satisfy baby until 3:00 or 4:00 A.M., requiring just one waking for you.

Reading Your Baby's Cues

Tempting as it is to give your baby a bottle every time he cries, using formula as a pacifier may lead to overfeeding. Learn alternative ways of comforting rather than automatically reaching for formula at the first whimper. Baby may need only holding, a playful interaction, a bottle of water when thirsty, a diaper change, or simply a change of activity. Bottlefeeding mothers actually need more of a variety of baby-comforting techniques than do breastfeeding mothers. Using breastfeeding as a pacifier is less likely to result in overfeeding (for an explanation, see the discussion of breastfeeding and obesity, page 249).

PREPARING FORMULA

Always remember to wash your hands thoroughly before preparing formula and baby food, and be sure all the equipment used in preparing formula is clean (see instructions on sterilizing, below). The feeding supplies you will need include bottles, nipples, and miscellaneous utensils.

Bottles. Start with four four-ounce (120-milliliter) bottles, and after you and your baby have decided on the favorite type of bottle and baby is taking more than four ounces a feeding, you may need as many as eight to ten eight-ounce bottles. Glass is easiest to clean, but breakable. Besides traditional bottles there are plastic nursers, holders with presterilized disposable bags that hold the milk and collapse as baby feeds, lessening air swallowing. For older babies there are clever bottles designed in a loop for baby to hold during self-feeding. We do not advise the use of these self-feeding bottles because they encourage baby to walk around holding a bottle and deprive baby of valuable social interaction during feeding.

Nipples. Latex and silicone nipples come in a variety of shapes and flow rates that are designed to deliver expressed breast milk, formula, or milk in a way that is most comfortable for your baby. For the full-time bottlefeeding baby, experiment with various types of nipples to see which one works best for your baby. If baby is both breastfeeding and bottlefeeding, see "Combo Feeding: Breast and Bottle," opposite.

To avoid baby's choking on a nipple, follow carefully the manufacturer's caution advice on the package. If the nipple becomes cracked or torn, discard it. "Some nipples

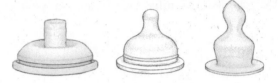

Three types of nipples (left to right): expandable nubbin, standard bulb-type, orthodontic.

come with a variety of hole sizes to fit the type of liquid and the age of the baby. The nipple hole should be large enough for formula to drip at one drop per second when you hold a full, unshaken bottle upside down.

IS BABY GETTING TOO LITTLE OR TOO MUCH FORMULA?

Signs that your baby may be getting too little formula are:

- slower-than-normal weight gain
- diminished urine output
- a loose, wrinkly appearance to baby's skin
- persistent crying

Signs that your baby is being fed too much at each feeding are:

- a lot of spitting up or vomiting immediately after the feeding
- colicky abdominal pain (baby draws his legs up onto a tense abdomen immediately after feeding)
- excessive weight gain

If these signs of overfeeding occur, offer smaller-volume feedings more frequently, burp baby once or twice during the feeding, and occasionally offer a bottle of water instead of formula.

Larger nipples and nipple holes are available for older babies.

If your baby is not getting enough liquid through the nipple, you can enlarge the nipple opening by using a needle approximately the same thickness as the hole size you desire. Heat the tip of the needle until red hot and insert the needle through the hole from the inside of the nipple. Pull the needle out of the nipple hole with a quick, straight pull. Repeat if the hole is not large enough. Attempt to enlarge the nipple hole in latex nipples only. Do not attempt to enlarge a hole in silicone nipples, as this may cause tearing.

Utensils. To prepare formula, have the following items on hand:

- punch-type can opener (for canned formula)
- bottle brush
- large pot (with a cover) for sterilizing
- clean towels or dishcloth

COMBO FEEDING: BREAST AND BOTTLE

Because of the health benefits of extended breastfeeding, many employed mothers choose to continue part-time breastfeeding. Here are some helpful tips on the art of "combo feeding" by both breast and bottle:

Choose a breastfeeding-friendly nipple. Try nipples that resemble, as much as possible, the shape of your areola and nipple. Use a nipple that has a *wide base* and gradually tapers down to the nipple, much like the shape your breast takes in your baby's mouth. Also, to ease the transition between breastfeeding and bottle feeding, choose a nipple with a slower flow, which baby is used to during breastfeeding.

Encourage proper latch-on. Be sure baby latches on to the bottle nipple the same way she latches on to your breast. Encourage her to open her mouth wide and to suck on the wide base and not just the top of the nipple. To prevent your nipples from getting sore while breastfeeding, don't let your baby learn lazy latch-on techniques while bottlefeeding. (See the illustrations on pages 130–131.)

Get the gas out. When making the transition from breast to bottle, some babies swallow more air. To minimize this nuisance, try using a bottlefeeding system that minimizes air swallowing, such as bottles with collapsible liners that keep the air out as baby feeds.

Ease the combo feeding transition. While most babies can switch back and forth between breastfeeding and bottlefeeding, some get very set in their ways of feeding. So, instruct baby's caregiver to feed your baby in a way that most resembles your baby's preferred pattern of breastfeeding. Warm the bottle nipple in warm water to make it more supple. Instruct the caregiver to interact with your baby during bottlefeeding in much the same way you do when breastfeeding. Let her watch you breastfeed while you show and tell her how to make eye contact and relate with your baby during the feeding. Remind your caregiver that feeding time is a time for social interaction. "Nursing" implies both comforting and nurturing, whether by bottle or breast.

Sterilizing

A dishwasher with a water temperature of at least 180°F (82°C) will adequately sterilize bottles and accessories. If not using a dishwasher, try the following sterilization process. (Sterilize six bottles, or a daily supply, at one time.)

- After a feeding, thoroughly rinse the bottle and nipple under warm water and leave them on a clean towel by the sink, ready for your next sterilizing session.

- Wash all the bottles and nipples in hot soapy water using a bottle brush and rinse thoroughly in hot water.

- Pad the bottom of a large pan with a towel or dishcloth. Immerse open bottles and nipples in the pan (place bottles on their side to be sure that they are filled with the sterilizing water) and boil for ten minutes with the pan covered. Allow to cool to room temperature while still covered. Place the bottles upside down on a clean towel with the nipples and caps alongside. Let the equipment dry.

Mixing Formulas

Use the following procedure to prepare liquid concentrate or powdered formula. Ready-to-feed formula can be poured directly into a sterile bottle with no mixing (before opening the can, thoroughly clean the top).

- Boil the water for five minutes, then let it cool.

- Align the six sterilized bottles in a row and pour the prescribed amount of cool boiled water into each bottle. (Theoretically, hot water could damage some of the nutrients in the formula.) Add the prescribed amount of liquid or powdered formula. For example, if using liquid concentrate in eight-ounce bottles, pour four ounces of boiled water in each bottle and add four ounces of liquid concentrate.

- Put nipples and caps on each bottle, shake well (especially for powdered formula), then place in refrigerator.

- Use refrigerated formula preferably within twenty-four hours, or a maximum of forty-eight hours.

The Right Mix

Never mix the formula in greater strength than the directions state. Always add the specified amount of water. Adding too little water makes the formula too concentrated for your baby's immature intestines and kid-

---

TIPS FOR QUICK AND EASY STERILIZING AND FORMULA PREPARATION

- Use disposable presterilized nurser bags to hold the formula in a plastic holder; this is convenient and minimizes air swallowing, as the bag collapses during the feeding.
- Use a dishwasher to sterilize bottles and nipples, and use ready-to-feed liquid formula. No water to boil, no extra sterilizing or measuring needed.

neys to handle, causing baby to get dehydrated. Sometimes your doctor may recommend overdiluting the formula during a vomiting or diarrheal illness. Overdiluting should not be done for more than a few days without your physician's advice, as overdilute formula does not provide enough calories for your baby.

BOTTLEFEEDING TIPS

To make feeding time pleasant for you and baby, here's how to get the most milk in and the most air up, and to do it safely.

Giving the Bottle

- Most babies enjoy their formula slightly warmed; run warm tap water over the bottle for several minutes. Shake a few drops on your inner wrist to check the temperature.

- To minimize air swallowing, tilt the bottle, allowing the milk to fill the nipple and the air to rise above the formula.

- Keep baby's head straight in relation to the rest of the body. Drinking while the head is turned sideways or tilted back makes it more difficult for baby to swallow.

- To lessen arm fatigue and present different views to baby, switch arms at each feeding or after burping midway through the bottle.

- Watch for signs that the nipple hole is too large or too small. If baby gets a sudden mouthful of milk and sputters and almost chokes during a feeding, milk flow may be too fast. Turn the full bottle upside down without shaking. If milk flows instead of drips, the nipple hole is too large; discard the nipple. If baby seems to be working hard and tires easily during sucking, and the cheeks cave in because of a strong suction vacuum, the nipple hole may be too small (as previously mentioned, formula should drip at least one drop per second).

- Know when to quit. Babies know when they've had enough. Avoid the temptation to always finish the bottle. If baby falls asleep near the end of the feeding, but has not finished the bottle, stop. Often babies fall into a light sleep toward the end of the bottle, but continue a flutter type of sucking. They have had enough to eat, but enjoy a little "dessert" of comfort sucking. Remove the bottle and allow baby to suck a few minutes on your fingertip.

Burping Baby

Besides the relaxing pat on the back, effective burping requires two actions: holding baby in an upright position and applying pressure on baby's tummy (parents often forget this latter step). With baby seated on your lap, lean her weight forward, with the heel of your hand against her tummy; firmly pat or rub baby's back. Or drape her up over your shoulder and firmly pat or rub her back.

If at first you don't succeed, try again in a while. If after a minute or two no burp appears, put baby down or carry her upright and go about your business. If baby is content, she doesn't need to burp. If, however, baby is not content after a feeding (squirming, grimacing, and groaning when you lay her down, or refusing to complete a feeding), take these signals to mean that baby needs to

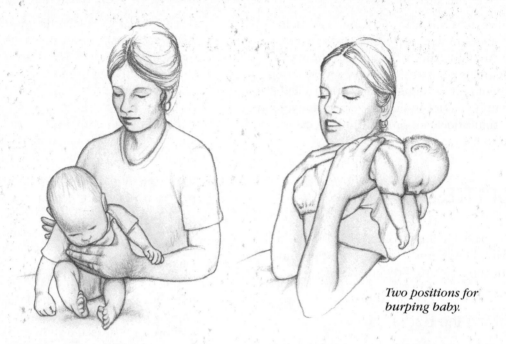

Two positions for burping baby.

burp. Snack-type feedings often skip a burp; big meals usually merit patience until baby burps. Some babies need to burp halfway through a bottlefeeding, or after finishing one breast, dubbed "burp and switch."

For nighttime burping, one or two minutes of sucking may not warrant a burp but a big feeding usually does. If you are not in the mood for nighttime burping, try putting baby down immediately after feeding. If she is content, no burp is needed. If she squirms as if uncomfortable, a trapped air bubble is probably causing discomfort. To avoid sitting up and going through the whole burping ritual, continue lying down but drape baby over your hip as you would over your shoulder. The need to burp lessens as baby gets older.

Try the *one-arm burp.* If you don't have time to sit and wait for your baby to burp, drape baby over your forearm so that your wrist presses against his tummy. Carry baby in this position while you stroll around the house. The only drawback is that spit-up may dribble onto your arm or the floor. (See the illustration of the colic carry hold on pages 402 and 403.)

Safe Feeding Tips

- If you question the safety of your tap water, use bottled water.

- *Do not microwave formula;* there is too great a risk of heating unevenly.

- It is all right to reuse leftover formula within a few hours if it is immediately refrigerated after the first use. Cap the bottle to keep the nipple clean. For *maximum safety,* however, do not reuse leftover formula, because bacteria may have been introduced through baby's saliva.

- If you are traveling and refrigeration is not readily available, presterilized, ready-to-feed four-ounce cans of formula are the safest and easiest. Powdered formula takes up less space, but use only if clean water is available. If taking along home-mixed formula, store it in insulated containers with a small ice pack.

- *Do not bottle prop.* Don't let your baby lie in a crib feeding himself with his own bottle. Leaving a baby unattended during feeding is potentially dangerous if the baby chokes and needs your help. Also, lying down during feeding allows milk to enter the middle ear through the eustachian tube which can trigger ear infections. (This is less true for breastfeeding.) Bottle propping deprives both you and your baby of the valuable social interaction that occurs during feeding.

- Lessen the number of nighttime bottles once baby has teeth. (See "Nightweaning Toddlers," page 360.)

WEANING BABY FROM THE BOTTLE

Like weaning from the breast, there is no rush. It is not unusual or abnormal for baby to still want a bottle at two years of age. Bottles bother adults more than toddlers. If you wean your baby to a cup early, be prepared to let him continue to use a pacifier to meet his sucking needs. The nighttime bottle is the most difficult to part with. Wean baby from nap and night bottles by a trick we call *watering down* (see page 364).

Continued use of bottles beyond eighteen months to two years can lead to two problems:

1. *Tooth decay.* If your toddler falls asleep with a bottle in his mouth, the unswallowed milk will remain on his teeth. The milk sugar can begin to cause tooth decay. To prevent this, remove the bottle before he falls asleep.

2. *Overbite.* Using a bottle beyond two years can begin to reshape the upper gum line and palate. This can lead to an overbite and buckteeth.

If your toddler is still using a bottle, ask your doctor to check his teeth for these changes. There is no set time that is best to wean every child off the bottle. Here are some suggestions to help you choose what time is appropriate for your child:

- When transitioning your baby from formula to whole milk, try giving whole milk in a cup only. This way, when baby is off formula, he's also off the bottle.

- Remember the toddler mind-set: Just try weaning a two-year-old off the bottle! Many parents find it easier to wean an infant between twelve and eighteen months before the stubborn streak sets in.

- If your toddler is a picky eater and not yet skilled in cup drinking, allow daytime bottles of milk or formula (a maximum of four eight-ounce bottles, about one liter) to ensure enough nutrition. When he is cup skilled and consistently eating a balanced diet of solids, gradually wean from bottle to cup.

- Have a "you can't walk around with your drink" policy. Discourage baby from walking around with a bottle. Some juice addicts cling to this sticky companion. Not only will there be trails throughout the house, but this habit, bad for nutrition and harmful to teeth, is hard to break.

- If baby has a love affair with the bottle and needs it for a pacifier, gradually "lose" the bottle and substitute other "pacifiers," preferably human ones.

A PERSON AT BOTH ENDS OF THE BOTTLE

The term "nursing" means comforting and nourishing, whether by breast or bottle. Feeding time is more than just a time for nutrition. It is also a time for special closeness. The mutual giving that is a part of breastfeeding should also be enjoyed during bottlefeeding. Besides giving your infant a bottle, give him your eyes, your skin, your voice, and your caresses. Baby will return to you more than just an empty bottle.

The special warmth of skin-to-skin contact can be accomplished by wearing short sleeves and partially undressing yourself and your baby when feeding. Hold the bottle alongside your breast as though it were coming from your body, and look into your baby's eyes. Interact with your baby during a feeding. You want your baby to feel that the bottle is part of you. Most babies, breastfed and bottlefed, feed better if you are quiet while they suck, but babies enjoy social interaction during pauses in the feedings. Watch your baby for signals that he wants to socialize during the feeding. Eventually you will develop an intuitive sense of your baby's feeding rhythm. Baby should feel that a person is feeding him, not just a bottle.

11

Introducing Solid Foods: When, What, and How

During a four- or six-month checkup, I expect the question, "Doctor, when should I start solid food?" One day I decided to take the initiative and ask an experienced mother of six, "How do you *know* when to begin giving your baby solid foods?"

"When he starts mooching!" she replied.

"Mooching?" I asked, a bit surprised.

"Yes," she went on to explain. "I wait for signs that he is interested. I watch him watch me eat. When his eyes follow my food as I move it from my plate to my mouth, when his hands reach out and grab my food and he is able to sit up in a high chair and join us at the table, I know it's time for the fun of solids to begin."

By her own experience, this wise mother discovered a basic principle of introducing solid foods — feed babies according to their own developmental skills rather than a preset calendar or clock. Babies' appetites and feeding skills are as individual as their temperaments. Let's feed them that way.

Over the past ten years infant-feeding practices have changed — for the better. No longer do we feed babies according to the calendar, stuffing cereal into the reluctant six-week-old and feeling we have failed if baby has not taken a full-course meal by six months. Today, infant feeding involves matching good nutrition with individual developmental and intestinal readiness, which varies widely from baby to baby. Reading the feeding cues of your baby, introducing solid foods gradually, and encouraging self-feeding all lead to that important principle of baby feeding: *creating a healthy feeding attitude.*

We have put the latest nutritional research on infant feeding together with what we have learned throughout thirty years of practice, and our own experience in feeding our babies. In this and the next two chapters we wish to present a style of infant feeding that will help you become more nutrition savvy, better enjoy feeding your infant, and have happier, healthier babies.

WHY WAIT?

You and your three-month-old are comfortably breastfeeding, and baby certainly seems to be getting enough to eat. Now comes the daily phone call from the family nutritionist — your mother. "What is he eating now, dear?" Silence. You've been caught! The jars of baby food that grandmother bought

INFANT FEEDING AT A GLANCE

Age	Food Sequence
Birth to 6 months	Breast milk and/or iron-fortified formula satisfies all nutritional requirements. Solid foods not nutritionally needed under 6 months of age.
6 months	Starter foods: bananas pears rice cereal applesauce
7 to 9 months	avocados mashed potatoes peaches barley cereal carrots teething biscuits squash pear and apple juice, prunes diluted sweet potatoes or yams
9 to 12 months	lamb, veal tofu poultry beans rice cakes peas egg yolk oatmeal cheese spinach yogurt
12 to 18 months	whole milk apricots cottage cheese grapefruit ice cream grape halves whole eggs strawberries beef tomatoes fish (salmon) pasta broccoli graham crackers cauliflower wheat cereal melon honey mango pancakes kiwi muffins papaya bagel

Food Presentation	Developmental Skills, Implications for Feeding
Breast and/or bottle	Designed to suck, not chew Rooting reflex; searches for food source Tongue-thrust reflex pushes out solid foods Sensitive gag reflex
Strained, pureed Fingertipful Small spoonful	Tongue-thrust and gag reflexes lessen; accepts solids Sits erect in high chair Begins teething
May drink from cup Finger foods begin Pureed and mashed foods Holds bottle	Thumb-and-forefinger pickup begins Fascination with tiny food morsels Begins mouthing chokable food and objects (parents beware!) Bangs, drops, flings Reaches for food and utensils Munches food
Lumpier consistency Finger foods mastered Bite-size cooked vegetables Melt-in-mouth foods Holds trainer cup	Self-feeding skills improve Holds bottle and cup longer Points and pokes, smears, enjoys mess High-chair gymnastics increase Tries to use utensils, spills most
Participates in family meals Eats chopped and mashed family foods Begins self-feeding with utensils	Has prolonged attention span "Do it myself" desire intensifies Tilts cup and head while drinking; spills less Holds spoon better, still spills much Begins walking — doesn't want to sit still and eat Picks at others' plates

INFANT FEEDING AT A GLANCE *(continued)*

Age	Food Sequence
18 to 24 months	Eats toddler-size portions of: sandwiches stews nutritious puddings sauces dips smoothies toppings shakes spreads pâté soups Toddler food "language": avocado boats O-shaped cereal cooked carrot toast sticks wheels cookie-cutter cheese blocks sandwich broccoli trees canoe eggs

are still unopened. Baby has not seemed interested, and you do not feel he is ready. You smoothly change the subject, defending your choice not to enter the race for solids just yet. (When this confrontation happens in my practice, I advise parents, "Make your doctor the scapegoat. Tell grandmother that Dr. Bill advised you to wait a while longer.")

Baby's tongue movements and swallowing skills are the first clues to delaying solid foods. In the early months, babies have a tongue-thrust reflex that causes the tongue to automatically protrude outward when any foreign substance is placed upon it. This may be a protective reflex against choking on solids given too early. Between four and six months this tongue-thrust reflex diminishes. Also, prior to six months of age many infants do not have good coordination of tongue and swallowing movements for solid foods. An added sign that babies were not designed for early introduction to solid foods is that teeth seldom appear until six or seven months, further evidence that the young infant is primarily designed to suck, rather than to chew.

Not only is the upper end of baby's digestive tract not designed for early solids, neither are baby's insides. A baby's immature intestines are not equipped to handle a variety of foods until around six months, when many digestive enzymes seem to click in. Pediatric allergists discourage early introduction of foods especially if there is a strong family history of food allergies. Research shows that starting solids before six months increases the risk of allergies. Maturing intestines secrete the protein immunoglobulin IgA, which acts like a protective paint, coating the intestines and preventing the passage of harmful allergens (cow's milk, wheat, and soy are common examples of foods causing aller-

Food Presentation	Developmental Skills, Implications for Feeding
Grazes — deserves title "picky eater" Nibble tray Weans from bottle Uses spoon and fork	Molars appear — begins rotary chewing Spoon-feeds self without spilling much Learns food talk, signals for "more," "all done" Wants to eat on the run — needs creative feeding to hold attention at table Has erratic feeding habits

gies when introduced early). This protective IgA is low in the early months and does not reach peak production until around seven months of age. As the intestines mature, they become more nutritionally selective, filtering out offending food allergens. Babies whose systems tend to be allergy-prone actually may show delayed willingness to accept solids — a built-in self-protective mechanism.

FEEDING SOLIDS: SIX TO NINE MONTHS

Breast milk or commercial formula with iron or a combination of the two contains all the essential nutrients your baby needs for the first six to nine months. Consider solid foods as an addition to, not a substitute for, breast milk or formula. For a breastfeeding baby, it's best to start solid foods slowly so they don't replace the more nutritious breast milk.

Ready-to-Eat Signs

Baby may start *begging* — reaching for the food on your plate, grabbing your spoon, looking at you hungrily, and mimicking feeding behaviors such as opening her mouth wide when you open your mouth to eat. Sometimes babies are more interested in the utensils than the actual food. If your baby shows interest in watching you eat, try offering her just a spoon to play with (preferably a sturdy plastic spoon — they make less noise when banged). If baby is content with the spoon, then the toy is desired more than the food. When baby continues showing interest, it's time for the fun to begin. Also, the ability to sit up in a high chair and pick up food with thumb and forefinger are other signs that baby is ready for solids.

First Feeding

Start with solids that are the least allergenic (see list on page 271) and the closest to breast milk in taste and consistency. Examples of favorite first foods include mashed ripe bananas or rice cereal mixed with breast milk or formula. (See "Constipation When Starting Solids," page 224.)

Place a fingertipful of banana (mashed to soupy) on baby's lips, letting her suck your finger as she usually does. Once she is introduced to the new taste, gradually increase the amount and thickness of the food, placing a glob toward the middle of baby's tongue. Watch baby's reaction. If the food goes in accompanied by an approving smile, baby is

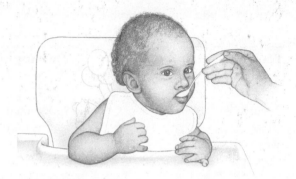

By age six months, many babies are ready to start taking strained or pureed solid foods from a spoon.

ready and willing. If the food comes back at you accompanied by a disapproving grimace, baby is not ready.

If baby spews the glob back at you, don't take this first impression personally. Your infant has not yet learned the developmental skill of sealing the mouth shut, sweeping the food from front to back, and then swallowing. If your baby just sits there confused, her mouth open, with a glob of food perched on her tongue, her persistent tongue-thrust reflex is giving the developmental clue to shut the door and come back later.

Progressing with Solids

Beginning with rice cereal or bananas as a test dose, progress from a fingertipful to a half teaspoon to one teaspoon, then a tablespoon, then around two ounces, or half a jar. Advance from soupy to pasty to lumpy consistency. Remember, your initial goal is to *introduce* baby to the new taste and touch of solids, not to stuff baby. Gradually vary the texture and amount to fit the eating skills and

---

FIRST SPOON

We advise that baby's first "spoon" be your finger. It is soft, at the right temperature, and by this stage baby is very familiar with its feel. Your finger also knows if food is too hot. Few babies like to begin their feeding life with a silver spoon in their mouth. Metal holds the heat in, so each bite takes longer if you have to blow to cool food that is too hot. A hungry baby finds this infuriating! A coated baby spoon is a good starter utensil. Use shatterproof plastic bowls that can survive battering on the high-chair tray and numerous tumbles to the floor.

appetite of your baby. Some like solids of thinner consistency and want a larger amount; some do better with thicker solids and smaller amounts. Expect erratic eating habits. Your baby may take a whole jar one day, but only a teaspoon the next.

Keeping a Favorite-Food Diary

We have found it helpful to make a food diary with four columns on a page. In the first column list the foods that baby seems to like; in the second column, foods that you have found by trial and error that baby does not like; in the third column, possibly allergenic foods and the signs of allergies; and in the fourth column, the techniques you have learned to get more food into your baby with the minimum of hassles. The food diary helps you learn your baby's food preferences and capabilities at each stage of development and is another way of getting to know and enjoy your baby. In case your baby may be intolerant of or allergic to a certain food, space each new food at least a week apart and keep a diary of which foods baby may be sensitive to or simply doesn't like. Also, the timing and progression of solids is much slower in the allergic baby. (Food allergies are discussed in detail beginning on page 267.)

FAVORITE FIRST FOODS

rice cereal	peaches
barley cereal	applesauce
bananas	carrots
pears	squash
avocados	sweet potatoes

How Much to Feed

After baby eagerly accepts the first fingertip-ful of food, gradually increase the amount. Remember that tiny babies have tiny tummies, about the size of their fists. So don't expect baby to take more than one fistful of food at one feeding. Expect erratic eating patterns. Baby may eat a couple tablespoons one day and only one the next.

When to Feed

Offer solids at the time of the day when your baby seems hungriest, bored, or when you both need a change of pace. Choose a time of the day that is most convenient for you, since a little mess is part of the feeding game. Mornings are usually the best time for offering solids to formula-fed babies, because you have the most time with your infant and usually do not have to worry about preparing a meal for the rest of the family. If breastfeeding, offer solids when your milk supply is lowest, usually toward the end of the day. Feed your baby solids between breastfeeding. Solid foods may interfere with absorption of valuable breast milk iron if both solids and breast milk are fed at the same time.

Grazing. Since babies have no concept of breakfast, lunch, and dinner it makes no difference whether they receive vegetables for breakfast, or cereal and fruit for dinner. If you have a mental picture of your baby sitting still in a high chair eating three square meals a day, forget it! Babies don't sit still very long in one place even to play, let alone to eat. Allow your baby the fine art of *grazing*. Remember, tiny eaters have tiny tummies. Nibbling throughout the day is nutritionally better than eating three big meals. Three squares a day is more of an adult pattern, and,

CONSTIPATION WHEN STARTING SOLIDS

Many infants become constipated when solid foods are introduced. Interestingly, the usual starter foods — bananas and rice cereal — may cause constipation in most infants. So why start baby off on these foods at a time when constipation is already a risk? Tradition. Rice cereal and bananas have always been recommended as baby's first foods. If your baby starts to show signs of constipation when starting solids, back off on whatever food you began with, and give strained or pureed prunes or peaches (or any other fruit listed on the previous page). When the problem resolves, slowly re-introduce other foods, while continuing with the fruit. You will learn what your baby needs to keep her regular.

for that matter, even for us it is not as healthy as more frequent, smaller meals. (See "Try the Nibble Tray," page 254.)

Forget fast feeding. Try to time baby's feedings for when you are not in a hurry. Infant feedings are very time-consuming. Babies dawdle, dabble, spew, spatter, smear, drop, and fling.

FEEDING STRATEGIES

To get more food into your baby than onto the floor, mix together your child's developing skills with a large pinch of patience and sprinkle in a few laughs. Here are some tips we have learned for getting more food into our babies with fewer hassles.

Enjoy table talk. Eating is a social interaction. As you offer your baby solids, consider that he may be thinking, "Something new is coming from someone I love and trust." Talk about both the food and the procedure so that baby learns to relate the words with the type of foods and the interactions that follow. Here is an example from the Sears family table: "Stephen want carrots . . . open your mouth!" as I would approach Stephen's mouth with the solids-laden spoon. As I asked Stephen to open his mouth, I also opened my mouth wide, and he mimicked my facial gestures. Eager eyes, open hands, and open mouth are body language clues that baby is ready to eat.

Show and tell. To entice the reluctant eater to eat, model enjoyment. Capitalizing on baby's newly developing social skill — mimicking her caregivers' actions — feed yourself in front of baby, but in an exaggerated way, slowly putting a spoonful of baby's food into your mouth. With big wide-open eyes showing how much you enjoy the taste, overreact, saying "Mmmmm, good!" Let baby catch the spirit and want to do likewise.

Open mouth, insert spoon. Wait for a time when baby is hungry and in a mood for facial gestures and interaction. As you engage your baby face-to-face, open your mouth wide and say, "Open mouth!" Once your baby opens the "door," put the food in.

Use lip service. Try the "upper lip sweep." As you place a spoonful of solids in your baby's mouth, gently lift the spoon upward, allowing the upper lip to sweep off the food.

Observe stop signs. Pursed lips, closed mouth, head turning away from the approaching spoon, are all signs that your baby does not want to eat right now. Perhaps at this time baby wants to play, sleep, or simply is not interested or hungry. *Don't force-feed.* Some babies eagerly take solids by six months, while others show little interest as late as nine to twelve months. You want your baby to develop a healthy attitude toward both the food and the feeding.

Avoid nighttime stuffing. Cereals are often advised as fillers, something to feed your baby to lengthen the intervals between breastfeeding or bottles and to encourage baby to sleep through the night. Not only does this filler fallacy seldom work, it may create problems in appetite control at an early age, thus contributing to eventual obesity. Baby may need other forms of interaction between bottlefeedings, not just to be filled up. Remember that milk, either breast

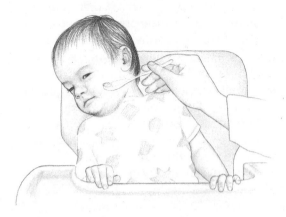

This baby is obviously not wanting to eat right now. Don't force the issue.

or formula, is still the most important nutrient at this stage. Avoid the urge to fill your baby up with solids before bedtime in a desperate hope that baby will sleep through the night. As tired parents, we, too, have considered this temptation. Controlled studies have shown, however, that infants who are fed solids before bedtime do not sleep through the night any sooner than infants who do not get the before-bed stuffing.

Encourage self-feeding. Around six months babies begin to develop two exciting skills that, when perfected, will make feeding much easier: the ability to sit up well in a high chair or on your lap and the ability to reach for food in front of them. Some babies simply hate having food come at them on a spoon and resist solids until you figure out that Mr. Independent wants to do it himself. Place a bit of mashed banana within grabbing distance on his table or high-chair tray. Around six months babies pounce on anything of interest placed in front of them. You will notice your baby capture this enticing material in his fist and gradually zero in on his mouth. By nine to ten months baby will be using his thumb and index finger to pick up small tidbits. In the beginning stages of finding his mouth, baby may have more misses than hits, resulting in much of the food being splattered over his cheeks or on the floor. As one mother of a messy self-feeder put it, "The floor has a more balanced diet than my baby does." It helps to remember that at this stage baby doesn't need the solid food — feeding is still in the explore category.

Get the messy feeder to clean up his act. To keep baby from grabbing at the spoon, sending the contents flying, give him something to hold on to, another spoon or even a toy. Don't ever punish him for making a mess or wanting to be part of the action. If you are really intent on getting something into your baby, gently hold both his hands in your free hand while you "chat him up" or even sing his favorite ditty to distract him from wanting to "help" too much. Expect baby to treat solids as toys. He's feeding his intellect while you are more intent on feeding his body. Don't fret! Your breast milk has all the nutritional bases covered. You can afford to let baby have his science lesson. When the flinging and spitting escalate, simply take the food away. When he's really hungry, instinct will take over, and he'll realize the food will do wonders to satisfy that big empty spot in his tummy.

Help your baby develop an interest in solids. Capitalize on a new social skill that develops between six and nine months — baby's desire to mimic the actions of her caregivers. Let your baby watch you eat and enjoy food. Teach by example: Prepare a small amount of infant food, such as rice cereal or mashed bananas, and take a bite yourself as you exclaim, "Ummmmmm gooooood!" Some babies at this age are somewhat reluctant to try anything new. Take a few bites of any new food yourself. Let baby catch the spirit by watching you enjoy this new food.

Rotate foods. Infants become bored with too much of the same food. Expect your baby to refuse previous favorites periodically. Take this as a sign that baby needs more variety in the menu.

Avoid mixed foods. Introduce single foods rather than several foods mixed together. In case baby is allergic to or dislikes a food, offering a single food makes it easier to identify the culprit. Once you know certain foods are OK, you can combine them in one meal. In fact, a little dollop of fruit on the tip of a spoonful of meat or vegetables can sometimes get the less favored taste past the sentry.

Pass on the salt; skip the sugar. Parents, you are the taste makers of the next generation. If your infant grows up accustomed to sweetened and salted foods, it may be difficult to kick this taste later on.

FEEDING SOLIDS: NINE TO TWELVE MONTHS

The previous stage was mainly to introduce your infant to solids — to get baby used to the transition from liquids to solids, from sucking to mouthing, and chewing food. Most beginning eaters dabble a bit with foods, eating only a small amount of a few select solids. Breast milk and/or formula make up about 90 percent of their diet.

In the later part of the first year, baby's swallowing mechanism greatly matures. The tongue-thrust reflex is nearly gone, the gag reflex diminishes, and swallowing is more coordinated. This allows a gradual progression from strained or pureed foods to mashed and coarser and lumpier foods. Advance the texture of solid food — but not too fast. Going too slowly deprives baby of the chance to experiment with different textures and prolongs the strained baby food stage. Advancing too quickly causes baby to retreat from new foods and new textures for fear of choking.

New Skills — New Foods

At this stage babies enjoy more variety and volume of solids. Solid foods become a major component of the infant's diet, often making up around 50 percent of baby's nutrition after one year of age. (This is an average; many breastfed babies are still at the 80–90 percent milk level at one year.) During this stage new developmental milestones bring about new feeding patterns. The thumb-and-forefinger pincer grasp, more highly evolved now, allows baby to pick up small morsels. Babies often show a preoccupation with any newly acquired developmental skill. Consequently, babies develop a fascination for small objects. Pick up on this new desire by presenting your baby with baby-bite-sized morsels. The fun of finger foods begins.

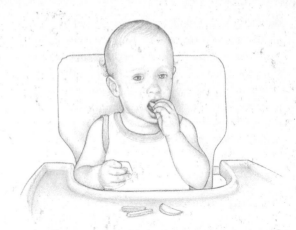

As baby's manual dexterity develops, finger foods take on greater appeal.

Finger Foods

To encourage picking up and eating rather than messing and smearing, place a few pieces of O-shaped cereal, cooked diced carrot, rice cake, or baby-bite-sized pieces of soft fruits on the high-chair tray. Babies also enjoy firmer finger foods for teething, such as teething biscuits. Harder foods, especially teething foods, should have a melt-in-the-mouth texture, dissolving easily while being gummed. We noticed that our babies were fascinated with a pile of cooked spaghetti placed within easy reach. The ability to pick up with thumb and forefinger enables baby to pick up one strand, shell, or elbow at a time. Pasta picking holds baby's meal attention longer than most foods. Some of the pasta may even make its way to the mouth. If worried about allergies, wait until one year to introduce wheat products such as zwieback, bagels, and pasta. If you know

your baby tends toward allergies, you can buy wheat-free teething biscuits and pasta made with rice.

The ability to pick up food also has its hassles. Food and utensils become interesting objects to bang, drop, and fling. This does not necessarily mean rejection of the food or the feeding but reflects baby's natural and normal need to explore new ways to use the newly developed skills of picking up, dropping, and throwing. When it gets too messy for you, simply end the feeding.

Pointing and Dipping

Besides developing thumb-and-forefinger pickup, around ten months babies are using their index finger for poking and social directing — giving cues to their caregivers. Baby is likely to poke into a new food as if dipping in and tasting it. Capitalize on this skill by making dip. Avocado or guacamole dip (without the salt and heavy spices) is a nutritious favorite at this stage. Remember, each new developmental skill has its nutritional benefits and humorous nuisances. While babies will use their poking finger to dip into food and suck the food off their finger, expect the young artist to begin body painting and finger painting with the food on the high-chair tray. Enjoy this developmental skill while it lasts. And feel free to stop the meal if baby is no longer eating.

Feeding Strategies

Now that you have introduced your baby to the different tastes and textures of his favorite solids, here are some tips gleaned from our family feeding experiences:

Respect tiny tummies. Offer small helpings in frequent feedings. Since babies' tummies are about the size of their fists, they seldom take more than two to four tablespoons of a food at any one meal. Don't overwhelm baby with a whole pile of food on her tray. Instead, begin with a small fist-sized dollop and add more as baby wants more.

Gradually increase variety and texture. For beginning solid eaters, fruits and vegetables should be strained. As babies gain eating experience, they can advance to pureed foods, then to foods that are finely minced. Most babies can begin to accept chopped foods by one year of age.

Avoid pressure tactics. Never force-feed a child, as this can create long-term unhealthy attitudes about eating. Your role is to select nutritious foods, prepare them well, and serve them creatively, matched to baby's individual capabilities and preferences. Baby's role is to eat the amount he wants at the time, according to his needs, moods, capabilities, and pref-

erences. Feeding children is similar to teaching them to swim — you need to find the balance between being too protective or restrictive and not vigilant or selective enough.

Dr. Bob notes: If your baby shuns eating, try a bit of group encouragement. Sit baby in a high chair. Let everyone start eating, but don't give baby anything. She will feel left out and want some food. When she starts reaching for some food, give her something off your plate. Let her think it's your food, even though it may be her own food on your plate. When she starts eating, don't suddenly put a whole plate in front of her. Let her keep asking for more, and give her only one or two bites at a time. This way, baby feels in charge of deciding to eat on her own.

Expect erratic feeding habits. There may be days when your baby eats solids six times, or she may refuse solids three days in a row and only want to breastfeed or take a bottle.

Teach table manners. Babies are born clowns. When a baby drops a utensil or a glob of food, everyone quickly reacts. Baby soon realizes that he is in control of this game and continues to put food everywhere but in his mouth. Shoveling is a familiar dinner-table-clown game. Sometimes the otherwise adept self feeder becomes impatient, shovels up a whole handful of food, and splats the palmful of food half into his mouth and half on his face. Baby continues to gorge and smear until his clowning gets the expected audience reaction. Laughter not only reinforces this habit but can be dangerous since baby may laugh with a mouthful of food, take a deep breath, and choke.

The ability to stimulate caregivers to react to one's antics is a powerful enforcer of

SAFE TODDLER (ONE YEAR AND OLDER) FEEDING TIPS

- Avoid stringy foods such as celery and string beans.
- Pick out fish bones before mashing fish. In canned salmon, mash the bones.
- Safe and natural frozen teethers are bananas or any melt-in-the-mouth frozen food.
- Avoid commercial *white*-bread preparations; they form a pasty glob on which baby could choke.
- *Spread* nut butters well, instead of offering baby a chokable glob.
- Cut meat and poultry *across the grain* and into tiny fingertip pieces rather than large chokable chunks.
- Check the chunks. Babies' front teeth are for biting only. The molars — chewing teeth — don't appear until after the first year. Babies still gum rather than chew.
- Offer finger foods only under supervision and when baby is seated, not when reclining or playing.
- Scatter only a few morsels of finger foods on baby's plate or tray at one time. Too much food in a pile encourages whole-handed gorging rather than individual pickup bites.
- Hot dogs are neither a nutritious nor safe food for *babies.* A bite of a whole hot dog is just about the size of a baby's windpipe, and baby may choke. Healthy nitrate- and nitrite-free hot dogs are a favorite of *toddlers,* and they can be safe if sliced *lengthwise* in thin, noodle-like strips. Even these "healthy" hot dogs can be high in sodium, so limit them.

SAFE AND FAVORITE FINGER FOODS

O-shaped cereals
rice cakes (unsalted)
diced carrots (well cooked)
whole wheat toast (remove crust)
whole wheat bagel
scrambled eggs
french toast

cooked peas (dehulled)
pear slices (very ripe)
apple slices (cooked well)
pasta pieces (cooked)
tofu chunks
green beans (well cooked, no strings)
avocado dip or chunks

CHOKABLE FOODS

nuts
seeds
popcorn kernels
hot dogs (whole or chunks)
hard beans
hard candy

raw carrots
raw apples
whole grapes
unripe pears
stringy foods
meat chunks

baby's emerging sense of competence. Enough is enough, however. Reacting too quickly to the messer and flinger only encourages this mealtime clown to continue his performance. Whether you laugh or scold, either way baby takes this as a reaction from the audience, and the performance continues. No comment is the best way to keep this little ham off the stage. If his antics get out of hand, assume he's not hungry and remove his food. Don't expect him to sit still as long as older children can. Even at this early age table manners are learned by example. If he sees the other children (or adults) laughing with a mouthful of food, flinging food, banging utensils, and enjoying all of it, this little imitator will do likewise. Also, remember to praise good manners.

Minimize the mess. Each new developing skill has its nutritional benefits and humorous nuisances. Baby's newly developing thumb and forefinger pincer grasp and finger pointing stimulates him to want to pick up tiny morsels of food and feed himself, yet it also creates an opportunity for more messes. Allow baby the luxury of messing around a bit with his newly discovered utensils. Believe it or not, baby is actually learning from this mess. While some food makes its way into the mouth, other pieces scatter. Food flinging, dropping, and smearing are usual mealtime antics parents can expect to deal with. Allow a certain amount of mess, but not when it gets out of control. Too much food on a baby's tray leads to two-fisted eating and major mess making. To discourage food flinging and give the food a fighting chance to make it into baby's mouth, put a *few* pieces of O-cereals, cooked carrots, pieces of rice cakes, and any other bite-size pieces of fruits and vegetables that baby likes on his tray. Then, refill as needed. Placing a whole pile of food in front of baby is inviting a mess.

Settle the squirmer. This trick worked for one of our babies who would constantly windmill her arms during feeding. Use three plastic spoons — one spoon for each of her hands to occupy them and one for you to feed her. Also, try this toy trick. Put toys with suction cups on a high-chair tray so she can play with them with her hands while you spoon food into her mouth. Sometimes when babies open their mouths to suck on toys, this primes them to open their mouths to receive food.

Make feeding fun. Play games, such as the spoon-airplane game. Say "Here comes the airplane" as the spoon makes its dive into baby's mouth.

Overcome lip lock. To relax tight lips that are refusing a feeding, back off and over-enjoy the food yourself. Model the excitement by replaying the old reliable "Mmmmmm goooood!" As your baby watches you open your mouth and savor the food, he may catch the spirit and relax his mouth and his attitude. Use one of your child's favorite foods as a teaser. As he opens his mouth for his favorite food, quickly follow with the food you wanted him to try.

Use camouflage. Cover more nutritious but less liked foods with one of baby's favorites. Try dabbing a thin layer of applesauce (or other favorite) on the spoonful of vegetables. Baby gets the applesauce on his tongue first and then a scoop of the more nutritious but less liked food on top of it. If he still hates it, forget it for a while.

Trick tiny taste buds. The taste buds for sweet flavors are found toward the tip of the tongue; the taste buds for salt are on the sides of the tongue; the taste buds for bitter are at the back of the tongue. In the middle of the tongue, the taste buds are more neutral. So it is wise to place a new sweet food on the tip of the tongue, but a new less sweet food on the neutral area in the middle in order to give the food a fighting chance of going into baby instead of coming back out. Veggies, for example, have a better chance of being willingly swallowed if placed on the middle of the tongue rather than on the tip of the tongue, except perhaps for sweet ones, like sweet potatoes.

Give your baby a bone. Baby can graduate from a nearly empty chicken bone (sliver bone removed) to one with a decent amount of meat left on it (still no sliver bone). It has great play value (for banging, gnawing on, waving, transferring from hand to hand) to buy you a few more minutes of savoring your own food, and baby may actually eat some of the chicken.

Forgive food fears. It is normal for some babies to fear new foods. Expect your baby to explore a new food before she eats it. Allow your baby to become familiar with the new food before actually tasting it. One way to encourage the cautious feeder is to place a bit of the food on baby's own index finger and guide his own fingerful of food into his mouth.

Enjoy the lap of luxury. If your child refuses to get in or stay in his high chair, let him sit on your lap and eat off your plate. If baby begins messing with your food, place a few morsels of food on the table between baby and plate to direct his attention away from your dinner.

Share a plate. Let baby eat off your plate. Sometimes babies just don't want to eat like a baby; they'll reject both baby food and baby plates. Around one year of age, babies enjoy sitting on parents' laps and picking food off their plate, especially mashed potatoes and cooked, soft vegetables. Try putting baby's food on your plate and trick the little gourmet into eating his own food.

Assist in self-feeding. Around one year of age babies enter the "do it myself" stage and may want to feed themselves with a spoon. Most parents find it much easier to feed a baby than to let baby take over the job with her own utensils. Compromise is needed here. A trick we have used with the determined self-feeder is to do the job together. The parent holds the spoonful of food, and when baby grabs the spoon, mom or dad continues to hold on and helps baby guide the spoon into her mouth. Take advantage of baby's desire to mimic you at this age. When he sees you using a spoon properly, baby is more likely to try it too. (For more feeding strategies, see "Nourishing the Picky Eater," pages 252–261.)

MAKING YOUR OWN BABY FOOD

Good nutrition, or the lack of it, can affect the health and behavior of your child. It is worth spending a couple of hours each week to prepare your infant's food. You know what's in it, and you can customize the texture and taste to your baby's palate. Before your baby's impressionable taste buds get spoiled with sugared and salted packaged foods, get your

infant used to the natural taste of freshly prepared foods. Besides, fresh foods taste better.
(See "Shape Young Tastes," page 242.)

Healthy Cooking

Before serving or cooking, wash fruits and
vegetables well. Scrub them with a vegetable
brush. Trim stringy parts and tough ends. Pit,
peel, seed, and remove anything that could
cause choking. Trim excess fat off meat and
poultry.

Steaming fruits and vegetables preserves
more of the vitamins and minerals than boiling. Recapture some of the lost nutrients by
adding a bit of the steaming liquid to the
food, or save it for making soups and sauces.
Also, try the following tips to make baby's
food as healthful as you can:

- Don't add salt or sugar — there's no need
  to. You may add a bit of lemon juice as a
  preservative and a natural flavor enhancer.

- Soften dried legumes (peas and beans) for
  cooking by boiling for two minutes, then
  allowing to stand for an hour, rather than
  the usual custom of soaking overnight,
  which depletes them of some nutrients.

- Bake vegetables such as potatoes and
  squash in their skins.

- Avoid frying and deep-frying, which adds
  unhealthy fats to foods.

Packaging and Storing
Homemade Baby Food

Store your homemade food in the freezer.
Allow the food to cool slightly before freezing
in small portions.

WHAT YOU NEED TO MAKE YOUR OWN BABY FOOD

- [ ] Food processor and/or blender
- [ ] Food mill
- [ ] Hand-cranked baby-food grinder
- [ ] Roasting pan
- [ ] Vegetable steamer
- [ ] Egg poacher
- [ ] Saucepan with lid
- [ ] Cutting board
- [ ] Ovenproof glass cups
- [ ] Fork and potato masher
- [ ] Fine-meshed strainer
- [ ] Vegetable brush and peeler
- [ ] Measuring cups and spoons
- [ ] Sharp paring knife
- [ ] Ladle
- [ ] Spatula
- [ ] Grater
- [ ] Colander

FOR STORING AND FREEZING

- [ ] Ice-cube tray
- [ ] Storage jars (4-ounce/120-milliliter)
- [ ] Small freezer bags
- [ ] Cookie sheet
- [ ] Waxed paper
- [ ] Freezer tape
- [ ] Marking pen
- [ ] Muffin tin

- An ice-cube tray stores ideal infant-sized portions. Pour the freshly cooked and pureed food into the tray, cover with cellophane wrap, and freeze.

- After freezing, remove the frozen food cubes from the tray and store the cubes in airtight freezer bags. You can then remove one serving-sized cube at a time when needed.

- An alternative to the handy cube-sized serving is the cookie-sized portion. On a cookie sheet lined with waxed paper, place heaping tablespoonfuls of the pureed baby food, or slices of cooked food, in rows. Freeze until solid. Peel off the food "cookies" or slices and freeze them in tightly sealed bags.

- Once babies graduate from cookie- and cube-sized portions, store the food in recycled commercial baby-food jars, small jelly jars, or plastic one-serving containers. Be sure not to fill the jars to the brim, as food expands as it freezes.

- Label all foods with the contents and date and put the most recently frozen foods behind the previously frozen foods, just like they do at the supermarket. Home-made baby foods can safely be kept frozen for three months.

Thawing and Serving Baby Food

Frozen foods should not be defrosted at room temperature for long periods of time. When you're ready to use frozen baby food, try these tips.

- For slow thawing, place one serving, or a whole day's worth, in the refrigerator to thaw for three to four hours.

- For fast thawing, use an electric warming dish, or place the frozen cube or uncovered jar in a heatproof dish and place in a small saucepan. Fill the pan with water to a level a bit below the rim of the thawing dish. Thaw and warm over medium heat and stir food occasionally to promote even heating.

- Before serving baby's food, be sure to stir it well and check to be certain no portion is too hot for the baby. I always instinctively touch the food to my upper lip each time I load another spoon. A bite of too-hot food can teach baby not to trust the material coming at him on the spoon. Your finger would know better.

- Because microwave warming may leave hot pockets in the food and burn your baby's mouth, we do not recommend it. If you choose microwave warming, use the low setting, be extra careful in stirring, and always sample for even heating before serving to baby.

- To avoid wasting, only spoon-feed baby from the portion you think she will eat. Add more to her dish with a clean spoon if she wants more. You can refrigerate the unused portion for up to two days, but only if saliva has not been introduced.

Some babies never eat "baby foods," and all this preparation information can be bypassed if your baby tolerates a lot of texture, delays solids, hates spoon-feeding, or goes straight to eating finger foods. Some mothers really get into making baby food; others just go with family fare for baby's meal and use a fork to mash.

COMMERCIAL BABY FOOD

Commercial baby foods do have some advantages as a convenience item. They are relatively economical, sanitary, ready to serve, packaged in baby-portioned jars, reusable for refrigerator storage of leftovers, and are staged in graduated textures as baby's chewing and swallowing skills increase. If you choose to feed your baby a steady diet of commercial baby food, call the manufacturer at its 800 number and ask the following questions:

- Does the food contain pesticides, and how do they police pesticide residues?
- How fresh are the fruits and vegetables that are used?
- How long a shelf life is allowed?
- Does the food contain additives?

Consumer questioning increases the standard of commercial baby food. Admittedly, we are purists. We believe parents should be advocates for their babies' nutrition.

BRING OUT THE CUP

"Introducing" the cup implies making the change from bottle or breast to cup gradually and smoothly. Going from sucking to sipping requires a completely different mouthing orientation and better coordination in swallowing.

Baby's Cup Runneth Over

Because baby's tongue-thrust reflex may not be completely gone at this stage, the protrud-

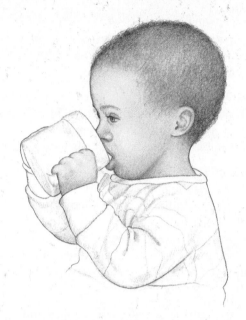

A trainer cup with a tight lid and small spout can be a good starter cup.

ing tongue may interfere with a tight lip seal, so that some of the liquid will flow over the tongue and dribble out the corners of the mouth. Most babies cannot master a good cup seal until after one year of age. Besides being dribbly, cup feeding is still a bit of a nuisance at this stage, as most babies have not yet mastered the art of gently putting the cup down. They are more likely to throw the cup on the table or floor or place it down sideways rather than gently set it down upright. Developmentally, baby will want to explore the joys of dumping. Here's how to minimize cup nuisances:

- Hold the glass or cup for your baby until he learns how to handle a cup himself.
- If baby dribbles too much out of a regular cup, then use a trainer cup with a tight lid and small spout.

- Use a cup that is weighted on the bottom so it doesn't tip over easily.
- Use a plastic two-handled cup that is easy to grab and hold.
- Make sure the cup has a wide base for greater stability.
- Protect baby's clothing with a large absorbent or waterproof bib.
- Put a *small* amount of formula or juice in the cup at any one feeding.

When to Introduce the Cup

There is no magic age for introducing the cup. Even a newborn can be taught to lap out of a very bendable plastic cup. If introducing a cup early, around five or six months, it is necessary for you to hold the cup at first, gradually introducing a few drops of milk between baby's lips and stopping frequently to allow swallowing. Observe stop signs that baby has had enough or is uninterested. When babies are able to sit up by themselves without using their hands for support (usually between six and eight months), they often want to "do it myself" and hold the cup without your assistance. Then you will need to use a cup with a lid.

Most breastfeeding mothers prefer to bypass the bottle stage completely and progress directly from breast to cup. If your breastfed baby still resists a cup by the end of the first year, and you want to encourage weaning, try the following get-to-love-the-cup tricks: To market the cup as fun, give your baby a plastic play cup as a toy. To overcome cup fear, encourage your baby to watch everyone around the table enjoy their own cup. Place baby's cup within grabbing distance on the table and notice that as you reach for yours, baby reaches for hers. Chalk up another dinner table win. Put diluted juice in the cup at first, instead of the suspiciously strange white stuff.

What to Drink

Besides the right foods, babies need the right fluids. Here's how to begin.

Juicy Advice

When to begin? Introduce diluted juice when your infant is able to drink from a cup, which in most cases is close to nine months of age.

What juice? White grape juice is the most friendly to tiny intestines because its sugar profile makes it easier to be absorbed. Pear, apple, and grape are also favorite starter juices. Some infants develop abdominal pain and diarrhea after drinking too much juice such as prune, pear, and apple. In excess (more than 12 ounces a day), the sugar profile of these juices may have a laxative and irritating effect on the colon. Orange, grapefruit, and lemon juice are too acidic and are usually refused by or upset baby. Vegetable juices, while more nutritious than fruit juices, are usually not a baby's favorite beverage, except for carrot juice.

How much? Because juice is less filling than breast milk or formula, infants can consume a much larger quantity without feeling full. Recommended amounts of 100 percent fruit juice are:

- 6 to 12 months: 4 ounces per day
- 1 to 4 years: 6 ounces per day

Dilute juice with at least an equal amount of water. Consider juice as a delivery system for extra water, which your baby needs once she is eating solid foods.

Be label savvy. Always serve juice that says "100 percent juice" on the label. Avoid juice "drinks," "cocktails," or "ades," which may contain as little as 10 to 20 percent juice with lots of added sweeteners, such as sugar and corn syrup.

Avoid nighttime juice bottles. Don't put your baby or toddler down to sleep sucking on a bottle of juice. When a baby falls asleep, saliva production and the natural rinsing action of saliva slows down, allowing the sugary juice to bathe the teeth all night and contribute to tooth decay, a condition called "juice bottle syndrome." If your baby is hooked on a nighttime juice bottle, remove the bottle promptly as soon as baby falls asleep and brush her teeth as soon as she awakens in the morning. Each night dilute the juice with more and more water until baby gets used to all water and no juice — a trick we call "watering down."

Don't Drink Your Milk (Yet)!

The Committee on Nutrition of the American Academy of Pediatrics recommends that breast milk or formula be continued for at least one year, and to avoid cow's milk as a beverage until at least one year (longer if your infant is allergic to dairy products). It is not wise to introduce a potentially allergenic drink at the same time that your baby's intestines are getting used to a variety of solid foods.

If you are no longer breastfeeding, use an iron-fortified formula until at least one year and longer if your infant is allergic to dairy products. Infant formulas are much better

---

FIRST DAIRY FOODS

Instead of introducing cow's milk, if your child does not have a family history of dairy allergies or is generally not an allergic baby, you may try dairy products such as yogurt, cheese, and cottage cheese between nine months and a year. Yogurt gives all the nutritional benefits of milk but with fewer problems. Yogurt is made by adding a bacterial culture to milk. This culture ferments the milk and breaks down the milk lactose into simple sugars, which are more easily absorbed — good to know when baby is recovering from diarrhea. Milk proteins are also modified by the culturing process, making yogurt less allergenic than milk. Most infants enjoy yogurt around nine months. Sweeten plain yogurt using your own fresh fruit or no-sugar-added fruit spreads rather than using the heavily sweetened fruit-flavored yogurt. Don't use honey until baby is at least one year old.

---

suited to infants' nutritional needs than is cow's milk. Formulas are much closer to the composition of human milk and contain all of the necessary vitamins. Most contain additional iron supplements that are so necessary at this age. Formulas are more expensive than cow's milk, but by the time you add the cost of additional vitamins and iron, the cost of formula is only slightly more. Perhaps thinking of formula as "milk" will lessen your urge to switch to cow's milk. (See page 261 for a more detailed discussion of the pros and cons of cow's milk.)

A Note About the Compulsive Drinker

Toward the end of the first year most bottle-fed babies consume around a quart (thirty-two ounces/one liter) of formula each day and get about half of their nutrition from solid foods. What about the baby who is a compulsive formula drinker, consuming forty to fifty ounces a day, and wanting more, but is not interested in solid foods and appears to be gaining excessive weight? For some suggestions on dealing with this, see "Seven Ways to Trim Baby Fat," page 249.

For the compulsive breastfeeder and apparently obese baby who still wants to breastfeed all the time but refuses anything else, parents need not worry. Breast milk naturally becomes lower in fat by the second half of the first year. As your baby becomes an active toddler, he will most likely burn off the excess baby fat.

12

Ten Tips for Becoming Your Family's Nutritionist

Parents, you have a nutritional window of opportunity in your child's first few years to shape her tastes into lifelong healthy eating habits. Here are ten tips from the Sears family's baby-feeding kitchen that will give your infant a smart nutritional start.

1. FEED YOUR BABY SMART FATS

Babies need a "right fat" diet, not a low-fat diet. Fats have gotten a bad rep lately, and "cholesterol" is another bad word in adult nutrition. Unfortunately, the low-fat, no-cholesterol craze has been carried over into infant feeding. Babies need fats — lots of them. Human milk, our nutritional standard, contains 40 to 50 percent of its calories as fats and — would you believe? — is also rich in cholesterol. A balanced diet for infants should contain at least 40 percent of its calories in the form of fats, and 30 to 40 percent for toddlers. Without fats babies won't grow well. Here are the nutritional reasons that your baby needs enough of the right fats:

- Fats are the body's largest storage batteries for energy. Each gram of fat provides nine calories, more than twice that of carbohydrates and proteins.

- Growing brains need smart fats. The brain grows faster during the first years of life than at any other time. It uses 60 percent of the total energy consumed by the infant, and the brain itself is 60 percent fat. Also, fats provide the major components of the brain cell membranes and the myelin sheath that insulates the nerves in the brain and spinal cord, enabling nerve impulses to travel more efficiently throughout baby's growing body.

- Fats are the basic components of important hormones and are valuable parts of cell membranes, especially red blood cells.

- Fats act like ferry boats for the absorption and transport of vitamins A, D, E, and K.

- Fats make food taste good. Babies enjoy the "mouth feel" of fat in food.

- Fats are the most nutrient-rich food, packing in the most calories in the smallest volume. This nutritional perk is important for toddlers since they are by nature picky eaters and consume small amounts at each feeding.

As you can see, fats do good things for baby, as long as we provide this little brain and body with the right kinds of fats, in the right proportions. In choosing the healthiest fats, consider the source.

Best Fats for Babies

Not only should infants get 40 to 50 percent of their calories from fats, they should eat the right variety of fats. In addition to breast milk, the best fats for babies (and also for children and adults) come from marine and vegetable sources. Ranked in order of nutritional content they are:

- seafood (especially salmon)
- flax oil
- avocados
- vegetable oils
- nut butters (because of possible allergies, delay peanut butter until after *two* years)

The top three sources of fats (breast milk, seafood, and flax oil) are rich sources of omega-3 fatty acids, which are essential for optimal brain growth. In addition to these smart fats, babies also need a variety of other fats in their diet.

Saturated Fats for Babies

These fats come primarily from animal sources such as meat, eggs, and dairy products. During the first two years of baby's life, parents should not keep their infant's diet thin in saturated fats (remember that human milk fat is 44 percent saturated fat). Older children, adolescents, and adults should avoid foods high in saturated fats because they contribute to an increased risk of adult heart disease, presumably because sat fats raise cholesterol. The moral of this fat story is feed baby a diet rich in saturated fats but gradually lower the amount of sat fats (meat, eggs, and full-fat dairy products) as your child gets older. Foods that have predominantly saturated fats include the following:

- meat
- poultry
- full-fat dairy products
- eggs
- butter
- chocolate
- cocoa butter
- palm and palm kernel oils
- coconut oil

Bad Fats for Babies

While it is nutritionally correct to say there's no such thing as a bad fat for babies, artificial processing of natural fats can make a good thing bad. Read labels, watching for the word "hydrogenated" — the only bad fat. Hydrogenated fats (also called "trans fatty acids") are produced by artificially processing vegetable oils to make them like saturated fats. Used to extend the shelf life of foods and give some packaged and fast foods a fatty, oily taste, the artificially processed fats raise blood cholesterol. In our opinion, these artificially made factory fats have never been proven safe for babies, and new insights have shown they are certainly not healthy for adults. These sinister fats are often tucked into these commercial foods:

- candy bars
- chips
- cookies and crackers
- deep-fried fast food
- doughnuts
- french fries
- shortening
- some peanut butters

Look at the fine print on labels. Shun foods whose ingredients list contains the words "hydrogenated" or "partially hydrogenated." Some healthier products have recently started proudly displaying labels that say "Contains no trans fatty acids."

2. FEED YOUR BABY THE BEST CARBS

Every baby is born with a sweet tooth. But, unfortunately, sugars have been getting a lot of bad nutritional press. Every possible malady has been blamed on sugar. Babies do need sugars, lots of them. But they need the *right sugars.* Here's the difference between healthy sugars and unhealthy ones.

Infants and children are natural sugarholics. Kids crave sugar because they need a lot of energy, mental and physical. Sugars are the body's main energy fuel. Each molecule of sugar is like a tiny power pack, energizing each cell to do its work. Sugars come in two forms, *simple* and *complex* (we like to call them *short* sugars and *long* sugars; you have probably heard them also called simple and complex carbohydrates, or sugars and starches). Each type behaves differently in the body.

Sweet Facts About Sugars

Nutritionally speaking, there is no such thing as a bad sugar. It's how it is served and what it's combined with that determine whether it's "good" or "bad." All sugars are good for babies, but some are better than others.

"Bad" Sugars

The least good of the sugars go by the names glucose, dextrose, and sucrose — the sweet-tasting stuff that is in the white granules in the sugar bowl, candy, icings, and syrups. Because it's cheap and sweet, this is the sugar most added to commercial foods, like catsup. A small amount of these sugars won't bother a child, but too much of these sugars can become bad. Let's take a ride with these sugars from the mouth into the bloodstream to see how they behave in the body.

These sugars are called simple, or short, sugars because they contain only one or two molecules. Because they are so small and simple, they require little or no digestion in the intestines. So as a spoonful of sugar hits the intestines, it immediately enters the bloodstream, and here's where the roller coaster ride begins.

The high blood sugar from a rush of this refined-sugar meal triggers the release of *insulin,* the hormone needed to escort these sugars into the body's cells. The sugar is rapidly used, causing the blood-sugar level to plunge into a sugar low (also known as hypoglycemia or sugar blues). This low blood sugar triggers stress hormones that squeeze stored sugar from the liver, sending the blood sugar back up. The ups and downs of the blood-sugar level and the hormones scrambling to smooth the ride result in roller-coaster-like behavior in your child. To witness this sugar ride in action, watch the antics of a bunch of icing-faced kids at a birthday party. Tame them if you can. These sugars also merit the label "sweet nothings," because nearly all of the natural vitamins and minerals have been refined out. For this reason, they have been dubbed "empty calories." Avoid letting your child indulge in these sweet nothings. They do nothing for him. Enough of these ups and downs. Give your child sweet somethings. (See "Fiber and Carbs — Partners in Health," page 243.)

Better Sugars

The *fructose* sugars, primarily from fruits, are better. These sugars are sweet tasting and better than the syrups and frostings above. We call these sources of quick energy "better" because they do not excite the hormone roller coaster like their sweeter relatives on top of the birthday cake do. Blood-sugar swings and consequent behavior swings are much less dramatic with an orange than with a candy bar. Milk sugar, or lactose, also behaves better in the body because it doesn't rush into the bloodstream as fast as the refined stuff. Another credit fructose and lactose have is the company they keep. Unlike the megadoses of concentrated sugar in the granular sweets, fruit and milk sugars enter the intestines along with so many other nutrients that the release into the bloodstream is not so fast.

Best Sugars

Complex polysaccharides, better known by grandmother's term "starches," are the best sugars. They are found in pasta, legumes, potatoes, grains, seeds, and nut butters. These nutrients enter the intestines as a

---

HEALTHIEST SUGARS

- apples
- beans and legumes
- breast milk
- dairy products (especially plain yogurt)
- fresh fruit
- pasta (whole-grain)
- potatoes
- soybeans
- sweet potatoes
- vegetables
- whole grains

---

long line of simple sugar molecules holding hands. Through digestion they are allowed to enter the bloodstream one by one, like a time-release energy capsule. These super sugars provide slow, steady energy and give the feeling of fullness longer, without the high and low feelings of the fast-acting sugars.

3. PERK UP THE PROTEINS

Proteins are "grow foods." Like the structural steel of buildings and the metal meshwork in concrete, proteins provide structural elements to every cell in the body. Proteins are responsible for growth, repair, and replacement of tissue. They are the only nutritional element that can duplicate itself. Tissues grow by piling millions of proteins on top of each other until each organ has reached full growth, after which they replace one another when worn out or injured.

While proteins are necessary grow foods, parents seldom need to worry that their baby isn't eating enough protein. During the first year, an infant's total protein needs can be met with breast milk or formula. Even during the second year, when toddlers typically become picky eaters, it's hard not to get enough protein. During the first two years an infant needs about 1 gram of protein per pound of body weight per day. The total daily protein needs of a twenty-pound toddler could be met by any of the following: a cup of yogurt and a glass of milk; a peanut butter sandwich on whole-grain bread and a glass of milk; two servings of whole-grain cereal and a cup of yogurt; two scrambled eggs with cheese; or a fish sandwich. As you can see, for most children, getting enough protein is not a worry. Foods that pack in the most protein are:

- seafood: especially salmon
- dairy products: cottage cheese, yogurt, cheeses, milk
- legumes: soybeans, tofu, dried peas, chick- peas, dried beans, lentils
- meat and poultry
- eggs
- nut butters
- whole grains: wheat, rye, oats, rice, corn, barley, millet

4. SHAPE YOUNG TASTES

Infants who enter childhood with a sweet, fatty, or salty taste in their mouths are likely to continue with these cravings throughout childhood and probably into adulthood. Infancy is the only time in your child's life when you can curb the candy. Junk foods shared by fellow toddlers, sugary birthday parties, and even chocolatey trips to grand- mother's house are normal nutritional insults awaiting your home-fed toddler. But here's a story that may be hard for you to swallow. Years ago we had a theory that if young taste buds and developing intestines were exposed to *only* healthy foods during the first three years, the child might refuse junk food later. Sound like pie in the sky? Read on.

We tried this experiment with our own children and encouraged it in our pediatric practice. For the first three years we gave our children only healthy foods. We kept out of our diet added salt, table sugar, and unhealthy fats. Our sixth infant, Matthew, was the most junk-food deprived. What happened when Matthew went out into the sugar-coated world of birthday parties and candy giving? Of course he had sticky fingers and icing on his face, *but he did not overdose.* That's the difference. Halfway through the mound of icing or chocolate delight, Matthew would slow his partaking to a stop and convey the "I don't feel good" signs of yucky tummy. Now our children know to scrape off the frosting and just eat the cake. At even as young as three years, children can make the food connection: "I eat good food — I feel good; I eat bad food — I feel bad." Health- food-primed babies seldom overindulge, and that's the best you can hope for in raising a healthy body — a child and later an adult who avoids excesses.

Here's how to shape your baby's tastes in the right direction:

- Avoid foods with added artificial sweeteners and lots of sugar and corn syrup.

GO FISHING!

Seafood, especially salmon and albacore tuna, is a rich source of protein and brain-building omega 3's. Unfortunately, most American infants and children do not get enough seafood in their diets. To lessen the risk of mercury contamination from seafood, eat wild fish, such as Alaskan salmon and Alaskan halibut. (Top fish for concerns about mercury contamination are shark, king mackerel, swordfish, and tilefish. See our website, www.AskDrSears.com, for fish/mercury updates.)

To shape young tastes toward seafood, at around one year of age gradually introduce tiny bits of salmon and tuna, perhaps camouflaged in a tuna or salmon salad or in pasta and sauce or in sandwiches. Helping your child enjoy fish is good preventive medicine. Studies show that the populations that consume the most seafood have the lowest risks of nearly all the most serious diseases, such as heart disease, stroke, diabetes, cancer, and arthritis. And, don't forget those growing brains. Next to mother's milk, seafood is a top brain food.

- Avoid foods that contain hydrogenated oils.
- Serve more fresh foods and fewer canned and packaged foods.
- Serve whole grains (e.g., whole wheat instead of white bread).
- Avoid foods with colorings and additives.

5. FILL UP WITH FIBER

Fiber, the undigestible portion of starches and fruits, is a natural laxative, helping remove food waste products from the intestines. Crunchy and chewy foods, such as whole grains and legumes, are the best examples. Fibers function as intestinal sponges and brooms. As sponges, fibers absorb water and unneeded fats from other foods, adding bulk to the stool, slowing the absorption of food, and giving the body a longer feeling of fullness. Other fibers sweep the waste products downstream to be more easily eliminated. In adults, adequate fiber diets help prevent many intestinal disorders and may even lower the risk of colon cancer. In children, the main role of fiber is to soften the stools, speed the transit time of waste products through the intestines, and ultimately prevent constipation — a condition common in toddlers. For fibers to do their intestinal clearing job, a child must drink lots of fluid. The best sources of fiber are vegetables (such as potatoes) with skins, whole grains, whole wheat bread, apples (with the skin), prunes, pears, apricots, beans, brown rice, whole-grain pasta, oatmeal, beets, eggplant, squash, and legumes. As a good fiber source for our family we sprinkle flaxseed meal (branlike flakes) on a more tasty cereal. *Whole* is the key to fiber. Peeling fruits and vegetables and refining grains remove much of the fiber — another reason for leaving foods the way they are grown or picked.

Fiber and Carbs — Partners in Health

Here's a valuable nutrition tip for parents to remember: A good carb is a fiber-filled carb; a bad carb is a fiberless carb. High-fiber foods that also contain carbohydrates and sugars are better for your child's behavior than high-sugar, low-fiber foods. Fiber mixes the food into a gel and slows the absorption of the sugar from the intestines. This steadies the blood-sugar level and lessens the consequent ups and downs of behavior. Many cookies and packaged goods are high in sugar yet low in fiber, a combination that does not favor pleasant behavior.

6. VALUE YOUR VITAMINS

In addition to the big three — proteins, fats, and carbohydrates — vitamins are a valuable ingredient in your child's diet. Unlike the big nutrients, these micronutrients do not directly supply energy to your baby's body, but they help the food your baby eats work better, and all the body systems work better. As the name implies, they vitalize the body. We cannot function without these life-sustaining helpers. Our bodies need thirteen vitamins: A, C, D, E, K, and the eight members of the B team — thiamine, niacin, riboflavin, pantothenic acid, biotin, folacin, B-6, and B-12.

Go for variety. Vitamin-conscious parents, relax. No matter how picky your eater is, it is unlikely your child suffers from any vitamin deficiency. Many foods contain such a variety of vitamins that even picky eaters are bound to pick up enough vitamins over a short period of time. Giving your child a *variety* of foods ensures enough vitamins.

Vitamin storage. Some vitamins (A, D, E, and K) are stored in the body fat, so if your

DOES YOUR INFANT NEED SUPPLEMENTAL VITAMINS?

Consider vitamin supplements a *drug* to be prescribed, in correct doses, by your doctor. Megadoses of vitamins, touted as cure-alls for many adult diseases, should not be given to children.

Unless their doctor determines otherwise, exclusively breastfed term infants do not need extra vitamins. Human milk contains all of the essential vitamins. As long as your infant is getting enough milk, he or she is getting enough vitamins. Commercial formulas also contain all the essential vitamins, provided your infant consumes the right amount of formula each day. When your infant averages formula consumption of thirty-two ounces (about one liter) a day, extra vitamins are unnecessary unless he needs extra nutrition — for prematurity, for example. When your infant drinks less than this amount of formula each day, supplemental vitamins are advised, depending on the consistent intake of solid foods.

Because of the erratic diets of most toddlers, pediatricians usually recommend a daily multivitamin/multimineral supplement beginning around one year of age and continuing until the child eats a consistently balanced diet. (For current recommendations on vitamins and other supplements, see www.AskDrSears.com/supplements.

child goes on a periodic veggie strike, he will survive on last month's vitamins. Other vitamins (C and the B team) are not stored in the body very long and need frequent boosts.

Fragile vitamins. Some vitamins, especially C, are weakened or destroyed by processes such as boiling. Steaming and microwaving preserve the most vitamins in cooked food. Fresh is best, followed by frozen; canned foods have the lowest vitamin count.

Yellow vegetables — yellow skin. Yellow vegetables (squash and carrots) contain carotene, which if eaten in excess may give a yellow or orange tint to the skin. This harmless condition, termed carotenemia, is often confused with jaundice, which also gives a yellow color. Carotenemia colors only the *skin* yellow, whereas jaundice also gives a yellow color to the whites of the *eyes*. Simply cutting down on the yellow foods takes away the yellow skin color.

7. MIND YOUR MINERALS

Like vitamins, minerals are micronutrients; your child's body needs only a small amount to stay healthy. Minerals get into foods from the soil, and into seafood from the ocean. Calcium, phosphorous, and magnesium, the big three minerals, help build strong bones. Iron and copper build blood. Zinc boosts immunity. Sodium and potassium (called electrolytes) regulate the body's water balance. Honorable mention is given to the smaller members of the mineral family, called trace elements, which help fine-tune the body's functions: iodine, manganese, chromium, cobalt, fluoride, molybdenum, and selenium.

Deficiencies of these minerals and trace elements are rare, except for iron, since they are found in all the same food sources as vitamins. The two most important members of the mineral team are iron and calcium. (Calcium sources are discussed on page 262.)

8. PUMP UP BABY'S IRON

Iron is an important mineral for the proper functioning of all vital organs. Its main use is to build hemoglobin, the substance in red blood cells that carries oxygen. During well-baby checkups, usually between nine and fifteen months, the doctor should check your baby's hemoglobin by taking one drop of blood from a finger stick. An infant's hemoglobin normally ranges from eleven to thirteen grams. If the hemoglobin is below eleven, the infant is termed "anemic," or has "low blood." If the anemia is due to insufficient iron, this condition is termed "iron-deficiency anemia." Signs and symptoms of this problem are irritability, slow growth, diminished appetite, fatigue, and a generally pale appearance, especially noticeable on the earlobes and lips and beneath the fingernails. New insights into iron requirements show that infants and children with long-term iron-deficiency anemia are at risk for delayed intellectual development.

To understand how your baby can become iron deficient, let's follow this interesting mineral through the body. During baby's life in the womb the mother gives him a lot of extra iron, which is stored in the tissues of his body and in the hemoglobin of red blood cells. (While term babies are born with a large supply of reserve iron stored in their bodies, premature infants need iron supplements beginning at birth.) As old red blood cells are used up and disposed of by the body, much of the iron is recycled into new blood cells. As the iron in the blood is used up, the iron stores in the body portion out enough iron to keep baby's blood hemoglobin normal. If no dietary iron were to come in, these stores would be used up by six months. This is the nutritional rationale for giving babies iron-rich milk, either breast milk or iron-fortified formula, beginning at birth, or at least within the first few months. Here are some guidelines for avoiding iron deficiency.

Breastfeed your baby for as long as you can. The special iron in your milk has a high bioavailability, so 50 to 75 percent of it is absorbed, but only 4 to 10 percent of iron in other foods, such as iron-fortified cereals and formulas, gets into your baby's blood. In studies breastfed infants had a higher hemoglobin value at four to six months than infants who were fed an iron-fortified formula.

Avoid cow's milk for infants; limit it for toddlers. Cow's milk (which is very low in iron) should not be given as a beverage to infants under one year of age. Besides being a poor source of dietary iron, excessive cow's milk can irritate the lining of your infant's intestines, causing tiny losses of iron over a long period of time, further contributing to iron-deficiency anemia. Also limit your toddler's cow's milk consumption to no more than twenty-four ounces (710 milliliters) a day.

If formula feeding, use iron-fortified formula. Give your bottlefed infant iron-fortified formula, preferably beginning at birth, but at least by four months of age. Continue iron-fortified formula for at least one year, or until your infant has adequate alternative dietary sources of iron.

Combine foods wisely. Some foods help and others hinder iron absorption. Feeding solids just before or right after breastfeeding can diminish absorption of the valuable iron in breast milk. For this reason, if your baby is iron deficient, space the feeding of solid foods and breastfeeding by at least twenty minutes. Here are some iron helpers: Vitamin C–containing foods (fruits and juice) are iron enhancers, meaning they increase the iron absorption from other foods. Orange juice with a meal can double the amount of iron absorbed from the food. Drinking milk with a meal can decrease the amount of iron

BEST IRON SOURCES FOR BABIES

- breast milk
- iron-fortified formula
- iron-fortified cereals
- prune juice
- tomato paste
- tofu
- chili con carne with beans
- lentils
- soybeans
- beans (kidney, pinto)
- turkey
- fish

Iron requirements: Babies and children need around one milligram of iron per pound (0.5 milligram per kilogram) of body weight per day. If your doctor finds your baby iron deficient, baby will need around 6 milligrams of iron per pound every day for several months.

absorbed from the other foods. Nutritionists believe that animal protein foods contain a "meat factor" that improves the absorption of vegetable iron eaten at the same time as meat. The best co-helpers are meat and vitamin C–containing foods eaten together at the same meal, for example, spaghetti with meat and tomato sauce, hamburgers and coleslaw, or a turkey sandwich and orange juice. Another good combination is fruit and iron-fortified cereal.

9. MAKE EVERY CALORIE COUNT

Toddlers have tiny tummies, about the size of their fists. Add this anatomical fact to the temperament of a busy toddler who doesn't want to sit still for anything, especially eating, and you have a recipe for a "picky eater." (We discuss the picky eater in Chapter 13.) Encourage *grazing*. Offer your toddler nutrient-rich foods, those that pack a lot of nutrition, in frequent, small doses.

10. RAISE A LEAN BABY

There once was a time when a plump baby was sure to win approval from grandmother. Now, fat is out; lean is in.

Are fat babies destined to become fat adults? Not necessarily, but there is a heavy tendency. A fat infant has a higher chance of becoming a fat child who has an even higher chance of becoming a fat teenager who has an even greater chance of becoming an obese adult. An obese infant has a one in five chance of remaining heavy at age five to eight

> ### TOP NUTRIENT-RICH FOODS
>
> Consider these nutrient-rich foods that toddlers are most willing to eat:
>
> - avocado
> - broccoli
> - brown rice
> - cheese
> - eggs
> - fish (salmon)
> - kidney beans
> - nut butter spreads
> - oatmeal
> - pasta (whole grain)
> - sweet potatoes
> - tofu
> - turkey
> - yogurt

years. An obese child has twice the chance of becoming an obese adult. An obese teenager has sixteen times the risk of becoming an obese adult. Fat children grow up with a physical, psychological, and emotional disadvantage, in addition to having a higher risk of adult diseases, such as heart disease, stroke, and diabetes. Medical studies show that leaner people live longer and healthier lives.

Some babies are more prone to obesity than others. Here are the main risk factors to consider.

It's in the Genes

Infants are at risk of obesity from what's in the genes and what's on the plate. Adopted children tend to follow the weight trends of their biological parents more than those of their adoptive parents. If both parents are obese, the child has an 80 percent chance of becoming obese; if one parent is obese, a 40 percent chance. If neither parent is obese, the child has only a 7 percent chance of being fat. Rather than saying that babies inherit obesity, it is more correct to say that they inherit a *tendency* toward obesity.

It's in the Body Build

Besides inheriting a tendency toward fatness or leanness, babies also inherit specific body builds, which are more or less prone to obesity.

Lean and tall "banana" body types (ectomorphs) are taller and lighter than average on the growth chart. Ectomorph babies, recognized even at birth by spindly "piano fingers" and long, slender feet, put more calories into height than weight. Persons with ectomorph body types seem to burn off more calories and better adjust their food intake to their activity level. If they eat a lot, yet don't gain weight, they are likely to be the envy of their calorie-watching friends.

Stocky babies (mesomorphs, or "apple" body types) have average height and weight, and both height and weight are near the same percentile on the growth chart. These square-shaped babies have a greater tendency toward obesity than their rectangular ectomorph buddies.

Endomorphs ("pear" body types) are short and wide. Of the three body builds, these babies have the greatest chance of becoming overweight or obese. Because of their pear-shaped contour, they carry excess weight the least attractively.

Not all babies are pure body types; some have features of all three.

During a well-baby exam, parents often ask, "Do you think our baby will grow up to be fat?" I am usually able to give them an educated guess by looking at the body builds of the parents and child. If mother and father are both lean, and baby has an ectomorph body type, it is safe to say, "Your child will probably be able to eat all the nutritious food she wants and not get fat." Because of this child's body build and heredity, she will probably not be fat. But if two short, round parents holding a short, round baby ask the same question, I would counsel these parents that their baby does have an increased tendency to obesity and that they should begin preventive measures even in infancy.

It's in the Temperament

Babies get fat not only by eating too many calories, but also by not burning enough off. Active, fidgety babies tend to burn more calories and have a lower risk of obesity. Easy, mellow, and quiet babies tend to burn fewer calories. "Sitters" tend to have an increased risk of obesity, which is accentuated if this sedentary temperament is prevalent in other family members. A long, lanky, wiry, active baby with similar parents has a slim chance of becoming fat.

Baby Thins Out

Most babies are most chubby around six months of age. Between six and eight months, as babies begin to sit up, crawl, and play, they begin to lean out. From one to two years even more leaning out occurs. Babies walk, run, climb, and earn the name "picky eater." Between the first and second birthdays most babies lean out even more, putting more calories into height than weight. It seems as if baby is finally growing into his oversized skin. Gone are the plump baby pictures of the earlier months. A slimmer toddler emerges. Often parents' weight worries change from "Doctor, is he too fat?" to "Doctor, is he too thin?" Cherish these grabbable baby rolls while you can. They will soon disappear.

Being "lean" means having the right percentage of body fat for your individual body type. Lean should not be confused with skinny (which is often unhealthy) or lanky (which describes a person's basic body type). Every child can be lean and trim; not everyone can, or should, be thin and lanky.

"Lean" is one of the most important health words you can know, since leanness equates with a lower incidence of just about every serious adult disease: heart disease, stroke, diabetes, and cancer. In the last decade childhood obesity has reached epidemic proportions and is now considered by both the surgeon general and the American Academy of Pediatrics one of the most concerning childhood health problems.

Seven Ways to Trim Baby Fat

1. Give baby custom-calorie milk. Breastfeed. We believe breastfeeding lessens the risk of obesity for these reasons:

- Breast milk contains the recently discovered satiety factor, a sort of built-in calorie counter that signals a full feeling toward the end of a feeding. The natural stop-eating factor in breast milk imprints on the infant the feeling of when he or she has had enough to eat — a feeling some older children and adults never learn.

- By varying his sucking style, the breastfed infant is more in control of the calorie content of the milk by the way he sucks. When hungry, baby gets high-calorie milk; when thirsty or needing only comfort, baby gets lower-calorie milk. When the breast is "empty" but baby needs continued sucking, very little milk is delivered. Not so the formula-feeding baby. No matter how the infant sucks, the high-calorie stuff keeps right on flowing. (See page 117 to learn how the fat and calorie content of breast milk change according to the needs of baby.)

- Recent studies comparing breastfed and formula-fed babies show that after the first four to six months, breastfed babies begin to "lean out" sooner than their formula-fed peers, as they gain proportionately more height than weight.

- Formula-fed babies tend to get solid foods earlier and gain proportionately more weight than height, suggesting an early tendency away from leanness.

- A breastfeeding infant is more in control of her feedings, how much and how often she eats. A breastfeeding mother is more likely to watch the baby for cues, and since she can't count ounces, she learns to trust baby's feeding signals. A bottlefeeding mother, on the contrary, can take control of the feeding away from the baby. She is able to count ounces and watch the clock. She can override an infant's automatic hunger control by urging the baby to take "just a little bit more." As a result, baby may come to expect that "stuffed feeling" after a meal and eventually seek out this feeling as part of her normal eating pattern. That's why it's important for bottlefeeding mothers to learn to read baby's hunger and satiety cues. Research shows that formula-fed infants, if allowed to determine for themselves how much formula to drink, can self-regulate their total daily calories quite well. In a study of six-week-old infants, babies who were given a diluted, lower-calorie formula drank more to make up for the less filling formula.

- It's tempting to allow a toddler to walk around with a bottle just to "keep him quiet." Offering formula at every peep may condition the infant to connect food with comfort. Breastfeeding conditions the child to connect comfort with a person.

Dr. Bill notes: In our pediatric practice, we occasionally see an exclusively breastfed baby who is "overweight" on the growth chart. Because exclusively breastfed babies nearly always "lean out" toward the end of the first year or during the second year, we advise the parents neither to worry nor to change baby's pattern of feeding.

2. Watch for lower-calorie cues. Not all cries are for food. Being held may alone sometimes pacify the upset baby; playing may entertain the bored baby. Oftentimes, crying or fussing babies are thirsty, not hungry. Formula-fed infants and infants eating solids early get more concentrated feedings, and consequently they need more water. Sometimes offer water instead of milk, formula, or food. It's noncaloric. If unable to appease the compulsive formula drinker with plain water, consult your doctor about feeding your baby fewer calories. In recent years, formula manufacturers have introduced follow-up formulas that contain slightly less fat and fewer calories, much like the difference between whole milk and low-fat milk.

3. Delay solids. Besides formula feeding, the early introduction of solids adds to the obesity risk. Forcing solids early in hopes of getting baby to sleep through the night not only seldom works (see page 324) but also is an unwise feeding habit. If your baby has risk factors for obesity, when you do begin solids, begin with the most nutrient-rich foods, those that pack the most nutrition in the fewest calories, such as vegetables rather than fruit and whole grains over refined grains. (Go to a nutrition store to buy whole-grain baby cereal.)

4. Respect tiny tummies. As we've said before, babies' tummies are about the size of their fists. Next time you fill a bottle or place a heaping plateful of food in front of your toddler, put them next to his fist and notice the mismatch. A leaner approach is to dole out smaller portions and refill as necessary. Avoid the temptation to insist your child clean his plate. Your job is to prepare nutritious food and serve it creatively. How much he eats is up to your child. In our experience toddlers rarely get fat from eating too much *nutritious* food.

5. Trim unhealthy food fat. While you don't have to overfocus on fat during the first two years, don't ignore the potential problem either. Besides introducing your baby to a variety of foods during this time, you are also helping your infant develop a *taste preference*. It is unhealthy for your baby to enter childhood with a craving for fatty foods. Here's how to trim unnecessary fats:

- Forget the frying. Bake or broil instead.
- Trim excess fat from meats and poultry. Children love crunchy and greasy chicken skin. You don't have to pare away every crunchy morsel of fat, but trim the excess.

- Defat the dairy. Except for the compulsive, obese milk drinker, we do not recommend the use of low-fat milk and certainly not skim milk after your baby is off formula (see "Milk Tips," page 263, for explanation). You can pare the fat from other dairy products. Babies love butter. Substitute healthy spreads, such as nut butters or avocado spread. Get your infant used to low-fat cheeses, yogurt, and cottage cheese.

- Slow the fast foods. Avoid packaged fat-laden snacks and high-fat fast foods.

- As discussed on page 239, avoid foods that contain artificial fats, such as hydrogenated or partially hydrogenated oils.

6. Serve fiber-filled carbs. Too much of the wrong sugars can produce obesity. High doses of sugar, corn syrup, and other sweeteners that are added to packaged foods and drinks already low in fiber can simply feed a baby's sweet tooth. As a result, the child can eat or drink an excess amount, since fiberless foods are less filling. (For an explanation, see "Fill Up with Fiber," page 243.)

7. Get baby moving. Rarely do you have to take your baby out purposely for exercise. Most awake babies are in constant motion anyway. There is the classic story of Jim Thorpe, the famous Olympic athlete. When he tried to mimic the constant motion of an infant, he tired out after an hour, but the baby kept right on going. Some mellow babies, however, are content to be visually stimulated. They lie and look rather than wiggle and crawl. The plumper the baby, the less baby likes to budge; and the cycle of inactivity and obesity continues. Encourage your mellow baby to be an active toddler. Crawl with the beginning crawler, take walks together, play chase (and chase your toddler away from the T.V.), and run around in the yard playing games.

13

Feeding the Toddler: One to Two Years

The table is set. You corral your busy eighteen-month-old into his high chair and proudly present him a plate heaping with painstakingly prepared cuisine, and, of course, containing all the basic food groups. And, to show off your thriving toddler, you have invited the grandparents. Everybody cleans his plate and praises the chef. But what about Junior? His plate is still full, except for a few holes in the potatoes from well-aimed pokes and a few dozen squashed peas scattered about to remind everyone there is a baby at the table. Your baby is utterly uninterested in your beautifully served meal. Meanwhile, grandmother remarks: "Well, he does look a little thin" — a put-down of your mothering. Your child is "starving," and your mothering is on the line. Want to avoid this scene? Read on.

NOURISHING THE PICKY EATER

"Doctor, my child is such a picky eater." I must have heard this complaint a thousand times before I realized that toddlers merit this feeding title for a reason. A knowledge of toddler behaviors and growth patterns will help you understand why most one-to-two-year-olds pick and peck. During the first year, babies eat a lot because they grow a lot. The average infant triples his birth weight by one year, but the normal toddler may increase weight by only one-third or less between the first and second birthdays. Also, many toddlers grow proportionally more in height than weight, as they use some excess baby fat for energy. This normal toddlerhood slimming down may further increase parents' worry that their child is not getting enough to eat. A toddler's eating habits change because her growth patterns change.

Changes in emotional and motor development also bring about changes in eating patterns. Toddlers do just that — toddle! They don't sit still to do anything, especially to eat. They are too busy to interrupt their relentless explorations around the house to sit still for long. *Grazing* — small, frequent feedings — is more compatible with your baby's busy schedule. Many nutritionists believe this may be the healthiest way to eat anyway. And in another respect, the term "picky eater" is well deserved. The thumb-and-forefinger pickup, a motor skill that is refined toward the end of the first year, also influences toddler eating patterns. Baby delights in practicing this important new skill by picking up small bits of edible items from his plate or high-chair tray, or by reaching to your plate. These are all the reasons toddlers are supposed to be picky eaters.

Dr. Jim notes: *Feeding is one of the few things toddlers can take control of. I remind parents that most of us were picky eaters, and we grew up just fine.*

Not in the Mood for Food

Erratic eating habits are as characteristic as the many mood swings of normal toddler development. Your child may eat well one day and eat practically nothing the next. He may adore fresh vegetables one day and refuse them the next. As one parent said, "The only thing consistent about toddler feeding is the inconsistency." This patternless eating is normal, though worrisome. If you average your baby's food intake over a week or month, you may be surprised to find his diet is more balanced than you thought. Toddlers need an average of between 1,000 and 1,300 calories per day from one to two years, but they may not eat this amount every day. One day they seem to eat nearly nothing, but make up for it the next. Nutritional intake seems to balance out over a period of time. One mother solved this nutritional balancing act: "When her appetite is low, I only serve her one food item, and a different one at each meal. Instead of worrying about serving her a balanced meal, I concern myself with a balanced *week*."

Parents' Role — Toddler's Role

As parents of eight we admit that with our first children we did not look forward to mealtime, especially when they were toddlers. We felt responsible for their every meal, what they ate, how much they ate, and worried that we had failed if they didn't finish everything we gave them. Now, the pressure is off. We learned *it was our job to buy the right food, prepare it nutritionally, and serve it creatively; then our job was over.* We now relax and leave the rest up to the child. How much he eats, when he eats, and if he eats are mostly the child's responsibility (admittedly, with some encouragement and structuring from us). Once we relaxed and felt less pressured at mealtimes, we enjoyed these special times with our children, and, in fact, they seemed to eat better and enjoy it more.

When we had so many children to feed, it was difficult enough getting them all to the table. We seldom had energy left to get them to eat. It was up to them not to go hungry. We tried to develop a balance between being pushy and negligent in feeding our toddlers. We tried to go with the flow of their needs and moods. Nobody wins the forced-feeding battle. Too much pressure leaves everyone exhausted and creates unhealthy feeding attitudes. It is normal to camouflage foods, bribe, play feeding games such as airplane and mommy-take-a-bite-baby-take-a-bite, and so on, as long as we lighten up a bit in our desire to fill up our babies. After feeding children for thirty-five years, we take neither the credit nor the blame for how much our children eat.

GETTING YOUR TODDLER TO EAT

Don't take baby's rejection of your lovingly prepared pureed carrots personally. Be flexible about your child's own style. If your child gives you stop signs that he has had enough food, it's time to call it a meal. With that in mind, here are a number of tips and observations that will help you get more food into your baby and take the pressure off you.

Try the Nibble Tray

One of the most novel ideas we have come up with to nourish our babies and take the hassles out of parenting is the *nibble tray.* It makes grazing easy, and thus is perfect for most toddlers' preferred eating style.

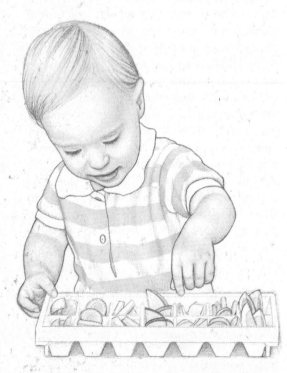

A "nibble tray" has real toddler appeal.

Assembling the nibble tray. Here's how to prepare the Sears family nibble tray:

- Use an ice-cube tray, muffin tin, or purchase a compartmentalized plastic dish with suction cups to attach it to a low table or high-chair tray. Put bite-sized portions of colorful and nutritious foods in each compartment of the nibble tray — sometimes we call this arrangement a rainbow lunch.

- Be sure to reserve a compartment for a nutritious dip.

- Call these foods childlike names that your two-year-old understands, such as

  - avocado *boats* — a quarter of an avocado sectioned lengthwise
  - cheese *blocks*
  - banana *wheels*
  - broccoli *trees*
  - little O's (O-shaped cereal)
  - *sticks* — cooked carrot or whole wheat bread
  - *moons* — peeled apple slices (with or without peanut butter)
  - *canoe* eggs — hard-boiled-egg slices cut up to look like canoes
  - *shells, worms, logs,* and so on — different shapes of cooked pasta

Place your baby's own tray on your baby's own table. As your toddler makes his rounds through the house and passes by the table, he will often stop, nibble a bit, and continue on his way. Teach him to stand by the table while he chews and swallows.

➤**SAFETY NOTE:** *To prevent choking, do not let your toddler run and play with food in his mouth. (See "Chokable Foods," page 229.)*

If your toddler continually spills the tray or throws it on the floor, he is too young to be allowed to nibble alone and may need supervision during the feeding. By two years of age many children can be taught that the tray stays at the table and is not to be dumped, dropped, or carried around the house.

Nibble tray for two. If your child is not enthralled with your creative nibble tray, put the tray between you and nibble together. All that may be needed is for your baby to catch the spirit of how fun it is to pick and choose from the colorful assortment displayed before him. Exaggerate your delight in nibbling from the tray by giving your child it's-fun-to-eat signals. Our children took to grazing from nibble trays so much that we began grazing with them.

Dress It Up

Dip it. Toddlers like to dip and dunk. Dipping less favored foods, especially veggies, in a favored dip is a sure winner. Dip tips:

- guacamole (with or without the spices)
- nutritious salad dressing
- cheese sauce
- yogurt, plain but flavored with honey and/or fruit concentrate
- pureed fruit or cooked vegetables flavored with a little salad dressing
- chickpea puree (hummus)
- cottage cheese dip
- tofu puree

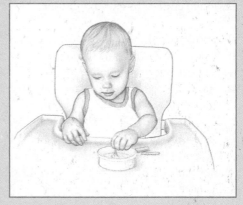

Smear it. Toddlers and young children are into spreading — or is it smearing? Let them smear nutritional spreads: avocado spread, cheese spread, meat pâté, peanut butter, vegetable sauce, pear or other fruit concentrates. Spread onto crackers, bagels, toast, or rice cakes.

Toddler toppings. Putting nutritious familiar favorites on top of new and less desirable foods is a way to broaden the finicky toddler's menu. Top toppings are melted cheese, yogurt, cream cheese, guacamole, pear concentrate, tomato sauce, meat sauce, applesauce, and peanut butter.

Make It Easy to Eat

Easy foods. Respect the fact that small children have small tummies and less well-developed chewing and swallowing skills. Cut foods in bite-sized pieces. Make pâté out of foods that are hard to eat, such as meat. Puree and spread it on a favorite cracker. A winner is equal parts cooked pureed meat and cottage cheese blended together.

Drink your meal. Make "smoothies" of yogurt blended with fresh fruit if your child refuses to eat but prefers to drink. With straws to make drinking more fun, some toddlers make less of a mess, some more.

Keep it small. Don't overwhelm your child with a plateful. Dole out minimeals a bit at a time and refill the plate when your child signals for more.

Encourage Grazing

Encourage nutrient-rich foods, those that are packed with a lot of nutrition for each calorie. Fruits have a low nutrient density, juice even less, and sweets the lowest. Nutrient-rich foods are especially important for the toddler who is as active as a rabbit but eats as little as a mouse. Children with picky eating habits tend to eat small volumes, so the key is nutrient-rich foods and frequent feedings. (See the list of nutrient-rich foods on page 247.)

Seating and Serving

Sit-still strategies. To fix your toddler in the high chair and restrain her from climbing out, use a safety belt. Never leave a child unattended while she is sitting in the high chair. Here's how one mother harnesses her escapee: "I keep coming at him with small spoonfuls of food. The rapid-fire method of feeding holds his attention and keeps him still. Before he knows it, the meal is finished, and I let him down. I'm able to get more food into him with fewer protests. I don't give him time to protest between bites." Moving or dangling feet make the toddler move more and eat less. Encourage your toddler to sit at a child-size table with his feet planted on the floor while eating alone. When he eats at the family table, place a box under his feet.

Shelf space. Reserve a low shelf in the refrigerator for your two-year-old's food and drink and leftover nibble trays. Your child may often go to the refrigerator and bang on the door to give you mealtime signals. Be sure the refrigerator or pantry shelf is low enough so that your child can reach in and grab her own food and drink when she wants it. When a toddler is ready to self-serve without a splattered mess varies from child to child. But encourage it. Also, reserving the

SEARS FAMILY SMOOTHIE

Here's a Sears family recipe for a smoothie we give our children nearly every school-day morning. It's a nutrient-rich, perfectly balanced, tasty way to get toddlers to try new foods they often shun. We call it "School-ade."

- 2–3 cups milk or soy or rice beverage
- 1 cup yogurt
- 1 banana
- 1 cup frozen blueberries
- ½ cup each of your favorite fruit, frozen (e.g., organic strawberries, pineapple, papaya, mango)
- 2 tbsp. flaxseed oil or 4 tbsp. flaxseed meal
- 4 ounces tofu
- 2 tbsp. peanut butter
- cinnamon and/or nutmeg to taste
- 1–2 servings of a multivitamin/multimineral chocolate or vanilla-flavored protein powder (See www.AskDrSears.com, *Baby Book* updates for brand recommendations.)

Blend until smooth. Serve immediately, while the mixture still has a bubbly milkshake-like consistency. Serve yourself first. Put on your "yum-yum — good!" face, which encourages your child to want to share what you're drinking. Make the smoothie together. Enjoy!

The above recipe makes enough for two hungry adults and a child.

Optional Variations

- For adults and older children, substitute flaxseed meal for flaxseed oil. The meal consists of ground flaxseeds, which contain the oil in addition to fiber and other nutrients. Some toddlers may find the consistency of the meal too grainy.

- Add 2 tbsp. of wheat germ or oat bran. These are valuable nutritional additions, but they may give the smoothie a blander taste and a grainier consistency.

- Add 1 tbsp. of honey for a sweeter taste.

- Add contents of 2 capsules of DHA oil (e.g., Neuromins) if your family shuns seafood. (Use a pin to make a hole in the capsule and squeeze the oil out.)

child's own shelf helps you keep track of how much your little consumer eats.

Table manners. Pleasant things go on at the table, consequently good behavior is expected there. This is the mind-set you wish your child to develop. Mealtime is special time, and the family table is a special place for good fun, good talk, and good food. Strain and tension should not be served up along with the food — this is not the time to bring up problems. Model good behavior between adults and between older children. If a toddler witnesses fighting and food flinging, she will view the family table as a battle-ground and join in. Even a baby as young as one year of age can catch the spirit of a meal-time prayer and happy conversation around the table.

The lap of luxury. Expect times when your child refuses to get in or stay in the high chair. Let him sit on your lap and eat off your plate. As honorary president of the Sears family mess-control club, Martha has found it helpful to push her plate just beyond baby-grabbing distance and place a few morsels of her food on the table in front of baby, between baby and plate. This keeps the lap baby's hands out of your plate. Enjoy this lap-sitting stage; it soon will pass.

Make Meals More Interesting

Mommy's little helper. Let your child make her own food. Use cookie cutters and create designs with cheese, bread, pasta, and sliced meats. A mother we know puts pancake batter in a squeeze bottle and lets her child squeeze the batter onto a griddle (not hot) in fun shapes, such as hearts, numbers, or letters, sometimes even spelling the child's name. Children are more likely to eat their own creations.

Open the surprise. Kids love surprises. A marketing ploy of seasoned veterans in the toddler feeding game is to let the child open the package of food or take the foil off a previously frozen kiddie meal, revealing compartments of colorful surprises. Play you-be-the-mommy by allowing her to open individual servings (not hot ones, of course), encouraging baby to want to serve herself. This also increases the likelihood that she will actually want to eat it.

Change the menu. Be flexible in your feeding styles and menus. If the serving technique continues to fail, change the menu. Try different techniques and food varieties. Keep and improve what works; trash what doesn't.

Pizza for breakfast? The concept of "breakfast, lunch, and dinner" has very little meaning to a child. If your child is fixed on eating pizza in the morning and fruit and cereal in the evenings, go with it. Better than not eating at all. As your child gets older, don't feel you have to be a short-order cook, always fixing her preferences that are different from the family menu. There will come a time when your child is expected to eat what the rest of the family does. A less-than-favorite menu starts to look pretty good when a five-year-old is presented with the alternative of making his own peanut-butter sandwich. Then again, peanut butter on whole wheat is a complete protein. Ever think of putting the green beans on the peanut-butter sandwich?

More Feeding Strategies

Overcoming lip lock. Ever spend precious hours preparing your one-year-old's favorite food, only to sit down at the table, scoop up a spoonful of a tasty morsel, and meet Mr. Tight Lips giving you the "No way I'm going to eat, mom" sign? You have two choices: Advance with better weapons or retreat from the battle. Try the following strategies: Sometimes it helps relax tight lips by simply backing off from the feeding, going about your business, or continuing to enjoy the food yourself. As your baby watches you open your mouth and eat with relish, he may catch the spirit and relax his attitude. Use one of your child's favorite foods as a teaser. Offer a spoonful of a proven winner. As the door

FAVORITE TODDLER SNACKS

avocado dip	dried fruit
yogurt dip	100% juice and nectar
rice cakes	healthy cookies
meat pâté	deviled eggs
crackers	fruit-and-yogurt
peanut butter	smoothies
apple slices	baby carrots, cooked

opens, follow up with the food you wanted him to have in the first place. Mr. Tight Lips may be giving you the message that he is not hungry, not in the mood to eat, and wants to do something else. Sometimes the best approach is simply to realize the door is closed, back off, and come back another day.

Keep the camera ready. One day when I was writing, Martha called from the kitchen, "Quick, take a picture before I get mad." Stephen had pulled an open box of cereal off a low shelf. There he sat, covered from head to toe with cornflakes, wallowing in his grainy mess and eating it — the boy was hungry!

Model excitement! To market unfamiliar or less favorite foods, first eat the food yourself while you use all the verbal and body language you can muster up to show your child how good it is. Or place the food in front of your child and ask for a bite of the food yourself (he may enjoy holding it out for you to eat) followed by the old reliable "mmmm-mmm gooooood!"

The grass is always greener on the other plate. Suppose your child has a thing about cauliflower, and this becomes your food challenge of the week. You have tried camouflaging it with sauce, dipping it, giving it a different name, and the cauliflower sits there, uneaten. Sit close to your child and put the cauliflower on your plate while you replay the old "mmmmmmm goooood" tune. To your amazement your child may pick the cauliflower off your plate. If not, enter the cauliflower in a new contest at a later date. You might try associating it with broccoli, which most kids love because of the tree shape — you can have green trees and white trees.

No two meals are the same. Toddlers are inconsistent in their eating habits. You may find one day your child wants to feed herself, the next day she wants you to feed her. On a day that you are not sure which way to go, use two spoons, one for your child and one for yourself. Sit with her while she eats. Sometimes she simply wants you to keep her company while she eats but to leave her alone to feed herself. Other days she may want you to entertain her and use your spoon to feed her. Sometimes we play the game, "You take a bite with your spoon, and mommy gives you a bite with her spoon." Toddler may add, "And I give mommy a bite."

Changing Habits

Putting the brakes on the binge. Sometimes a child may go on an eating binge, overdosing on a favorite food, not wanting anything else. One mother described how she solved this problem: "When we give her any food or drink that we want to decrease her intake of, we often tell her it's the last one — 'All gone, no more!' This avoids her harping for more." But if the binge food is a nutritious one (like a peanut-butter sandwich), there is no reason to withhold it.

Food fixations. This feeding mind-set used to drive us bananas, until we realized how to swallow it. Sometime between two and three years of age, expect your child to be very set in the patterns of food he expects to be served. If he has in his mind that peanut butter must be on top of the jelly and you put jelly on top of the peanut butter, be prepared for an ungrateful protest. Don't interpret this as your child's being stubborn, manipulating, or controlling. It is simply a passing stage. A young child's developing mind goes through stages in which he has a preconceived idea about the order of things. Peanut butter must be on top of jelly; the reverse is unacceptable. Grin and spread it. Enduring these whims is a piece of cake. Wait until you later go shopping for clothes.

Voting down veggies. Every day I hear, "Doctor, he won't eat his vegetables." Vegetables usually require more creative marketing than other foods. Here's the pitch:

- Use veggies as finger foods, letting your child dip them in a favorite dip, cheese sauce, or dressing.

- Camouflage the vegetables with a favorite sauce. Peanut-butter sauce is actually quite good on cauliflower.

- Play dress up: Adorn the vegetables with favorite foods, for example, tomatoes laced with cottage cheese.

- Hide the vegetables in favorite foods, such as rice, cottage cheese, or avocado dip.

- Steam the vegetables. They're more flavorful that way.

- Make designer veggies — try veggie art, colorful faces with olive-slice eyes, tomato ears, a cooked-carrot nose, and so on.

EATING OUT WITH A BABY OR TODDLER

The adage "Children should be seen and not heard" was possibly coined by a restaurant owner. Here's how to make dining out with a toddler an enjoyable, or at least a tolerable, experience.

If possible feed your child before going out. Or order a quick child's meal as soon as you arrive at the restaurant. A hungry child is more likely to be unruly.

If you're planning an evening out and your sitter cancels, you can make it an evening for three. Time your dinner reservation when baby is likely to be tired. A long drive to the restaurant may lull her to sleep. Take the sleepy baby, still in the car seat, and quietly place the baby–car seat package underneath your restaurant table. Or request a booth and lay the sleeping babe on one side.

If baby's sleeping time and your eating time don't match, here are some strategies. Take along baby's favorite finger-food snacks. For the high-chair baby, bring soft, noiseless toys and plastic utensils. We have found that wearing our baby in a sling is the easiest way to quiet and contain the young restaurant goer. Seek out restaurants that show a "children welcome" atmosphere. Shun a restaurant that doesn't have high chairs. A final tip: Choose a table off to the side so baby is not the center of attraction and stimulated to entertain the audience.

- Put on your best vegetable face. Food likes and dislikes are contagious. Let your child see how much you and the rest of the family enjoy eating veggies.

- Disguise vegetables in soups and sauces. Juicing, grating, grinding, and pureeing help unwanted veggies slide down easier. Zucchini pancakes are a big hit at our house, as are carrot muffins.

- If you sincerely feel that family life cannot go on without vegetables, let your child help you plant a vegetable garden. Have your child dig up or pick the ripe vegetables, wash them, and help prepare them. Veggies from the little farmer's home patch at least have a fighting chance.

Take the pressure off. Pressure tactics make feeding harder, not easier. Don't force-feed, as this can create long-term unhealthy attitudes about food and feeding.

CHOOSING THE RIGHT MILK FOR YOUR TODDLER

Is cow's milk the perfect food? Yes and no. Yes, for baby cows. No, for baby humans. For toddlers who are not intolerant of or allergic to dairy products, milk is a one-stop shop for nutrition. It contains nearly all the basic nutrients that the toddler needs for growth: fats, carbohydrates, proteins, vitamins, and minerals. The main value of dairy products is their reasonably balanced nutrition, especially at a time when toddlers are notoriously picky eaters. While it is true that there is nothing in milk that cannot be gotten just as well (and sometimes better) from other food sources — vegetables, legumes, and seafood — a realistic fact of feeding is that toddlers usually eat or drink dairy products in larger and more consistent amounts than other foods. The problem with all this good stuff in milk is that it was designed for the growth of calves, not babies.

A Closer Look at Cow's Milk

Baby cows grow much faster than baby humans, and this is the problem with cow's milk. It contains too much stuff. Cow's milk contains excessive mineral content (e.g., salt and phosphorus), in much higher concentrations than in human milk or infant formulas. Why could too much of this good stuff be bad for babies? The body's waste-disposal system is geared to handle what is called the renal solute load, which is simply the hard stuff that the body does not need, usually excess proteins and minerals. If the kidneys are presented with foods that contain high renal solute loads (cow's milk is two to three times higher than human milk or infant formulas), they must work harder to eliminate this excess. The excess is especially tough on the system in the early months, when an infant's kidneys are still immature.

Besides these excesses in cow's milk, the likelihood of allergy is another reason that the American Academy of Pediatrics Committee on Nutrition advises against using cow's milk as the primary beverage in infants *under one year.* Allergists estimate that if cow's milk is given to babies under three months of age, approximately 25 percent will later become allergic to milk. (See the discussion of intestinal closure, page 120, for an explanation of the association of early feeding and later food allergies.)

Cow's milk contains very little iron, a necessary ingredient of the rapidly multiplying red blood cells of the growing toddler, and its overconsumption by toddlers can contribute to iron-deficiency anemia (see page 245).

Types of Milk

Milk is labeled according to its fat content. Whole milk is what comes from the cow. It contains 3.25–4 percent fat and twenty calories per ounce (an ounce equals about thirty milliliters). Two percent (low-fat) milk has some fat removed and contains fifteen calories per ounce. Skim milk has practically all of the fat removed and contains eleven calories per ounce. Since fat has received so much bad press lately, shouldn't infants drink lower-fat milk? No! Low-fat and skim milk deprive the growing infant of valuable fat nutrients.

Goat's milk. The nutritional qualities of goat's milk are similar to those of cow's milk,

SOURCES OF CALCIUM

Where does baby get enough calcium? What about the toddler who will not drink milk or is allergic to milk and other dairy products? In North America calcium deficiency is rare, because some calcium is present in most foods. The recommended daily value for calcium for infants and children is 800 milligrams per day. Drinking three cups of milk will supply a child's daily calcium requirements. Consider the following sources.

Best Dairy Sources	Calcium Content*
yogurt, 1 cup	415 mg.
milk, 1 cup	300 mg.
cheddar cheese, 1 oz. (1-inch cube)	200 mg.
macaroni and cheese, 1 cup	200 mg.
cottage cheese, 1 cup	155 mg.

Best Nondairy Sources	Calcium Content*
sardines, 3 oz.	371 mg.
calcium-fortified orange juice, 1 cup	300 mg.
chickpeas, 1 cup	300 mg.
spinach, 1 cup	272 mg.
kale and collards, 1 cup	179–357 mg.
tofu (firm), 3 oz.	190 mg.
broccoli, 1 cup	177 mg.
rhubarb, 1/2 cup	174 mg.
salmon (canned), 3 oz.	167 mg.
refried beans, 1 cup	141 mg.
blackstrap molasses, 1 tbsp.	137 mg.
figs, 5	135 mg.
almond butter, 2 tbsp.	86 mg.
dried apricots, 1 cup	59 mg.
dried beans (cooked), 1 cup	50–100 mg.

*The calcium contents are average values, depending on type of packaging and other such factors. For fish (sardines and salmon) the calcium content varies with the amount of mashed bone in the fish. Greens (kale and collards), though high in calcium, are usually unpalatable for infants, but they may be chopped and disguised in casseroles.

Sources: "Nutritive Value of Foods," USDA Home and Gardens Bulletin No. 72 (US. Department of Agriculture, 1981) and Food Values of Portions Commonly Used, by A. De Planter Bowes and H. H. Church (Lippincott, 1998).

and the caloric content is the same. Because the structure of its protein and fat is different, some children may find goat's milk easier to digest than cow's milk. Goat's milk contains only trace amounts of the allergenic casein protein alpha S1, which is the protein found in cow's milk. Goat's milk contains more essential fatty acids than cow's milk does and a greater percentage of short- and medium-chain triglycerides, the type of fats that are more easily digested. An agglutinin, which causes fat globulins to cluster, is present in cow's milk but absent in goat's milk. Most goat's milk produced in the United States today is pasteurized and antibiotic-free, and the goats are not given any milk-enhancing hormones like the bovine growth hormone (BGH) in some brands of cow's milk. Because goat's milk contains less than 10 percent of the amount of folic acid contained in cow's milk, be sure that the goat's milk you use is supplemented with folic acid. (For more information see www.meyenberg.com.)

Yogurt. Perhaps an even better toddler food than beverage milk, yogurt is made by adding *Lactobacillus* bacterial cultures to milk. These cultures act like digestive enzymes, coagulating the milk proteins and transforming milk lactose to lactic acid. With its less allergenic milk protein and more digestible lactose, yogurt is tolerated by some toddlers who are allergic to beverage-milk protein or intolerant of milk lactose.

Yogurt is an ideal toddler food because you can do so much baby stuff with it: spreads, dips, icings, pudding, and as a healthy substitute for cream in recipes, sour cream on potatoes, and in sauces and custards.

Lactase milk (Lactaid). Lactase milk is made by adding the enzyme lactase to milk. This breaks the lactose down into simpler sugars, allowing them to be more easily digested by children who are lactose intolerant. As an alternative, the enzyme lactase can be purchased as a tablet or drops that you add to regular milk.

Imitation milks. "Nondairy" creamers, for example, are made with corn syrup, vegetable oils, emulsifiers, stabilizers, flavorings, and occasionally contain components of milk such as sodium caseinate. *These are not milk substitutes and should not be used as a beverage for infants and children.*

MILK TIPS

- Buy organic cow's milk, which is free of antibiotics and added bovine growth hormone (BGH).
- Avoid cow's milk as a beverage for children under one year of age. Use breast milk and/or iron-fortified formula instead.
- Skim milk is not recommended for toddlers.
- Use whole milk for toddlers.
- Consider low-fat milk for children over two years of age.
- Low-fat milk may be used from eighteen months to two years if the child is a compulsive milk drinker.
- For most toddlers, limit milk to 24 ounces (3 cups) a day.
- Be aware of the symptoms of a subtle milk allergy or intolerance.

SWEET TOOTH SIPPING

What about toddlers walking around with bottles and sippy cups? Toddlers need a lot of fluids, approximately one and one-half ounces per pound per day, mostly in the form of milk, formula, or water. Allowing your toddler to sip frequently on a bottle or cup increases the likelihood that she will get enough fluids. Yet, constant sipping on a bottle or a cupful of syrupy or acidic beverages can cause tooth decay. If your toddler likes to toddle around the house with a sippy cup, fill it with water only, please. Take this opportunity to shape the toddler's tastes for drinking plain water instead of always sweet beverages.

IS YOUR CHILD EATING ENOUGH?

"Doctor, I don't think he eats enough" is a guaranteed concern sometime between the first and second birthdays. The question is, Does baby eat enough to satisfy mother or grandmother (no child eats that much!) or himself? Try this step-by-step approach to becoming your child's own nutritionist.

Step One: Plot Your Baby's Progress on a Growth Chart

Using a growth chart, record your toddler's height and weight. Your doctor does this routinely at each well-baby visit, and you might request a copy of the two years' growth chart at your baby's one-year checkup and ask how to plot future growth on it. Growth charts are not infallible guides to infant nutrition, but they are a place to start.

If your toddler plots near the top of the chart in height and weight, you certainly don't have to worry about his nutrition. Chances are your child is getting enough of the right stuff to eat. If your child has been consistently around the same percentile line all along, seldom is there cause for nutritional concern. Take heredity into account in growth-chart plotting. If a baby has two petite parents and is in the twenty-fifth or even the tenth percentile, he probably belongs there. Babies with different body types plot differently on the chart. Ectomorphs (slim) may plot above average in height and below average in weight. Mesomorphs (stocky) tend to center around the fiftieth percentile in both height and weight. Endomorphs (short and wide) show a somewhat higher weight percentile than height. All of these variations are normal.

A gradual fall to a lower weight percentile over several months is a common occurrence. We call this "leaning out." This happens most noticeably between six and twelve months, when baby is learning to crawl, and between twelve and eighteen months, when baby is learning to walk and run. During these periods, infants burn off a lot of their baby fat. So don't be surprised at your baby's one-year checkup to see that she has gone from a chunky ninetieth percentile to a leaner fiftieth percentile on the weight curve. And do not be alarmed at the eighteenth-month checkup if your already slim toddler has gone from the twenty-fifth percentile down to the tenth percentile. Your health care provider will track your baby's growth closely and determine if any dramatic decline in percentile could be a sign of inadequate nutrition.

In the year 2000, new growth charts were developed that allow for the different growth patterns of breastfed and formula-fed infants. The older U.S. growth charts were based completely on Caucasian, formula-fed, middle-class infants living in Ohio. The new U.S. charts reflect the growth patterns of a more racially and economically diverse population. They take into account that breastfed infants and formula-fed infants grow differently during the first year of life. One-third of the infants and children used to compile the new growth data were breastfed. (For more on growth charts, see page 446.)

Step Two: Examine Your Toddler for Signs of Nutritional Deficiency

In addition to looking at the chart, look at your child from head to toe. Here are the most obvious signs of nutritional deficiencies:

- *Hair:* brittle, easily plucked, dry, wirelike, sparse
- *Skin:* wrinkled and loosely attached to muscle, dry, flaky, easily bruised especially in areas not usually exposed to falls, spiders (broken blood vessels in the skin), irregular pigmentation, delayed healing, areas of thickened or thinned skin, pale
- *Eyes:* dull and lusterless, bloodshot, night-blind, fatty deposits in the nasal corner, dark circles underneath
- *Lips:* fissures at corners of the mouth that heal poorly, pale, swollen
- *Gums:* bleeding, spongy
- *Teeth:* cavities, brittle
- *Tongue:* smooth, fissured, pale
- *Nails:* thin, concave, brittle

TODDLER NUTRITIONAL NEEDS AT A GLANCE

- 1,000–1,300 calories per day average*
- protein needs: 1 gram per pound per day
- ideal balanced nutrition:
  50–55 percent carbohydrates
  35–40 percent fats
  10–15 percent proteins
- vitamins and minerals
- water
- vitamin and fluoride supplements if prescribed†
- frequent feedings best; allow grazing

Use only as a guide; calorie needs vary considerably according to preferences and development.

†*Vitamin supplements are rarely necessary in breastfeeding infants; thirty-two ounces of formula contain the daily requirements of vitamins for term infants. Fluoride supplements are recommended according to the amount of naturally occurring fluoride in your tap water and how much water your child drinks.*

- *Bones:* bowed legs, prominent ribs
- *Feet:* swollen (edema)

Step Three: Record a Dietary History

Prepare your child's food record. Record the type of food eaten, the amount, and the number of calories in each serving. Complete the food record for seven straight days and total the number of calories each day. It is normal for a child's food record to vary from day to day. This is why a *weekly* average is more accurate. As a rough guide, an infant should average 50 calories per pound per day (about 23 calories per kilogram). For example, the average 20-pound one-year-old needs around 1,000 calories per day. Some days he may eat 700 calories, on other days 1,300. Don't expect to be accurate to the last calorie. Even professional nutritionists aren't. If your toddler eats a weekly average of around 1,000 to 1,300 calories per day, chances are he or she is getting enough. This figure includes the calories obtained from milk, so if your child is still breastfeeding a lot, the number of calories from food would be somewhat lower.

The Right Kind of Food

Determining if your child is getting enough calories is Nutrition 101. If you want to graduate to level 202, determine if your child is getting not only the right amount of food but the right *kind* of food. This means taking your food record and breaking down each food serving into the percentage of proteins, carbohydrates, and fats. Total the number of grams of proteins, carbohydrates, and fats each day, and then do a weekly total. Balanced nutrition would give these weekly percentages: carbohydrates 50–55 percent, fats 35–40 percent, and proteins 10–15 percent. Don't expect a balanced day. Shoot for a balanced week.

The Wisdom of the Body

Usually a calorie count suffices to determine if your child is getting enough nourishment. Studies have shown that if presented with a buffet of nutritious foods, toddlers will, over a period of time, naturally eat the right balance of foods. Nutritionists believe that the body has an inner sense of wisdom in craving the right balance of nourishment. Besides doing the calorie count, using the food-balance calculation is a valuable exercise in learning about your child's eating preferences and principles of good nutrition.

AIDS FOR RECORDING A DIETARY HISTORY

Resources for Your Nutritional Calculations

The Complete Book of Food Counts, by Corinne T. Netzer (Dell, 1988).

Food Values of Portions Commonly Used, by A. De Planter Bowes and H. H. Church (Lippincott, 1998).

"Nutritive Value of Foods," USDA Home and Gardens Bulletin No. 72 (U.S. Department of Agriculture, 1981).

Measuring Tools You Will Need
- [ ] One set standard measuring spoons
- [ ] One set standard measuring cups
- [ ] One standard glass measuring cup

Equivalent Measures

3 teaspoons = 1 tablespoon

16 tablespoons = 1 cup

2 tablespoons = 1 fluid ounce

Step Four: Look for Other Circumstances Affecting Your Toddler's Growth

Expect a leveling off of growth, especially weight, during a prolonged or recurring illness, such as diarrhea or frequent bouts with colds. Appetite lags and the nutrition that would have gone into growth is redirected into healing. Anticipate a period of catch-up growth when your child is well. Between nine and eighteen months, crawling and walking slow down weight gain but not height gain, as your toddler normally begins to "lean out."

Besides medical and developmental reasons, emotional setbacks may slow growth and diminish the appetite. If something happens to upset the parent-infant relationship (for example, untimely weaning, premature mother-infant separation, marital disturbances, family crises), the baby may fall down a few notches on the growth chart. One of the most fascinating areas of research is the need that some infants have for a close parent-infant attachment in order to achieve optimal growth — that is, to thrive. We foresee the day when researchers will uncover biochemical links between nurturing and growth. (See the discussion of high-need babies, page 369, and "The Shutdown Syndrome," page 446, for a further explanation of the relationship between attachment and growth.)

Step Five: Obtain a Complete Medical and Nutritional Evaluation

If after going through the preceding steps, you suspect your toddler is undernourished, consult a nutritionist for an evaluation of your child's food record and obtain nutritional counseling. The nutritionist will examine your child's food diary and, using a computer program, analyze the nutrient content of what your child has eaten, mainly average intake of calories, proteins, carbohydrates, fats, vitamins, minerals, and fiber. Comparing these values with the recommended dietary allowance, or optimal values, for your child's age, the nutritionist will advise you how to make up for deficiencies, if any.

Besides an examination of your toddler's nutrition, a thorough medical checkup may uncover reasons for his undernourishment. There may be physical and emotional reasons that he is underweight. Your doctor may obtain laboratory tests to determine if your child is getting enough protein, iron, vitamins, and minerals.

FOOD ALLERGIES

Food allergies are great masqueraders. I've heard just about every imaginable problem attributed to food allergies. Sometimes food allergies are overdiagnosed, depriving the child of nutritious and fun foods; other times food-related problems are ignored. Somewhere between these two extremes lies the truth about food allergies.

What "Allergy" Means

"Allergy" comes from two Greek words: *allos* (other) and *ergon* (action). So an allergic person shows an unexpected or different action, or reaction. Medically, the term "allergy" is used to describe the reaction that occurs when the body's immune system reacts to an allergen.

A SAMPLE TODDLER MENU

The following list summarizes the components of a balanced daily menu for the average twenty-five-pound, eighteen-month-old toddler. Choose from the five basic food groups (see page 149) to ensure balanced nutrition. (One serving of fruit, vegetables, and grains ranges from one-fourth to one-half cup. The serving size of meat and of legumes is two ounces.)

- 1,000–1,300 calories per day
- three cups of whole milk or dairy equivalent (or breastfeeding *at least* three to four times a day)
- three to four servings of grains
- two to three servings of vegetables
- two to three servings of fruit
- one serving of legumes
- one serving of meat, fish, or poultry
- three to four ounces of healthy snacks

Food	Amount	Calories
egg *or*	1	
iron-fortified cereal	½ cup	80
toast (with margarine or butter)	½ piece	55
milk	1 cup	160
orange slices	½ orange	35
cheese pizza *or*	1 slice	
peanut butter sandwich	½	150
broccoli tree	1	20
milk	1 cup	160
green seedless grapes	10	30
cheese chunk or slice	½ ounce	50
fish sticks	2	100
biscuit (two inch)	½	50
green beans	10	15
pasta	1 cup	150
rice-and-raisin pudding	⅓ cup	130
		1,185

A food *intolerance* is often more difficult to diagnose than a food allergy. The term "intolerance" is used when a food affects the body in an undesired way that does not involve an immune response, such as lactose intolerance or hyperactivity to sugars or additives. Some food intolerances, such as lactose intolerance (caused by a missing enzyme in the intestines, resulting in abdominal discomfort and diarrhea in reaction to milk products) are fairly objectively diagnosed. Other intolerances — of sugars and food additives, for instance — are more subjective and difficult to prove. Any food can be blamed for intolerance.

A third term, *hypersensitivity,* means the same as "allergy." All three terms (allergy, intolerance, and hypersensitivity) can be lumped into the simple term "food sensitivities," meaning a certain food causes a child not to feel right and act right, or certain organs not to function right.

Here's an example of how allergies work. Babies Allison and Danny each drink a glass of milk. Allison smiles for more. Danny's skin blushes; his nose and eyes water. He may even sneeze, wheeze, or have frequent diarrhea. Danny's observant mother quickly blacklists milk. Danny is allergic to milk; Allison is not.

What's different in the bodies of these two babies? Every food, especially of animal origin, contains proteins called *antigens* (allergens, if we are allergic to them). These suspicious proteins enter the bloodstream and are recognized by the body as foreign intruders who were not born there. The body's immune system perceives these alien bodies and mobilizes its own protein troops called *antibodies.* The fight begins. When the antigens and antibodies come together for battle, the effects invade certain parts of the body — the target organs — usually the lining of the breathing passages, intestines, and skin. Reactions resembling tiny explosions release chemicals that cause the allergic signs. The best known of these released chemicals is histamine (hence the allergy medicines called antihistamines), which disturbs the tissues, causing blood vessels to leak fluid (runny nose and puffy, watery eyes) and to dilate (rash). Sometimes muscles of the breathing passages go into spasms (wheezing).

Baby Allison's body, however, is not bothered by milk. Even though milk antigens get into her bloodstream, and she may even

---

COMMON SIGNS OF FOOD ALLERGIES*

Respiratory Passages	**Skin**	**Intestines**
runny nose	red, sandpaperlike facial rash	mucusy diarrhea
sneezing		constipation
wheezing	hives	bloating, gassiness
stuffy nose	swelling in hands and feet	excessive spitting up
watery eyes		vomiting
bronchitis	dry, scaly, itchy skin (mostly on face)	intestinal bleeding
recurring ear infections		poor weight gain
persistent cough	dark circles under eyes	burnlike rash around anus
congestion	puffy eyelids	abdominal discomfort
rattling chest	lip swelling	
	tongue soreness and cracks	

Many of the symptoms can also be signs of inhalant allergies. See page 698 for a discussion of this problem.

make antibodies to milk, signs of the antigen-antibody battle do not occur or are less obvious. She is not allergic. Why some babies are allergic and some are not is not well understood. Mostly, it's in the genes.

Allergic Signs to Look For

Signs and symptoms of food allergies are as unique as baby's fingerprints. The most obvious signs occur at three sites: the breathing passages, the skin, and the intestines (see box on page 269). These kinds of signs are the most common and easily identified. Others are more subtle, and the offending food more difficult to pinpoint. These symptoms affect the central nervous system or brain:

crankiness	headaches
anxiety	sore muscles and joints
night waking	irritability
crying	hyperactivity

The battle signs differ in severity; some occur immediately or within minutes; others are delayed for several hours or days. Baby Susan may eat an egg in the kitchen and break out in hives by the time she toddles into the family room, or she may develop a rash days later. Food allergies also range in severity. You may be rushing your wheezing child to the nearest emergency room within minutes after he eats a strawberry, or he may develop only a nuisance type of rash that needs simply a tincture of time and an over-the-counter antihistamine.

Food allergies, unlike fingerprints, change. Most lessen as the child gets older; some occasionally worsen; many disappear entirely. Some children show a shift in food allergies: They lose their allergy to tomatoes and can

again hit the catsup bottle, but may develop an allergy to mustard. Some allergies occur every time the child eats a certain food; others are cyclical, related to the quantity and frequency of the food. Food allergies also show a threshold effect, meaning that each child has a certain level of sensitivity to a particular food, and some allergies are dose related. For example, some children may wheeze or develop hives after eating only a fingertipful of peanut butter. Others do not show obvious allergies to peanut butter if they limit this food to one sandwich a week.

Tracking Down Hidden Food Allergies

If your child is showing signs of food sensitivity, here are guidelines to help you identify the culprit(s).

Step One: Keep a Food Record

Record everything your child eats for four days, including all meals and snacks.

Step Two: Try the Elimination Method

From the list of the foods your child most commonly eats select the most suspicious allergen, probably one of the "big eight": dairy products, wheat, egg whites, peanut butter, corn, citrus fruits, soy, or food additives. Start your elimination at a time when other factors do not cloud the detection of food allergies. Avoid, for example, holiday times, birthdays, or other celebrations, and wait until pollen season or home remodeling is finished. The most common offender seems to be dairy products, so you may decide to start there if you have no other hunches to go on. It is not the easiest food to eliminate because it comes in so many

MOST- AND LEAST-ALLERGENIC FOODS

Most-Allergenic Foods

berries	dairy products	shellfish
buckwheat	egg whites	soy
chocolate	mustard	sugar
cinnamon	nuts	tomatoes
citrus fruits	peas	wheat
coconut	peanut butter	yeast
corn	pork	

Least-Allergenic Foods

apples	dates	raisins
apricots	grapes	rice
asparagus	honey	rye
avocados	lamb	safflower oil
barley	lettuce	salmon
beets	mangoes	squash
broccoli	oats	sunflower oil
carrots	papayas	sweet potatoes
cauliflower	peaches	turkey
chicken	pears	veal
cranberries	poi	

Read Labels

Potentially allergenic foods may be listed under another name in packaged foods. The most common are:

- wheat flour: durum semolina, farina
- egg white: albumin
- dairy products: whey, casein, sodium caseinate

Careful label reading will help you discover what you are eating:

- Cocoa mixes, creamed foods, gravies, and some sauces contain milk.
- Noodles and pasta contain wheat and sometimes eggs.
- Canned soups may contain wheat and dairy fillers.
- Most breads contain dairy products.
- Margarine usually contains whey.
- Hot dogs, cold cuts, and "nondairy" desserts contain sodium caseinate.
- For persons who keep kosher, the word "parve" on a label means the food does not contain milk or meat.

MAKING A FOOD-ALLERGY CHART

Keeping a written record will help you discover if there is a connection between your child's allergic symptoms and foods in his daily diet. Here's a sample:

Possible Allergenic Food	Signs and Symptoms	Results After Elimination	Notes
Milk	Runny nose, diarrhea, watery eyes, cough, awakened three times at night	Nose dried up, cough lessened, frequency of diarrhea lessened, awakened once	Couldn't tolerate milk, but yogurt and cheese OK

When trying to pinpoint the source of trouble, start with single-ingredient foods, milk, for instance. Bread, noodles, and luncheon meats may contain multiple potential allergens, making isolation of a single offender difficult. Under the food column write the first food to be isolated.

Focus on the most objective signs — rashes, changes in bowel patterns (diarrhea or constipation), respiratory symptoms. Chart the most troublesome signs and symptoms. If you are an observant person, you may include some general behavior signs, such as irritability and night waking.

Under the results column, record the change in these signs and symptoms after the food is omitted. Be as objective as you can; remember, any new "treatment" can have a placebo effect because you are expecting to see results, perhaps partly because of all the trouble you are going through. In the notes column, chart additional observations or anything you want to remember.

Keep a record of all foods eaten daily so you can recall what was eaten when, in case symptoms change.

delightful forms (milk, yogurt, cheese, sour cream, ice cream). But cow's milk protein *is* the leading allergen.

For a period of two weeks (three weeks if you're not in a hurry) eliminate this food and chart your observations (see "Making a Food-Allergy Chart," above). If you do not see any change, go on to another suspicious allergen, continuing until you have exhausted the list.

Step Three: Challenge Your Findings

When you have tracked down the culprit, to be sure the disappearance of the symptoms is not just coincidental, reintroduce the suspicious food into your child's diet and see if the concerning signs and symptoms reappear. Remember, an allergic reaction does not imply a lifelong allergy. Children outgrow most food allergies. When reintroducing foods, gradually introduce a small amount of the food, and increase the amount every three or four days to see if the signs and symptoms reappear.

Some children are allergic to a food only if they overdose on it or eat it every day. Toddlers are prone to food jags during which they crave only one food for a week and then won't touch it for months. *Rotation diets* — spacing the suspicious foods every four days — may lessen the allergy.

A quicker way to relieve the symptoms may be preferable if your child is very allergic (sneezing, hives, frequent colds, ear infections, poor weight gain, frequent night waking, abdominal pain). Eliminate all eight of the foods previously mentioned for a period of one week or until you see changes (maybe as long as three weeks). Then reintroduce one food each week to see if the symptoms reappear. If so, that food goes on the no-no list for at least four months, then slowly try small amounts again. "But what can my child eat?" you ask. During this time your child may eat fresh vegetables (except corn, tomatoes, and peas), fresh fruits (except berries and citrus), avocados, rice, barley, millet, poultry, and lamb. It is wise during this time to also avoid junk foods, nitrites, and other allergenic foods. This would be a great way to get the whole family on a healthier program.

Medical Help for Allergies

How much time and energy you are willing to devote to elimination diets depends upon how severe your infant's allergies are. If they are simply a nuisance and do not particularly bother the baby, by the time you go through all of the elimination diets your child will probably have outgrown the allergy anyway. If, however, your child is truly bothered by food allergies, it is worthwhile, in consultation with an allergist knowledgeable about food allergies, to do whatever is necessary to identify the food allergens.

Blood tests called RAST tests are helpful but not 100 percent diagnostic of food allergies. These tests measure the level of antibodies in your child's blood to certain foods. If your child has a very high level of antimilk antibodies, this at least helps you in identifying milk as a possible allergen. Skin tests for children over three are also helpful in identifying food allergies. It is true, however, that laboratory tests should only be used in conjunction with the preceding elimination diet and observational charting. If your child has a high level of antimilk antibodies but exhibits absolutely no symptoms of milk allergy, then it is seldom necessary to treat only on the basis of a lab test. Food allergies, like most nuisances of infancy and childhood, lessen or disappear in time. (See the Food Allergy and Anaphylaxis Network (FAAN) website, www.foodallergy.org.)

PESTICIDES: HOW TO KEEP THEM OUT OF THE MOUTHS OF BABIES

An apple a day may not keep the doctor away. After researching the pesticide issue, we felt like moving our family to some unpolluted area (if there are any left), planting our own garden, milking our own cows, and drilling for clean water. Instead, we realized that there are ways to not only live with this problem but clean up the food we feed our children. The following information is not meant to scare, but to inform and motivate parents to take action about a potentially serious problem that affects today's children and our future grandchildren.

Why Food Chemicals and Children Don't Mix

Poisoning our own food with pesticides is bad enough, but the special eating habits and growth patterns of children pose the following additional hazards:

- Children's eating habits are different from those of adults. They eat proportionally more contaminated food on a volume-per-weight basis than adults. Infants and children consume much more fruit and juices than do adults. They also do not eat the variety of foods that adults do, often binging on applesauce, for example, three days at a time. The Natural Resource Defense Council (NRDC) estimates that young infants consume three times more apple juice than adult women consume.

- Today's children will be exposed to toxic chemicals over a longer time, so they face greater health risks as adults. Researchers believe that *prolonged* exposure to a toxic chemical may have a cumulative effect.

- Researchers believe that the rapidly dividing cells of an infant and a child are more susceptible to the carcinogenic effects of pesticides.

- Could the neurotoxic pesticides be more damaging in the first two years of life, when the child's brain is growing at its fastest rate?

- An infant's immature liver may have a limited capacity to detoxify chemicals.

- Children, especially infants, have proportionally more body fat than adults. Pesticides are stored in fat.

In 1990 the NRDC released the results of the most comprehensive analysis ever conducted on pesticide residues in children's food. This study identified sixty-six potentially carcinogenic pesticides in foods that a child might eat. The researchers estimated that children have four times as much exposure as adults to eight of these carcinogenic pesticides. In 1998 a nonprofit organization called the Environmental Working Group analyzed FDA, EPA, and USDA data on pesticides in food and concluded that over one million children consumed more than the "safe" adult amount.

Food Laws — Do They Protect Children?

The answer is no. What is legal may not be healthy, and it is astonishing what is legal in the pesticide–food growers industry. Usage and labeling of pesticides is monitored by the Environmental Protection Agency (EPA). The amount of pesticide residue in foods is periodically tested by the Food and Drug Administration (FDA). Here's why the current laws and these agencies don't protect the apple your child eats.

How Pesticides Are "Tested" and Presumed "Safe"

Animals are given various amounts of pesticides and tested for the effects of these chemicals. Besides obvious effects such as life or death, paralysis, and growth retardation, the tissues are examined for microscopic evidence of damage. Once a level is found that causes no *identifiable* damage, that level is extrapolated to humans as the "maximum acceptable level" or "tolerance level" or "safe level" — the level of pesticide residue in a food that is legally acceptable. However, what is safe in the animal and legal for the committee may not be healthy for the human. We cannot rely on these studies for the following reasons:

- The process of extrapolating animal results to humans is plagued with errors. How do you measure the intelligence of a rat?

- Short-term effects, not long-term damage, are measured in these studies. Our concern in children is the small amount of pesticide residue accumulating over a long period of time and causing damage years later, perhaps even in the next generation.

- The EPA-allowed levels are for adults and are based on food-consumption habits of adults in the 1960s. The agency's recommendations do not take into account eating habits of children, who eat proportionally more produce per pound of body weight than adults.

- These studies are artificially done. How animals are tested is not the way humans eat. Usually one or a few chemicals are tested on an animal. In reality a child may ingest a hundred different pesticides. Chemicals have a *synergistic* effect, meaning that when put together, chemicals may have a more harmful effect than when used singly. Pesticides A and B may pass if tested separately in different animals, but put them together in the same animal and

they may take on harmful qualities. The gradual piling up of many chemicals over long periods of time is the basic concern that is not being measured. We believe it is worthless to label any chemical poison "safe."

- Independent studies are usually better than EPA tests. The EPA does batch testing. If you blend one hundred pounds of potatoes and test the batch, you get an average pesticide level. But what if only a few potatoes contain most of the chemicals and the child eats one of these "hot" potatoes?

- Inert ingredients get by. In studying exposure levels the FDA doesn't consider the health effects of inert ingredients. These are labeled "inert" because they have no pest-killing action, not because they are harmless. Inerts, however, can be dangerous. The EPA has recently identified 110 inerts as hazardous, but there are no food standards or tolerance limits for inerts. Also, the FDA does not monitor food for inert ingredients. Pesticide manufacturers consider inerts trade secrets and usually do not list them on package labels.

A Pesty Issue

The EPA laws require that pesticides have no more than the minimal allowable levels in foods while considering the need for an "adequate, wholesome and economical food supply." The EPA weighs the cancer risk of a pesticide against its economic benefits. In plain language, they will accept a cancer risk in a food if it keeps the price down and the supply up. Putting such a price tag on health has been criticized by the National Academy of Sciences and the NRDC. Are we a nation that cannot afford healthy food for our children?

What You Can Do

By now you may have concluded that government agencies are more concerned with politics than health. Parents, don't expect help from the government. Food producers lobby more than parents; babies and children don't vote. The logical conclusion we come to, based on the preceding evidence, is to ban all carcinogenic or neurotoxic and other harmful toxins from food and milk, and eventually this ban should filter down to cleaner water. This drastic step would be costly to food growers and to the six-billion-dollar-a-year pesticide industry, but it can be done. Here's how.

Just Say No!

Don't buy poisoned food. Consumer pressure, especially from parents, has corrected many medical and social problems; it can also clean up our food. The food chain of consumer pressure is very simple: Parents demand pesticide-free food at the store, the store only orders pesticide-free foods from the food growers, and the food growers are, therefore, required to stop using pesticides. We believe that this is the only "law" that will work. Why? Because the motive is pure: to protect the health of ourselves and our children. Any government motive is laced with residues of pleasing most of the people most of the time. Allow a little bit of cancer in return for a little bit of pesticides in return for a happier food grower. This keeps most voters happy, except the nonvoters most at risk, our babies and children.

Buy Organic

Look at the label on a jar of commercial baby food and you will see the effects of consumer pressure. Labels read "no salt, no sugar, no preservatives." Now only one "no" is missing — no pesticides. Baby-food manufacturers claim that they no longer use Alar-containing apples and they have reduced the pesticide content far below legal limits. Commendable, but not enough! Parents, use your purchasing power to send baby-food manufacturers a clear message — you want pesticide-free food.

Initially expect to pay a higher price for pesticide-free food. You're paying the grocer now instead of the doctor later. If all food growers were required — by consumer pressure and by law — to grow safe food, they would find a less expensive way, and the cost would decrease.

Look for the label "certified organically grown food." This certification means that food is grown according to strict standards with third-party verification by an independent organization or state government agency. Certification includes on-farm inspections, soil and water testing, and careful record keeping. Certified-organic farmland must be free of agrichemical use for three years. Unless you know the farmer, this certification is your best insurance that the food you are paying for is truly organic.

Other Things You Can Do

You have a right to expect that legal food is safe food. Vote for laws that fill the loopholes

---

RISKY FOODS

When it comes to foods that have no peel and have rough, difficult-to-clean surfaces (such as strawberries), always buy organic.

in existing EPA and FDA monitoring and their ability to detect pesticides. Here are some specific ways you can influence the safety of food:

Wash fruits and vegetables. Washing produce in a diluted solution of water and dish detergent (one-quarter teaspoon to a pint of water) may remove some surface pesticides. Rinse well. Even careful washing may not remove all surface residues, and it can't remove pesticide residues that remain inside the produce.

Buy domestically grown produce in season. Imported produce often contains more pesticides than domestically grown and may contain pesticides that are banned from use in the United States. Require your supermarket to label produce with its country of origin. By buying domestic you interrupt the "circle of poison." American chemical manufacturers export banned pesticides and the stuff comes back in the produce.

Avoid fish from contaminated waters. Check with your local health department for information on which fish from which waters to avoid.

Avoid food containing nitrites and nitrates. Examples of these are cured meats, such as lunch meats, hot dogs, and bacon. Nitrite-free foods can be found in nutrition stores and through food co-ops.

Have your tap water tested. Periodically test your water for hazardous chemicals, such as PCBs. Your local water department, EPA, or private laboratories can check water samples. Bottled water may be safer.

Write to your elected officials. The short-term answer to the pesticide problem is simply don't buy it. Food-buying cooperatives can help lower the cost of organically grown foods. The long-term solution is to pass laws ensuring pesticide-free foods.

Join with others. Become a member of organizations that are not alarmist but have a genuine concern for feeding our children pesticide-free food. Such an organization is the Natural Resources Defense Council, 40 West 20th Street, New York, NY 10011, (212) 727–2700 (tel.), (212) 727–1773 (fax), www.nrdc.org. Send for or read on-line their publication *Putting Children First: Making Pesticide Levels in Food Safer for Infants and Children.*

III

Contemporary Parenting

At the very time when more parents are realizing the importance of being close to their babies, social and economic pressures are competing with this attachment process. Two-income parenting, single parenting, colicky babies, sleepless nights, and special-needs babies are just a few of the situations facing today's parents. Parents are busy and are likely to get busier. The good news is that there are more resources available to help parents meet these challenges. To make parenting life easier, the next several chapters present ways to keep attached while keeping busy — a contemporary juggling act to prevent a distance from developing between parent and child. Here is attachment parenting in action.

14

Babywearing: The Art and Science of Carrying Your Baby

As long as I carry my baby, he's content," mothers of fussy babies in our practice would say. After hearing parents extol the benefits of carrying their babies, we decided to study how this parenting style, so useful in other cultures, could be part of our own parenting repertoire. Here is the story of babywearing — how it changed the lives of parents and babies in our practice and how it can change yours.

NEW SUPPORT FOR AN OLD IDEA

In many other cultures parents wear their babies; in our culture we wheel our babies, then park them somewhere. Infant development specialists who travel throughout the world studying infant-care practices have repeatedly observed that babies who are carried in a variety of cloth-type slings or front packs seem more content than infants who are kept in cribs, playpens, strollers, prams, and plastic seats. The mother of a patient of ours visited the island of Bali, where she witnessed a ground-touching ceremony. The Balinese babies are carried, or worn, for the first six months of life. The mother or some other caregiver in the extended family wears the baby all day long, and baby is put down to sleep next to the mother. The baby literally does not touch the ground for the first six months, at which time a ground-touching ceremony is held, and for the first time the baby is put down on the ground to crawl and learn freestyle movements.

For a number of years we have researched infant-care studies and found general agreement that babies behave and develop better when they are carried a lot. Years ago, while attending an international parenting conference, we interviewed two women from Zambia who were carrying their babies in slings that matched their native dress. We asked them why women in their culture wear their babies most of the time. One woman replied, "It makes life easier for the mother." The other woman volunteered, "It's good for the baby." These women went on to relate the feelings of "completeness" and "value" that babywearing gave them. Women in their culture don't have the benefits of books and studies about mothering hormones. What

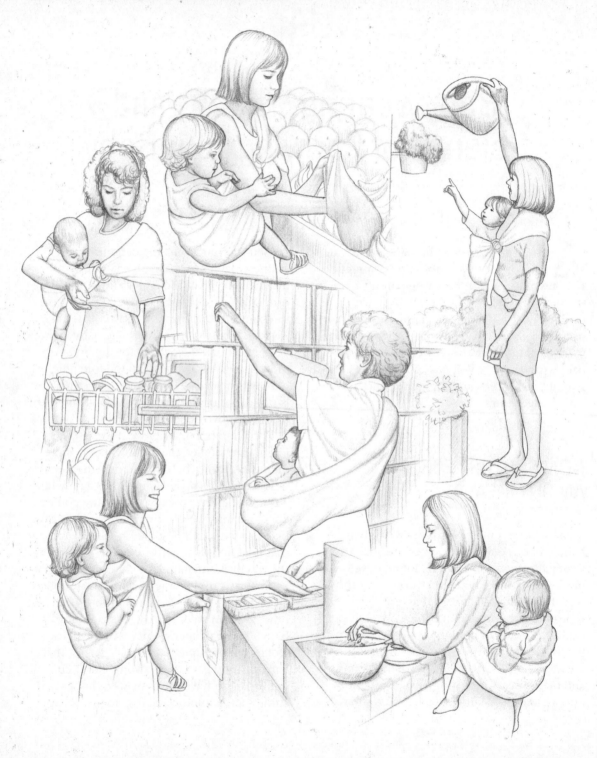

they have is centuries of tradition that have simply taught them that something good happens to women and their babies when the babies are worn.

Doesn't every parent in every culture have these two simple desires: *to make life easier for themselves and to make life better for their baby?* Babywearing does both.

Encouraged by these observations, in 1985 we began our own personal study on the beneficial effects of babywearing on babies and their parents. Since that time we have logged miles of wearing our own babies and have kept precise records as we experimented with various carrying styles. We have advised parents to carry their babies as much as possible, beginning right after birth. We have asked them to try out a variety of baby carriers and choose the one most comfortable for themselves and their babies.

To the mothers we now say, "Try to get used to wearing your baby in a sling-type carrier just as you would wear one of your favorite items of clothing." At their baby's first checkup, usually at one week, we show the new parents how to wear their baby. During their personal course on babywearing, we advise each parent to ex- periment with various carrying positions, to find the one that is most comfortable and allows baby to mold to the contours of the parent's own body; we encourage them to shift carrying positions to match baby's development.

This is why we call it babywearing. Now, to teach you how this practice can make your parenting life easier and enhance the devel- opment of your baby, here are the results of our studies and your own course in baby- wearing.

THE BABYWEARING MIND-SET

In case you are wondering how much parents should carry their babies, cer- tainly parents have to put down their babies sometimes! In fact, it is impor- tant to take a balanced approach to babywearing. But this style of parent- ing means changing your mind-set regarding what babies are really like. You may envision your picture-book baby lying quietly in a crib, gazing pas- sively at dangling mobiles, and picked up only to be fed and played with and then put down; you may think that "up" periods are just dutiful intervals to quiet your baby long enough to put him down again. To understand baby- wearing, reverse this view: Carry your baby much of the time, and put him or her down for longer nap times, night- time, and to attend to your personal needs. Take a balanced approach to babywearing. Allow baby to enjoy down periods and freestyle move- ments on the carpet, but pick her up when she signals the desire to be car- ried. You will note an interesting con- trast in behavior. "Down" babies learn to cry to get picked up; "up" babies learn noncrying body language signal- ing their need to get down. The amount of holding time naturally decreases as your baby increases in age and motor skills. Even your toddler, however, may show occasional high- need periods when he or she wants to be picked up and worn.

CHOOSING THE RIGHT BABY CARRIER

Early in our study we realized one of the reasons Western mothers did not wear their babies much was that the baby carriers then available were not easy to use. One of the reasons that mothers in other cultures wear their babies so much is that they fabricate a sling-type carrier that looks like part of their garments and, in fact, usually is. We encouraged mothers either to find or create a carrier that would be comfortable for them and easy to use and that would keep their baby from fussing. As we were exposed to a whole parade of babywearing mothers, we observed what types of carriers and styles of wearing worked for most parent-baby pairs most of the time. After years of watching babywearing parents, we came to the same conclusion that mothers in other cultures have known for centuries and Western mothers are now beginning to discover — a *sling-type* carrier works the best. In selecting a sling-type carrier look for the following features.

Safety. The most important feature of any baby carrier is safety. The sling must both *support* and *contain* the baby.

Comfort. A baby carrier must be comfortable for both parents and baby. A well-designed carrier should distribute the baby's weight on the adult's shoulders and hips, not the back and neck. The sling should be comfortably padded over all pressure points, especially along the wearer's back and shoulder and wherever the edges of the carrier press against baby's torso and legs.

Versatility. Choose a carrier that you can use from birth to at least two years of age, thus making it unnecessary to purchase a series of carriers as baby gets older. Fussy, colicky babies are seldom content to be carried in the same position all the time. Carriers that flatten baby against mother's chest are often too restrictive for a baby who, like all of us, is more content being stimulated by a 180-degree view of the world around him. The illustrations in this chapter show the versatile positions of a sling-type carrier.

Ease of use. A fact of human nature is that if something is not convenient to use, we won't bother with it. Fathers, especially, shy away from carriers that have sets of buckles and straps. A well-designed sling-type carrier can be adjusted with baby inside, with one hand, without disturbing the baby. Another important feature of a well-designed carrier is that you should be able to easily and safely slip out of the carrier, leaving baby still inside — a useful maneuver while putting baby down if you want, once baby is asleep.

Suitability for feeding. One thing we often hear from mothers is that they have to remove their babies from a carrier in order to breastfeed. With a sling-type carrier, however, you can easily and discreetly breastfeed your baby while she is still in the sling. A hungry baby can be quickly attached before having to fuss for a feeding and can quietly drift off to a satisfied sleep while still in the sling. Using the sling carrier as a shield allows you to meet baby's need to feed at those inopportune times when you just can't get to a quiet, private place or when you don't have a place to sit down (such as standing in line at the grocery store).

Consult experienced babywearers for advice on which carrier to select and how to use it. Borrow and test-wear various carriers before settling on the best one for you and your baby. You are not only selecting a carrier, you are investing in a parenting style. Baby carriers are nurturing devices, and sling carriers make rediscovering the lost art of wearing the baby easier for parents — and good for the baby.

▶ **BABYWEARING HELP LINE:** *For information about where to purchase baby slings, see "Baby Carriers" in "Resources," page 745.*

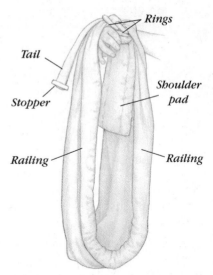

Parts of a sling.

HOW TO WEAR YOUR BABY: A PERSONAL COURSE

Each baby has his or her individual preference on how to be carried, and each babywearer has his or her preference on how to carry the baby. Because the sling-type carrier has enjoyed worldwide use for centuries and is the one we have used for our personal research, we suggest the sling as standard apparel for your course in babywearing. (The following general instructions apply to most sling-type carriers. They may vary according to the design of the carrier.)

Initially parents may feel uncomfortable wearing their newborn because baby seems scrunched down too far in the sling. Remember, your baby was scrunched in the womb, so she is used to this secure feeling. Being curled up is a natural position for a newborn. Colicky babies especially are comforted by rolling into a little ball and drawing their legs up onto their abdomen.

The following is a step-by-step approach to wearing your newborn.

PUTTING ON THE SLING

Decide which shoulder you wish the sling to rest on. Hold the baby sling where the tail passes through the rings and place it over your head, letting it come to rest on your shoulder and across your chest. For the standard position, have the tail in front and the shoulder pad on your shoulder. For a newborn, put the sling on "backward" (with the shoulder pad in front, and rings and tail at top of shoulder) so that your newborn's head can rest on the shoulder pad as a pillow.

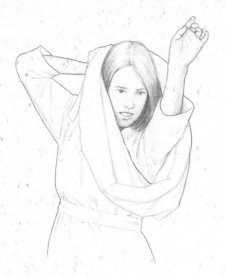

Putting on a baby sling.

Adjusting the sling. You can adjust the size of the sling by simply pulling on the tail, creating a snugger fit. The smaller the infant and/or the babywearer, the longer the tail will be. Holding baby's bottom while you adjust the size of the sling lessens the weight on the sling, making adjustment easier.

➤*PUT IT IN GEAR! As soon as baby is nestled securely and comfortably in the sling, start walking immediately; babies usually associate being nested in the sling with movement. If you stand still too long after putting baby in the sling, he may fuss.*

CRADLE HOLD (SHOWN HERE FOR NEWBORNS)

The cradle hold and its variations are useful from birth and throughout the first year.

1. Put the sling on "backward" for babies under about 10 pounds.

2. While supporting baby's back and head, align baby in the direction you wish him to be in the sling, open the sling, and slide baby's body into the sling while lowering the back of his head into the pocket formed by the shoulder pad and padded railings of the sling.

3. Rest baby's head on the shoulder pad as a pillow.

4. Adjust the size of the sling.

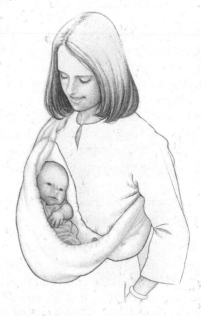

Upright cradle hold, newborn; sling is in "backward" position.

Variations of the cradle hold. In the first month or so, for a snugger fit on a newborn, place her head toward the ring buckle. Some babies enjoy riding higher in the sling, semi-upright; others prefer nesting more horizon-tally especially when asleep; some enjoy the wraparound position, facing toward your body as when breastfeeding. Other variations of this hold are described later in the chapter.

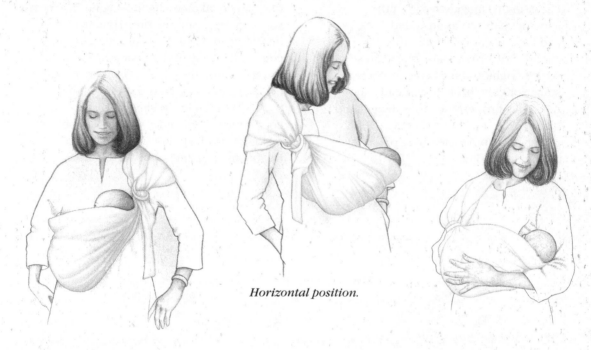

Horizontal position.

Semiupright position.

Breastfeeding position.

SNUGGLE HOLD

This carrying position is useful from birth to six months. During the first two months, the snuggle hold usually works best if the sling is put on in the backward position, using the shoulder pad as an added support for baby's back and head and taking up the slack in the sling. As baby grows and seems to fill the sling more, try putting on the sling in the regular position, with the pad on your shoulder. Experiment to find the position that works best for you and your baby.

1. Put on sling in the backward position.

2. Hold baby against your left shoulder with your left hand. With the right hand, pull the edge of the sling out and up over baby.

3. Bend over slightly, holding baby's back with your right hand, and with your left hand pull baby's feet down under and out-side the lower railing of the sling, or, if baby is still so young that he likes tucking

his feet up close to his body, leave baby's feet nestled inside the sling.

4. Adjust the snugness of the sling so that baby is securely nestled against your chest. In the snuggle position the shoulder pad acts as an added back and head support for the tiny baby. Be sure the lower railing is snug against baby's thighs and the upper railing snug along the back of his head and neck. In a properly secure snuggle hold, baby will seem to be sitting in a little pouch, just above the lower padded railing of the sling.

Some babies need the sling to be very snug or they don't feel securely held. If after adjustment the sling still feels too large in the snuggle hold, try the following: (1) The upper edge will usually have much more slack that can be taken up by tucking it underneath your arm opposite the ring. Hold that arm tightly against your body to secure the upper edge of the sling under your arm so that it sits snugly around the back of baby's head and neck and all the slack is transferred to your back. (2) Cinch in the sling so that the lower edge snugly cups under your baby's bottom, making sort of a pouch — enabling baby to sit on the inner railing of the sling.

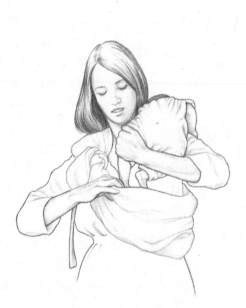

Easing baby into the snuggle hold.

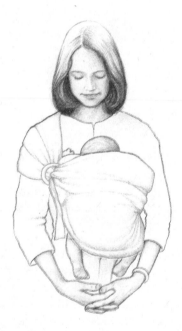

Snuggle hold.

KANGAROO CARRY (FORWARD-FACING POSITION)

Between three and six months (earlier in some babies) your baby may prefer the kangaroo carry, or forward-facing position. Once baby has developed good head control and a curious personality, he may find the cradle and snuggle holds too confining and want to see more. The kangaroo position is usually preferable for very active babies who are quieted by the stimulation of the 180-degree view. If your baby is one of those "archers" who fusses and stiffens out as if attempting back dives while you are trying to wear him in either the snuggle or the cradle hold, the kangaroo carry may be the answer.

To determine whether your baby is ready to be carried facing forward, try the following: Without the sling, hold your baby against your chest with her head and back resting against your chest, your arms underneath her legs, bending her thighs upward to touch her abdomen. This is one of the colic curl positions (see page 403). Start walking and revolving a bit side to side, giving your baby a full 180-degree sweeping view. If your baby likes this position, she is probably ready for the kangaroo carry.

Six-month-old babies love the forward-facing carry. Started early, some babies may enjoy this forward-facing position for up to a year or longer.

Use your sling as follows for the kangaroo carry:

1. Support baby facing forward with one arm under her legs and her back against your chest.

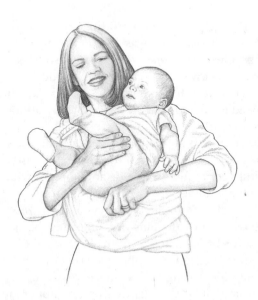

Easing baby into the kangaroo carry.

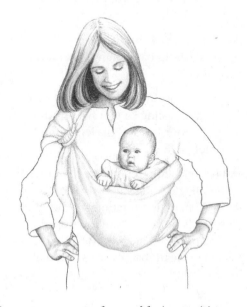

Kangaroo carry, or forward-facing position.

2. With your free hand hold the edge of the sling outward, forming a pouch.

3. Slide baby down into the pouch, bottom first, either with her back resting directly against and sliding down the front of your chest or nestled in the crook of your arm. Most babies sit cross-legged at the bottom of the pouch. Some older babies enjoy being flexed so much that their feet protrude over the edge of the sling.

Sidesaddle carry. This is a variation of the forward-facing position. Slide baby down into the pouch, bottom first as in the kangaroo carry. Next turn baby's feet toward the side opposite the rings and nestle his head in the sling pocket a few inches beneath the rings.

HIP STRADDLE

Between four and six months, or when baby can sit without support, your baby may like to be carried on your hip (see illustration on next page). Try the following steps:

1. Most parents prefer to wear their baby on the hip opposite their dominant hand; wear your baby on your left hip if you are right-handed, for example.

2. With your left hand (if you are right-handed), hold baby high up on your shoulder.

3. Using your right hand, pull baby's feet through the sling so that his bottom rests on your hip and his legs straddle your left side.

4. Adjust the sling to have the lower padded railing resting snugly behind baby's knees and the body of the sling across his buttocks. Pull the upper railing of the sling upward so that it fits snugly beneath baby's arms and high on his back.

Some babies like to play the game of arching themselves backward shortly after being put in the hip straddle. It is all right for baby to lean away from your body to some extent; he doesn't have to be held in as tightly as in the snuggle hold. Try giving your baby a toy, or engage your baby in immediate eye-to-eye contact to lessen this nuisance, convincing him that he wants to be close to you rather than push away from you.

Shifting positions from the hip straddle. Baby can be shifted easily from the hip straddle to the *safety hip carry* by shifting baby backward so that her legs straddle the back of your hip, rather than the side, and her head is behind your shoulders. This position is a favorite for the toddler, especially if you are doing something in front of you and wish baby to be safely out of the way. Baby can still peer around your side and observe what you are doing.

To shift from the hip carry to the *cradle hold* for breastfeeding or comforting, bring baby's back leg to the front alongside the other one, and swing both legs over to the ring side, letting baby cradle across your front. Pull up extra fabric from the upper railing so that your entire front area is covered for private feeding.

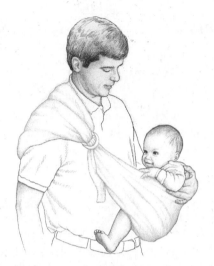

Hip straddle.

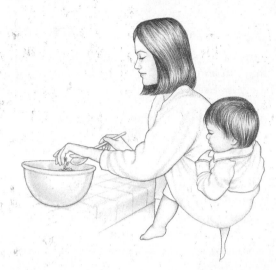

Safety hip carry.

The real fun of babywearing, for you and your infant, is experimenting with various positions and carrying styles to find the ones that work best for you and your baby. The earlier you begin wearing your baby (preferably begin in the newborn period), the better baby will become accustomed to the sling. Even infants six months old or older can be taught to enjoy the sling, but it often takes some creative wearing styles to get the older first-time sling baby to get used to being in a carrier.

THE BABYWEARING FATHER — BECOMING A SHAREHOLDER

As a father and certified babywearer, I feel that it is important that a baby get used to father's handling, too. Father has a different rhythm to his walk, a difference that baby learns to appreciate. The snuggle hold and neck nestle are favorite wearing positions for father.

The neck nestle. Place the baby in the snuggle position and lift him up a bit until his head nestles into the curve of your neck. You will have found one of the most comforting and calming holding patterns. In the neck nestle dad has a slight edge over mom. Babies hear not only through their ears but also through the vibration of their skull bones. By placing baby's head against your voice box, in the front of your neck, and humming and singing to your baby, the slower, more easily felt vibrations of the lower-pitched male voice often lull baby right to sleep. As you rock and walk with your baby, sing a calming song such as "Old Man River."

SAFE BABYWEARING

Baby carriers made by reputable manufacturers have been safety tested, but there are human elements that must be accounted for. Observe the following safety tips when wearing your baby:

- While you are getting used to wearing your baby, support her with your hands. As you go through the learning phase of babywearing, holding your baby with your hands becomes instinctive — like embracing your protuberant abdomen while pregnant. After you become a baby-wearing veteran, you can safely carry your baby in the sling with one or both hands free.

- When baby is tiny and in the cradle position, rest one arm (usually the one opposite the side with the shoulder pad) along the top rail of the sling. This added protection contains baby while you are getting used to the sling.

- While carrying baby in the forward-facing position, keep one hand on baby until you and baby feel secure with this method of wearing.

- In the hip carry, be sure the top rail of the sling is pulled up over baby's back at least as high as baby's shoulder blades. The archers like to practice their back dives when carried in this position. Containing baby in the sling discourages this action.

- Older babies like to squirm and sometimes even stand in the sling. Carefully support your baby during these antics.

- Do not wear baby while cooking at the stove, cycling, or riding in a moving vehicle. Baby carriers are not substitutes for an approved car seat.

- Avoid sudden twisting. Babies can fall when a mother suddenly turns to do something (such as rescue another child from danger) and "forgets" she is wearing her baby. As a precaution, try this safety rehearsal: Suddenly twist your upper body to grab something, and at the same time embrace your baby with your other arm. After you have frequently rehearsed this reaction, you will instinctively clasp your baby with one hand while lunging with the other.

- When wearing your baby and stooping over, bend at the knees, not at the waist, and hold baby in the sling with one hand while picking up something with the other.

- Toddlers, while being worn, are at your reaching level and can grab dangerous or breakable objects off shelves. Keep an arm's distance away from potential hazards.

- When going through doorways or around corners, be careful that baby's body does not stick out past your arm and strike the wall or doorjamb.

- Don't drink hot beverages when wearing baby, although wearing her while eating is all right.

- Watch baby closely if bottlefeeding in the sling, since the bent position may cause some babies to spit up.

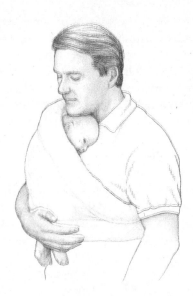

The neck nestle, a favored position of babywearing fathers.

Another attraction to the neck nestle is that baby feels the warming air from your nose on her scalp. (Experienced mothers have long known that sometimes just breathing onto baby's head or face will calm her. They call this "magic breath.") Our babies have enjoyed the neck nestle more than any of the other holding patterns, and I have, too. Dads, become a *shareholder* in the family art of babywearing.

The warm fuzzy. For a uniquely male variation of the snuggle hold, place baby's ear over your heart — bare skin to bare skin. The combination of the rhythm of your heartbeat and movement of your chest, plus the feel of abdominal breathing and the rhythm of your walk, introduce baby to the uniqueness of being worn by dad. If baby falls asleep during the warm fuzzy (as usually happens), lie down with your baby and drift off to

sleep together (see "Wearing Down to Sleep," page 295).

For a father to be comfortable wearing his baby and a baby to respond to dad's babywearing techniques are real bonuses for mothers of high-need babies. It helps prevent mother burnout. Here is a common scenario a mother of a high-need baby recently shared with me:

"I love our new baby, but he is one of these high-need babies and I need to wear him constantly. He was wearing me down and I was burning out. My husband feels very insecure in calming fussy babies and for this reason I was reluctant to release our baby to him during those trying fussy times. The sling was the answer. After my husband got used to wearing our baby, and I saw that our baby liked it, I felt more comfortable releasing our baby to him. Initially I would hover over my husband to make sure our baby would stop fussing but as soon as he proved himself as a competent babywearer I felt a sense of relief. Even though I wear our baby most of the time, just having my husband share this beautiful experience gives me a much-needed break."

My own experience is similar. I felt a real high the first time I put Stephen in the neck nestle and snuggled him securely against my chest for a walk. As we strolled together, I felt a sense of completeness. Sometimes I wore him for hours at a time. I felt right when we were together and not right (or complete) when we were apart. These are feelings usually reserved for the mother-infant pair. I wanted a piece of this babywearing action, too. The more I wore Stephen, the more comfortable we both became at trying different wearing positions. The more he liked it, the more I liked it, and the more we enjoyed being together.

OTHER BABYWEARERS

While infants enjoy being worn by their parents best, babies will adapt to substitute caregivers better if worn in the sling they are used to. "Home" to a baby can be in the sling. Brian, a toddler in our practice, calls his sling "my little house."

Babywearing and Baby-sitters

Parents of high-need babies often confide to us that they are afraid to leave their baby with anyone because no one else can comfort these special babies. High-need babies who are accustomed to being worn are more easily comforted by a baby-sitter who wears them. Barbara, a busy mom whose only hope of survival was to wear her high-need baby, relates this story. "Jason is so happy when he is in the sling that I feel comfortable briefly leaving him with a sitter. Sometimes if I'm in a hurry, I greet the sitter at the door, transfer Jason to her while in the sling — sort of like the transfer of a baton in a relay race — and she takes over the wearing. He forgets to fuss, and I feel better knowing his routine is not disrupted."

Babywearing by Siblings

When we adults wear babies, we model for our other children that big people carry little people. Children and grandchildren are later likely to adopt the style of parenting that they received or witnessed when young. For example, our own children have sometimes "worn" their dolls in homemade baby slings because they have witnessed us wearing babies so often. The effect of role modeling on children's views of the mother-infant relationship was brought home to us one day when our then six-year-old daughter Hayden was asked by her teacher to draw a mother and baby. She drew the two as essentially one person. She recognized that, at least in the early months, mothers wear babies, and the two are inseparable.

Babywear in Day Care

To ensure that your baby gets a lot of holding time, especially if you have a high-need baby, instruct your day-care provider on how to wear baby in a sling. Impress upon her how much happier and better behaved are "sling babies." The following is a "prescription" I often give parents to present to their day-care providers:

SEARS FAMILY PEDIATRICS
William Sears, M.D., James Sears, M.D., Robert Sears, M.D., Martha Sears, R.N.

NAME *Baby Erin*

Rx *To keep baby content, wear baby in a sling at least 3 hours a day.*

REFILLS *as needed*

Wm. P. Sears M.D.

Special Groups: Teens and Marines

Teenage girls often enjoy wearing babies, but this style of baby care is not easy to model to teenage boys. Here's how our son Peter at fourteen years old got hooked on wearing his then two-month-old brother, Stephen. Martha was asked to give a talk to a group of military wives at a local U.S. Marine base. The topic was how to get their husbands to share in more baby care. Martha offered to provide slings in a camouflage pattern. We did, and the dads loved wearing their "baby marines." Peter, who was into army things anyway at that time, couldn't wait to put on the camouflage sling and wear his baby brother. It is important that boys develop tenderness. How heartwarming it is to see men and boys care for little babies.

WEARING DOWN TO SLEEP

It's 9:00 P.M. and you're tired but baby isn't. Nestle baby in the sling and stroll around the house until he falls asleep. This is what we call wearing down.

First-time parents may have been led to believe that the way a baby goes to sleep is that at some preassigned time they put the half-awake baby into the crib, kiss him on the cheek, turn out the lights, and leave the room. Baby peacefully drifts off to sleep without much bother. This happens only in books and movies, or for everybody else's baby, but seldom in real life. Most babies want to or need to be nursed (comforted) down to sleep in a caregiver's arms. Babywearing allows the infant to make the transition from an awake state to sleep more easily.

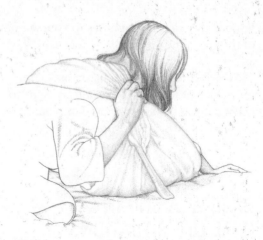

After "wearing down" — babywearing your baby to sleep — gently slip yourself out of the sling and leave the sling on baby as a cover.

When you feel that baby is ready to go to sleep (or you are ready for her to go to sleep), wear her in the sling in the position that you have found to be least stimulating and most sleep inducing. Walk around the house. Try breastfeeding while moving. When your baby is in a state of deep sleep (recognized by a motionless face and limp limbs) lower yourself onto the bed until she is lying down and you can gently slip yourself out of the sling. Allow baby to remain on the bed in the sling, using it as a cover. If baby sleeps best on her side, tuck the sling between baby and bed to keep her from rolling over. Although asleep, baby may still seem restless while you are wearing her down (this is called REM — or rapid eye movement — sleep, a lighter state of sleep in which baby is likely to awaken if you put her down and try to sneak out of the room). If this happens, keep your baby in the snuggle hold and lie down with her on your chest while she is still in the sling. The rhythm of your heartbeat and breathing motion will lull baby into a deep sleep, after which you can roll over and slip yourself out of the sling, and your baby will usually stay asleep.

Wearing down is particularly useful for the reluctant napper. Sometimes it helps to leave baby in the snuggle hold on your chest so you can both drift off to sleep together.

BABYWEARING IN REAL-LIFE SITUATIONS

Breastfeeding While Babywearing

In the last twenty years the majority of mothers have chosen to breastfeed their infants. Babywearing allows breastfeeding on the move so that busy mothers can more easily nurture their babies with the best nutrition, yet continue their active life-styles.

Advantages

It's convenient. Breastfeeding while babywearing makes life easier for the mother of a marathon nurser, a baby who in the early months wants to nurse constantly, such as a baby who is going through a growth spurt. Breastfeeding while wearing allows mother to be on the go and get things done around the house while meeting her infant's breastfeeding needs. It's convenient outside the house, too. If you are shopping with the baby and need to feed in public, private breastfeeding is very easy while wearing baby. Because baby feels comfortable in the sling, he is content feeding there, even in a public place. Martha has spent a few hours of babywearing and breastfeeding in the checkout line at the grocery store. Breastfeeding in the sling is

especially convenient in restaurants and similar places where being a baby may not always be socially acceptable. Patrons in a restaurant would much prefer a discreetly breastfeeding baby to an annoying, screaming baby. Additionally, babies who are worn in public places tend to fuss less and are therefore more welcome — especially in a society that has heretofore traditionally not welcomed babies everywhere.

It organizes problem suckers. Some babies breastfeed better on the move, especially those problem suckers who need movement to organize their sucking. Tense babies (those with a suck problem called tonic bite) and back archers often breastfeed much better in the sling because of the organizing effect babywearing has on their entire physiology. As the baby's whole body relaxes, so do the suck muscles. For babies who suck

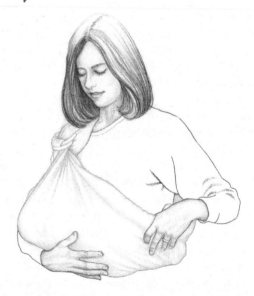

Babywearing allows for discreet, convenient breastfeeding.

better on the move, first position baby in the sling in order to achieve proper latch-on, and then quickly begin walking.

It helps mother to care for older siblings. Breastfeeding in the sling is especially valuable when there is a new baby and a toddler. By feeding the tiny baby in the sling, mother has the mobility to attend to the toddler also. As one mother said, "Breastfeeding our new baby in the sling gives me an extra pair of hands to play with and enjoy our toddler. This has done wonders to lessen sibling rivalry and allowed me to mother both children well."

It helps the slow-weight-gaining baby. In our practice, when a breastfeeding baby is showing a less-than-adequate weight gain and we have exhausted all possible reasons why, we have experienced amazing results by encouraging the mother to wear her baby at least several hours a day and breastfeed while doing so. Mothers report that babies feed more frequently and in a more relaxed way, and weight dramatically increases. This proves again what researchers have long known: Proximity to the mother encourages a baby to feed more frequently. In addition to this, it could be that the nearness of mother to baby enables and encourages mother to read and respond to baby's feeding cues more promptly. Also, because baby is always near the source of milk and comfort, he does not have to waste energy summoning mother; baby can use this energy to grow. (See related sections on premature and failure-to-thrive babies, pages 300–301.)

Babywearing Positions for Breastfeeding

The cradle hold is the usual breastfeeding position for a baby of any age. The sling itself, however, does not hold baby snugly enough

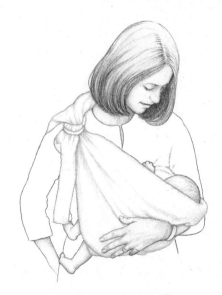

The cradle hold is the usual position for breastfeeding a baby in a sling.

at the breast to maintain latch-on. It is necessary to support baby with your free arm to keep him close to the breast. This is done with your arm alongside baby's head and back on the outside of the sling, and with baby positioned on his side so that he is facing the breast without turning his head. Your other hand can be slipped inside the sling in order to present the breast. Mother can continue to hold her breast for her baby, or if she needs a free hand, she can prop her breast with a cloth diaper or hand towel to keep it at the right level for baby, if needed.

The clutch hold. In the early months babies may prefer breastfeeding in the clutch hold. Using a modified snuggle hold, shift baby into a side cradle position, with his head in front of the breast and his legs curled up beneath the same arm. Mother can then use her arm on the side of the sling to hold baby's back

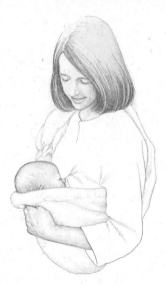

Breastfeeding in the clutch hold.

and head close to her breast and use the opposite hand inside the sling to help baby latch on. The clutch hold is particularly useful in the early weeks of breastfeeding while babies are learning how to latch on. Bending some babies in the clutch hold helps them suck better and maintain proper latch-on longer. This is especially true of the archer — the clutch hold may keep her from doing back dives during feeding.

Burping baby. To burp your baby, shift from the clutch or cradle hold to the snuggle hold so that baby is upright. The pressure of your chest against baby's tummy plus the gentle patting on baby's back (in addition to the snugness of this hold) will help baby burp.

Work and Wear

Babywearing fits in beautifully with complex life-styles. It makes life easier for the busy mother. Mothers in other cultures have fabricated various sling-type carriers because it is necessary to carry their babies with them when they work or when they are on the go. Mothers in Western cultures are also on the go, they just "go" differently.

Besides mothering eight children, Martha is a lactation consultant and taught breastfeeding classes. One day, just before a seminar, Matthew, who was then six months old, developed an ill-timed fussy period. Not wishing to cancel her class but more strongly not wanting to leave Matthew during a high-need period, Martha wore him in our sling while delivering a one-hour lecture to 150 pediatricians. After mother and baby finished "their" talk on the attachment style of parenting, one of the doctors came up to her and exclaimed, "What you did made more of an impression than what you said!"

Many mothers who have part-time jobs outside the home have been able to wear their babies at work. They call this "work and wear." Such jobs as selling real estate, shopkeeping, demonstrating products, and housecleaning lend themselves well to babywearing. Janice, a mother whose business involves cleaning houses a few hours a day, wears her baby in a sling while doing housework. A pediatrician friend wears her baby to work in her office. She often wears her baby during well-baby exams on her patients. Her office staff members wear her baby if she is examining a patient who might have a contagious disease. Work and wear helped her and her new baby to stay together yet allowed her to continue working in her profession.

Most employers are initially reluctant to allow mothers to wear their babies to work, but we encourage them to give it a fair trial. Employers often find that the babywearing mothers actually do a more productive job, since they so appreciate being given the opportunity to keep their babies with them. They make an extra effort to prove that they can do two jobs at once. One employer even found the baby to be an added attraction for his customers, as if they sensed that a centuries-old custom of working and wearing was being practiced in this store. The customers felt that something right was going on. Try it and see!

Wearing Out, Eating Out

How often have you said, "I'd love to go, but I've just had a baby." Some mothers go stir-crazy after a few months. There is nothing in the mother-baby contract that says you have to stay home and become a recluse after you have a baby. But a new mother is usually not ready to leave her baby to go out. Babywearing allows you to "have your baby and take it with you."

When our son Stephen was two months old, we were invited to a black tie formal affair. Rather than decline the invitation, as new parents usually do, we wore Stephen in a fashionable sling, and we all had a great time. With a few breastfeeding snacks, Stephen nestled peacefully in the sling during the three-and-a-half-hour affair. Stephen was not a disturbance, but he was often the center of attention. Onlookers initially had that puzzled expression, as if wondering, "What is that she's wearing?" The puzzlement turned to admiration. "Why it's a baby, how cute!" By the end of the evening, as the guests noticed how content we were with our babywearing arrangement, there was an air of acceptance throughout the room. Babywearing had achieved not only social approval but social admiration.

Here's another scenario: Shortly after the birth of a baby, dad says, "Honey, how about a date? Let's go out to dinner." Mom replies, "But we can't leave our baby." The answer to this dilemma? Babywearing. Babies are quiet in restaurants when worn in a sling. They seldom cry and are usually seen and not heard. Babies can breastfeed discreetly and are rarely disruptive to restaurant patrons.

Babywearing While Traveling

Wearing your baby in a sling provides a safe, protective environment for baby when you are shopping or traveling anyplace in which there are crowds. Walking through a crowded shopping mall or airport with a toddler in tow is nerve-racking when you consider what could happen if you let go of his hand even for a moment (or take your hand off his stroller and get distracted). Between the ages of one and two, when the infant begins to walk, dart out from your protective arms, and explore the environment, babywearing keeps the toddler close to your side in any situation where a free-roaming toddler may not be safe. Have you ever noticed that a pedestrian toddler's face is at the exact level that people hold their lit cigarettes? Busy shoppers or travelers often don't watch out for little people. Bring your baby or toddler up to a safe level and relax — he won't go anywhere without you.

Busy parents throughout the world are on the go, and babywearing makes traveling easier. During travel babies are constantly required to make the transition from one activity to another. With babywearing, transitioning (changing environments or going from wakefulness to sleep) is easier. While you are standing in line at the airport, a baby worn is safe, secure, and happy. If your baby fusses a bit on an airplane, wear her and walk around the plane so that she is attracted by the visual stimulation of the environment. When baby is ready to go off to sleep in a hotel room, wear her down onto a bed in the sling until she falls asleep. Home to a baby is where mother and father are, and the sling is a constant reminder of baby's "home." It makes adaptation to new environments easier and travel more pleasant for the whole family.

Here are some other uses for the sling while traveling:

As a pillow. For breastfeeding or just for laying baby across your lap, a folded-up baby sling makes a comfortable pillow. Fold the sling the way it came in the package, and you have a useful pillow.

As a changing pad. Place the sling on the floor or on a changing table (don't leave baby unattended on a table), place baby's head on the shoulder pad of the pillow, and presto! you have a comfortable diaper-changing surface. During changing, place a clean diaper under baby to protect the sling.

As a cover. The baby sling makes a convenient cover during travel for napping, discreet nursing, and warmth.

BABYWEARING IN SPECIAL SITUATIONS

For families with special circumstances and infants with special needs, babywearing eases some of the strains.

Wearing Twins

After the first few months, twins are usually too heavy to carry one in each arm. Baby-

wearing is the solution. Either wear one baby in the baby sling while holding the other in your arms (safer than two babies in arms in case you trip), or have two slings — one for each baby and parent. Besides being convenient for parents, twin wearing allows interaction between babies. As the parents are relating, so are the babies, because they are face-to-face rather than behind each other in a stroller.

Babywearing for Medical Benefits

Premature babies. A premature baby, especially one with medical problems needing weeks or months of intensive care, is deprived of those final weeks or months in the womb. Instead, baby must grow in an outside womb. The problem is that outside wombs are static. They don't move. Research has shown that a premature whose "womb" moves gains weight faster and has fewer stop-breathing (apnea) episodes. Specialists in newborn care have fabricated a variety of moving wombs, such as oscillating water beds.

A group of newborn-care specialists in South America made an ingenious discovery. Some hospitals could not afford incubators and all the technology needed to care for the preemies. They were forced to use the mother. These preemies were wrapped around their mothers in a slinglike wrap, a custom called packing. To everyone's amazement the babies thrived as well as or even better than the technologically cared-for babies.

The researchers concluded that the close proximity to mother helped the babies to thrive. Being close to mother enticed babies to feed frequently. Mother's warmth kept the baby warm; mother's movement calmed the baby, enabling the baby to divert energy from crying to growing. Mother's breathing movements stimulated baby's breathing, so that these babies had fewer stop-breathing episodes. Mother acted as sort of a respiratory pacemaker for baby's breathing.

As soon as a premature baby no longer needs oxygen and intravenous therapy and enters the growing phase, we encourage mothers to wear their babies as much as possible, the practice called kangaroo care. (For an explanation, see page 185.)

Failure-to-thrive babies. The infant who fails to thrive also benefits from babywearing. Some babies, for a variety of medical reasons, are very slow to gain weight, the condition called failure to thrive. In our pediatric practice, and for one of our own babies, we have used babywearing as a therapeutic tool to stimulate thriving. My doctor's orders to the parents are very simple: "Put your baby on in the morning and take him off at night. Wear him down for naps and to sleep. Wear him when you go out and about the house. Take long relaxing walks while wearing your baby. This will help both of you to thrive."

How does babywearing help babies thrive? Motion does good things for growing babies. It has a calming effect on infants. They cry less and therefore divert the energy they would have wasted on crying into growing. Also, proximity increases feeding frequency, another reason that babywearing stimulates growth. Frequent feedings are a potent stimulus for growth. Perhaps babywearing promotes growth hormones and body enzymes that enhance growth. This has been shown to be true in experimental animals. I believe that in addition to these growth-promoting effects babywearing helps babies thrive because of the organizing effect on the baby. The baby's overall biological system seems to work better when she is worn.

The handicapped baby. Parents often spend much time and money on infant stimulation techniques and better-baby classes when the best stimulation available at the lowest possible cost is right in front of them — babywearing. The handicapped baby especially profits from being worn. Picture the stimulation baby gets: He hears what you hear, sees what you see, moves like you move, because he is near your eyes, ears, and mouth. Baby is in constant touch.

Cerebral palsy babies who arch and stiffen are greatly helped by babywearing. The contoured, bent position of the cradle hold and kangaroo carry competes with baby's tendency to arch backward, and lessens this annoying back-diving posturing. (See "Babywearing Enhances Learning" on page 304.)

HOW BABYWEARING BENEFITS INFANTS AND PARENTS

During our study of the effects of babywearing on infants and parents, we noticed many benefits. Here's how this age-old custom of infant care brings some of them about.

Babywearing Organizes and Regulates the Baby

It's easier to understand babywearing when you think of a baby's gestation as lasting eighteen months — nine months inside the womb and at least nine more months outside. During the first nine months the womb environment regulates baby's systems automatically. Birth temporarily disrupts this organization. The more quickly, however, baby gets outside help with organizing these systems, the more easily he adapts to the puzzle of life outside the womb. By extending the womb experience, the babywearing mother (and father) provide an external regulating system that balances the irregular and disorganized tendencies of the baby. Picture how these regulating systems work. Mother's rhythmic walk, for example (which baby has been feeling for nine months) reminds baby of the womb experience. This familiar rhythm, imprinted on baby's mind in the womb, now reappears in the "outside womb" and calms baby. Mother's heartbeat, beautifully regular and familiar, reminds baby of the sounds of the womb as baby places her ear against her mother's chest. As another biological regulator, baby senses mother's rhythmic breathing while worn tummy to tummy, chest to chest. Simply stated, regular parental rhythms have a balancing effect on the infant's irregular rhythms.

➤ *THE WOMB LASTS EIGHTEEN MONTHS: Nine months inside mother, and nine months outside.*

Another way mother exerts this regulatory effect is by stimulating the regulating hormones in baby's developing adrenal and nervous systems. Researchers have shown that continued mother-infant attachment, such as babywearing provides, stimulates the infant to achieve quicker day-night regulation. They believe that mother's presence exerts a regulatory influence on the baby's adrenal hormones, which promotes night sleeping and day waking.

Mother's voice, which baby is constantly exposed to during babywearing, regulates baby's limb movements. In a 1974 study, video analysis of an infant's body movements while the mother was talking to her baby showed the baby moving in perfect synchrony with the inflections of mother's speech during her unique "baby talk." These synchronous movements did not occur in response to a stranger's voice. In essence, the mother's rhythmic movements and vocalizations "teach" the baby to put more rhythm into her movements, balancing out the usual newborn tendency toward irregular, uncoordinated, and purposeless movements.

Babywearing exerts a balancing effect on baby's *vestibular system*. This system, located behind each ear, helps keep a person's body in balance. For example, if you lean over too far to one side, the vestibular system signals that you should lean over to the other side to stay in balance. The system is similar to three tiny carpenter's levels, with one oriented for side-to-side balance, another for up and down, a third for back and forth. The "levels" function together to keep the body in balance. When carried, baby moves in all three of these directions. Every time baby moves, the fluid in these levels moves against tiny hairlike filaments that vibrate and send nerve impulses in the muscles of baby's body to keep him in balance. The preborn baby has a very sensitive vestibular system that is constantly stimulated because the fetus is in almost continuous motion. Babywearing "reminds" the baby of and continues the motion and balance he enjoyed in the womb.

What may happen if the baby does not have the benefit of a strong mother-infant attachment, spending most of his time lying horizontally in a crib, attended to only for feeding and comforting, and then again separated from mother? A newborn has an inherent urge to become organized, to fit into his or her new environment. If left to his own resources, without the frequent presence of the mother, the infant may develop disorganized patterns of behavior: colic, fussy cries, jerky movements, disorganized self-rocking behaviors, anxious thumb sucking, irregular breathing, and disturbed sleep. The infant who is forced to self-regulate before his time spends a lot of energy self-calming, wasting valuable energy he could have used to grow and develop.

Fussing and disorganized behavior is a withdrawal symptom — a result of the loss of the regulatory effects of the attachment to the mother. Babies should not be left alone to train themselves to become self-soothers, as some parenting advisers suggest. This style of detached parenting is not supported by common sense, experience, or research. Behavioral research has repeatedly shown that infants exhibit more anxious and disorganized behaviors when separated from their mothers. While there is a variety of child-rearing theories, attachment researchers all agree on one thing: In order for a baby's emotional, intellectual, and physiological systems to function optimally, the continued presence of the mother, as during babywearing, is a necessary regulatory influence.

Babywearing Reduces Crying and Colic

During the course of our study, parents in my practice would commonly report, "My baby seems to be content as long as I wear him." Babywearing parents of previously fussy babies related that their babies seemed to *forget to fuss.* Parents enjoyed their babies more because their babies were more content. Babies were happier because they had less need to cry. Families were happier, and I was happier because finally there seemed to be a way to reduce crying in fussy babies. Stimu-

lated by this new discovery of the old art of comforting, I wondered why babywearing reduced crying; also, did other pediatricians notice that carrying a baby reduced his crying?

In 1986 a team of researchers in Montreal reported a study of ninety-nine mother-infant pairs, half of which were assigned to a group that was asked to carry their babies in their arms or in a carrier for at least three hours a day. In the control, or noncarried, group, parents were asked to position their babies facing a mobile or pictures of a face when baby was placed in a crib but not to try to calm the baby by increased carrying. The infants who received supplemental carrying cried and fussed 43 percent less than the noncarried group. The unique feature of this carrying study is that mothers were encouraged to carry their infants throughout the day regardless of the state of the infant, *not just in response to crying or fussing.* The usual mode of carrying in Western society is to pick up and carry the baby *after* the crying has started.

We surveyed the writings of anthropologists who study infant-care practices in other cultures. These researchers uniformly agree that *infants in cultures that wear their babies cry less.* In the Western culture we measure our baby's crying in hours per day, whereas in other cultures it may be measured in terms of minutes. In Western culture we have been led to believe that it is "normal" for babies to cry an hour or two a day, whereas in other cultures this is not the accepted norm. Stimulated by the general agreement among infant-care researchers that increased carrying reduces crying (as well as observing this correlation in our own pediatric practice), the next question is *why?*

Babywearing reduces crying by its organizing effect on the baby's vestibular system, as previously described. Vestibular stimulation (rocking, for example) has been shown by long experience and detailed research to be the best cry stopper. Vestibular stimulation, as occurs during babywearing, soothes baby because it reminds him of the womb, allowing baby to click into the familiar experiences that were imprinted upon his developing mind during life inside the womb. The familiar overcomes the unfamiliar to which he is now exposed. This lessens baby's anxiety and lessens the need to fuss.

Because babywearing resembles the womb as closely as is humanly possible, it fulfills a style of parenting that baby would have anticipated and helps a new baby fit into her environment. This rightness of fit lessens the need to fuss. Baby is learning to fit into her outside womb as she did in the inside womb. We may erroneously regard birth as the end of an assembly line, producing a tiny adult immediately ready to adapt to the world. It helps if we regard the newborn as somewhat incomplete. Babywearing completes the attachment that baby was used to, giving her a sense of rightness. A baby feels valuable because of the way she is treated. *Wearing values the baby.*

Babywearing Enhances Learning

If infants spend less time crying and fussing, what do they do with the extra time and energy? We've already discussed how babywearing helps babies thrive and grow physically. It also helps baby's mental development. My own observation and that of others who study carried babies is that these babies do not sleep a lot more but actually show increased awake contentment time called quiet alertness. This is the behavioral

---

BABYWEARING HELPS BABIES CRY BETTER AND PARENTS COPE BETTER

In counseling parents of fussy babies, we strive for two goals: to mellow the temperament of the baby and to increase the sensitivity of the parents. Babywearing helps foster both of these goals. By creating an organized, womb-like environment, wearing lessens a baby's need to cry. Even when baby does cry, babywearing teaches her to "cry better." Parents, please remember it is not your fault that your baby cries, nor is it your job to keep baby from crying. The best you can do is not to let baby cry *alone,* and create a secure environment that lessens baby's need to cry. Babywearing helps you do this.

---

state in which an infant is most content and best able to interact with the environment. It may be called the optimal state of learning for a baby.

Researchers have reported the following effects of babywearing and quiet alertness: Carried babies show enhanced visual and auditory alertness. The stability of the infant's physiological system is related to the capacity for contented behavior during awake periods; simply stated, during the state of quiet alertness, the infant's whole system seems to work better.

The behavioral state of quiet alertness also gives parents a better opportunity to interact with the baby. When worn in the cradle hold, baby sees mother's face in the *en face* position. Notice how mother and baby position their faces in order to achieve this optimal visually interactive plane. Researchers have found that the human face, especially in this position, is a potent stimulator for interpersonal bonding. In the kangaroo carry, baby has a 180-degree view of her environment and is able to scan her world. She learns to choose, picking out what she wishes to look at and shutting out what she doesn't. This ability to make choices enhances learning.

Carried Babies Are More Involved

Another reason that babywearing enhances learning is that baby is intimately involved in the babywearer's world. Baby sees what mother or father sees, hears what they hear, and in some ways feels what they feel. *Wearing humanizes a baby.* Carried babies become more aware of their parents' faces, of the parents' walking rhythms and scents. Baby becomes aware of and learns from all the subtle facial expressions and other body language, voice inflections and tones, breathing patterns, and emotions of the babywearer. A parent will relate to the baby much more often, just by virtue of the baby's sitting there right under his or her nose. Proximity increases interaction, and baby can be constantly learning how to be human. Carried babies are intimately involved in their parents' world because they participate in what mother and father are doing. A baby worn while a parent washes dishes, for example, hears, smells, sees, and experiences in depth the adult world. He is more exposed to and involved in what is going on around him. Baby learns much in the arms of a busy person.

Consider the alternative infant-care practice, in which baby is separate from the mother most of the day and picked up and interacted with only at dutiful intervals. The voices he may hear in another room are not associated with anything happening to him. Because they have no meaning to him, he does not store them. He gets the message that they are neither important nor worth storing. For the infant who lives alone, normal daily experiences have no learning value for him and no bonding value for the mother. Because baby is separate from her, mother does not, as a matter of course, gear her activities and interactions as if baby were a participating second or third party. At best, baby is involved as a spectator rather than a player.

The babywearing mother, on the other hand, because she is used to her baby being with her, automatically gears her interactions to include the baby. The baby, in turn, feels that he is included and feels that he is valuable — a real boost to baby's emerging self-esteem.

How Babywearing Promotes Cognitive Development

To help the brain grow and develop, environmental experiences stimulate nerves to branch out and connect with other nerves. Babywearing helps the infant's developing brain make the right connections. Because baby is intimately involved in the mother's and father's world, she is exposed to and participates in the environmental stimuli that mother selects and is protected from those stimuli that bombard or overload her developing nervous system. She so intimately participates in what mother is doing that her developing brain stores a myriad of experiences, called *patterns of behavior.* These may be thought of as thousands of tiny short-run movies that are filed in the infant's neurological library to be rerun when baby is exposed to a similar situation that reminds

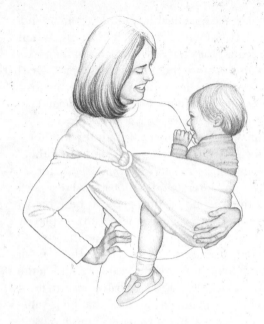

Wearing a toddler — having a conversation.

her of the making of the original "movie." For example, mothers often tell me, "As soon as I pick up the sling and put it on, my baby lights up and raises his arms as if in anticipation that he will soon be in my arms and in my world."

I have noticed that carried babies seem more attentive, clicking in to the conversation as if they were part of it. Babywearing enhances speech development. Because baby is up at voice and eye level, he is more involved in conversations. He learns a valuable speech lesson — the ability to listen.

Normal ambient sounds, such as the noises of daily activities, may either have learning value for the infant or disturb him. If baby is alone, sounds may frighten him. If baby is worn, these sounds have learning value. The mother filters out what she perceives as unsuitable for the baby and gives the infant

an "It's OK" feeling when he is exposed to unfamiliar sounds and experiences.

Parents sometimes worry that their baby won't learn to crawl very well if they carry him a lot. Even carried babies can get down and enjoy floor freedom and crawling. Actually, attachment-parented babies show enhanced motor development, perhaps for two reasons: the effect of attachment on nervous-system development and the extra energy they have that might have been wasted on fussing.

Babywearing Enhances Parent-Infant Bonding

The term "bonding" receives a lot of press, but is probably the least understood concept of parenting. Bonding is not instant intimacy. Bonding is a *gradual* process. Some parent-infant pairs achieve bonding more quickly and strongly than others. Babywearing accelerates the formation of this bond.

Babywearing Helps Mothers and Babies Get the Right Start

The way a mother and baby get started with each other often sets the tone for how successful the bonding relationship is going to be. Early in the newborn period we focus on what the mother does for the baby, as if baby minding were all a case of mother gives and baby takes. After thirty years as a pediatrician and thirty-five as a parent, I have grown to realize that the idea of this early give-a-thon is only partially true. Not only do the parents develop the baby, but the *baby develops the parents.* The ideal infant-care system — when it operates at its best — is a mutual giving, whereby all parties follow their mutual instincts to bring out the best in each other. Here's how the system works.

The mother (and to a lesser extent the father) has a biological instinct drawing her toward her infant; an innate desire to pick up, carry, nurse, and simply be with her baby. This is called mother-infant attachment. In some mothers this attachment comes naturally — mother's intuition. Other mothers feel a bit shaky in this intuition. Here's where the baby does his or her part.

Just as mothers have attachment-giving qualities, babies come wired with attachment-promoting qualities that stimulate in the mother the desire, and perhaps the need, to be near her baby. Cooing, sucking, smiling, and the beautiful round and alluring features of the baby all do something good to the mother. Within the mother are the so-called mothering hormones, specifically prolactin and oxytocin. The attachment-promoting behaviors of the baby stimulate these hormones to flow in the mother. Thus baby actually gives to mother a biological booster shot that in turn helps her give the baby the quality and quantity of mothering the baby needs — a mutual giving between two needy members of the biological pair. If we make an assumption that the higher and more consistent these hormones are, the easier mothering will be, it follows that a mother is well advised to adopt a style of mothering that keeps her hormones high. This is exactly what babywearing does. The continued presence of the baby is what keeps these biological systems active. Intermittent contact does not. Let's analyze this further.

Hormones have a biological measure of activity called a half-life — meaning the time required for one-half of the substance to be used up in the bloodstream. Some substances have a long half-life; others, a short one. Mothering hormones have a very short half-life — approximately twenty minutes. This means that in order for a mother to maintain a consistently high level, these hormones need to be stimulated around every twenty minutes. Babywearing causes this to happen. The continued presence, the frequency of feeding and touching, keeps mother's hormones high.

Babywearing Stimulates Attachment Parenting

When a mother wears her baby many hours a day, she gets used to being with her baby, and baby gets used to being with her. In a nutshell, bonding means *they feel right when together and unright when apart*. This mother is more likely to give an immediate nurturant response to a baby's cry, to continue to breastfeed more frequently and longer, and to sleep with the baby at night — a sort of nighttime babywearing. Margie, one of the babywearers in my practice, proudly exclaimed, "I feel absolutely addicted to my baby." This consistent hormonal stimulation is probably the biological basis for Margie's feeling. Martha says, "I miss my baby if she's been asleep too long in some place other than the sling."

Babywearing is even more important for the mother-baby relationship that is slow to start, either because of a medical condition causing temporary separation between mother and baby or a mother whose biological attachment system takes a while to click in. The extra closeness with your baby may be just what you need to get started.

The Next Step: Harmony and Competence

After mother and baby feel connected and complete, what's next? The net effect of babywearing may be summed up in one word — *harmony.* This beautiful term is what babywearing and bonding are all about. There are various dictionary definitions of "harmony," but the simplest, and the one I like best, is "getting along well together." Other definitions include: "an orderly and pleasing arrangement" and "an agreement of feelings or actions."

During the first month much of the mother-baby interaction is a learned response. Baby gives a cue, and mother learns what the best response is. After the pair has rehearsed this cue-response interaction hundreds of times, what initially was a learned response becomes an intuitive response. Mother naturally and intuitively gives a nurturant response, and the whole relationship operates in harmony.

The way bonding through babywearing helps mothers know and feel their babies' needs is best illustrated by how mothers in some cultures toilet their infants without the use of diapers. The mothers who constantly wear their babies learn to read them so intimately that the mother anticipates when the infant is about to urinate or defecate, picks the baby up out of the sling, holds the baby away from her, and baby does his or her thing and then is repositioned back in the sling.

Along with promoting harmony, babywearing promotes a sense of *competence* in baby and mother. Because a mother can read her baby's cues, she learns to respond effectively and meet her baby's needs; she feels fulfilled and somewhat amazed at her own increasing powers of observation. Mother and baby are so close that mother doesn't miss a cue. The cue-response network, although at first learned, eventually becomes intuitive. The mother feels very competent. The infant also develops a sense of competence because his

cues are interpreted correctly. He learns to cue better because of the consistent and appropriate responses his cues elicit in the mother. This mutual awareness, sensitivity, and competence are all enhanced by babywearing.

Carrying your baby a lot also helps you witness and enjoy your baby's quickly changing developmental skills — also important in developing the bond. The way your baby moves, the way he looks at you, the way he reaches and touches you, the way he reaches toward other persons and things all give you an enhanced appreciation for the daily changes that occur in the developing baby. In essence, mother and baby develop together. The understanding and appreciation for your baby's developmental skills are just one more aspect of cementing the bond.

Babywearing Overcomes Obstacles to Bonding

Not only does babywearing enhance bonding by promoting stimulation of mothering hormones, a mutual reading of each other's cues, and competence, it also helps mothers overcome many of the obstacles to bonding.

Postpartum depression. One of the main obstacles is postpartum depression. Postpartum depression is much less common in babywearing mothers than among other mothers. Perhaps this is due to several factors, including mother's hormonal stimulation and baby's reduced crying. Frequent hormonal stimulation, as previously discussed, causes mothers to have a consistently high level of maternal hormones instead of fluctuating ups and downs, as happens with infant care at a distance. From a biological standpoint, these mothering hormones have been shown to have a tranquilizing effect on mother, which may help ward off depression. Women I have interviewed often report that after using attachment activities such as wearing their babies they feel relaxed, as if they have learned to take advantage of the natural biological tranquilizing effect of the maternal hormones. Babywearing also prevents depression because a baby who is worn fusses less, so the mother feels more confident, less strained, and therefore less depressed.

But mothers take note: *The goodness of a baby is not a measure of your effectiveness as a mother.* Some babies cry a lot regardless of your style of mothering, so do not feel that you are not a good mother if your baby cries a lot. This is a reflection of the temperament of your baby and not your style of mothering. (For a complete description of how the amount of time a baby cries is due to the temperament of the baby, see Chapter 16, "Parenting the Fussy or Colicky Baby.") But a babywearing mother develops competence more quickly, which overrides the usual feelings of inadequacy that most new mothers initially experience.

Babywearing helps mothers be more discerning when they read books and magazines that promote mother-infant detachment, or parent-centered magazines. Over the last several years I have noticed that mothers who wear their babies a lot feel so competent that they are not bothered by well-meaning friends and relatives preaching, "You hold that baby too much; you're going to spoil her." They are resistant to parent-centered books and magazines that promote high-tech baby care, giving new parents the message that the outcome of their infant is directly proportional to the things they purchase for the baby — a so-called *enriched environ-*

ment. (Think about it. What environment could be richer for a baby than his parents' arms?) The parent-centered school of thought, which promotes a more restrained response to an infant's needs, becomes foreign to the internal programming of a babywearing mother. This advice does not feel right to her, or if she temporarily succumbs to this advice, her system rebels and she does not feel right afterward. Babywearing mothers intuitively feel that the best enriched environment to give their baby is the closeness of babywearing. They are able to resist high-tech advertising and settle comfortably into their high-touch style. Family-centered mothers of the babywearing set are more likely to develop the slogan "The *us* generation."

Babywearing Makes Life Easier for Busy Parents

Because we have a large and busy family, Martha and I enjoy our once-a-week dinner for two after the dust has settled and the younger children are in bed. Whenever we had a new baby, this usually turned out to be a dinner for three. If one of us wore the baby at the dinner table, baby was usually quiet, content, or, with Martha, breastfeeding, but not at all disturbing or interrupting. Also, the baby, if awake, was intimately involved in the conversation and all the goings-on without disturbing us.

In social situations babywearing allows uninterrupted socializing with guests; instead of your having to excuse yourself continually to go to another room and breastfeed or attend to baby, baby joins the group. What a beautiful sight to see a group of parents sitting around enjoying one another yet wearing their babies. When infants are old enough to be in the hip carry (usually four to six months), babies can make eye contact and engage in some form of baby communication while the parents talk.

BABYWEARING MAY CHANGE YOUR LIFE-STYLE FOR THE BETTER

Even a busy babywearing mother does not regard her baby as interfering with her life-style but rather enhancing it. Because she has become competent in the art of babywearing she finds ways to incorporate her baby into her daily tasks and desires, and an exciting cycle occurs: Babywearing enhances bonding, which stimulates the mother to want to be with her baby more. Because she wants to be with her baby, yet wants to or needs to have other pursuits, she finds creative ways to carry her baby with her while she does other things. This further enhances the bonding, as mother finds baby not at all inconvenient or disruptive, but enjoyable and completing.

Karen had planned to return to her career outside the home once her baby was six months old. She had been a perfectionist in her career and was used to doing everything right. She carried this professional attitude over into her mothering and wanted to do everything right for her baby. As part of the attachment style of parenting, she wore her baby several hours a day during the first six months. Essentially the baby went with her in every activity she did. After six months Karen and baby Jane were so bonded that Karen said to me, "I cannot return to my former job and leave my baby." She went on to state that there was something in her internal makeup that prevented her from separating from her baby. Acting on her conviction, Karen sought out and obtained employment that allowed her to "work and wear" her baby. (Mothers who cannot wear their babies to work can strengthen the bond by wearing their babies when away from work; see Chapter 17, "Working and Parenting.") Babywearing provides the circumstance that strengthens the bond, and because the bond is strengthened the mother seeks out a life-style that allows the babywearing bond to continue — another example of how babywearing does something good for the mother, for the baby, and for society.

As the parenting style of the new millennium, babywearing makes life easier for parents — and does good things for babies.

BENEFITS OF BABYWEARING

Because babywearing is an exercise in baby reading, it is a valuable attachment tool. Not only does babywearing benefit parents, it benefits babies.

Sling babies cry less. Both research and parents' observations show that carried babies cry less, perhaps because the sling provides a familiar motion that babies enjoyed while in the womb. Babywearing is particularly helpful to calm those "P.M. fussers," babies who seem to save up all their energy for a long blasted cry in the evening. We would plan ahead for this "happy hour" by putting baby in the sling and taking a long walk. The fresh air, the motion, and the visual attractions, such as moving cars, birds, trees, and kids playing in the park, all worked together to help baby forget to fuss.

Sling babies grow better. As we explained on pages 300–301, babywearing is particularly beneficial for babies who are premature or slow to gain weight. Motion and the proximity to a familiar caregiver help babies thrive. (Thriving does not only mean getting heavier and taller, it also means growing optimally: physically, intellectually, and emotionally.)

Sling babies learn more. Babies learn a lot in the arms of a busy caregiver for two reasons. Contented, carried babies spend more time in a state of *quiet alertness,* the behavioral state in which babies are best able to interact and learn from people and activities in their environment. Also, when worn in a carrier, baby is intimately involved in the world of the caregiver. She goes where you go and sees what you see. A sling baby sees the world from your viewpoint. Certainly, a sling baby learns more than one who is lying flat in a pram and looking up at the sky.

Sling babies talk better. Because a sling baby is up at voice and eye level, she learns the subtleties of body language and human expression. Baby is more involved in the conversation because she watches her caregivers talk. A speech pathologist and veteran baby-wearer in our practice shared her observations with us: "My husband and I used the sling from about one month to one year with both of our children. When they were able to sit upright in the sling, they began watching speakers use turn-taking and eye contact to communicate. By viewing the speaker's mouth up close, children learn to imitate correct speech movements for accurate articulation patterns. Sling babies start practicing words and sounds and store these memories at an earlier age. We feel that wearing our babies has greatly contributed to our children's abilities to communicate."

Enjoy the babywearing stage while it lasts. The time in your arms is a relatively short time in the total life of your child, but the memories of your touch and availability will last a lifetime. The Original Babysling is available at www.AskDrSears.com.

15

Nighttime Parenting: How to Get Your Baby to Sleep

From our knowledge of good sleepers we have isolated those factors that go into helping baby and parents sleep through the night. Here is a balanced approach to nighttime parenting which takes into account that tired and busy parents need to sleep and need their baby to sleep, yet respects babies' unique set of nighttime needs. Hence, we use the term "nighttime parenting," not just "how to get your baby to sleep." We want you to develop a style of nighttime parenting that helps you sleep better, helps your baby sleep better, and — the long-range goal — helps your baby develop a healthy sleep attitude.

Sleep is not a state you can force a baby into. A more appropriate approach is to create a sleep-inducing environment that allows sleep to overtake the baby — both in going to sleep and in staying asleep. Nor should getting baby to sleep be a mechanical process using insensitive techniques: "Let baby cry five minutes the first night, ten minutes the second . . . " and so on — a method that trains babies with less sensitivity than we train pets. Our goal is not only to get baby to fall asleep and stay asleep,

we want baby to regard sleep as a pleasant state to enter and a fearless state to stay in. You can't separate daytime and nighttime parenting. The 50 percent (or more) of the day that baby spends in sleep is not wasted time. It's a time when baby develops healthy and trusting attitudes about sleep — and about life.

As we were studying ways to help baby sleep better, we also surveyed various theories of how to get baby to sleep. We found all of them to be variations on one tired theme: *Let baby cry it out.* This insensitive dogma first appeared in baby books around 1900 and has carried over, with modern modifications, into every baby book thus far. Yet here are the sleepless facts: Sleep problems in babies — and adults — have reached epidemic proportions. There are now sleep-disorder centers in nearly every major city, yet the same forced-sleep techniques continue. It's time for a more humane approach. First we want to share with you some facts about infant sleep, and then we'll suggest a step-by-step approach to helping your baby develop a healthy sleep attitude — one that will carry over into healthy adult sleep habits.

FACTS OF INFANT SLEEP

Ever wish you could "sleep like a baby"? When you learn how babies really sleep — or don't — you won't wish an infant's sleeping habits on yourself. Imagining how babies sleep brings visions of peaceful, uninterrupted slumber. But here's how babies really spend their nights — and why.

No One Sleeps Through the Night

During the night, everyone — adults and babies — progresses through many stages and cycles of sleep. Let's first put you to sleep, and then your baby, to see how differently you both sleep.

As you drift into sleep, higher brain centers begin to rest and gradually shut down, enabling you to enter the stage of deep sleep, called non-REM (non–rapid eye movement) or quiet sleep, because the eyes are quiet. You are now in sound sleep. Your body is still, breathing is shallow and regular, your muscles are loose, and you're really zonked. After about an hour and a half in the deep-sleep stage your brain again begins to arouse with increasing mental activity from deep sleep into light sleep, or active sleep (called REM because during this stage of sleep the eyes actually move under the closed lids). During REM sleep we perform mental exercise, and the higher brain centers don't really sleep. You catch a few dreams, stir, turn over, adjust the covers, perhaps even fully awaken to go to the bathroom, return to bed, and descend back into deep sleep. This sleep cycle of light and deep sleep continues every couple hours throughout the night so that a typical adult may spend an average of about six hours in deep sleep and two hours in light sleep. So you don't sleep soundly all night even though you may think you do.

Babies Sleep Differently

While adults can go directly from wakefulness into the state of deep sleep rather quickly, babies can't. They first go through a period of light sleep before entering deep sleep. Let's now put your baby to sleep.

Babies Enter Sleep Differently

It's time for baby to go to bed. His eyelids droop, and he begins to nod off in your arms. His eyes close completely, but his eyelids continue to flutter, his breathing is still irregular, his hands and limbs are flexed, and he may startle, twitch, and show fleeting smiles — called sleep grins. He may even continue a flutterlike sucking. Just as you bend over to deposit the "sleeping" baby in his crib and creep quietly away, baby awakens. That's because he wasn't fully asleep in the first place. He was still in the state of light sleep when you put him down.

Now, try again. Rock, feed, pace, or use your proven bedtime ritual, but continue this ritual longer. Soon baby's grimaces and twitches stop; his breathing becomes more regular and shallow; his muscles completely relax. His previously fisted hands unfold, and the arms and limbs dangle weightlessly (the limp-limb sign of deep sleep). Now you can put baby down and sneak away, breathing a satisfying sigh of relief that finally baby is asleep.

> *Lesson one in nighttime parenting:*
> Babies need to be parented to sleep,
> not just put to sleep.

Why? Infants in the early months enter sleep through an initial period of light sleep lasting around *twenty minutes.* Then they gradually enter deep sleep, from which they are difficult to arouse. If you try to rush by putting baby down during this initial light sleep period, he will usually awaken. This fact of infant sleep accounts for the difficult-to-settle baby who "has to be fully asleep before I can put him down." In later months many babies can enter deep sleep more quickly without first going through light sleep. Learn to recognize your baby's sleep stages. During deep sleep you can move a sleeping baby from car seat to bed without baby awakening.

Babies Have Shorter Sleep Cycles

Stand adoringly next to the bassinet or bed and watch your nearly motionless baby in peaceful slumber. After about an hour she begins to squirm. She tosses a bit, her eyelids flutter, her face muscles grimace, she breathes irregularly, and her muscles tighten. Baby is reentering the phase of light sleep, and during this vulnerable period many babies awaken if any upsetting or uncomfortable stimulus occurs. You lay a comforting hand on your baby's back, sing a soothing lullaby, and over the next ten minutes baby drifts through this light sleep period and descends back into deep sleep. For the rest of the night? Not yet! Another hour passes and baby reenters light sleep, another vulnerable period occurs and perhaps another night waking. Babies have shorter sleep cycles than adults. In the early months, baby's sleep cycles are shorter, periods of light sleep occur more frequently, and the vulnerable period for night waking occurs twice as often as for an adult, approximately every hour. Most restless nights are due to difficulty *getting back to sleep* after waking up during this vulnerable period. Some babies have trouble reentering another stage of deep sleep.

Babies Don't Sleep as Soundly as Adults

Not only do babies go to sleep differently and have shorter sleep cycles and more arousal periods, they have twice as much light sleep as adults. This hardly seems fair to parents tired from daylong baby care.

> *Lesson two in nighttime parenting:*
> Babies sleep the way they do — or
> don't — because they are designed
> that way.

Survival Benefits

Suppose your baby slept like an adult. He could spend most of his night in deep sleep with only a few vulnerable periods of night waking and would resettle on his own after those. Sounds wonderful! Perhaps for you, but not for baby. Suppose baby was cold and couldn't awaken to signal his need for warmth; suppose he was hungry but did not awaken to communicate his need to eat. Suppose his nose was plugged and his breathing compromised, but he did not awaken to signal the need for help. We believe that babies are wired with sleep patterns to awaken easily in the early months when their nighttime needs are most intense but their ability to communicate them is most limited.

Developmental Benefits

Sleep researchers believe that light sleep is good for baby because it provides mental exercise. Dreaming during light sleep provides visual images for baby's developing brain. This autostimulation during sleep enhances brain development. One day as we explained the theory that light sleep helps babies' brains develop, a tired mother of a wakeful infant chuckled and said, "If that's true, my baby's going to be very smart."

But when will baby sleep through the night? The age at which babies settle — meaning they go to sleep easily and stay asleep — varies widely among babies. Some babies go to sleep easily but don't stay asleep. Some go to sleep with difficulty but will stay

---

TIRING FACTS OF INFANT SLEEP

- Babies enter sleep through REM sleep; they need help to go to sleep.

- Sleep cycles are shorter for babies than for adults, with more light than deep sleep.

- Babies have more vulnerable periods for night waking than adults; they have difficulty getting back to sleep.

- The medical definition of "sleeping through the night" is a *five-hour stretch.*

- Babies usually awaken two or three times a night from birth to six months, once or twice from six months to one year, and may awaken once a night from one to two years.*

- Babies usually sleep fourteen to eighteen hours a day from birth to six months, fourteen to sixteen hours from three to six months, and twelve to fourteen hours from six months to two years.

- Babies' sleep habits are more determined by individual temperaments than parents' nighttime abilities. It's not your fault baby wakes up.

- Stuffing babies with solids at bedtime rarely helps them sleep longer.

- It's all right to sleep with baby in your bed. In fact, sharing sleep works better than other arrangements for many families and may be more "normal" than baby's sleeping separately in a crib.

- You cannot force sleep upon a baby. Creating a secure environment that allows sleep to overtake baby is the best way to create long-term healthy sleep attitudes. The frequent-waking stage will not last forever.

Babies' night-waking habits and parents' perception of what constitutes a sleep problem vary so widely that "average" or "normal" amounts of night waking must be stated as ranges rather than in exact figures.

asleep. Other exhausting babies neither want to go to sleep nor stay asleep.

In the first three months babies' sleep habits resemble their feedings: small, frequent feedings, short, frequent naps. Tiny babies seldom sleep for more than four-hour stretches without needing a feeding. They have little respect for day or night schedules and usually sleep a total of fourteen to eighteen hours a day.

From three to six months most babies begin to settle. They are awake for longer stretches during the day, and some may sleep for five-hour stretches at night. Expect at least one or two night wakings.

As baby gets older, periods of deep sleep lengthen, light sleep lessens, the vulnerable periods for night waking decrease, and babies can enter deep sleep more quickly. This is called *sleep maturity,* and the age varies at which babies develop these adultlike sleep patterns.

Theoretically it sounds good, but why do they still wake up? Just as baby's brain is beginning to sleep better, the body wakes it up. Arousal stimuli, such as colds and teething pain, become more frequent. As babies go through major developmental milestones (sitting, crawling, walking, for example), they often awaken to practice their newly developing skills. Just as baby begins to sleep through these nighttime warm-ups, other causes of night waking, such as separation anxiety, remind you that parenting is an around-the-clock job. While you never completely go off nighttime call, expect night waking to lessen with time. Then a sibling arrives and intensive nighttime parenting starts all over again.

Now that you are familiar with the way a baby's sleep differs from your own, here is a step-by-step approach that has evolved from the approach we have taken with our eight little sleepers, and one that, in our experience in counseling hundreds of parents, works — most of the time.

STEP ONE: GIVE YOUR BABY THE BEST SLEEP START

To begin, take a look at your attitude toward sleep.

Develop a Nighttime-Parenting Mind-set

How do you regard a baby's sleep? Do you look at night as a time of relief from the constant attachment of baby during the day, a well-deserved baby break, when you can disconnect from baby? Is "sleeping through the night" at the top of your parent-achievement list? And if you are not rewarded with a perfect sleeper, have you failed Parenting 101? If you answer yes to the last three questions, consider another approach.

What you do with your baby at night is part of the whole parenting package, an extension of an attitude that says, "During the day I want my baby to feel close to me, to trust me. I want to carry these feelings of a healthy attachment into the night. I don't want my baby to feel disconnected from me at night." In other words, attachment is different at night than during the day, but there is still an attachment. The nighttime mind-set we want to steer you away from is that getting your baby to sleep through the night requires a list of gadgets and insensitive techniques that "break" baby of night waking.

This is a short-term gain and possibly a long-term loss. In breaking baby's night waking, you may also break other, more fragile connections with your baby.

Develop a Nighttime-Parenting Style That Works for You

Having a baby opens the door to a barrage of "experts," all advising you on how to get your baby to sleep, and sleep through the night at all costs. Because babies have varied temperaments, and families have varied life-styles, there is no *right way* to get a baby to sleep — only a *right attitude* about sleep.

Every baby comes wired with an overall temperament that affects how she sleeps. Every parent has a unique life-style and individual sleep habits that must also be considered. Develop a nighttime-parenting style that fits all of these individual needs. Try the approach that feels right for you, your baby, and your life-style, and if it's working, stick with it. If it's not, be open to trying other nighttime-parenting styles.

Good sleepers are partly born, partly made, never forced. We present various options for nighttime parenting and take a balanced approach to meeting the whole family's nighttime needs. One or more of these techniques will fit most families most of the time. Some parts of one method may fit better at one stage of baby's development and parents' life-style; other nighttime styles fit better at other stages. Our only request: *Be open to trying different nighttime approaches to see which one fits the sleep temperament of your baby and your life-style and sleep habits.* Being closed to any of the options may deprive you of the joys and benefits of certain parts of nighttime parenting and lead to long-term unhealthy sleep attitudes, and possibly long-term distancing between you and your child.

BEWARE OF SLEEP TRAINERS

Since the days when baby books found their way into bedrooms, a parade of sleep trainers have all claimed magic formulas to get babies to sleep. Most are just the old cry-it-out method in a new guise; few get to the real cause of the restlessness.

Be discerning about using someone else's "method" to get your baby to sleep. Before trying any sleep-inducing program, you be the judge. Run these schemes through your inner sensitivity scale. Weigh the pros and cons. Select what best fits your own family situation and seems right to you, eventually arriving at your own method.

The Attachment Style of Nighttime Parenting

The approach we have learned, by trial and error, that usually works for most families is the attachment style of nighttime parenting. It is what we used in our family, what we teach in our practice, and what experience, science, and plain common sense seem to validate. It is not radical or extreme; it's fundamental and simple. The best things in life usually are. The two elements of this style of nighttime parenting are (1) *organizing and mellowing* your baby's temperament during the day and (2) *sleeping close* to your baby at night.

Restful Days Promote Sleepful Nights

Most sleep disturbances result from an overall disorganization. Newborns are disorganized. Sleeping and feeding "schedules" are not in a newborn's initial plan. A baby's physiological systems seem irregular, and this disorganization lasts over a twenty-four-hour period. Organizing a baby during the day helps baby become better organized at night. Here's how to do it.

Feed on cue. Frequent cue feedings during the day tank up a baby, promoting better sleep at night. Babies who are rigidly scheduled during the day are more likely to become day sleepers and night feeders.

Wear baby during the day. Put your baby in a baby sling and carry your baby a lot during the day. Proximity promotes frequent feeding, closeness promotes calmness, and a calm baby by day is more likely to be a calm baby at night (see page 303 for the calming effects of babywearing). Your daytime parenting style and its effects on baby's daytime behavior carry over into nighttime sleep habits. An in-arms baby in a responsive caregiving environment learns trust and calmness. A less anxious baby during the day becomes a less anxious baby at night.

The effects of daytime attachment parenting on nighttime sleep habits are especially true for the baby who comes into this world fussy. These babies are notoriously restless sleepers. Mellowing a baby's fussy tendencies during the day carries over into a mellower baby at night. In essence, daytime attachment parenting gives baby the early message: There is no need to fuss — day or night.

What's in It for Parents?

Besides giving your baby a less anxious start by frequent feedings and holding, daytime attachment parenting gives you a good nighttime start. By interacting with your baby so frequently during feeding and wearing, you become *sensitive* toward your baby. You begin to know your baby during the day, and this carries over into your nighttime sensitivity, helping you to intuitively know: Where should baby sleep? How should I respond to her cries? What is the best way to parent her to sleep? Almost every sleep-training method is curiously silent on the topic "*Your* Baby's Nighttime Needs." Attachment parenting helps you fill this gap.

Your daytime parenting style allows this connection to flow into a nighttime connection. Sometime during the first month of attachment parenting you will naturally develop a nighttime-parenting mind-set, and for most parents that means sleeping close to their baby, not because they read it in a book, but because it feels so right to them. Attachment parenting is, after all, a continuum of life in the womb. As one mother put it: "Just because my baby is now all of a sudden born doesn't mean he should be separate from me in the crib — I just can't bring myself to put him in there."

Where Should Baby Sleep?

Wherever all your family members sleep the best is the right arrangement for you. Some babies sleep best in their parents' bed; some sleep well in their own crib in the parents' bedroom; other families prefer encouraging their baby to sleep in a separate room. Realistically, plan to juggle all these sleeping arrangements as you come to know your

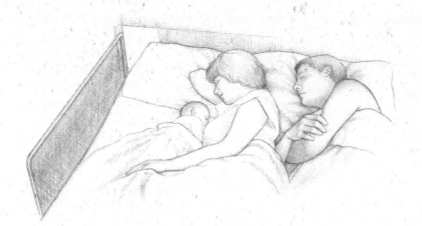

Sharing sleep is one way many parents respond to their baby's nighttime needs.

baby's nighttime temperament and needs. Sharing sleep with your baby is a practice we firmly believe in and highly recommend (see the detailed discussion beginning on page 329). The key to surviving night life with a new baby is to be open to trying various nighttime-parenting styles and settling on one that works — and to be open to changing styles as your baby's developmental needs and your family situation change.

STEP TWO: CONDITION YOUR BABY TO SLEEP

We repeat: Sleep is not a state you can force your baby into. Sleep must naturally overtake baby. Your role is to set the conditions that make sleep attractive and to present cues that suggest to baby that sleep is expected. Choose from the following sleep-tight tips those that are appropriate to your baby's age, stage of development, nighttime temperament, and your own life-style and sleep habits. And remember: Which sleep tips

work depends on your baby's temperament and stage of development. What doesn't work tonight may work next week.

We purposely omit what we call the "harden your heart" method, which preaches, "Put your baby down to sleep awake in a crib in her own room and let her cry herself to sleep so that she gets used to falling asleep by herself and won't always need to rely on you to get her back to sleep. When she awakens, don't go in to her. She will soon learn to put herself to sleep and back to sleep." We believe that, at least in the first six months, this method is unwise; you run the risk of losing your baby's trust, you may become insensitive to your baby's cries, and, in the case of infants with persistent personalities, it usually doesn't work.

Many of the following sleep-conditioning tips would be absolutely forbidden in the teach-your-baby-to-sleep-on-his-own books. How sad to deny a mother these simple pleasures for the sake of expedience. How even sadder to deny the baby valuable human touch in his journey to maturity. How can the hands-off approach do anything but weaken your bond?

Getting Baby to Fall Asleep

Parents often wear out before baby winds down. Here are ways to close those little eyes.

Make sure daytime is peaceful. A peaceful daytime is likely to lead to a restful night. Holding and soothing your baby a lot during the day mellows your baby into an easier sleeper at night. If your baby has restless nights, take inventory of unsettling circumstances that may be occuring during the day. Are you too busy? Is the day care and day-care provider the right match for your baby? Does your baby spend a lot of time being held and in the arms of a nurturing caregiver, or is he more of a "crib baby" during the day? We have noticed that babies who are carried in baby slings for several hours during the day settle better at night. (See Chapter 14, "Baby-wearing.")

Set consistent nap routines. Pick out the times of the day when you are the most tired, for example 11:00 A.M. and 4:00 P.M. Lie down with your baby at these times every day for about a week to get your baby used to a daytime nap routine. Napping with your baby helps you get some much-needed daytime rest rather than being tempted to "finally get something done" while baby is napping. Babies who have consistent nap routines during the day are more likely to sleep longer stretches at night.

Set consistent bedtimes. The older the baby, the more desirable are consistent bedtimes and rituals. Babies who have a reasonably consistent bedtime usually sleep better. Because of modern life-styles, rigid and early bedtimes are not as common or realistic as they used to be. Consider busy parents who often do not get home until six or seven o'clock in the evening. This is prime time for a baby; don't expect him to go right to sleep as soon as you get home. By the time you get home from a busy day at work, father, mother, or both may be eager for baby to go to bed early, rather than endure spending an evening with a cranky baby. If one or both parents are accustomed to arriving home late, then a *later* bedtime is more practical and realistic. In this situation give your baby a later afternoon nap so that baby is well rested during prime evening time with the busy parents.

Enjoy predictable bedtime rituals. Familiar bedtime rituals set your baby up for sleep. The sequence of a warm bath, rocking, nursing, lullabies, and so on, set baby up to expect sleep to follow. Capitalize on a principle of early infant development known as *patterns of association.* Baby's developing brain is like a computer, storing thousands of sequences that become patterns. When a baby clicks into the early part of a bedtime routine, she is programmed for the rest of the pattern that ends with drifting off to sleep.

Calm your baby down. A soothing massage or a warm bath is a solution for relaxing tense muscles and busy minds. (See infant-massage techniques, page 92, and bathing techniques, page 84.)

Wear your baby down. This technique worked best for our babies, especially one who was in high gear most of the day and had difficulty winding down. (See techniques for wearing down, page 295.)

Nurse your baby down. Going off to sleep at mother's breast is at the top of the natural-sleep-inducer list. Nestle up next to your baby and breastfeed him off to sleep. The smooth continuum from warm bath to warm arms to warm breast to warm bed usually leads to sleep. And bottlefed babies can also be nursed down to sleep.

Father your baby down. As stated earlier, "nursing" implies not only breastfeeding. Fathers can nurse down by their own uniquely male ways of soothing baby. It is wise for baby to get used to the sleep-inducing styles of both mother and father. (See suggestions for practical ways that fathers can comfort babies using the warm fuzzy, page 293, and our favorite, the neck nestle, page 291.)

Nestle your baby down. Your baby may be almost ready to fall asleep, but just doesn't want to be put down to sleep *alone.* After rocking, wearing, or feeding baby to sleep in your arms, lie down on your bed with your

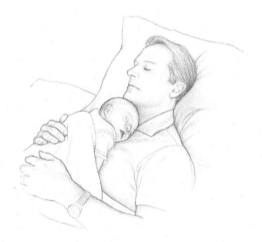

The neck nestle is a popular "fathering down" technique.

sleeping baby and nestle close until you are certain baby is sound asleep (or you are sound asleep). We call this the "teddy-bear snuggle."

Rock your baby down. A bedside rocking chair is near the top of your bedroom furniture list. Treasure these moments of rocking to sleep, as they are unique to the early years and soon pass.

Create a bed on wheels. Suppose you've tried everything. You are ready for bed, or are ready for your baby to go to bed, but she is not able to wind down. As a last resort put your baby in a car seat and drive while she falls asleep. Nonstop motion is the quickest sleep inducer. I call this "freeway fathering"; the before-bed ritual is especially practical for nighttime fathering and gives a tired mother a baby break. We also used this driving time for much-needed communication between ourselves as baby nodded off to sleep from the constant motion and hum of the car engine. When you return home and notice that baby is in a deep sleep, don't remove her immediately from the car seat or she will probably awaken. Carry the baby car seat into your bedroom and let baby remain in the seat as her bed. Or if baby is in a very deep sleep (look for the limp-limb sign), you might be able to remove her from the car seat and place her in her own bed without her fully awakening.

Try a mechanical mother. Gadgets to put and keep baby asleep are big business. Tired parents pay high prices for a good night's sleep. It's all right to use these as relief when the main comforter wears out, but a steady diet of these artificial sleep inducers may be unhealthy. One newspaper article extolled the sleep-tight virtues of a teddy bear, with a tape player in his stuffing, that sang or made breathing sounds. Baby could snuggle up to the singing, breathing, synthetic bear. Personally, we were not keen on our babies going to sleep to someone else's canned voice. Why not use the real parent?

➤ *WATCH FOR THE LIMP-LIMB SIGN.*
All of these tips for getting baby down will be thwarted if you try to sneak away while baby is still in the state of light sleep. Watch for a motionless face and dangling limbs, signs that your baby has entered the stage of deep sleep, and you can safely deposit your sleeping beauty into his or her nest and creep away. (See the illustration on page 402.)

Getting Baby to Stay Asleep

Now that your baby is finally asleep, here's how to keep him that way.

Tank up baby during the day. Help baby learn that daytime is for eating and nighttime is for sleeping. Some older infants are so busy playing during the day that they forget to eat and make up for it during the night by waking frequently to feed. To reverse this habit, feed your baby at least every three hours during the day to cluster baby's feedings during the waking hours.

Tank up baby before bed. Before you go to bed, or upon baby's first night waking, attempt a full feeding; otherwise, some babies, especially breastfed infants, enjoy nibbling all night.

Position baby for safe sleeping. Unless instructed otherwise by your baby's health care provider, place your baby down to sleep on her back for at least the first nine months. While babies are thought to sleep longer on their tummies, new insights into safe sleeping patterns have revealed that sleeping longer may not mean sleeping safer. (For an explanation, see "Put Baby to Sleep on His Back," page 641.)

Dress baby for sleep. Experiment with different ways of dressing your newborn at bedtime to see which coverings help your baby settle best. Many allergy-prone babies sleep better in 100 percent cotton sleepwear.

Moving beds. Some babies do not stay asleep after being rocked to sleep in a rhythmic motion and then put down on a static bed. The bed needs to continue moving. This is why the time-honored cradle works. After rocking your baby to sleep in your arms or in a chair, gently nestle your baby in the cradle and immediately continue your previous rocking motion at around sixty beats per minute, the heartbeat rhythm that your baby grew accustomed to in the womb. If you don't have a cradle, put quiet roller wheels or rocker springs on baby's bed and gently roll or rock it back and forth. In the early months some babies use both the cradle and the parents' bed, alternating between the two in settling. Often parents, intending to get a crib "one of these days," never get around to the purchase.

Laying on of hands. Ever notice that as soon as you release your sleeping baby onto her bed she immediately awakens, and you start the whole ritual all over? Or you may notice that as soon as you place your baby into the crib, she squirms and bobs her head up and down. Your baby is giving you the

> ## LONGER STRETCH OF SLEEP AT NIGHT
>
> Want your baby to sleep longer at night? Change how he sleeps during the day. In our family and in our practice, we have observed that babies who are fed frequently on cue and carried in a sling during the day sleep in a cat-nap pattern during the day and save their long stretch of sleep for the night.

signal that she is not in deep enough sleep to be left alone and is not ready to disconnect completely from your touch. Put one hand on the back of your baby's head and another on your baby's back. The warmth of a secure hand may be the added touch that is needed to help baby give up her silent protest and nod off to sleep. To add the finishing touches to this sleep-inducing ritual, pat your baby's back or bottom rhythmically at sixty beats a minute. Then remove your hands *gradually,* first one, then the other, easing the pressure slowly so not to startle baby awake. When laying hands on our babies we found it better to remove a hand very gradually, even allowing it to hover a bit above baby's body surface before backing off. Sometimes fathers, perhaps because they have larger hands, are more successful in this hands-on sleep-keeping ritual.

Leave a little bit of mother behind. If your baby is particularly separation sensitive, leave a little bit of yourself in baby's bed. One mother noticed that her baby settled better when she left her breast pad or nightgown in the cradle. Another mother left a continuous

tape recording of herself singing a bedtime lullaby.

Honor your partner with his share of nighttime parenting. It's important for baby to get used to father's ways of comforting and putting him to sleep (and back to sleep). Otherwise, mother burns out. A father's participation in nighttime parenting is especially important for the breastfeeding infant who assumes that "mom's diner" is open all night. (For suggestions, see "The Babywearing Father," pages 291–294, and "Wearing Down to Sleep," page 295.)

A quiet place to sleep. Most babies have an amazing ability to block out disturbing noises, so you don't have to tiptoe around and create a noiseless sleeping environment. Our first baby slept in a cradle next to my study. He slumbered through telephone rings, study noises, music, and all the ambient sounds of student life. Some babies startle easily at sudden noises and need a quieter sleeping environment. Oil the joints and springs of a squeaky crib. Put out the dog — before it barks. Take the phone off the hook or turn off the ringer. If guests are arriving, put a sign on the door: "Please enter quietly, baby is sleeping."

Get to baby quickly. Determine what your baby's nighttime temperament is. Is your baby a born self-soother who awakens, whimpers, squirms, and then resettles without bothering anybody? Or is your baby not a self-soother, who, if not promptly attended to, fully awakens, becomes angry, and is difficult to resettle? If you get to your baby quickly before he completely wakes up, you may be able to settle him back to sleep with a quick laying on of hands, a cozy cuddle, or a warm nurse. If you

SOUNDS TO SLEEP BY

Your baby has not exactly had the quietest sleeping environment during her nine months in utero. Baby may still need some background music to settle. So it is natural for babies to settle best with sounds that remind baby of the womb, such as

- running water from a nearby faucet or shower
- a bubbling fish tank
- recordings of mother's heartbeat and other womb sounds
- a loudly ticking clock
- a metronome set at sixty beats per minute
- tape recordings of waterfalls or ocean sounds

Other sounds that settle a restless baby are known as white noise — sounds that are repetitive, without meaning, that lull baby to sleep. Some producers of white noise are a vacuum cleaner, a fan or an air conditioner, and a dishwasher. We have known mothers who have worn out several vacuum cleaners during the course of the first year of getting their baby to sleep. (One finally realized she could accomplish the same result by tape-recording the vacuum cleaner sound.) Wearing your baby in a sling while vacuuming may be a winning combination. Some sensitive babies, on the other hand, startle at the sound of a vacuum cleaner.

You can also try continuous-play tape recordings. Make your own medleys of sleep-inducing sounds and songs that work. Lullabies of your own voice are at the top of the list.

In seeking out sleep-best music, remember that sleeping babies have selective musical tastes. Choose a medley of tunes that both soothe your baby and are easy listening to your ears. Babies settle better with classical music that has slowly rising and falling tempos, such as Ravel, Mozart, and Vivaldi (also Dvořák, Debussy, Bach, and Haydn). Babies prefer music that is simple and consistent, such as flute and classical guitar. Turbulent, nonrhythmic rock music is a proven night waker. Music boxes or musical mobiles with lullabies, such as Brahms, are other sounds that soothe. A relaxing and sleep-inducing CD is *Soothing Moments* by Livesay, available at www.AskDrSears.com.

---

parent your baby through this vulnerable period for night waking, you can often prevent him from waking up completely.

A full tummy, but not too full. You may be tempted to feed your baby a glob of cereal in hopes that a before-bed stuffing will keep him asleep. Studies comparing babies given cereal before bed and those given milk alone showed no difference in night waking. But, for tired parents, it's worth a try. Babies whose tummies are either too empty or too full will be more restless. Breastfeeding or a bottle of formula before you go to bed is usually enough to satisfy the infant. A glass of milk, a bowl of cut-up fruit, or a nutritious cookie is a good bedtime snack for the toddler.

STEP THREE: LESSEN CONDITIONS THAT CAUSE NIGHT WAKING

While some night waking is inevitable and the result of the temperament and developmental stage of your baby, there are many causes of disturbed sleep over which you do have some control.

Physical Causes

Teething pain. Even though you may not yet be able to feel baby's teeth, teething discomfort may start as early as three months and continue off and on all the way through the two-year molars. A wet bed sheet under baby's head, a telltale drool rash on the cheeks and chin, swollen and tender gums, and a slight fever are clues that teething is the nighttime culprit. What to do? With your doctor's permission, give appropriate doses of acetaminophen (see page 657) just before parenting your baby to sleep and again in four hours if baby awakens.

Wet or soiled diapers. Some babies are bothered by wet diapers at night; most are not. If your baby sleeps through wet diapers, there is no need to awaken her for a change — unless you're treating a persistent diaper rash. Nighttime bowel movements necessitate a change. Here's a nighttime changing tip: If possible, change the diapers just before a feeding, as baby is likely to fall asleep during or after feeding. Some breastfed babies, however, have a bowel movement during or immediately after a feeding and will need changing again. If you are using cloth diapers, putting two or three diapers on your baby before bedtime will decrease the sensation of wetness.

Irritating sleepwear. Some babies cannot settle in synthetic sleepwear. A mother in our practice went through our whole checklist of night-waking causes (see page 344) until she discovered her baby was sensitive to polyester sleepers. Once she changed to 100 percent cotton clothing, her baby slept better. Besides being restless, some babies show skin allergies to new clothing, detergents, and fabric softeners by breaking out in a rash.

Hunger. Tiny babies have tiny tummies, about the size of their tiny fists. A baby's digestive system was designed for small, frequent feedings, so expect your baby to need a feeding at least every three to four hours during the night for the first few months. As they grow older, babies may be so busy playing they forget to eat. To lessen nighttime hunger, tank up your baby with frequent daytime feedings.

Stuffy nose. In the early months babies need clear nasal passages to breathe. Later they can alternatively breathe through their mouth if their nose is blocked. Newborns are especially restless if their nose is congested. To deal with this, first clear the air (see "Environmental Causes," page 326). Next, to unstuff baby's nasal passages, see the suggestions on pages 98 and 665.

Baby too hot or too cold. Restless sleeping may be a sign that your baby is too hot or too cold. See page 88 for tips on how to dress your baby at night.

Environmental Causes

Fluctuating temperature and humidity. Provide a room temperature and relative humidity conducive to sleeping. In the early weeks, this means a consistent temperature and humidity. See page 88 for a discussion of how to maintain the proper sleeping environment in baby's bedroom.

Airborne irritants. Environmental irritants may cause congested breathing passages and awaken baby. Common household examples are cigarette smoke, baby powder, paint fumes, perfumes, hair spray, animal dander (keep animals out of an allergic child's bedroom), plants, clothing (especially wool), stuffed animals, dust from a bed canopy, feather pillows, blankets, and fuzzy toys that collect lint and dust. If your baby consistently awakens with a stuffy nose, suspect irritants or allergens in the bedroom. (See page 700 for suggestions on allergyproofing a bedroom.)

A cold bed. Placing a warm baby on cold sheets is a guaranteed night waker. Flannel sheets in cold weather, a lambskin, or a warm body preceding baby provide a toasty bed.

Unfamiliar sounds. A startling sound, especially a sudden, loud, unfamiliar noise, is likely to awaken a sleeping baby, particularly if it occurs during light sleep or during the vulnerable period for night waking, the transition from deep to light sleep. Don't feel you have to hush-hush and tiptoe around a deeply sleeping baby. In fact, consistent, familiar, womblike sounds may lull a baby to sleep. (See "Sounds to Sleep By," page 324.)

Hidden Medical Causes

Most babies wake up more frequently when sick, while some take advantage of the healing effects of sleep and sleep more during illnesses. If your baby is not only waking up frequently, but also seems to hurt and wake up in pain, consider a medical cause. Here are some of the common medical causes of painful night waking as well as some hidden causes of internal irritation that can awaken baby.

Gastroesophageal reflux. See page 388 for a full discussion of this most common medical cause of "hurting baby."

Colds. A baby with a cold awakens because of the congestion that blocks his breathing passages and the general discomfort that comes from colds. (See page 664 for the gen-

---

WHEN TO SUSPECT A MEDICAL CAUSE

Suspect a medical cause of night waking if

- baby awakens with sudden colicky-type abdominal pains
- a good sleeper suddenly becomes a restless sleeper
- baby has not slept well since birth
- there are other signs or symptoms of illness
- baby cries inconsolably
- your intuition tells you something's wrong
- no other cause is apparent

eral treatment of colds, particularly nighttime remedies.)

Ear infections. An ear infection is a painful cause of night waking. Suspect an ear infection as a cause of nighttime restlessness when the following occur:

- Your baby's sleeping patterns change from sleeping well to restlessness and waking.

- Your baby has a cold, and the discharge from her nose changes from clear and watery to thick and yellow, and the cold is accompanied by yellow drainage from baby's eyes.

For more about ear infections, see page 674.

Fever. Many germs produce a higher fever at night than during the day. If your child is ill during the day but does not have much of a daytime fever (yet he spiked a fever on previous nights), it is still wise to give your baby the appropriate dose of fever-lowering medicine before bedtime in anticipation of the fever going up at night, even though he may appear to have a normal temperature before going to bed. It is seldom necessary to awaken a sleeping child to take his temperature; just feel or kiss his forehead. Unless advised by your doctor, it is usually unnecessary to awaken a sleeping feverish baby to administer fever-lowering medicine.

Allergies and the resulting intestinal discomfort. Allergies and their effects can be hidden causes of frequent night waking. Food allergies head the list. Suspect a food or milk allergy as the nighttime culprit in the following situations:

- Baby's sleep is restless most of the night.

- Baby awakens with sudden, colicky pains, and you lay hands on a tense, gas-filled abdomen.

- Baby shows other signs of allergies: daytime colic, rashes, nasal congestion.

A recent discovery is that baby may be allergic to the cow's milk the breastfeeding mother drinks and may wake up more frequently as a result. (If you suspect a food or milk allergy, follow the elimination diet suggestions outlined on page 152.)

Pinworms. Common residents in many children's intestines, pinworms look like tiny pieces of white thread about a third of an inch long and may produce night waking in the older infant and child. Here's how these little parasites behave in your baby's intestines to cause night waking: The pregnant female travels down the intestines and out the rectum to lay her eggs, usually at night. This activity around the rectum causes intense itching that often awakens the child to scratch the egg-infested area around the anus, buttocks, and vagina. These eggs are picked up under the fingernails and transmitted to the child's mouth, to other children, or to other members of the household. The swallowed eggs then hatch in the intestines, mature, mate, and repeat the life reproductive cycle.

Here are clues for nighttime worms:

- itching and scratch marks around your baby's anus
- vaginal irritation and/or frequent urinary tract infections in girls
- other members of the family with confirmed pinworms
- worms seen by you

Pinworms may cause no symptoms or may be a painful, itching nuisance. If you suspect but can't confirm pinworms, here's how to tell: In the dark, spread your child's buttocks apart and shine a flashlight on the anus. If you see the tiny creatures, don't panic. A middle-of-the-night call to your doctor is not warranted; the worms can wait until morning. Sometimes you know they're there, but you can't see them. Place a piece of tape, sticky side out, on a popsicle stick or a tongue depressor and capture the eggs by pressing the sticky side of the tape against the anus at night. The tape test may also be performed immediately when your child awakens, before a bath or bowel movement. Take the tape to your doctor or a laboratory where it can be examined under a microscope for pinworm eggs, and the condition can then be appropriately treated.

Urinary tract infections. Any baby who suffers from frequent night waking, especially if accompanied by signs of poor growth, vomiting, and unexplained fevers, and who is not thriving well, should be evaluated for a possible urinary tract infection.

While it is true that night waking is more commonly due to behavioral causes than medical causes, consider the preceding hidden medical reasons for night waking. I have seen many babies who were too quickly assumed to have poor sleep habits and who were victims of the unsuccessful cry-it-out method who turned out to have one or more of the above medical reasons for night waking, which subsided once the cause was found and treated. Like fever and pain, night waking should be considered a symptom that needs the right diagnosis and treatment.

Developmental Causes

Expect the previously steady sleeper to begin night waking while going through a major developmental milestone, such as sitting up alone, crawling, and walking. You may be summoned to your baby's bed to find he has crawled to the side of the crib, pulled himself up, but is left standing and doesn't know how to get down, or is sleepwalking around the crib. Sometimes the beginning sleepwalker will sit up, half-asleep, then topple over to a rude awakening.

What is the reason for these developmental night nuisances? Probably, baby in some way "dreams" about his daytime accomplishments and tries to practice them at night while partially asleep. Three A.M. is no time to show off his new skills, and an appreciative audience is unlikely. If you find your baby sitting up in bed half-asleep but on the verge of toppling over, gently reposition her into her favorite sleeping posture before she fully awakens. If baby is disoriented and upset, comfort and resettle her to sleep.

Separation anxiety is another developmental reason for night waking. The eight-to-twelve-month-old, who was previously such a good sleeper, now awakens frequently at night and clings more frequently to you during the day. We believe this curious developmental phenomenon occurs because baby's body now tells him he has the capability to move away from mother and father, but his mind says, "You need to stay close." The normal daytime clinginess carries over into nighttime closeness as baby wakes up to connect with home base. (See discussion of separation anxiety, page 515.)

Emotional Causes

Ever had a stressful day followed by a restless night? Babies do, too. If your baby has a close attachment to you, and there's an overall family closeness, expect sleep disturbances when this harmony is interrupted by events such as separation, divorce, family strife, and hospitalization. Expect more night waking when your family's usual routines are upset, as during a move. If you are too busy during the day, expect baby to awaken for play and attention at night. If you and your baby have a close attachment, expect her to share your emotions. If you are upset, depressed, or wakeful yourself, expect similar emotional and sleep disturbances in your baby. As one mother in our practice put it, "When I've had a bad day and am restless at night, so is my baby. When I get hold of myself and am more calm during the day, my baby sleeps better."

Temperament and Sleep

You're among other new mothers all bragging about how "good" their babies are. The loaded question arises, "Is your baby sleeping through the night?" Not wanting to appear left out of this restful circle you hedge a feeble, "Well, almost." Your misery wanted some company, but all you got was a roomful of perfect mothers with perfect sleepers. Don't lose any more sleep over your friends' good babies. *The goodness of babies' sleep is not a measure of good mothering.* Besides, they're likely to be exaggerating their babies' nighttime goodness anyhow. Two mothers may be employing the same parenting style: One has a night waker; one doesn't. You may be blessed with a high-need baby (whom you will meet in the next chapter) who carries his daytime temperament into his night-waking habits. No two babies look the same, eat the same, or sleep the same. Babies awaken because of their temperaments, not because of your parenting abilities.

SLEEPING WITH YOUR BABY — YES? NO? SOMETIMES?

Is it all right to let your baby sleep in your bed? Yes! We are astonished how many baby books flatly put thumbs down on this most time-tested universal sleeping arrangement. Are they also against motherhood and apple pie? How dare self-proclaimed baby experts discourage what science is proving and veteran parents have long known — *most babies and mothers sleep better together.* Sleep sharing isn't for every family, and you are not less of a parent if you don't sleep with your baby. We simply want to validate this nighttime parenting practice as a healthy option for many families.

Our first three children slept in cribs. We were young parents, and all our friends' babies slept in cribs, so we joined the crib-and-cradle set. They slept fine, and we had no reason to consider any other sleeping arrangement. Then came our fourth baby, Hayden (you will meet this special child in the next chapter), who broadened our previously narrow view of nighttime parenting. In the early weeks and months Hayden slept in a cradle next to our bed. Around six months we moved her into a crib on the other side of our room. She began to awaken every hour each night. Martha would breast-feed and comfort her back to sleep, only to be summoned again by an anxious crib baby's cry. Finally out of sheer exhaustion one night, rather than Hayden's being dutifully returned to her crib, Martha and Hayden fell asleep together in our bed. Both awoke refreshed the next morning. Same routine the next few nights. Hayden was telling us she needed to sleep next to us. I consulted all the baby books. Big mistake. They all said no. Martha said, "I don't care what the books say, I'm tired, I need some sleep, and it works."

At this time we were writing our first book, *Creative Parenting,* in which we were stressing this point: *Parents, don't be afraid to listen to your baby.* Our own advice hit home. Hayden was telling us her nighttime needs, and we listened. She remained in our bed for the next two years, after which she gradually shifted to her own bed to sleep comfortably on her own.

Then we began to study why sleeping with babies works. At first we thought we were doing something unusual, until we surveyed other parents. Many others also slept with their babies; they just didn't tell their doctors or relatives about it. One evening we were at a party, and the subject of sleep (or a lack of it) came up. We confided (in a whisper), "We sleep with our baby." Our listener smiled, looked around to be sure no one could hear her, and said, "Me, too." Why should parents have to hide this beautiful style of nighttime parenting? That just doesn't make sense.

We initially had to get over all those warnings about manipulation and terminal nighttime dependency. You know, the long litany of you'll-be-sorry reasons. Well, we are not sorry; we're happy. Hayden opened up a whole wonderful nighttime world for us that we now want to share with you.

What to Call It

Sleeping with your baby has various labels: "Co-sleeping" sounds like something adults do, yet this seems to be the most popular term. The "family bed" conjures up visions of lots of kids squeezed into bed and dad somewhere on the couch or floor. We prefer to call this arrangement *sharing sleep,* because you share, as you will see, more than just bed space. You share sleep cycles, nighttime emotions, and lots of other good things that occur between persons in nighttime touch.

First, sharing sleep is more than an issue of where baby sleeps. It is a mind-set — a nighttime-parenting style that implies parents are open to trying various sleeping approaches and settling upon one that works for that stage of baby's development and parents' life-style. They are also flexible enough to shift to another nighttime parenting style as circumstances change. Every parent goes through nocturnal juggling acts until settling on a sleeping arrangement that works. Sharing sleep reflects an attitude of acceptance of your child as a little person with big needs. Your infant trusts that you, his parents, will continually be available during the night, just as you are during the day. Sharing sleep also requires that you trust your own intuition that you have made the best decision for yourselves and your baby.

Why Sleep Sharing Works

Babies go to sleep better. Especially in the early months, babies enter sleep via the light sleep stage, in which they need parenting to sleep, not just putting to sleep. Being held by, or lying down with, a familiar person in a familiar bed winds baby down more easily. Baby clicks into a familiar mental picture he has learned to love and trust. Being parented to sleep in the arms of father or on the breasts of mother creates a healthy go-to-sleep attitude. Baby learns not to resent going to sleep and not to fear staying asleep.

Babies stay asleep better. Put yourself in the sleep pattern of baby. As baby passes from deep sleep into light sleep, he enters a *vulnerable period* for night waking, a transition state that may occur as often as every hour and from which it is difficult for baby to resettle on his own into a deep sleep. You are a familiar attachment person whom baby can touch, smell, and hear. Your presence conveys an "It's OK to go back to sleep" message. Feeling no worry, baby peacefully drifts through this vulnerable period of night waking and re-enters deep sleep. If baby does awaken, she is sometimes able to resettle herself because you are right there. A familiar touch, perhaps a few minutes' feed, and you comfort baby back into deep sleep without either member of the sleep-sharing pair fully awakening.

Mothers stay asleep better. Mothers in our survey who shared sleep with their babies revealed they felt more rested the next day, although they might have awakened during the night to comfort their babies. These mothers and babies are in *nighttime harmony.* Baby's and mother's internal clocks and sleep cycles are in sync with each other. Frequently a mother notices, "I automatically awaken seconds before my baby does. When she starts to squirm I lay a comforting hand on her and she drifts back to sleep. Sometimes I do this automatically and I don't even wake up all the way." Not all mothers achieve this perfect nighttime harmony, but this is the best of both nighttime worlds: a full night's sleep and a contented baby.

Contrast this nighttime harmony with the crib-and-nursery scene. The separate sleeper awakens — alone. He is out of touch. First a squirm and a whimper. Still out of touch. Separation anxiety sets in, and baby cries. In time, baby's nighttime cries will awaken even the most long-distance mother. You jump up, stagger down the hall, and the night-comforting scene turns into a major operation. By the time you finally reach baby, his cries have escalated. He's wide-awake and angry. You're wide-awake and angry. The comfort that follows becomes a reluctant duty rather than an automatic response. It takes longer to resettle a crying, angry baby than it does a half-asleep baby, but finally baby is resettled in the crib. Now you're too wide-awake and upset to resettle easily. Also, because of long-distance sleeping, it is unlikely that mother's and baby's sleep cycles are in harmony. If baby awakened when entering light sleep but mother was still in deep sleep, out-of-sync night waking results. Being awakened from a state of deep sleep to attend a hungry baby is what makes nighttime parenting unattractive and leads to sleep-deprived mothers and fathers.

Breastfeeding is easier. Most veteran breastfeeding mothers have, for survival, learned that sharing sleep makes breastfeeding easier. Breastfeeding mothers find it easier than bottlefeeding mothers to get their sleep cycles in sync with their babies. They often wake up just before the babies awaken for a feeding. By being there and anticipating the feeding, mother can breastfeed baby back to a deep sleep before baby (and often mother) fully awakens.

A mother who had achieved nighttime-nursing harmony with her baby shared the following story with us: "About thirty seconds before my baby wakes up for a feeding, my sleep seems to lighten and I almost wake up. By being able to anticipate his feeding, I usually can start breastfeeding him just as he begins to squirm and reach for the nipple. Getting him to suck immediately keeps him from fully waking up, and then we both drift back into a deep sleep right after feeding." In this situation baby breastfeeds through the vulnerable period for awakening and then reenters the state of deep sleep. What might have happened if the mother and baby had not been within touching distance? The baby would have awakened in another room and cried loudly to signify his needs. By the time mother reached him, both mother and baby would be wide-awake and have difficulty settling back to sleep. (Note: There is no need to roll baby across your body to feed from the other breast. Instead, turn your upper shoulder toward baby to adjust the level of the upper breast.)

Mothers who experience daytime breastfeeding difficulties report that breastfeeding becomes easier when they sleep next to their babies at night and lie down with baby and nap nurse during the day. We believe baby senses that mother is more relaxed, and her milk-producing hormones work better when she is relaxed or sleeping. Mothers sometimes relate how their babies have gotten into the frustrating habit of wanting to breastfeed only when lying down with them. In counseling, we encourage these mothers to take seriously what their babies are communicating by this behavior, the babies' sensitivity to tension. Somehow babies know that if they can get their mothers to lie down, the milk flows better and the "ambience of the restaurant" is conducive to good digestion.

Sleep sharing fits in with busy life-styles. Sharing sleep is even more relevant for today's life-styles. As more and more mothers, of necessity, are separated from their baby during the day, sleeping with their baby allows them to be reunited at night. In counseling mothers who plan to go back to work within a few months of their baby's birth, we encourage them to consider sleeping with baby. This arrangement gives the baby and mother the closeness at night that they miss during the day. As an added benefit, the relaxing hormones produced when mother night nurses help her wind down from a busy day and enjoy a better night's sleep (see "Waking Up After Mother's Return to Work," page 353).

Slow starters can catch up. Sharing sleep is particularly valuable for the mother-baby pair who has had a slow start, and was unable to bond in the early newborn period because of a situation such as prematurity or another medical condition that separated mother and baby. Sharing sleep allows catch-up bonding. Also, sleep sharing helps parents, especially mothers, who have difficulty getting into parenting if the instinctive mothering feelings have been slow to come. Here's why: Mothering hormones may be slower to develop for some moms. Three conditions increase mothering hormones: sleeping, touching baby, and breastfeeding. A mother takes advantage of all three of these conditions when sleeping with her baby.

Babies thrive. Over our years of observing all the good things that happen to babies when they share sleep with their parents, one medical benefit stands out — these babies *thrive*. In fact, one of the oldest "treatments" for the slow-weight-gaining baby is taking baby to bed and breastfeeding. The health benefits of sharing sleep have been recognized for many years. A child-care book written in 1840, *Management of Infancy,* by A. Combe, states that "there can scarcely be a doubt that at least during the first four weeks and during winter and early spring a child will thrive better if allowed to sleep beside its mother and cherished by her warmth than if placed in a separate bed."

Perhaps someday science will confirm what experienced baby watchers have long known: Something good and healthful happens to babies (and parents) when they share sleep.

►**SPECIAL NOTE:** *The important issue in nighttime parenting is not where your baby sleeps but how responsive you are to baby's nighttime needs and how open you are to finding the best sleeping arrangement for your family.*

When It Doesn't Work

No one sleeping arrangement works for all families all the time. Sleep sharing may not work if it is started too late. Parents have tried everything, and baby still sleeps poorly. Reluctantly, months later, they take baby into their bed, but they really don't want him there. Also, if parents and baby have not begun life in the bed together, they are not used to each other's presence and their sleep cycles are not in harmony. They may wake up more.

Some babies and parents seem to have a critical sleeping distance; too far or too close increases their night waking. In the case where sleeping too close causes night waking in baby *or* parents, consider a co-sleeper, a criblike bed that attaches safely and securely to the parents' bed. A bedside co-sleeper allows you and baby to have your own sleeping space, yet it enables you to be within arm's reach of your baby for nighttime

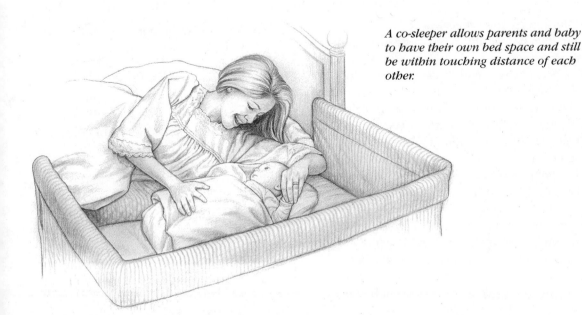

A co-sleeper allows parents and baby to have their own bed space and still be within touching distance of each other.

nursing and comforting. (For the best co-sleepers, see www.armsreach.com or call (800) 954-9353 or (818) 879-9353.)

HANDLING WORRIES AND CRITICISMS OF SLEEPING WITH YOUR BABY

Our longstanding advocacy of sleep sharing as an important aspect of nighttime parenting has made us aware of many of the questions about and criticisms of this approach. Here are some of the questions we most frequently encounter.

Fear of Dependency

I've heard that once baby gets in the habit, he'll never be able to go to sleep on his own. Am I creating a bad habit?

While initially this seems true, eventually your child will be able to go to sleep and stay asleep without your help. You're creating a *good* habit. The real question is, Which do you think your baby prefers: to drift off to sleep peacefully at his mother's breast or in his father's arms, or to soothe himself to sleep with a tasteless, emotionless rubber pacifier? The choice seems obvious, although a few babies, from the very beginning, prefer to approach sleep "Lone Ranger" style.

Consider the long-range benefits of sleeping together. One of the most precious gifts you can give your child is a vivid memory of happy childhood attachments. What a beautiful memory it is for a child to recall how he was parented to sleep in the arms of his mother or father or to recall how he awakened in the mornings surrounded by people he loved rather than in his private room in a wooden cage, peering out through bars. We will always remember how happy our children were when they awakened. Every time we looked over at our baby sleeping next to us, we saw a contented look on her face that said, "Thanks, mom and dad, for having me here." You're building intimate memories that last a lifetime.

Becoming a Self-Soother

I've heard that if baby is used to going to sleep at my breast or in dad's arms, when he wakes up he will expect the same thing and won't be able to get

---

GET BEHIND THE EYES OF YOUR BABY

Many kids ago we learned an important parenting principle when confronted with the dilemma of how to respond to our children in certain situations. Get behind the eyes of your baby and imagine you were a baby. What would you need, and how would you want your parents to react? If you were a baby, would you rather sleep alone in a dark, quiet room behind bars or nestled close to your favorite people in the whole wide world, inches away from your favorite cuisine and comforted by the familiar scent, sounds, and movements of the people you trust? Ah, night life is good!

himself back to sleep without us. Is this true?

True, true — and so what? This is a valid observation of nighttime attachment parenting. But your baby is a baby a very short time, and this is a stage when you are building foundations of trust. Consider what may happen if a baby wakes up alone and is forced, before his time, to become a self-soother.

The style of parenting called self-soothing, which is creeping into the "Let's have babies conveniently" mind-set, emphasizes techniques of teaching babies how to comfort themselves — by leaving them alone or setting them up to devise their own methods — rather than allowing babies to rely on mother or father. On the surface this sounds so convenient and liberating, but watch out for shortcuts, especially in nighttime parenting. This school of thought ignores a basic principle of infant development: A need that is filled in early infancy goes away; a need that is not filled never completely goes away but recurs later in "diseases of detachment" — aggression, anger, distancing or withdrawal, and discipline problems. We have a practical rule of thumb for you to consider: During the first year, an infant's wants and needs are usually one and the same.

Nighttime offers a special time for closeness, whether you actually share sleep with baby or not. Martha has fond memories of her nighttime parenting of Peter (now Doctor Pete), who was our last baby to sleep in the nursery. Here's her story:

"In the first few months I attended to Peter's needs for feeding rather mechanically two or three times a night: Baby cried, I got up and trudged down the hall, picked baby up, sat in the rocker, and did what it took to get him back to sleep — usually a twenty-minute feeding, and more time spent methodically changing the poopy diaper, gave him a second "top off" feed, gingerly placed him back in his cradle, slipped out quietly, and eagerly returned to my own warm bed (this was in the winter). What amazes me is that I never once thought of taking him to bed during the night! After several more months of this (and feeling quite desperate some nights if he woke again before I even got back to sleep) he finally got to where he would only wake up once each night. I would look forward to this nighttime togetherness because I was no longer so exhausted and I could begin to appreciate what I was doing — being with my baby with the whole house asleep, no interruptions or distractions — just the two of us. I learned not to try to rush him so I could get back to sleep. I would take him

---

A BABY NEEDS TO HAVE NEEDS

It is a natural, appropriate, and desirable part of development for a baby to be dependent. *A baby needs to have needs.* A baby who's forced into independence (to become a self-soother) before his time misses the needs stage. A baby needs first to learn to bond to *people* before *things.* If a baby can't have needs, who can? If the parents can't fill those needs, who will? Later in life you may be very distressed to see who or what will be used to fill needs that went unmet in infancy.

from his crib and go into the family room, get really comfortable and snug in a giant beanbag, turn on some quiet music, and spend an hour in this special place I had carved out of my busy life. It was so special to be alone with my baby that I would often continue to sit and hold him long after he was asleep. This was an important bonding time, and I didn't even know it."

An Unusual Custom?

Isn't sleeping with your baby an unusual custom?

Sleep sharing is not unusual or abnormal. I was once asked by a national TV network to consult on a show about children's sleep problems. The producer, learning that I favored babies sleeping with their parents, asked, "Dr. Sears, how many parents do this new thing?" Puzzled about what she meant by "this new thing," I realized that she was talking about sharing sleep. I informed her that the *new* thing was sleeping separately.

Cultures that do not have the "benefit" of experts regard sharing sleep as a natural continuum from mother's womb to mother's breast to mother's bed. They never even consider any alternative. The mother of a patient of mine studied family sleeping habits on the island of Fiji, as a research project for the World Health Organization. Fijian babies sleep next to their parents until weaning. The native women were surprised that the researcher even asked where babies sleep and said, "Is it true American mothers put their babies in cages at night?" Fortunately, we don't export our parenting ideas.

A separate nursery is a strange concept to most of the world's parents. In a survey of

186 traditional societies throughout the world, mother and baby shared a bed in most cultures, and none of the societies studied endorsed the Western separate nursery. We have broken a worldwide sleeping tradition, and we are losing sleep.

Suppose we spend an afternoon at the library reading about sleeping customs and sleeping advice throughout the world. If you select books from the anthropology section, all regard sleep sharing as the normal standard of parenting, like breastfeeding and holding a baby. What's all the fuss about babies in parents' bed? That's where they belong, say anthropologists.

Not so the medical and psychology books, which conjure up all sorts of reasons that this time-tested sleeping arrangement, present from the beginning of mankind, is all of a sudden wrong. That such a natural human custom should be controversial is ridiculous. In reality sleep sharing is following the same trend as breastfeeding. In 1950 breastfeeding was controversial! Now as more and more parents discard experts' taboos, breastfeeding has returned, and its relative, sleep sharing, is making its rightful comeback.

May Never Leave

We enjoy sleeping with our baby, and it's working for us, but should we worry? Our friends warn us that we'll be sorry we let our baby into our bed. She'll never want to leave.

You won't be sorry, and she will want to leave. True, your baby will not one day announce, "I'm ready now. Please get me my own bed and my own room." You are years away from that. As with so many parenting questions, look at it from your baby's viewpoint. Get under your baby's covers and imagine how she feels about her cozy quarters. Of course baby won't want to leave. She fits where she is. Why hurry a baby into independence? A child's needs that are filled early will eventually go away; a child's needs that are not filled leave an empty space that can come back later as anxieties. It is not your job to make your child nighttime independent, but rather to create a secure nighttime environment and feeling of rightness that allow your child's independence to develop naturally. The important fact is that for now you enjoy this arrangement and it's working for you. When the time comes, your baby will wean from your bed just like all the other weanings.

Doctor Says No

We would like to have our new baby sleep with us, but my baby's doctor advises us not to. I'm confused. Who is right?

There are three questions you should *not* ask your doctor: "Where should my baby sleep?" "How long should my baby breastfeed?" and "Should I let my baby cry?" Doctors do not study the answers to these questions in medical school, and much of their advice likely comes from their own personal experience as mothers and fathers, not as professionals. You are putting doctors on the spot when you ask them where your baby should sleep. Doctors are trained in the diagnosis and treatment of illness, not in parenting styles. If you want to sleep with your baby and feel that your baby, your husband, and you will all sleep better with this nighttime-parenting

style, this is the right decision for your family. Also, you will find that most doctors are becoming increasingly flexible about parents sleeping with their babies. Family doctors, pediatricians, and psychologists are now realizing that they will not have to spend so much time correcting sleep problems (or emotional problems) later if they spend more time helping a baby create a healthy sleep attitude in the early months.

Might Ruin Our Sex Life

The idea of sleeping with our baby sounds appealing, but how do we do that and still have a normal sex life?

Sex and babies do mix, but as in choosing a name, mom and dad must agree on having baby in their bed. If mother wants to, but dad doesn't, he may resent baby (and his wife) and feel he has to compete with baby for nighttime attention. It's up to the mother to not let the "baby's coming between us" scene occur. Talk it out. Before deciding on this arrangement and periodically during the early months, have an "Is it working?" chat. Be sensitive to each other's feelings.

Tiny babies are too young to notice and are not aware of lovemaking, but as baby gets older, parents may be inhibited by another person in bed, even though sound asleep. You could move the sleeping baby into another room or you could move to another room.

An alternative to putting baby to sleep in your bed is to put baby in his own bed or crib first and then bring him into your bed after the first waking. If baby is sleeping in your bed when the mood hits, you'll discover that every room in the house is a potential love chamber.

Time your intimacy. Day's-end, before-sleep sex is not the only way for couples to be together. Besides, during the early months most mothers are too tired by nighttime to do anything but sleep. As one mother put it, "I need my sleep more than he needs sex." If baby in the bed is a bit of a turnoff, enjoy mornings, afternoons, or any other time when baby is napping elsewhere.

Nighttime Privacy

I've read a lot about sleeping with a baby. Many of my friends let their babies sleep in their beds, but quite honestly I don't want our new baby in our bed. We have four other children, and by the time evening comes I've had enough of kids. I want some time alone with my husband. Am I a neglectful mother because I don't want to sleep with my baby?

No, you are not being a neglectful mother. You are a wise mother to have a realistic appraisal of your nighttime needs. Just as a breastfeeding mother is not better than one who bottlefeeds, a mother who shares sleep with her baby is not better than one who doesn't. It sounds as though you honestly feel that for your particular family situation it is necessary for you to have this special time with your husband at night to nurture your marriage, recharge your own batteries, and be a more effective mother by day. Our advice is to choose whatever sleeping arrangement works best for all members of the family. Don't feel pressured into a nighttime-parenting style that you don't believe in simply because your friends endorse it. Besides, you may have a baby who is not very separation sensitive at

night and may sleep quite well in his own crib or in his own room.

Easing Baby Out

How shall we handle it when it's time for our child to leave our bed?

You will probably be ready for your child to leave your bed before *she* is ready. Weaning from your bed is like weaning from the breast. Do it *gradually.* Between two and three years, most children accept weaning from your bed.

To ease your child from your bed into her own, try this two-step transition. First, make a fun trip to the store to let your child pick out her "big-girl bed" or "special bed." (In dealing with children you'll get a lot of mileage out of the term "special.") Place this special bed (or just a mattress) next to your bed. You may need to either lie in your bed next to her or sit or lie next to her as you parent her off to sleep. Expect her to want to crawl back into your bed when she wakes up at night. You can either allow this or place her back in her bed and "shush" or comfort her back to sleep. Second, once she feels comfortable sleeping in her own bed, move her bed into her own or a sibling's room. Getting her to accept this arrangement may take a few months. Lie down with her in her room and parent her back to sleep with a story, back rub, and some cuddle time. Then set nighttime rules. Keep a sleeping bag or futon at the foot of your bed and explain that if she wakes up, she can come in, but she must "tiptoe as quiet as a mouse and not wake up mommy and daddy because we need our sleep, otherwise we'll be a cranky mommy and daddy the next day."

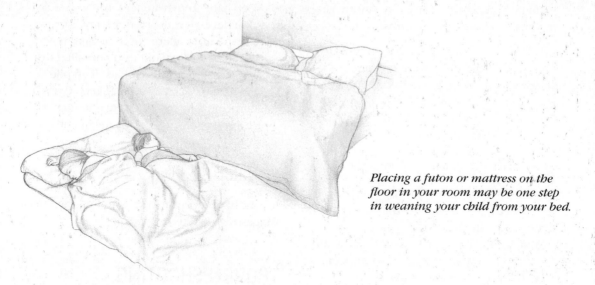

Placing a futon or mattress on the floor in your room may be one step in weaning your child from your bed.

Certainly by three years of age children can understand that nighttime is for sleeping and everybody needs to sleep. Eventually she will spend more time in her own bed and come into your room only during times of stress, such as illness, a move, or any of life's little upsets that can disturb a child's sleep. Don't worry, your child will eventually leave your bed.

Dr. Bill notes: *During an office visit with an eight-year-old boy, I asked him why he occasionally crawled into his parents' bed. Proudly he replied, "Because my parents are in it!" That said it all.*

SLEEP SAFETY

Whether your baby sleeps in your bed, a crib, or a combination of these arrangements, be sure to provide your baby with a safe sleep-ing environment. Take the following safe-sleep precautions:

- Place baby to sleep on his *back*. Alternatively, you can place baby on his side (preferably the left side) in certain situations, such as if baby suffers from reflux, but only if advised by your doctor.

- Don't put an infant under nine months to sleep on her tummy unless there is a doctor-recommended reason for doing so.

- Don't put baby to bed on a soft surface, such as a waterbed, beanbag, or any other squishy surface that could obstruct baby's breathing passages.

- Don't leave baby sleeping alone unsupervised in a carriage. An older child may caringly, but unsafely, snuggle a stuffed animal next to baby's head. Also, carriage mattresses tend to be less cared for than other bedding, and they tend to collect dust and other allergens. Clean them as needed.

Carriages are a common site of smothering in babies, second only to cribs.

- Don't use deep-pile (more than one-and-one-quarter inches or three centimeters) sleeping mats, such as lambskin. These not only collect dust and other allergens, but also can obstruct baby's breathing passages, especially if they get wet from drool or spit-up.

- Don't cover baby's head after the first day or two. This is a baby's primary path of normal heat loss. Covering the head risks overheating the baby. (Very premature hospitalized babies often need their heads covered to maintain their body temperature, but the medical staff monitors this.)

- Never smoke in the room where baby sleeps. Smoke irritates baby's sensitive breathing passages.

- If you must smoke, wear a smoke-free nightgown if baby sleeps with you, and take a shower before bed to get the smell of smoke out of your hair. Ditto this precaution for dad.

- Be particularly vigilant when traveling, since baby will be sleeping in an unfamiliar and potentially unsafe environment. Bring along a portable crib or a roll-out safe-sleeping mat. These are safer sleeping alternatives than soft adult mattresses, such as the ones used on sofa beds or rollaways in motels. If you are using a hotel-provided crib, do a safety check (see page 603).

- Be equally vigilant when putting baby to sleep in a carriage. Observe the same precautions as you would anywhere else. Place infant to sleep on her back or side, and remove any potentially dangerous objects from the carriage.

- Keep baby's environment as fuzz-free as possible, especially if your baby is prone to respiratory allergies. Besides removing stuffed animals, avoid using bedding that is likely to collect lint, such as deep-pile lambskin or fuzzy wool blankets. Hypo-allergenic mattresses and mattress covers are available for allergy-prone infants.

Safe Crib Sleeping

If your baby sleeps in a crib, follow the safety suggestions listed on page 603.

TROUBLESHOOTING: SOLVING YOUR BABY'S SLEEP PROBLEMS

If you've been through all the nighttime-parenting steps and your baby is still a restless sleeper, here's what to do:

- First, decide if night waking is a problem. Is it simply a nuisance that you can live with until your baby is old enough to get to sleep without your help? (Most eventually can.) Or is night waking interfering with your baby's optimal development and daytime behavior? Are you so tired the next day that you don't enjoy daytime parenting and are becoming increasingly resentful of nighttime parenting — and of your whole child? In short, are you ready to resign at bedtime?

- Go through the checklist of possible causes of night waking (see page 344). Match the most likely solutions to the causes, and one by one try these solutions

SAFE CO-SLEEPING

Parents often worry about rolling over onto their baby during the night. Sleep sharing is safe. Mothers we have interviewed on the subject of sharing sleep notice they are so *physically and mentally aware* of their baby's presence even while sleeping that they feel they would be extremely unlikely to roll over on their baby. And if they did, baby would put up such a fuss they would awaken in an instant.

Fathers, on the other hand, do not enjoy the same keen awareness of baby's presence while asleep, so it is possible that they might roll over on baby or throw out an arm onto baby.

The following precautions will help you share sleep safely:

- Place babies to sleep on their backs.

- Place baby between mother and a guardrail (available at baby-furniture stores or in catalogs) or push the bed *flush* against the wall and position baby between mother and the wall, not between the parents (see illustration on page 319). Toddlers tend to turn 360 degrees during the night and often awaken father if sleeping between the parents. Be sure there is no crevice between the bed and wall or the guardrail and mattress. Fill in any gaps with a rolled-up baby blanket.

- Do not sleep with your baby if you are under the influence of any drug that diminishes your sensitivity to your baby's presence, such as alcohol or tranquilizing medications.

- Avoid overheating from overbundling. This may occur if baby has been bundled appropriately to sleep in his own bed and then is brought next to a warm body as an added heat source (see signs of overheating, page 642).

- Use a big bed with few sleepers. Too small or too crowded a bed space is also an unsafe sleeping arrangement for a tiny baby. For example, it is unsafe for a father or a sibling to fall asleep with a tiny baby on a couch. Baby may get wedged between the back of the couch and the larger person's body. A queen- or king-size bed is a must for safely sharing sleep with a baby. Avoid letting an older sibling sleep with a tiny baby.

- Do not sleep with baby on a very wavy water bed. He may sink down too far in a crevice between the mattress and the frame or alongside mother. Don't leave a tiny baby on a wavy water bed alone. His neck muscles aren't strong enough to clear his face out of the sinking surface and he may suffocate. Firm or "waveless" water beds are safer, providing you make sure all crevices are filled.

- Take precautions to prevent baby from rolling out of bed, even though it is unlikely, especially when baby is sleeping next to a parent. Like heat-seeking missiles, babies automatically gravitate toward the parent. But to be safe, especially if baby is sleeping alone in your bed, use a guardrail.

until you find something that works. You may need to try different solutions at different stages of your baby's development or during life-style changes.

- If you have excluded all the causes of night waking on the list, realize there is no quick fix. It may take a few weeks to improve your baby's sleeping habits. Remember your long-range goal: *to help your baby develop a healthy sleep attitude.* While babies need some consistency in bedtimes and rituals, get your baby used to a *variety* of sleep associations that help her get to sleep and stay asleep without always relying on the same parenting-to-bed props.

Healthy Sleep Associations

A key to understanding your baby's wakefulness is understanding the concept of sleep associations — the persons, things, and events that a baby associates with going to sleep and getting back to sleep. We all have our favorite sleep associations: a book, a warm bath, music, and so on. But the difference between adults and babies is that an adult is able to go back to sleep when awakened without the same prop that was used to get to sleep. When you awaken during the night you can usually resettle simply by changing positions or fluffing your pillow. On the other hand, when babies awaken, they cannot get back to sleep without the same crutch that put them to sleep. When an infant or a child achieves sleep maturity, they are able to resettle, like an adult, without needing the same persons or props that helped them go to sleep.

Consider the implications of the sleep-associations concept. If your baby is used to being rocked, fed, massaged, cuddled, that is, *parented to sleep,* when she awakens she will expect and/or need the same warm and human touches to get back to sleep. If, on the other hand, you put a baby into a crib, alone, and do not help her go to sleep, she will learn to put herself to sleep by her own props. Then when she awakens at 3:00 A.M., she will be able to get back to sleep without your help.

This basic sleep fact has birthed two dissenting schools of nighttime parenting: One school believes a baby should be *parented* to sleep; the other teaches that a baby should be *put* to sleep. Whether to parent or to put is the basic nighttime question. Our approach combines *both.* We believe that for a baby to develop a healthy sleep attitude, she must first go through the parenting-to-sleep stage and ease into the put-herself-to-sleep stage. To force a baby to become a self-soother before her time risks a baby's developing a fear of sleep and sets baby up for long-term sleep problems. It also deprives babies and parents of an important period of growing together, when babies develop trust and parents develop sensitivity. Most babies who have been attachment parented to sleep and given responsive nurturing back to sleep gradually learn to get themselves back to sleep without anybody's help.

Some babies, however, get to enjoy night nurturing, increase their desire (or need) for it, and by two years of age show no inclination to give up their nighttime desires. This is especially true with busy babies and busy parents. Nighttime is quiet time. Baby has mom or dad all to herself and, especially if breastfeeding, will "milk" this quiet time for

---

NIGHTTIME PARENTING TIP

If you resent going to bed because it's work rather than rest, that's a clue you need to make some changes. Otherwise, you'll become so sleep deprived that you won't be able to function during the day.

---

all she can get. What was initially a need becomes a habit, which becomes a nuisance and escalates into parental resentment. In this situation nighttime parenting has gotten out of balance and gradual night weaning is necessary.

Should Baby Be Left to Cry It Out?

New parents often say to us, "I saw a technique on television that advised parents to let their baby cry longer and longer each night until he learned to fall asleep on his own. This approach doesn't feel right to me. Does it work?"

This advice has been around for nearly a hundred years, and each decade we see baby books advising variations of this sad theme. Going to your baby after five, then ten, then fifteen minutes of crying may sound humane or reasonable, but the result is usually the same: a strung-out mother and an angry baby, who will eventually exhaust himself to sleep — but at what price? We wish to put the cry-it-out approach to sleep — forever. We have written articles about the cry-it-out controversy, debated it on national television, and, for the benefit of tired but vulnerable parents, we have thoroughly researched what

is at the top of our hit list of bad baby advice. Here's what we found.

Doesn't Feel Right

To learn how parents feel about this question, we surveyed three hundred mothers. One of the questions was: What advice do you get from friends and relatives about what to do when your baby awakens at night? The most common advice was "Let baby cry it out." We also asked mothers how they felt about this advice. Ninety-five percent of the mothers replied, "This advice doesn't feel right." Our conclusions: 95 percent of mothers can't be wrong, and there is real confusion created by the advice a mother hears and what she feels.

It Sells

We interviewed publishers and TV producers who print and air this approach. Their defense: "It sells. Parents want quick recipes and quick results." Moms and dads, there are no quick fixes, no crash courses on baby calming and baby sleeping. Like all good long-term investments, creating a lasting healthy sleep attitude (our goal in this chapter) requires the gradual step-by-step approach we propose.

We are not saying that the cry-it-out approach is always wrong, doesn't work, and you should never use it. Instead, we wish you to be careful about jumping right into this method before you deeply understand its ramifications and have carefully considered less drastic alternatives. The following discussion will help you do just that.

Why Mothers Can't

First understand what is in a baby's cry. A baby's cry is designed for the thriving of a baby and the development of the parent.

A CHECKLIST FOR TIRED PARENTS

Night-Waking Causes

- [ ] Separation anxiety
- [ ] New skill being practiced
- [ ] Temperament — a high-need baby
- [ ] Family upsets
- [ ] Move to another house
- [ ] Depressed parents
- [ ] One parent away from home
- [ ] Irritating sleepwear
- [ ] Teething

- [ ] Wet or soiled diaper
- [ ] Diaper rash
- [ ] Hunger
- [ ] Stuffy nose
- [ ] Too hot
- [ ] Too cold
- [ ] Nasal irritants
  - cigarette smoke
  - perfume
  - powder
  - hair spray
  - animal dander

- dust, lint
- fumes
- [ ] Milk or food allergy
- [ ] Noisy bedroom
- [ ] A cold
- [ ] Ear infection
- [ ] Fever
- [ ] Gastroesophageal reflux
- [ ] Pinworms
- [ ] Urinary tract infection

What to Do

- [ ] Sleep close to baby
- [ ] Wear down in a sling
- [ ] Nurse down
- [ ] Massage before bed
- [ ] Rock
- [ ] Cuddle up
- [ ] Use the neck nestle
- [ ] Try a warm fuzzy: dad's chest
- [ ] Lay on hands

- [ ] Use a swaying cradle, rolling crib
- [ ] Bathe in warm water
- [ ] Warm the bedsheets
- [ ] Play soothing music
- [ ] Use white-noise sounds
- [ ] Play back-to-the-womb sounds
- [ ] Feed before bed

- [ ] Take a car ride
- [ ] Try a mechanical mother
- [ ] Put cotton sleepwear* on baby
- [ ] Schedule a doctor's examination

Cotton fire-retardant sleepware is now available.

Let's look again at that laboratory experiment we described in Chapter 1, which measured a mother's biological response to her baby's cry. When baby cries, the flow of blood to mother's breasts increases, accompanied by an intense urge to pick up and nurse (meaning comfort) her baby. No other signal triggers such strong emotions in a mother as her baby's cry. This is the reason mothers confide, "I just can't stand to hear my baby cry."

So the first arrow we shoot at this so-called scientific method is: *The cry-it-out advice goes against a mother's basic biology.*

Feeling Guilty

One morning I received a call from a weepy mother whose baby was waking up frequently. She had seen the cry-it-out approach seductively packaged and delivered on television. She opened her call, "I've been trying it. It didn't work and this morning we're both a wreck. Am I a bad mother? I feel so guilty."

I reassured her, "You're not a bad mother. You're a tired mother. Your overwhelming desire to get some sleep pressured you to succumb to so-called expert advice over your own intuition." I went on to explain, "As a result you set off an internal alarm that is shouting 'Not right.' This feeling of unrightness is what you call guilt. This means that you are a *sensitive* person. This inner sensitivity is your fail-safe signal. Listen to it. It won't fail you." I worry more about the mothers who are *not bothered* by their baby's nighttime crying.

Breaking Baby's Night Waking — And More

By breaking baby from waking up, does mother break other valuable connections? Suppose, despite her feelings of guilt and intuitively knowing the cry-it-out approach is not for her, a mother persists because she is advised to. Nights of crying continue, but each night baby cries less and mother's tolerance increases. Finally baby's night crying no longer bothers the mother, and baby begins to sleep longer. See, it works. Wrong! Would you toilet train your baby by forcing him to stay on the potty until he goes?

By persisting with the cry-it-out approach, the mother breaks her trust in herself and her trust in her baby's signals. She desensitizes herself, and *insensitivity* is what gets a mother into trouble. Baby loses trust in his mother's availability and ability to comfort him and loses trust in his own ability to influence her comforting behavior to meet his needs. Perhaps he senses that he is now a less valuable person. Sensitive parents overnighting with friends who have trained their babies to sleep alone report that these babies do cry for help during the night. They are dismayed to learn that the parents simply do not hear their babies crying.

The sensitive connection that mother and baby had when mother was bothered by the cry is now broken. Because both baby and mother have less trust in each other and in themselves, the parent-infant connection is devalued from an atmosphere of trust to that of mistrust, which will carry over into other aspects of their relationship. More detachment will follow, and this mother will buy into a parenting mind-set that a few weeks earlier would have been foreign to her.

Missing the Real Cause of Night Waking

This nighttime "hands off, let baby resettle on his own" approach has other flaws: It keeps parents from searching for the real causes of night waking and seeking out more sensitive and long-term solutions. It presumes the only reason baby wakes up is that he is "spoiled." He has not learned to put himself to sleep because you always help him. If you didn't help him get back to sleep, he would have to learn self-comforting techniques. What's the implication? It's your fault your baby wakes up, which is not true.

Cindy, a sensitive and very attached mother, consulted me about her one-year-old's recent change from a restful sleeper to

THE DETACHMENT SNOWBALL

Mark and Kelly were first-time parents who were blessed with a high-need baby — especially at night. They were sensitive and responsive parents, but one day a friend gave them a cry-it-out book, with the admonition, "Now you'll be tempted to give in, but harden your hearts and in a few nights he'll sleep." As their one-year-old baby screamed, these sensitive parents stood sweating and hurting outside his door, afraid to go in and "break the rules." Each night baby's night waking decreased, as did the parents' attachment. Baby *cried in* a feeling of mistrust and *cried* the sensitivity right *out* of the parents. Previously Mark and Kelly had taken baby Matthew with them everywhere because they wanted to and it felt wrong to leave him. Well, it was now easier to leave him. Getaway weekends extended to getaway weeks. A distance developed between parents and baby. More was cried out of the family than only night waking.

a restless night waker. She opened by saying, "I know my baby, he's waking for a reason. Something's wrong and I'm not going to let him cry it out, as my friends advise me." I gave Cindy the checklist of causes of night waking. By the process of elimination she identified polyester sleepwear as the nighttime irritant. The night she changed baby to all-cotton sleepwear, her baby again slept well. The cry-it-out advice often covers up medical causes of night waking. In our pediatric practice, we frequently see infants who wake up at night because they hurt, often from a medical condition such as gastroesophageal reflux (see page 388).

This is why you can't separate daytime parenting from nighttime parenting. A mother who starts off practicing attachment parenting becomes so sensitive to her baby that the whole cry-it-out approach is foreign to her parenting mind-set, and she intuitively seeks out the reasons for her baby's night waking and finds more sensitive solutions. A mother who buys into a more restrained style of parenting, however, is more easily lured into the cry-it-out approach. It is not so foreign to her mind-set, and she may more easily succumb to it.

Sink or Sleep

In teaching a baby to swim, you don't throw him in and force him to sink or swim. Likewise, you don't just put a baby in a crib alone and expect him to go to sleep. You first build baby's confidence that water is not something to be afraid of, then you help baby create an attitude that water is pleasant to be in. Then you teach swimming skills. Learning to sleep is a nighttime discipline and skill that begins with learning not to fear sleep; next baby discovers that sleep is a pleasant and not a lonesome state to enter (and reenter); and finally you teach baby the skills to maintain sleep.

Two Mothers' Stories

For some babies with easy temperaments, the cry-it-out approach may work, at least on the surface. For high-need babies (whom you will meet in the next chapter) it seldom works. By not responding to a baby's cries, you are not really teaching the baby to sleep; you are teaching your baby that crying has no communicative value. By not "giving in" to your baby you are teaching him to give up. We have great difficulty with the wisdom of this approach. It is night training, not nighttime parenting. We train pets — we parent children. Consider these parents' stories.

Laurie, an exhausted but attached mother of a night-waking baby, in desperation succumbed to the restraint advice.

"I plugged my ears and let him cry. Soon my husband had to hold me down, as I deeply wanted to go pick him up. My baby's cries got louder and louder and finally I couldn't stand it any longer and went to him. Boy, was he mad! I'll never do that again."

Another failure of the cry-it-out approach was shared with us by a mother who was advised to let her night-waking baby cry:

"I couldn't stand it any longer, and finally I went in to nurse him back to sleep. We both sat there in the rocking chair crying together, and it took me twice as long to nurse him back to sleep than if I'd gone to him immediately. The next day he was clinging to me all day long.

"As I read the 'cry book' I had to memorize when to soothe the child, when to hold him, how to act around him, when to put him to sleep, how many seconds I could comfort him, etc. Sure parenting is a learning game — but not like that! Parenting shouldn't end up a science. It should be natural, guided with intuition. I am sure the cry-it-out advice is not right for me — for us."

Alternatives to the Cry-It-Out Approach

Rather than the cold turkey approach to letting baby cry it out or the measured (and less inhumane) approach of letting baby cry with intermittent comforting, consider the following modifications of these approaches — ones that maintain parent-infant trust and the mutual sensitivity between babies and parents.

Like weaning from the breast, when to ease baby out of your bed and resort to a variety of sleep props varies from baby to baby and according to parents' life-styles. We are concerned about the rigid approach the cry-it-out books take. A whole list of do nots permeate this approach. For example, "Do not give in and pick up baby." The only do not in our approach is "Do not *rigidly* follow anyone's method but your own." Babies are too valuable and individual for that. Instead, here are some basic suggestions from which you can build your *own* helping-baby-sleep approach.

Be Flexible

If you pick a system from a book, you don't have to buy into it 100 percent. You can try part of an approach, keep what works, discard what doesn't. Each time you try a sleeping method, you build a nighttime *experience file*. It's not as if night waking will go on for years if you don't break it in the next two nights. Each month that you try something, you are wiser, and baby is more mature. Time is on your side. The rigid cry-it-out approaches require you to use the system 100 percent. This is not right. How can anyone write something for general readership that is 100 percent right for your individual baby? *Easing* into a system of sleep training makes baby less alarmed by a change of nighttime management.

Use Baby as a Barometer

Use your baby to gauge whether your approach is working, not someone else's schedule in a book. If it isn't working, pull back and try a month later. A problem we have with many of the cry-it-out approaches is that they ignore the baby's input. Your baby is a *partner* in your approach. Consider your baby's daytime behavior as a barometer. If you are thrilled with baby's behavior and don't get any vibrations that baby is disturbed or that your sensitivity is weakened, go on to the next step of nighttime weaning. If, on the contrary, early symptoms of premature detachment occur (anger, distancing, clinginess, tantrums), pull back and alter your course.

Kim and Allen were sensitive nighttime parents, but the consistent night waking of their two-year-old high-need baby, Jeremy, was getting to them. Parents were tired; baby was tired. A change of nighttime routine was definitely needed. These parents had practiced the attachment style of parenting. They knew their child, and the child trusted his parents. Now when Jeremy awoke, instead of rushing to immediately comfort him, they would give him time and space to resettle by himself. They put no time limit on how long to let him cry and set no rigid rules on "not giving in." They played each night by ear. If Jeremy's cries had a panic sound that touched their red-alert button, they trusted themselves to respond. Each night they waited a bit longer, and when they did go to comfort Jeremy they gave a simple "It's OK" message. Also, the parents increased their daytime attachment to Jeremy. They used their baby

as a barometer of whether their method was working. If Jeremy showed any daytime upset or became more distant from them, they would pull back on their nighttime-weaning pace. They did not let themselves become insensitive. Within two weeks Jeremy slept longer, as did the parents.

Why did this work? First, the parents and child had built the foundation of trust and sensitivity. Second, the parents did not lock themselves into a rigid schedule on how long they would let their baby cry. Baby became a partner in the approach as they eased him into nighttime independence.

Take Baby Steps

Vicky and Jack were sensitive parents of a nine-month-old night-waking baby, Michelle. A friend gave them a cry-it-out book that laid down an insensitive schedule of how long to let her cry. After two nights of cry it out, Vicky noticed the following changes in their baby. "She cried a lot all day. Sometimes she was more clingy; other times she was distant. Something we had before was gone." Jack concluded, "She doesn't trust you anymore."

These parents consulted us, asking for help in fixing their child's daytime behavior. Here's what we advised: "You see by your baby's negative daytime behavior that you pushed her too far too fast. You wisely realize that your baby's emotional well-being and your trusting relationship are at stake. She is not ready for such a giant step. Going from your bed to a crib in her own room with no or only partial response from you was too much. So you tried it — that's OK — and you see you need to back off. Give yourselves a few nights to get back in harmony, then consider taking some smaller steps that you all can live with. First, since she's been waking hourly, there could be a physical cause for the night waking. Go through the checklist of possible night-waking causes. Next, have your husband lull her to sleep after you've nursed her, and have him put her down asleep in her crib — or your bed if you choose to go a little slower. Then on her first waking you decide if you or your husband should comfort her back to sleep. When you are ready for bed, go ahead and take her into your bed at the next waking and nurse — it's easy to nurse once or twice at night — *you* decide. Ask your husband to alternate dealing with her as she awakes. Several nights of this should be all it takes for a return to a nighttime regimen that you can handle."

What We Did

Here is what we did if our babies showed persistent night waking. First, we regarded teaching a baby how to sleep as nighttime discipline. Just as we programmed ourselves against spanking as a daytime discipline technique, we vowed we would not use the cry-it-out approach as a nighttime discipline technique. This mind-set meant that we were highly motivated to find the real *cause* of our baby's night waking and seek, by trial and error, alternative approaches. Just as spanking keeps a parent from learning the real cause of a child's misbehavior and finding a more appropriate method, so the cry-it-out approach keeps parents from finding the real cause of the child's night waking and trying healthier alternatives.

Next, we decided on just how much night waking we could handle, making allowances for changing situations (illness, moves, and so on). For example, at nine months we could handle one to two night wakings and easy resettlings or an occasional bout of more-frequent night waking about every three weeks. More than that (unless baby is sick) meant we put "the system" into effect — meaning we went through our checklist of night-waking causes and altered the middle-of-the-night response accordingly.

One night twenty-month-old Matthew woke up wanting to nurse — for the third time in three hours. "Neee," Matthew said. "No," Martha responded. "Neee," Matthew said louder. "No!" Martha said louder. I awoke at the peak of this "neee-no" dialogue and realized that Matthew had pushed Martha too far.

Martha had trained Matthew to be satisfied with her body next to him, but not always with an available breast. Sometimes a pat or a back rub would do, or just holding him extra close as he struggled and fussed. Then he would gradually get the message "no nurse" and would give up and go back to sleep. On this occasion, yet another approach seemed in order; it was my turn to take over as comforter. The important point is to use a *variety* of comforting techniques that satisfy baby's need to relax.

Dad as a Co-comforter

While nighttime purists might advise the mother to just "keep on nursing; he'll grow out of it," this does not work for some parents. Lack of sufficient sleep undermines even the most committed parents. It's an advantage to moms for dads to develop comforting skills early on, so when the nighttime crises hit, the buck doesn't stop with mom. When our babies were fussing in my arms, Martha was comfortable. If the crying was escalated, she resumed the role of primary comforter. *We did not persist with a failing experiment.* This is different from the cry-it-out approach, in which the baby is not allowed to have any effect on the parents.

Beth and Ed practiced the attachment style of nighttime parenting, and it worked. Baby Nathan awoke every few hours during the night, but Beth nursed him back to sleep. Both were in nighttime harmony and reasonably well rested the next day. While most babies of this style gradually lengthen their sleep stretches as they get older, Nathan continued his frequent night-nursing requests. At eighteen months of age, he still wanted to nurse every two to three hours at night. What began as nighttime parenting evolved into nighttime turmoil. Beth began to resent Nathan's night nursing and, because she was tired the next day, was not a sensitive daytime mother. Dad was a blur at work. They went through the checklist of night-waking causes and solutions, but nothing worked. Clearly Nathan had associated going to sleep with breastfeeding. He was hooked. When he awakened, he would settle for nothing but the breast to get him back to sleep.

Nathan needed to learn other associations to gradually wean from frequent night nursing. I saw Beth and Ed in counseling, and we went through the following steps.

Recognizing the problem. The first step, and sometimes the hardest, is for sensitive and responding parents to realize they have a problem that needs a solution. "Just continue to meet your baby's needs and he'll outgrow it" wasn't working. In this instance, the parents sincerely felt that their baby's continued night feedings were no longer a need but a preference. So the first hurdle was for the parents to come to grips with the reality that a change in nighttime-parenting style was needed.

Teaching baby different sleep associations. Instead of Beth nursing Nathan to sleep every night, I advised Ed to "father-nurse" Nathan to sleep. Ed wore his baby in a sling in the neck nestle position (see page 291), walked, rocked, and sang to Nathan. When his baby was asleep he lay down with him on a futon next to their bed for ten to fifteen minutes, until he was sure Nathan was in a deep sleep.

Using father as comforter. Like clockwork, two hours later Nathan awakened and expected an instant breast. Instead, Ed became the pacifier, trying to comfort Nathan with the least amount of fuss. Sometimes only a pat on the back was needed. Other times, Ed would walk, rock, and neck nestle Nathan back to sleep.

Initially, Nathan didn't buy this change of nighttime management. He fussed — but he did not fuss *alone*. He was in dad's arms. Nathan would plead for "num-nums," but on each night waking, Ed would reaffirm: "Mommy go night-night, Daddy go night-night, num-nums go night-night, and Nathan go night-night." Nathan got the picture that when it's dark everyone sleeps — including num-nums. A couple of nights dad couldn't pacify Nathan, and Beth came to the rescue in the middle of the night. After a week Nathan consistently settled for dad, even though this was not his preference. After two weeks Nathan only awakened once. And after a month he slept for seven-to-eight-hour stretches.

From Mom to Dad to Soothie

Bill and Susan were caring and responsive parents, day and night. At eighteen months, baby Natalie began frequent night waking. These parents had decided they would do everything possible to help Natalie develop a healthy sleep attitude. As a child, Susan had feared sleep and vowed, "I don't want her growing up like me, afraid of sleep." But Susan was three months pregnant with her second baby and didn't have the energy to get up with Natalie — and she had the wisdom to recognize this. Bill parented Natalie to bed. He lay down with her on a mattress in her room or sometimes on a futon at the foot of their bed. Natalie snuggled to bed with daddy on one side and her favorite teddy bear, Bear-bear, on the other. As they drifted off to sleep, dad would frequently interject "Night-night, Natalie, and night-night, Bear-bear." When baby was asleep daddy would pick up baby (and Bear-bear) and put them into the crib or sometimes let them sleep on the futon. When Natalie awoke crying in the other room, dad would go in and pat her back, put her arm around Bear-bear, and "night-night" them back to sleep. After a while when Natalie awoke she would reach over and snuggle with Bear-bear and put herself back to sleep.

Nighttime purists may be offended by teaching a baby to use T. Bear as a pacifier instead of mommy or daddy. But there are family circumstances (pregnancy, illness, working schedules) in which the parents are worn-out, and for them a substitute nighttime parent is a salvation. Besides, like all healthy weaning, a gradual weaning from the real parents to a soothie (a teddy bear, a blanket, a doll) is a normal part of a child's sleep maturity. Every age has its props.

Consider a Physical Cause

If after trying these techniques your baby is still night waking, consider a physical cause. Because of the emphasis on bad habits as a cause of night waking, parents and doctors forget to search for physical causes. Seek consultation with your doctor about the possible physical causes of your baby's night waking. (See "Hidden Medical Causes," page 326.)

FREQUENTLY ASKED QUESTIONS ABOUT SLEEP PROBLEMS

The following are real-life nighttime-parenting situations that we have encountered in our mail, on our website, www.AskDrSears.com, or in personal nighttime counseling. We have also experienced most of these situations ourselves.

BABY AND MOTHER ARE OUT OF SYNC

Our two-month-old wakes up every couple of hours. I can't stand to let him cry, but by the time I do get to him and nurse him he's upset and so am I. It's taking me longer to resettle him and get back to sleep myself. My baby doesn't seem tired the next day, but I'm exhausted. What's wrong?

You and your baby are out of nighttime harmony with each other, and you need to be within touching distance. Remember, your baby has shorter sleep cycles than you do. Around every hour, as he ascends from the stage of deep sleep into light sleep, he goes through a vulnerable period for night waking. Some babies wake up during these vulnerable periods; others do not. It sounds as if you have a light sleeper who wakes up each time he changes sleep cycles. He wakes up during his light-sleep cycles while you are aroused out of your deep-sleep cycles. The *way* a person wakes up, not the frequency of waking, causes sleep deprivation. This is the reason you are more tired than your baby.

Try these steps to achieve nighttime harmony with your baby: Take baby into your bed either initially or after the first night waking and breastfeed him to sleep. On the next waking first try just patting him or placing your hand on his head or back, because he may not be hungry. If he needs to suck he'll let you know. After a week or more of this you will notice that you and your baby are beginning to get your sleep cycles in sync with each other, so that as your baby enters the state of light sleep and starts to wake up, so do you. You can then roll over and feed or pat your baby through this vulnerable period for night waking. You will both drift back into the state of deep sleep without having fully awakened. Eventually your baby won't wake at each change of sleep cycle because just your closeness will smooth his transition from deep to light and back to deep sleep without his waking at all.

SLEEPS TOO MUCH?

Can an infant sleep too much? My baby is four and a half weeks old, and I have to wake him up to feed him every three to four hours. Is this normal?

Oh, how many mothers would love to have your "problem"! Sleep patterns in infants are extremely variable. Babies with easy temperaments tend to be easy sleepers; high-strung infants are often frequent wakers. But it's possible for excessive sleep to keep an infant from thriving. "Thriving" means more than just getting bigger, it means that your baby is developing to his fullest potential physically, mentally, and emotionally.

Babies are born with attachment-promoting behaviors (such as crying) that cue their caregivers to the quantity and quality of touch and feeding they need in order to thrive. Infants who sleep too much may not initiate interaction, so you have to do it (as you've been doing when you wake him up to feed).

We suggest that you continue to schedule your baby's feedings at least every two to three hours during the day, but let him wake you at night. Be sure to have him weighed frequently by your doctor to be sure he is gaining enough weight. Because they are not demanding babies, heavy sleepers often do not get enough to eat. This is why you are wise to take charge of the feeding routine and continue to awaken your baby for meals every two to three hours during the day.

In addition to ensuring that your baby gets adequate food, it's also important to make sure he gets enough touch. Demanding babies often cry if somebody doesn't hold them, but easy babies often sleep right through potential holding times. One way to address this is to wear your baby around the house in a baby sling at least a couple hours a day to provide touch and stimulation.

In the meantime, enjoy your full night's sleep while it lasts!

WAKES UP AS SOON AS I PUT HER DOWN

Our six-month-old baby won't go to sleep by herself. I know she's tired when she falls asleep in my arms. But as soon as I put her into her crib and try to tiptoe out of the room, she wakes up and screams.

Try this nighttime-parenting style: Comfort your baby to sleep as you are now doing, but for a longer time, until she has drifted through the state of light sleep (you can recognize if she is still in this state by facial grimaces, partially clenched fists, muscle twitches, fluttering eyelids, and overall tense muscle tone). Lie down with your baby on your bed or anyplace that allows both of you to snuggle close to each other if you are breastfeeding. If you are bottlefeeding, a rocking chair works well. Nurse (either breast or bottle) your baby until you notice that the signs of light sleep are no longer present and she has slumbered into the state of deep sleep, which you can recognize by her almost motionless face, regular breathing, still eyelids, and especially the limp-limb sign — arms dangling weightlessly at her sides, hands open, and muscles relaxed.

After your baby shows signs of reaching deep sleep, you can put her down. Try having the crib sheet warm if she startles awake. Or you may find that you need to lie down with her on your bed to keep her asleep until you can ease away. In this case you will wind up with her sleeping in your bed, which may be what she really needs for a while anyway.

WAKING UP AFTER MOTHER'S RETURN TO WORK

I have recently returned to work, and my four-month-old has begun to wake up more frequently. I'm still breast-feeding him part-time. I'm up and down all night trying to resettle him into his crib. I'm so tired that it's hard to work the next day. Help!

This is a common nighttime nuisance when mothers return to work. We frequently hear of the following scenario: Mother picks her baby up at the baby-sitter's and the baby-sitter boasts, "My, what a good baby. He slept all day." Your baby may be tuning out the baby-sitter during the day and sleeping in order to save his prime waking time to be with you at night. You may feel that your baby is deliberately getting his days and nights mixed up. Remember that babies do what they do for a reason. They don't wake up purposely to annoy or deprive you of sleep.

Your baby is probably telling you, "Mommy, I need more time with you." Here's how to give your baby more touch time and yourself more sleep: Take him into your bed and enjoy sleeping side by side. Snuggle next to each other and enjoy the nighttime closeness. You may find that he awakens less, and even if he does continue to awaken, it will be much easier to resettle both of you if you are in closer touching distance. Some night feeding is necessary in order to keep up your milk supply if you are away from him during the day, and we recommend that you continue to breastfeed after returning to work. Your bond will be stronger because of it. As an added benefit, night feeding allows the natural sleep-inducing substances present in your milk to help baby sleep and gives you a higher level of the natural tranquilizing hormones that help you unwind. Take advantage of these sleep inducers and enjoy sharing sleep with your baby. You are likely to have a better night's sleep and a better day's work — besides giving your baby a special nighttime touch.

DAYS AND NIGHTS MIXED UP

Our newborn likes to sleep a lot during the day but wakes up a lot at night. How can we reverse this habit?

Many newborns come into the world with their sleep-wake cycles established for day sleeping and night waking. In the womb, babies sleep when mom is awake, mainly because motion lulls babies to sleep. And, babies awaken and kick when mom goes to sleep. Here's how to teach your baby that daytime is for feeding and interacting, and nighttime is for sleeping.

During the day, wake your baby for a feeding every two to three hours, so that she does not sleep longer than a three-hour stretch. Interact with her with eye contact and touch after each feeding for as long as she can stay awake. The more often you feed and interact with your baby during the day, the longer stretches she is likely to sleep at night.

WAKING UP TO PLAY

Our baby sleeps with us, and we really enjoy it, but sometimes he wakes up in the middle of the night bright eyed and bushy tailed and ready to play. Initially this was funny, but now we're tired of it. How can we stop this habit?

Your baby needs nighttime conditioning. He needs to learn that a bed is for sleeping, not for playing. We solved this semiamusing nighttime nuisance by "playing dead." When our baby woke up eager to play, we pretended that we were still asleep and ignored his desire to play. Lie quietly with your eyes closed and preferably with your back to baby. This is tough to do, since your baby will probably start pawing at you and crawling all over you trying to get attention, especially since you initially encouraged him. If you persist long enough, though, he will eventually get bored and also get the message that nighttime is for sleeping and not for playing.

NAPTIME PARENTING

Our two-year-old just doesn't seem to need a nap, but I need a break. Do two-year-olds need naps? How can I get her to nap so that I can get something done?

Yes, most two-year-olds need naps, and their parents need them to need naps. In the first year most babies need at least a one-hour nap in the morning and a one-to-two-hour nap in the afternoon. Between one and two years most babies have dropped the morning nap, but still require a one-or-two-hour afternoon nap. Most children require at least a one-hour afternoon nap until around the age of four. Sleep researchers feel that napping does have restorative value. Some children and adults actually fall asleep more quickly and sleep more efficiently during a short nap than they do during the night.

Here are ways to encourage the reluctant napper. Plan a car ride around naptime and your toddler is almost sure to fall asleep. Or nap *with* her. Even if your child doesn't want to nap, she may need a little downtime. Choose a consistent time of the day (preferably a time when you're the most tired) and set your child up for a nap. Take her into a dark, quiet room, turn on some soft music, nestle together in a rocking chair, or lie down on a bed. Set aside a special quiet time every day, during which you read a story together or give her a massage to condition her into a nap.

My ten-month-old refuses to take a morning nap and usually doesn't get more than a half-hour nap during the day. How much of a nap do babies need?

Both babies and parents need naps. Ten-month-old babies need at least a one-hour nap in the morning and a one- to two-hour snooze in the afternoon. Between one and two years, some babies drop the morning nap but still require one in the afternoon.

You can't force your baby to sleep, but you can create conditions that allow sleep to overtake him. Try the following:

Nap with baby. You probably look forward to your baby's naptime so you can "finally get something done." Resist this temptation. Naps are as important for you as they are for your infant.

Establish a routine. To get him on a predictable nap schedule, set aside time in the morning and in the afternoon to nap with

him. This will get your baby used to a consistent pattern.

Set the scene. A few minutes before naptime, cuddle your baby in a dark, quiet room. Play soft music and nestle together in a rocking chair, or lie down on a bed. This will set him up to expect sleep to follow. Once he's in a deep sleep you can ease him into his crib, continue napping with him, or slip away.

We have a two-and-a-half-year-old and a six-month-old. How can I get them to nap at the same time?

This is a challenging situation, since toddlers and infants have different sleep patterns and different needs, and the mother of both a toddler and a baby has a reason to be doubly tired. First, try to get them on a similar nap schedule. At least once a day try to get them to sleep at the same time. What helped us when we were trying to get our baby to nap at the same time that we were chasing down a busy toddler was the trick of creating a "nap nook." Try a large box with a cutout door, a card table with a blanket over the sides, or a mat under a grand piano. Settle your older child into his "special place" reserved just for napping. Once he's asleep, you can then lie down with your baby wherever it's most comfortable.

Try napping with your baby and toddler. Pick a consistent time during the day when you are the most tired. Lie down on your bed and feed or cuddle your baby to sleep on one side while singing your toddler to sleep on the other. If your toddler is reluctant to give in to a nap, put your infant in a sling and stroll around until he falls asleep. Then entice your toddler into the bedroom for a sleep-inducing story and music. Market this as quiet time. Two-year-olds are old enough to understand the concept of daily "quiet time." Eventually your toddler may actually look forward to these special snuggle times with mom, and you'll get a much-needed nap yourself.

One of the most difficult parts of parenting is realizing that you can't always be all things to all of your children. Parenting is a juggling act in which you try to give each child what he needs according to his stage of development and your energy level. Although mothers often seem to defy many laws of mathematics, you just can't give 100 percent to each child all the time. You may need to call in some reserves. In this case, you might get your two-and-a-half-year-old involved in a playgroup for a few afternoons each week or hire a teen to baby-sit your toddler after school. When possible, mom and dad can do shift work. Dad takes the older child while mother naps when the baby naps.

NIGHT WAKING IN PREVIOUSLY GOOD SLEEPER

Our one-year-old used to sleep through the night, but now he's waking up every night. He stands up and rattles his crib. Why is he doing this, and what should we do?

Anytime a previously sound sleeper wakes up, consider what's new in baby's development or in your family situation that would cause night waking. Expect night waking when babies achieve a major developmental skill such as sitting up, crawling, or walking. Babies seem to awaken to "practice" this new skill. Your beginning walker may walk around his crib half-asleep and awaken when he bangs into one side.

Try to resettle your crib walker with a minimum of fuss. First, try to get him back to sleep without taking him out of the crib — soothing words, a pat on the back, a lullaby — and as he sinks back down onto the mattress continue to pat his back around sixty beats per minute in gradually diminishing touches until he's fast asleep.

SQUIRMS TOO MUCH IN OUR BED

We enjoy having our three-month-old sleep in our bed, but now she's beginning to squirm so much that nobody's getting any sleep. Help!

Some babies, and parents, are too sensitive to sleep snuggled against a warm body. They need some space. Some babies seem to have a critical sleeping distance from parents: too close and they wake up, too far and they also wake up. Try putting just the right distance between you and your baby at night. Place a rolled-up blanket or a foam bolster between you and baby. These props may cushion the contact on your back from your nighttime squirmer. If a few feet more of distance is needed, try a co-sleeper (see page 333) or put her crib adjacent to your bed. In this way baby has her own bed space, and you have yours, but you are still within close touching and nursing distance.

TOO NOISY AT NIGHT

We want to sleep with our new baby, but it isn't working. She's too noisy, and I'm too aware of her presence. She sleeps great, but I don't, and my husband wakes up every time she whimpers. Will she grow up insecure if we don't sleep with her?

The fact that you are responsive enough even to consider sleeping with your baby indicates that you are nurturing parents, and it's likely that your baby will grow up secure even if she sleeps separately. Sharing sleep is just one part of the overall style of attachment parenting.

Wherever all family members sleep the best is the right arrangement. Sometimes it takes a few weeks for parents to get used to sharing sleep, especially dads. Give this arrangement a thirty-day free trial.

If it still isn't working, try gradually increasing the distance between you and baby until you both are not awakened by her nighttime noises. Place her between you and a guardrail, not between you and your husband (see illustration on page 319). Or try putting her crib next to your bed. If you are still supersensitive to her sounds, put her crib or cradle at the foot of your bed or across the room. As the weeks pass, you'll gradually discover a comfortable sleeping distance. Giving some time to adjust to this new little person in your night life is important. Things worthwhile are rarely achieved instantly. Soon you will get used to these normal sounds. While a silent bedroom is impossible with a new baby, you can block out some noises by playing a continuous tape of soothing environmental sounds such as running water and ocean waves.

HOW MUCH SLEEP?

My daughter is thirteen months old and sleeps from ten at night to seven or eight in the morning. She also has one or two forty-five-minute naps during the day. Is this enough sleep? How much sleep should she be getting?

Most thirteen-month-old babies sleep eleven to twelve hours a day, including naps, so your daughter is probably getting enough sleep. If she seems well rested, this may be enough sleep. But if she seems tired or irritable or nods off to sleep frequently during the day, she needs more sleep. While the optimal amount of sleep varies greatly from child to child, below is a chart of average sleeping times for children at different ages.

AFRAID TO SLEEP ALONE

Our eighteen-month-old awakens every two hours. By the time I get to his room, he is standing up in the crib reaching out for me. As soon as I try to put him back down, he clings to me. But he used to sleep so well. Should I just let him cry it out?

No! There's a better solution. Between twelve and eighteen months a baby's normal separation anxiety intensifies. He becomes clingy during the day and more aware of his separation and loneliness at night (see "Separation Anxiety," page 515, for a detailed explanation). Don't be afraid to listen to your baby. You are neither spoiling him nor being manipulated. He needs to be parented through this high-need stage rather than

Age	Hours of Sleep per Day
birth to 3 months	14 to 18
3 to 6 months	14 to 16
6 months to 2 years	12 to 14
2 to 5 years	10 to 12

have you succumb to the trust-shattering and insensitive cry-it-out approach.

Your baby is telling you that he can't sleep alone. He misses you. Here are your options. You can continue going in every time he wakes up and offer periodic "It's OK" reassurances; but you're going to be very tired, and this nighttime nuisance is going to wear thin after a while. Or you can get right to the heart of the problem and provide nighttime company. Move a mattress or a roll-away bed into your baby's room and lie down next to his crib when he goes to sleep. Then leave. Sometimes having a parent there when baby goes to sleep is enough to pacify the night waker. If he continues to awaken, you and your husband can try taking turns sleeping in his bedroom — if you sleep well there. Or move his crib into your bedroom. Or let him sleep at the foot of your bed on his crib mattress or a futon on the floor.

When this nighttime separation-anxiety period lessens, gradually ease baby back into his own room, or leave him in yours for a few more months if this arrangement is working. Playing musical beds is a normal and passing stage of nighttime parenting.

"NURSING" BABY TO SLEEP AT DAY CARE

My six-month-old daughter will be entering day care part-time, and I'm concerned about naptime. At home she either nurses to sleep or I take a drive with her. How can I teach her another way to go to sleep?

Talk to your childcare provider about how he or she can create an environment for your daughter that mimics her home environment as closely as possible. It will also be less con-fusing for your baby if the childcare provider can use a parenting style that's similar to yours.

Even if your infant can't be nursed to sleep, she can still be lulled to sleep in the arms of her childcare provider. Nursing is about comforting, not just breastfeeding, especially at this age. Anyone can nurse a baby to sleep in this sense. Explain to the childcare provider that your infant is used to being nursed to sleep and that you would like her to go to sleep in the caregiver's arms, either by rocking, singing, or with someone lying next to her, if possible.

A nap-inducing trick that works well in day care is "wearing down." Show the childcare provider how to wear your baby in a carrier — preferably a sling-type carrier — as naptime nears. Babies love to fall asleep in a sling. Once your baby is in a deep sleep, the childcare provider can ease her out of the sling and into the crib. (See "Wearing Down to Sleep," page 295, and "Babywear in Day Care," page 294.)

NURSING ALL NIGHT

Our six-month-old sleeps with us, and she used to wake up once or twice a night to breastfeed. I could handle that, but now she wants to nurse all night. I feel like a human pacifier. I'm exhausted.

You are right. Your baby is using you as a pacifier — "pacifier" meaning "peacemaker." But the human pacifier can wear out, and baby needs to learn that there are nighttime pacifiers other than breastfeeding. First, let's get into your baby's mind to understand why she does this. During the first six months your baby has developed a familiar mental picture:

Distress is followed by comfort. When she's hungry, thirsty, lonesome, anxious, teething — relief is spelled B-R-E-A-S-T. By reflex you give her the breast within seconds of her wakening. Perhaps your baby needs a few minutes to resettle by herself without the breast.

First, increase her feeding during the day. Between six and nine months, babies are often so busy playing they forget to feed. But at night hunger pangs overcome, especially when the all-night diner is so convenient. At least every three hours during the day take her into a quiet, unstimulating room and get down to the business of feeding. Offer solids two to three times a day. Baby needs to learn daytime is for playing and feeding; nighttime is for sleeping.

When she awakens, instead of breastfeeding her by reflex, try nursing her back to sleep without breastfeeding. Use calming techniques that work with the minimal amount of fuss and arousal:

- Lay on hands and pat her tummy.
- Hold her securely and cuddle awhile.
- Try a nighttime lullaby to accompany either of the above soothers.
- Treat teething pain (see page 497).

JUST SAY NO

I'm trying to wean our eighteen-month-old from night nursing, because I'm wearing out. But she's not buying it, and I'm not a good martyr.

This baby is an older relative of the previous one. As we've said before, babies are takers, and parents are givers. That's a realistic fact of nighttime life. But like many aspects of parenting, this is a question of *balance*. Sometimes babies become "overtakers."

Some mothers, because they are sensitive and giving, continue letting baby drain them until they give out. This scene is not what attachment parenting is all about. Fortunately, it sounds like you have a realistic appraisal of how much you can give and when to stop. That's part of maturing as a giving parent.

If you continue the nighttime-parenting level that you are resenting and from which you are becoming too exhausted, you will carry this resentment — and your tiredness — into your daytime relationship with your baby and your spouse, and the whole family will lose. For suggestions for dealing with all-night nursers, see the boxes on pages 360–363.

WAKES UP FOR BOTTLE

Our fifteen-month-old won't go to sleep without his "ba-ba." Then he wakes up twice during the night screaming for his bottle. I'm getting to hate "ba-ba," and I wish he did.

Babies like to feed off to sleep either by breast or bottle. And, in fact, many toddlers need a before-bed feeding to set aside their hunger until morning. There are a couple of problems with night bottles. Baby always associates going to sleep with the bottle, just as the breastfeeding baby associates sleep with breastfeeding. As we've stated elsewhere, an important fact of sleep is called sleep associations: The object or person baby associates with *going* to sleep is the same prop baby expects in order to get *back* to sleep. The key to keeping babies asleep is giving them various sleep associations so that they don't get hooked on one.

NIGHTWEANING TODDLERS:

11 Alternatives for the All-Night Nurser

Frequent night nursing is characteristic of high-need babies. They regard it like going to their favorite restaurant. The ambiance is peaceful, the server is familiar, the cuisine is superb, and they love the management. Ah, life is good! Who can blame the all-night gourmet?

Before seeking a solution to the problem, ask yourself how much of a problem the frequent night nursing is. This stage of high-level night nurturing will pass. Both you and your baby will someday sleep through the night. On the other hand, if you are sleep deprived to the degree that you are barely functioning during the day, you are resenting your nighttime parenting style (and your baby), and the rest of your family relationships are deteriorating, you need to make some changes in your nighttime feeding schedule. Here is a parenting principle we learned many kids ago: IF YOU RESENT IT, CHANGE IT!

Even if you can't get your baby to sleep through the whole night, you can help him cut back on nighttime nursing, making the situation more tolerable for you. Try these solutions for dealing with all-night nursing:

1. Tank your baby up during the day. Toddlers love to breastfeed, yet they are often so busy during the day that they forget to nurse, or mom is so busy that she forgets to nurse. But at night, there mom is, only inches away, and baby wants to make up for missed daytime nursings.

(This is a common scenario when a breastfeeding mother returns to work outside the home.) Finding more time to nurse during the day may make the breast less needed at night.

2. Increase daytime touch. Wear your baby in a sling or otherwise give your baby more touch time during the day. When babies get older, it's easy to greatly decrease the amount of touching time without realizing it. All-night nursing can sometimes be a baby's signal reminding mothers not to rush their baby into independence. As a child develops a healthy independence, she leaves and comes back, lets go and clings, step by step until she is going out more than she is coming back. Many mothers have noticed that babies and toddlers show an increased need for nursing and being held right before they begin a new stage of development, such as crawling or walking.

3. Awaken baby for a full feeding just before you go to bed. Rather than going off to sleep only to be wakened an hour or two later, get in a feeding when you retire for the night. This way, your sleep will be disturbed one fewer time, and (hopefully) you'll get a longer stretch of uninterrupted sleep.

4. Get baby used to other "nursings." Try wearing baby down to sleep in a baby sling. After baby is fed but not yet asleep, wear him in a baby sling around the house or around the block. When he's in a deep sleep, ease him onto your bed and extricate yourself from the sling. This is a good way for dad to take over part of the bedtime routine. Eventually your baby will associate father's arms with falling asleep, and he'll be willing to accept comfort from dad in the middle of the night as an alternative to nursing. Other ways to ease your baby into sleep without nursing him include patting or rubbing his back, singing and rocking, or even dancing in the dark to some tunes you like or lullabies you croon.

5. Make the breast less available. Once your baby has nursed to sleep, use your finger to detach him from the breast. Then pull your nightgown over your breast and sleep covered up. A baby who can't find the nipple quickly may just fall back to sleep. If you can stay awake long enough to put the breast away, he may not latch on again so soon.

6. "Nummies go night-night." Between twelve and eighteen months, your child has the capacity to understand simple sentences. Program your toddler not to expect to be nursed when she awakens, saying, for example, "We'll nurse again when Mr. Sun comes up." The key is to get baby to associate "it's dark outside" with "the kitchen is closed," except, perhaps, for the initial nursing down to sleep. Also, consider nursing in a rocking chair and no longer nursing in the bed so that she no longer associates the bed with nursing.

Expect to have several rough nights. Remember, though, that you are there for her and not letting her cry by herself. This won't damage your trust relationship, because you are still there.

When you nurse her to sleep (or have the first or second night nursing), the last thing she should hear is "mommy go night-night, Daddy go night-night, baby go night-night, and nummies go night-night" (or whatever she dubs her favorite pacifiers). When she wakes during the night, the first thing she should hear is a gentle reminder, "Nummies are night-night. Baby go night-night, too." This program may require a week or two of repetition. Soon she will get the message that daytime is for feeding and nighttime is for sleeping. If "nummies" stay night-night, baby eventually will too. To reinforce this teaching, here is an idea we got from several moms: Put together a picture book of babies sleeping without a breast nearby. Several times during the day review these pictures and talk to her about how the babies sleep without "nummies."

7. Offer a sub. High-need babies are not easily fooled; they don't readily accept substitutes. Yet, it's worth a try. Remember, nursing does not always mean breastfeeding. Honor your husband with his share of night "nursing," so your toddler does not always expect to be comforted by your breasts. This gives dad a chance to develop creative nighttime fathering skills and the child a chance to expand her acceptance of nighttime comforters.

Martha notes: One of the ways we survived a toddler who wanted to nurse frequently during the night was for me to temporarily go off night call. Bill would wear Stephen down in a baby sling, so he got used to Bill's way of putting him to sleep. When he woke up, Bill would again provide the comfort Stephen needed by rocking and holding him in a neck nestle position, using the warm fuzzy and singing a lullaby. After three or four nights of father nursing, Stephen was back to nursing only once or twice. Babies may initially protest when offered father instead of mother, but remember, crying and fussing in the arms of a loving parent is not the same as crying it out. Dads, realize that you have to remain calm and patient during these nighttime fathering challenges. You owe it to both your wife and baby not to become rattled or angry if your baby resists the comfort you offer.

Try this weaning-to-father arrangement on a weekend, or another time when your husband can look forward to two or three nights when he doesn't have to go to work the next day. You will probably have to sell him on this technique, yet we assure you that we have personally tried it and it does work. Be sure to use these night-weaning tactics only when baby is old enough and your gut feeling tells you that your baby is nursing at night out of habit and not out of need.

8. Increase the sleeping distance between you. If the above suggestions do not entice your persistent night nurser to cut back, but you still feel you must encourage him to do so, try another sleeping arrangement. Try putting him on a mattress or futon at the foot of your bed, or even in another room with a sibling. Dad or mom can lie down beside baby to comfort him if he awakens. Mom can even nurse, if necessary, and then sneak back to her own bed if continued closeness seems to encourage continued waking.

9. Just say no! When our son Matthew was twenty months old, Martha felt desperate for sleep if awakened more than two times. I often woke up to the following: "Nee" (his word for nurse) . . . "No!" . . . "Nee!" . . . "No!" . . . "Nee!" . . . "No, not now. In the morning. Mommy's sleeping. You sleep too." A firm but calm, peaceful voice almost always did the trick. You can manage to stay peaceful in this situation when you know you are not damaging your very secure, attachment-parented child.

10. Sleep in another room. If your baby persists in wanting to nurse all night, relocate "Mom's All-Night Diner" to another room and let baby sleep next to dad for a few nights. He may wake less often when the breast is not so available, and when he does wake, he will learn to accept comfort from dad. Use this "move out" technique as a last resort.

11. Let baby be the barometer. When trying any behavior-changing technique on a child, don't persist with a bad experiment. Use your baby's daytime behavior as a barometer of whether your change in nighttime parenting style is working. If after several nights of working on night weaning you feel that your baby is her same self during the day, then continue with your gradual night weaning. If, however, she becomes more clingy, whiny, or distant, take this as a clue to slow down your rate of night weaning.

Babies will eventually wean, and someday they will sleep through the night. This high maintenance stage of nighttime parenting will pass. The time in your arms, at your breast, and in your bed is a relatively short while in the life of a baby, yet the memories of love and availability will last forever.

Parents also get into a sort of nighttime rut. The bottle or breast works so well that they stick to it. This is OK if you're going to offer the same prop every time baby wakes up. But if you want baby to learn to resettle himself without "ba-ba," offer a variety of go-to-sleep props. For example, give him his bottle in a rocking chair, then help baby snuggle to sleep with one arm around a teddy bear and the other around mommy or daddy. When he awakens, cuddling the bear may be enough to resettle him.

WON'T WIND DOWN

Our nine-month-old just won't wind down. We know he's tired, but he won't give up. How can we get him to go to sleep without so many hassles?

You can't force a baby to go to sleep; but here are some sleep-inducing hints that allow sleep to overtake your baby: Avoid before-bed activities that rev up baby. An evening wrestle with daddy is OK, and may burn off excess energy, but not just before bedtime. A warm bath, a soothing massage,

quiet music, calmly looking at two or three books you keep just for bedtime, are time-tested winding-downers.

What works best in our family is wearing down. Suppose around eight-thirty you are marketing sleep, but baby is not buying it. Place baby in a sling-type carrier and wear him around the house, or around the block in warm weather, while singing a slow, repetitive tune like my favorite, "Old Man River." Add a touch of the neck nestle, and it's "night-night." (See related sections on wearing down, page 295, and the neck nestle, page 291.)

BEDTIME PROCRASTINATOR

Our two-year-old doesn't want to go to bed until nine or ten o'clock. We're tired after a day's work, and we're ready to go to sleep before he is. What time should a two-year-old go to bed?

Every family needs to arrive at a bedtime that gets baby enough sleep *and* enough quality time with the parents. Early bedtimes were more common years ago when rural families

NIGHTTIME BOTTLE SAFETY

Going off to sleep with a bottle of milk, formula, or juice can damage the teeth — a condition called bottle mouth (see page 500). To ease baby off the nighttime bottle, try *watering down:* Gradually dilute the bottle contents with increasing amounts of water until baby figures out it's not worth waking up and fussing for a bottle of water. Also, *don't bottle prop.* Though it is tempting to leave a bottle in the crib for a 3:00 A.M. self-serve, don't! Not only does this practice contribute to tooth decay, baby can choke on the contents, with no one there to help.

went to bed early and got up early. If you both work outside the home during the day, expect your baby to want a later bedtime. Picture this situation: Mom and/or dad return home from work around 6:00 P.M. expecting baby to be ready for bed by 8:00 P.M. That gives you two hours with baby, and it's anything but quality time. The time before bedtime is often a cranky period for baby, not the best time of the day for you to enjoy being with him.

Consider this alternative. Have the caregiver give baby a later afternoon nap so that he is well rested and fun to be with when you arrive home. Opt for a later bedtime. Make evening time prime family time.

Bedtime rituals are the salvation of tired parents. Babies, like adults, are creatures of habit. Before-bed rituals condition baby to recall a mental picture that when a certain activity begins (warm bath, wearing down, massage, story, and cuddle), sleep is soon to follow. The older the child and the busier the daytime parents, the longer the bedtime procrastination. Children have a way of extracting from parents the very thing they have the least of — time.

Dr. Bob's tip: After spending a month of wasting two hours each evening trying to nurse Andrew down to sleep at eight P.M. (he would keep squirming and waking up), we just let him stay up with us. The afternoon nap left him happy and playful, and he would roam around the house as we all enjoyed our evening together. Then we would all go to bed together at eleven P.M., and Cheryl and baby would sleep until nine or ten A.M. No time was wasted, and we got some time together as a couple (when Andrew was happy on his own) and as a family. This works only if baby is happy during the evening and mom does not have to get up early.

WON'T GO TO BED

Our baby won't go to bed before midnight. What do we do?

Take charge! You are the parents, and that gives you the privilege of deciding what bedtime needs to be for your family. Try these suggestions:

• Push the afternoon nap back to an earlier time so that baby is truly tired. If baby naps too much or too late in the day, he may not be tired enough to be a student in your slumber school.

- Stick to a bedtime ritual — winding down and wearing down, brushing teeth, a lullaby, and lights out — so that baby expects sleep to follow this routine.

- Try the cuddly approach: Lie down next to baby with a lullaby tape, give him a massage, lay on a comforting hand. Try whatever you can think of to get baby to relax and enjoy this new way of being together. Remember, he is used to being up in his bright and stimulating world or playing with someone. Now you are asking him to give in to sleep.

- Try the adult-in-charge approach. If despite all your soothing strategies baby still protests succumbing to sleep, calmly but firmly lay hands on baby, saying, "It's OK . . . go to sleep . . . go night-night." You communicate that this is sleep time and your only agenda for the moment is to usher the two of you into dreamland.

- "Play dead." If, even after you minister to him, baby still fusses and fumes, use your final ploy — pretending to sleep. Lie next to baby and play dead (see "Waking Up to Play," page 354). Baby will eventually wind down and join you in slumber. It may take a week or two, but eventually baby will get the message that this is the routine in your home.

- Bore him to bed. If your toddler has been away from you during the day or is going through a stage of separation anxiety, he may not want to separate from you at night and turn off at a preassigned bedtime. If you sense that your child is not tired or will definitely not go to bed on his own and you yourself are not ready to go to bed, simply do the preparing-for-bed ritual and then go about your adult agenda. Eventually you will notice baby crumpled sound asleep in the middle of the living room floor. Let baby crash wherever he wishes. Pick him up and place him in bed. Sometimes during the second and third year, children go through periods of separation anxiety where they do not want to drift off to sleep without you. Snuggle down together in front of a soothing video. I have spent many nights with our babies watching *Lady and the Tramp*. Actually, I got to enjoy this special time.

DELAYING THE EARLY RISER

Our two-year-old wakes up at sunrise and comes into our room. Then he wakes us up to play. How can we get him to sleep in?

Through the open shade comes the first ray of morning sunlight and wakens your little rooster. Here's how to catch an hour or so more sleep. Put blackout drapes in your baby's sleeping room. Lay down rules for noiseless waking with the older siblings. Leave a box of fun toys, and even an occasional surprise toy, at baby's bedside to entice him to stay in his room and play quietly by himself. A nibbly snack on a bedside table may tide the hungry baby over until breakfast. If baby persists in coming into your room (in the morning or during the night), lay down some entry rules: Put a sleeping bag at the foot of your bed with the admonition "quiet as a mouse." Show your child how to quietly slip into the sleeping bag for some extended sleep.

These going-to-sleep-and-staying-asleep techniques are temporary strategies. Your child will eventually learn to leave your bed, go to sleep and stay asleep on her own, and adjust to a regular bedtime. As with the other aspects of attachment parenting, the need to be parented to sleep lasts such a short while, but your message of love and security lasts a lifetime.

16

Parenting the Fussy or Colicky Baby

Some babies enter the world with unique qualities that early on merit labels such as "fussy." These challenging babies will extract from their caregivers every ounce of patience and creativity and will leave all those who have had the privilege of caring for them a bit wiser and more sensitive. Let's now meet these special little persons.

FUSSY BABIES

Our first three babies were so easy that we wondered what all the fuss was about difficult babies. Enter Hayden, our fourth, who turned our relatively peaceful home upside down. Hayden came wired differently. What worked for our other babies, she didn't buy. For eating and sleeping, the term "schedule" was not in Hayden's vocabulary. She was a constantly in-arms and at-breast baby. She wailed when we put her down, settled when we carried her — usually. Playing pass-the-baby became a Sears family game. Hayden spent hours being passed from arms to arms. When Martha's arms gave out, I held her.

Wearing her in a baby carrier usually worked, but not always.

If we tried to leave her for a much-needed baby break, she was inconsolable. The family motto became "Everywhere that Bill and Martha went, Hayden was sure to go." Hayden was glued to us day and night, and she carried her daytime fussiness into the night. She vehemently rejected the crib; she could only sleep next to a warm body in our bed. The crib, which had comfortably housed our first three babies, soon found its way to a garage sale. The only consistent behavior from Hayden was her inconsistency: What worked one day didn't work the next. We were always trying new ways of comforting her. "Demanding" became her label, and she wore it well.

Our feelings toward Hayden were as erratic as her behavior. Some days we were sympathetic; some days we were exhausted; other days we were just confused and angry.

If she had been our first baby, we would have felt it was our fault and wondered what we were doing wrong. But by this time we were experienced parents, so we knew it wasn't us! Then we were bombarded with conflicting advice: "You carry her too much." "You're spoiling her; just let her cry." "She's

WHAT'S IN A NAME?

In this chapter you will meet three types of babies who merit three different titles: fussy babies, high-need babies, and colicky babies. While all three share many similar features and respond to similar comforting techniques, they are different.

Fussy babies is the general tag that is given to babies who fuss to be picked up but are easily comforted and satisfied as long as they are held. These babies cry and protest for a variety of reasons during the first few weeks but then mellow out as they get used to life outside the womb.

High-need babies is a kinder and more descriptive term than "fussy babies." These babies crave physical contact. They like to be held constantly and will protest loudly when put down. They are supersensitive, intense, have difficulty self-soothing, and can be very demanding and draining on parents. High-need babies are, however, generally happy when their needs (as *they* perceive them) are met. These "Velcro babies," as we dub them, are blessed with persistent personalities that encourage parents to keep working at a caregiving style until they find the one that works.

Colicky babies don't just fuss, they hurt! A colicky baby will scream inconsolably for hours, or will generally be unhappy and appear to be hurting in the evening or all day every day, no matter how much soothing, bouncing, and holding you do. Oftentimes, as you will soon learn, they hurt because of a medical cause. In the Sears Family Pediatric Practice we seldom use the term "colicky baby"; we prefer a more accurate term, the "hurting baby." This term motivates both parents and doctor to keep searching for a reason baby hurts and to come up with a comforting solution.

It's not as important to tag your baby with the right term as it is to understand why your baby fusses and to learn what you can do about it.

manipulating you." We fielded these attacks on our parenting styles by carrying on with what worked and what felt right. Lesson number one in parenting this type of baby: *Babies fuss primarily because of their own temperament, not because of your parenting abilities.*

Within weeks after her birth we knew we had a special baby with special needs who needed a special kind of parenting — and we were determined to give it to her. But how?

We believed that Hayden would thrive if we developed a more sensitive and creative parenting style. But it was tough. We could have nicknamed Hayden "More." She needed more of everything, especially holding and nursing, except sleep. We soon learned that Hayden was not the standard baby, and standard baby advice wouldn't work for her. Once we viewed her not as a behavioral problem to be fixed but as a personality to be nurtured, living with her became much easier.

A High-Need Baby

One of our earliest confusions was how to describe Hayden. We didn't like the usual terms "difficult" and "fussy." These were negative and demeaning. Besides, they implied one or both members of the parent-infant pair were failing: Something was wrong with the baby or something was wrong with the parents, and we didn't accept that. We kept justifying Hayden's behavior and our parenting styles by saying, "She has a high level of needs," and we had heard many other parents with similar babies say the same. One day the light went on. "Let's call her a *high-need baby.*" We lived with this term for a while and tried it on many other babies and parents. It fit, and we stayed with it. This term was the turning point of our acceptance and appreciation of Hayden.

Redefining Hayden in more positive terms helped us focus on her exciting qualities rather than her inconvenient ones. Our job was to accept rather than squelch Hayden's unique personality, appreciate her special traits, and channel those traits into behaviors that would work for her, and for our family. We learned to open ourselves up to be flexible enough to keep working at a style of parenting that helped all family members thrive. The parents who are most frustrated by high-need babies have difficulty unloading the baggage of a *control mind-set.*

"High-need baby" says it all. It's a term that accurately describes why these babies are so demanding and the level of parenting they need. It's a positive, uplifting term, sounding intelligent and special. It relieves the guilt from parents and gives these special babies the recognition they deserve. Parents of fussy babies, don't you feel better already?

"But she'll outgrow it," friends kept reassuring. Yes and no. Once we understood and accepted the baby we had and adjusted our parenting styles accordingly, life with Hayden became easier. But her needs didn't diminish with age; they only changed. She graduated from a high-need baby to a high-need toddler to a high-need child and a high-need teen. She was slow to wean from her three favorite places of security: bed, breast, and arms. But she did wean. How did we discipline her? Sensitively.

Twenty-four years later Hayden is a wonderfully creative, deeply sensitive, and delightfully exuberant person who is caring and giving to others and to us. What Hayden taught us:

- Babies fuss primarily because of their own temperament (meaning their basic tendency to behave a certain way), not because of their parents' parenting abilities.

- Every baby comes wired with a level of needs, and requires a certain level of parenting for all members of the parent-infant relationship to bring out the best in one another.

- To accept and appreciate that high-need babies have unique temperaments and require a unique style of parenting. She taught us to be more *sensitive,* a quality that has carried over into our professional, social, and marital relationships.

What we taught Hayden:

- Her caregivers are responsive to her needs.

- She has value (it's OK to have needs).

• Her caregiving world is a warm and trusting place to be.

We have gathered from our own experience and from hundreds of high-need babies (and their surviving parents) many insights on why babies fuss and what to do about it. Here are the strategies that work for most babies and parents most of the time.

Features of High-Need Babies

To help you recognize if you are blessed with a special type of baby, here are the most common characteristics mothers note in describing their high-need babies.

"Supersensitive." High-need babies are acutely aware of their environment. They are easily bothered by changes in their secure and predictable environment and do not readily accept alternatives. They startle easily during the day and settle poorly at night. This sensitivity enables them to form deep attachments to trusted and consistent caregivers, but don't expect them to readily accept strangers or baby-sitters. They have selective tastes and definite mind-sets. This sensitive personality trait, which may seem exhausting early on, is likely to profit the baby when older. These babies are more capable of forming deeper and more intimate relationships.

"I just can't put him down." Lying peacefully in a crib and needing to be picked up only for feeding and changing — this is not the profile of a high-need baby (or of most babies). Motion, not stillness, is a way of life for these babies. These are in-arms, at-breast babies who seldom accept much down time in a crib.

"Not a self-soother." This baby is not known for his ability to self-soothe. Parents confide, "He can't relax by himself." Mother's lap is his chair, father's arms and chest his crib, mother's breasts his pacifier. These babies are very choosy about inanimate mother substitutes, such as cuddlies and pacifiers, and often forcefully reject them. This expectation of a higher standard of soothing is a personality trait that enables a high-need baby to become a people person rather than a thing person — a forerunner to developing the quality of intimacy.

"Intense." "He's in high gear all the time," observed a tired father. High-need babies put

---

THE HIGH-NEED BABY — A BLESSING OR A TRIAL?

One day we were comparing our babies' temperaments when we realized that high-need babies have a good thing going for them. Consider which baby gets the higher standard of care and the most out of life. The high-need babies get held more because they demand it. The high-need babies get taken more places because they are difficult to leave with anyone else. And who gets more touch, more hands-on comforting, more time at breast, and cozier sleeping quarters? These babies fly first-class. Which parents know their babies best? Which parents have, for survival, developed more creative parenting styles? You guessed it. Parents of high-need babies get the prize. As a matter of fact, we believe that all infants have some traits of the high-need baby.

a lot of energy into what they do. They cry loudly, laugh delightedly, and are quick to protest if their "meals" are not served on time. Because they feel things more deeply and interact more forcefully, these babies are capable of forming deep and lasting attachments and are disturbed if these attachments are broken. These babies are likely to become enthusiastic individuals. Of the many labels these babies receive, we have never heard them called boring.

"Wants to nurse all the time." Expect a feeding schedule to be foreign to this baby's mind-set. She will try to marathon breastfeed every two to three hours around the clock and enjoy long periods of comfort sucking. Not only do these babies feed more often, they suck longer. High-need babies are notoriously slow to wean and usually breastfeed into the second or third year.

"Awakens frequently." "Why do high-need babies need more of everything but sleep?" asked a tired mother, groaning. They awaken frequently during the night and seldom reward parents with a much-needed long nap during the day. You may feel that your baby has an internal light bulb that cannot easily turn off. Perhaps this is why these babies are often labeled "bright" as older children.

"Unsatisfied, unpredictable." Just as you figure out what your baby needs, expect a change of plans. As one exhausted mother put it, "Just when I think I have the game won, baby ups the ante." One set of comforting measures works one day but fails the next.

"Hyperactive, hypertonic." These babies squirm a lot while being held, until you find their favorite holding position. Nursing nuisances are frequent as these babies arch their backs and attempt to do back dives while feeding. "There's no such thing as a still shot," remarked a photographer-father of his high-need baby. While holding some high-need babies, you can feel their muscles tense.

"Draining." Besides putting their own energy into what they do, these babies use up parents' energy, too. "He wears me out" is a frequent complaint.

"Uncuddly." These are the most difficult high-need babies, because they don't always accept the old standby of constant holding. Whereas most babies melt into the arms and mold into comfortable positions while being held, the uncuddly baby arches his back, stiffens his arms and legs, and withdraws from intimate holding. Most tiny babies crave physical contact and settle when held tightly; uncuddly babies are slower to soften into a comfortable nestle in parents' arms. Eventually most do if the mother persists in her efforts to bond, offering baby a safe, firm holding place that baby can give in to.

"Demanding." Babies with high needs have high standards and have a strong personality to get what they need. Watch two babies raise their arms as a "Pick me up" gesture to their parents. If parents miss the cue, the mellower baby may put his arms down and begin to satisfy himself in play. Not so the high-need baby, who at the unacceptable thought that the parent missed his cue will howl and continue his demands until he is picked up.

Be prepared for this demanding personality trait to set you up as a target for destructive advice such as, "She's manipulating you." Consider for a moment what would happen if the high-need child were not demanding. If baby had a strong need but did not have a strong temperament to persist until the need was met, perhaps baby would not thrive to her full potential. The demanding trait of a high-need baby may be a forerunner of the later label "the strong-willed child."

Exhausted parents often ask, "How long will these traits last, and what can we expect as he grows?" Don't be too quick to predict the person your child will become. Some difficult babies show a complete turnabout in personality later in childhood. But in general, the needs of these babies do not lessen; they only change. While these early personality traits may sound somewhat negative and initially cause parents to feel a bit discouraged, as life with a new baby progresses most parents who adopt our approach to the high-need baby change their tune to include more positive labels, such as "challenging," "interesting," "bright." Those same qualities that at first seem to be such an exhausting liability often turn out to be an asset for the child and the parents *if* the cues of the high-need baby have been accurately read and appropriately responded to. The intense baby may become the creative child; the sensitive infant, the compassionate child. The little taker may later become the big giver.

WHY BABIES FUSS

Now that you have met this special person, how do you handle the high-need baby? To learn how to parent these special babies, you first need to understand why babies fuss. Very simply, babies fuss for the same reasons adults fuss: They hurt, either physically or emotionally, or they need something.

Babies Fuss to Fit

While in the womb, the preborn baby fits perfectly into his environment. Perhaps there will never be another home in which he fits so harmoniously — a free-floating environment where the temperature is constant and his nutritional needs are automatically and predictably met. In essence, the womb environment is well organized.

Birth suddenly disrupts this organization. During the month following birth, baby tries to regain his sense of organization and fit into life outside the womb. Birth and adaptation to postnatal life bring out the temperament of the baby, so for the first time he must do something to have his needs met. He is forced to act, to "behave." If hungry, cold, or startled, he cries. He must make an effort to get the things he needs from his caregiving environment. If his needs are simple and he can get what he wants easily, he's labeled an "easy baby"; if he does not adapt readily, he is labeled "difficult." He doesn't fit. Fussy babies are poor fitters, who don't resign themselves easily to the level of care they are being given. They need more, and they fuss to get it.

Missing the Womb

Another reason babies fuss is that they miss the womb environment they once had. Baby expects life will continue as before, but things are not right and he does not feel right. Baby wants to adapt to his new environment and has an intense desire to be comfortable. The conflict between wanting comfort and not being able to achieve it causes inner stress and outward behavior that is termed "fussy." Baby's fussings are pleas to his caregivers to help him learn what makes him feel right, a sort of "Give me my womb back" plea until he is old enough to develop his own self-comforting measures.

Suppose a baby doesn't miss the womb attachments because he still has them. Immediately after birth baby is placed on the warmth of mother's abdomen, nourished physically and emotionally by her breasts, worn nestled in a sling by day, and snuggled next to parents at night. Baby has no need to fuss. His womb attachments are still there, birth having changed only the way these attachments are expressed.

What about the baby who enters a different caregiving world? Instead of a warm and familiar body he gets the plastic-box treatment in a nursery. Instead of a warm breast he gets a silicone nipple. Instead of constant holding and frequent feedings he stays in the box and is held and fed on a convenient schedule. Even his sleep is disturbed. Instead of the warm body he had been used to for nine months he's in that plastic box. He has two choices. He can settle for a lower-level "womb" and become a "good baby," or he can protest that his new home is not to his liking. The more he fusses the more he gets picked up and held. The more he fusses the more he gets fed. He learns to demand to be fed "on demand." Even in the first day or two of life he merits the label "the fusser." At night he fusses until, out of desperation, he is taken into his parents' bed. Finally after weeks of fussing to fit, baby learns that fussing is a way of life. That's the only language that gets him the level of care he could have been automatically given before demanding it. This baby, a victim of what we call the poor-start syndrome, has learned to fuss.

The Need-Level Concept

All babies need holding, feeding, stroking, and other responsive attachment behaviors, but some need more than others, and some babies communicate their needs more. It was while trying to figure out why some of our babies behaved differently although they received the same level of care that we came up with the need-level concept. We believe that every baby has a certain level of need, which, if met, enables baby to reach his full potential, emotionally, physically, and developmentally. It also stands to reason that every baby would come with a corresponding temperament to be able to communicate this level of need.

Suppose a baby has medium needs that must be met in order for him to feel he fits. He fusses only a little and gets held and soothed just the right amount to keep the fussiness in check. This baby may be labeled an "easy baby." Suppose he needs a lot of holding. He continues to fuss when he's put down so he gets held more, sort of like a baby who demands an upgrade from coach to first class. This baby receives the label "demanding." But once in first class (lots of holding, frequent feedings, and day and night attachments) he fusses less and less. He's now where he fits, and there is no longer a need to fuss. Both babies are normal, both fit, and one is not better than the other. They just have different levels of need and a corresponding temperament to get their needs met.

A Sense of Oneness

The demanding baby who "cries whenever I put her down" needs to continue her sense of oneness with the mother. Before birth this baby had a oneness with the mother. After birth mother knows the baby is now a separate person, but baby does not feel separate. Baby still needs to feel connected to mother, birth having changed only the manner in which this connection is expressed. This baby will protest or fuss if her attachment to mother is disrupted. She needs to continue the attachment a bit longer, and fortunately she has the ability to demand this. If this baby's needs are heard and filled, she fits; she is in harmony with her environment. She feels right. When a baby feels right, her temperament becomes more organized, and she becomes a "more settled" baby.

Glued or Unglued

Mothers often refer to this sense of oneness as "My baby seems glued to me." They also use the term "unglued" to describe the way their babies crumble when they lose this sense of oneness with their environment. Nancy, a mother who had worked long and hard to develop a strong attachment bond with her high-need baby, told us, "When my baby becomes unglued and seems to be falling apart, I now feel I can pick up the pieces and glue him back together. It has been a long, tough struggle, but I am finally beginning to cash in on my investment."

MATCHING BABIES AND PARENTS

While it is true that babies begin to fuss primarily because of their own temperament, not because of the parents' skills, parents are not completely off the hook. How quickly parents pick up on their baby's need level and how sensitively they respond can influence the intensity of baby's fussing and whether or not their baby's demanding temperament is channeled into desirable or undesirable personality traits. Babies need a central attachment figure to organize their behavior; this person is usually mother. Without this organizing influence, baby remains disorganized, and fussy behavior results. This means changing our mind-set from regarding newborns as separated persons to viewing the mother-baby relationship as one. For some high-need babies outbursts of fussy behavior, commonly called colic, are withdrawal symptoms resulting from the loss of the regulatory influence of mother as an organizer.

Bringing Out the Best in Your High-Need Baby — And Yourself

Child-care specialists have long debated the nature versus nurture question: whether it's primarily a baby's genes or his home that determines how an infant behaves. It's really both. Baby's temperament isn't a blank slate onto which caregivers can write a set of rules that will cause the baby to act any way they wish. Neither is a baby's temperament permanently cast in cement. While all babies come equipped with a certain temperament, the caregiving environment can influence a child's personality (how a baby feels and reacts in certain situations). One of the most exciting new areas of research is the awareness of how the quality and quantity of mothering and fathering can affect a child's personality.

An even newer and more exciting area of research is the way the temperament of a

HANDLING CRITICISM OF YOUR PARENTING

Early in your parenting career, expect to be on the receiving end of well-meaning advisers giving you the subtle (and sometimes not-so-subtle) message that their way is better than yours. This is especially likely to be the case if you are blessed with a high-need baby. You may feel that criticizing your way of parenting is like attacking your personhood. Here are some ways to cope with criticism:

Lessen your exposure. Nothing divides friends like a difference of opinion regarding parenting styles. Surrounding yourself with like-minded parents is the best way to avoid criticism.

Be confident. Confidence is contagious. When a would-be adviser is about to pounce, exude conviction. ("It's working for us.")

Consider the source. The attachment style of parenting may threaten the person who believes otherwise. You may push guilt buttons. They wish they had the courage to follow their own instincts as you have.

Respect your parents. Most criticism is likely to come from your parents or in-laws. Remember, they grew up in the "spoiling" era, when some parents placed more trust in experts than in themselves. Acknowledge that times and experts change. Admit that in another time and place you might have used a different approach yourself. Tell them you think you turned out pretty well! Assure them that your "new and radical ways" are really old ways tried and true. Grandmother had her shot; now it's your turn. To make

grandparents your allies, focus on issues where you do have something in common. Try to understand your parents' feelings. Every time you do something with your child that is different from the way they did with you, they may take it as implying that you are raising your baby better than they raised you.

Defend your child. Most people don't understand a high-need child. To them a baby who needs to be held a lot is simply spoiled. You may have to do a bit of educating. But avoid giving the impression you think your way is the only way and their way is wrong. Convey to your criticizer that you respect her way of child raising if it is working for her, and ask her to respect your way as long as it is working for you.

Don't set yourself up. Getting involved in a discussion about the "big three" (discipline, extended breastfeeding, and sleeping with your baby) is like waving a red flag in front of people with a different mind-set. Stress that parenting styles are a matter of personal choice and take care not to preach judgments that one style may in all circumstances be better than another. If you have developed a healthy balance in all the aspects of attachment parenting, the ease with which you go about your parenting and the behavior of your children will be your best witnesses.

Use "the doctor" as a scapegoat. Sometimes it is wise to take the heat off

(continued)

yourself and make the point that you have researched your approach to parenting and modern research validates what you are doing. You may want to add, "My doctor advised me that for our family situation and the temperament of our baby this parenting style will work best for us." In some cases you may have to let the information in this book be your "doctor." But don't overwhelm people with quotes from the literature, for then you may be criticized for doing things too much by the book.

baby affects the parents. A mother of a high-need baby once confided to us, "Our fussy baby absolutely brings out the best and the worst in me." This is certainly true. Just as babies come wired with different temperaments, mothers and fathers also start out with varying levels of nurturing abilities (depending on how they themselves were nurtured). For some mothers, nurturing is automatic and is proportional to the need levels of their babies. Other mothers are slower to match their responsiveness to the need level of their babies and require a boost. Baby provides that boost. Both mother and baby are endowed with mutual temperaments that, if they get the right start, bring out the best in each other.

Baby's Temperament — Parents' Responsiveness

As we've said, every baby is born with a certain level of need. To help them convey the level of care they need, babies possess attachment-promoting behaviors (APBs), those "irresistible" qualities and behaviors that draw the caregiver toward the baby and promote responsiveness: smiling, cooing, clinging, eye gazing. The strongest of these APBs is the baby's cry.

Every parent, especially the mother, begins his and her parenting career with a certain level of nurturing abilities. The key to parenting the high-need baby is to match the nurturing abilities of the parents with the need level of the baby. The infant becomes an active participant in shaping the parents' behavior so they can fit into a style of parenting that brings out the best in their baby and themselves. Here's how this matching system works.

The Matchup: Easy Baby Plus Responsive Mother

The Outcome: This combination is usually a good match. Mother is likely to be delighted with her baby's behavior because mothers tend to feel that the "goodness" of their babies reflect their goodness as a mother (which is not always true). Because easy babies are less demanding, they do not have the forceful attachment-promoting skills to initiate a high level of interactions with their caregivers. For example, since they don't fuss when put down they may be held less. But the intuitive and responsive mother realizes that her baby may need more than he demands and makes up for this by *initiating interactions with her baby.* Mother takes the initiative and in so doing helps baby develop more readable cues, and the mother-baby pair's communication operates at a higher level.

The Matchup: Easy Baby Plus Restrained Mother

The Outcome: This may not be a good match, and a strong bond may not develop. Because the mellow baby is not very demanding, mother may interpret her baby's behavior as "He doesn't seem to need me much." As a result, this mother may seek more challenging interactions outside of her life with baby. She may devote relatively little energy to developing creative interactive skills. In this match, not only does mother fail to bring out the best in the baby, but the baby does not bring out the best in the mother. Sometimes this match leads to the *delayed fusser,* a baby who starts out easy and then around four to six months (or whenever mother's energies are diverted) shows a turnabout in personality. He becomes a fussy baby and releases a burst of attachment-promoting skills to demand a higher level of interaction with his caregivers. It's important for parents to be open to their baby and pick up on a sudden shift of behavior as a signal to shift their parenting style.

The Matchup: High-Need Baby with Good Attachment-Promoting Skills Plus Responsive Mother

The Outcome: This is usually a good match, and a strong bond develops. Mother and baby are likely to bring out the best in each other. Baby gives a cue, and mother, because she's open to her baby's cues, responds. Baby enjoys the response and is then motivated to give more cues because he has learned that he will get a predictable and rewarding response. The result is that mother and baby grow accustomed to each other. Even when she is confused and may not be able to read her baby's cues easily and identify the needs, mother experiments with different responses until she finds one that works. Baby learns to communicate better, mother learns to nurture better, and the relationship operates at a high level, as baby and mother become mutually sensitive to each other. Because mother is able to listen better, baby learns to cry better and develops nonfussing ways of communicating her needs.

The Matchup: High-Need Baby with Poor Attachment-Promoting Skills Plus Responsive Mother

The Outcome: This can also be a good match, but it is more difficult to achieve than the preceding one. Labeled "uncuddlers" or "slow-to-warm-up infants," these babies may appear to be easy babies, but in reality they are high-need babies in disguise. Instead of demanding close contact, fussing to get picked up, and melting gratifyingly in your arms, these babies withdraw from snuggling. They need to be held and nurtured but do not have the attachment-promoting skills to communicate this. Because baby doesn't gush forth appreciation of her efforts, mother may not feel gratified with her mothering and may seek alternative sources of fulfillment away from baby. The pair drifts apart. But a mother may approach her non-cuddler in a better way. With the help of *interaction counseling* mother learns to read baby's more subtle cues. She experiments with various baby-soothing interactions until she finds baby's preference. Mother woos her baby into cuddling. She initiates interaction, arriving at the right balance, knowing when to come on strong and when to back off. Eventually baby likes being held, and parents like holding baby. Consequently, baby develops better attachment-promoting skills, and parents develop more baby-reading skills. The pair fits.

The Matchup: High-Need Baby Plus Restrained Caregiver

The Outcome: This situation is at the highest risk for not becoming a good match. This is a lose-lose situation. Neither baby nor mother brings out the best in the other. This baby has good attachment-promoting skills and starts life by demanding the level of care he needs. The mother, however, instead of being open to baby and following her intuition (even shaky intuition gets more steady if practiced), buys into a more restrained style of parenting. She makes a science out of parenting and succumbs to detachment advice: "He's manipulating you." "Let him cry it out. You're making him too dependent." "You're spoiling him." Mothers of high-need babies, beware of advice that suggests you restrain yourself from responding to your baby. If you are getting lots of this kind of advice, you're running around with the wrong crowd of advisers. The restraint advice will tear down a mother-baby relationship because it confuses new mothers who are particularly vulnerable to any advice that promises to work. Beware especially of quick and easy solutions that suggest adhering to rigidly scheduled feedings and periods of crying. This seldom works for any baby, but it can be especially disastrous for the high-need baby. A mother is using so much energy trying someone else's method that she has little left for experimenting with *her own* comforting skills for *her own* baby.

What happens to baby? A high-need baby whose signals are not falling on receptive ears and arms may respond in two ways. Baby may fuss more and fuss louder until finally someone holds and attaches to him. Eventually baby will break through the restraint-parenting barrier, convincing parents to try a more nurturing approach, but not without a cost. Baby may expend so much energy fussing that little is left for overall development. He may not thrive. Or baby may give up, shut down his signals ("See, it worked, he finally shut up," some misguided adviser may conclude), and withdraw into himself, attempting to survive emotionally on a variety of self-soothing habits.

SOOTHING THE FUSSY BABY

Exhausted parents will try everything. And that's the key — *try everything.* Most soothing actions can be grouped into four categories:

- motions that mellow
- sounds that soothe
- sights that delight
- touches that relax

Calming fussiness is not only what you do to or for baby, it requires some parent training, too. All the calming techniques we discuss are aimed at four goals:

- mellowing the temperament of the baby
- easing the discomfort of the baby
- improving the sensitivity of the parents
- making living with a fussy baby easier for parents

Attachment Parenting Calms Babies

This high-touch style of cue parenting (reading and responding to baby's cues) lessens a baby's need to cry. Attachment parenting is an intuition-building style of parenting that also boosts parents' sensitivity, helping them to cope better with a fussy baby and to persevere, detectivelike, to find the cause and the treatment. Practice either the whole package or as many of the following attachment concepts as you can. The three parenting activities that have been shown to calm fussy babies best are feeding frequently, responding quickly to baby's cries, and carrying baby a lot.

Feeding baby frequently. Studies have shown that babies who are fed frequently cry less. In fact, cultures that have the fewest fussy babies feed their babies every fifteen minutes. This may sound like the "Velcro mother and baby," especially to Western parents of the three-to-four-hour-feeding-schedule mind-set, but it works.

Responding promptly to baby's cries. Studies have also shown that babies whose cries are promptly responded to cry less.

Wearing your baby. Stacy, an experienced baby settler, related her success: "I put him on in the morning and take him off at night. As long as I carry him in the sling, he's calm." While few mothers and fathers can carry their babies constantly, wearing your baby in a baby sling tops the list of womb-duplicating baby soothers. (See Chapter 14, "Babywearing," for a thorough discussion of how this age-old custom helps keep babies from fussing and calms them when they do.)

In essence a mother who is a frequent feeder, quick responder, and babywearer is more likely to have a contented baby.

A GOOD CRY

Ever have an occasion when your baby or child is crying and nothing works to stop her? Take heart! It's not your fault she is crying; nor is it your urgent responsibility to stop the cry. In fact, research has shown that crying is a healthy part of the recovery process — a physiologic aid to releasing stored stress. Tears produced to wash away irritants in the eye and those secreted as an emotional outlet have different chemical compositions. Emotional tears contain breakdown products not found in irritant tears, namely stress hormones, which increase during painful experiences.

These fascinating findings indicate there may be a physiologic basis for the expression "to have a good cry." Grief and hurt may be released through tears. Why be so quick to get babies and children to hold back their tears? Frantic hushing and admonitions like "Stop crying," or "Big boys don't cry," train children to stifle pent-up emotions that, by a good cry, could be carried down the river of tears. Lucky is the child who feels the freedom to cry without rebuke. Wise is the parent who gives a supportive presence. There is a big difference between allowing your baby to cry (without panic on your part!) and leaving her to cry alone and uncomforted. Give your child the message, "It's OK to cry; I'm here to help you."

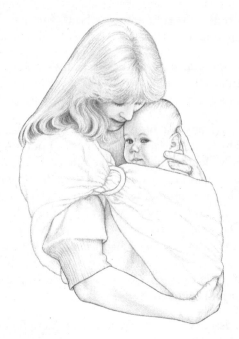

Babywearing can have a calming effect on fussy babies.

Slings, Swings, and Other Things

Dancing with your baby snuggled close to you provides the kind of rhythmic motion and comforting contact that infants like. Most parents soon learn to improvise their own dance routines to cope with a fussy baby. For some parent-tested techniques and ideas, see "The Colic Dance," and "Colic Carries," page 401. Here are some other effective baby soothers.

Swings. The table is set for your long-awaited dinner for two. But there's a fact of new-parent life that your childbirth instructor didn't tell you. Babies fuss most from 6:00 to 8:00 P.M. Surviving parents call this "happy hour." The quiet dinner for two may be an event of your childless past. Enter an auto-

matic mechanical swing. Baby swings while parents eat. Dinner music it's not, but, in addition to the motion, the monotonous ticktocking of the swing (or some swings come with a lullaby at a slight additional charge) helps to soothe baby. At the twist of your wrist, you wind baby up, or down, for the next course.

Sometimes all the fuss-fixing projects in the world will not convince baby to settle for anyplace but your arms. A dinner for two becomes a dinner for three. Mother holds and feeds baby cradled in her lap, while dad serves and even cuts up mother's meat. Sometimes even the best-laid dinner plans go astray during baby's fussy time. While not at all romantic, shift eating is sometimes the only path to fussy-hour survival. Mom eats while dad paces with baby and vice versa.

Play ticktock. Dan, a chiropractor father of a fussy baby, came up with this fuss fixer. Hold baby at his hips and swing him upside down at sixty beats per minute, like the pendulum of a grandfather clock. According to chiropractic research, upside-down swinging has a calming effect. Don't hold a baby under six months upside down by the feet or legs because of the possibility of dislocating baby's hips. Holding baby at the hips is safest. Perhaps one reason ticktocking works is that baby has been upside down for months inside mother — another good womb memory.

Magic mirror. For a baby over the age of two months, here is a scene that has pulled us through several fussy ordeals. Let baby reflect on her antics. Hold baby in front of a mirror to witness her own performance. If the image itself does not turn off the tizzy, as an added touch place her bare feet against the surface of the mirror. We have seen our frantic baby settle within seconds after seeing

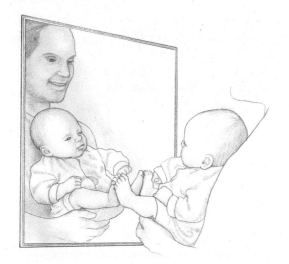

Magic mirror.

caregiver, and the moving attractions of cars, trees, and kids playing in a park will often help baby forget to fuss. A morning walk helps start the day on a fuss-free note. A late afternoon walk can detour the evening fusser.

Feeding on the move. Some babies settle easier and feed better on the move. Settle your infant in the baby sling and take a walk around the house or around the block while feeding. (See techniques of breastfeeding while babywearing, page 296.)

Sounds that soothe. See page 324 for a list of musical medleys and household sounds that soothe fussy babies.

Right Touches

Skin-to-skin contact ranks right after motion on the baby-calmer list. Here are a few of baby's favorite touches.

Infant massage. There are times when massage may be a fuss saver. If baby has predictable fussy times (usually late afternoon and early evening), get into a massage routine just *before* the usual fussy time. Untensing baby before "happy hour" may entice baby to forget to fuss. Abdominal massage can be a colic favorite. Use the "I Love U" (see page 403 for technique) to give the right touch before the expected evening blast.

Nestle nursing. Curl up, womblike, around your baby and snuggle, skin to skin, off to sleep.

The neck nestle. (See the explanation and illustration on pages 291 and 293.)

herself in the mirror, as if so distracted by what she sees that she forgets to fuss.

Moving attractions. Sometimes the mover wears out before the fusser, and you need a baby-calming break. Baby may settle for watching moving things rather than being on the move herself. Place baby upright in an infant seat and set her before a bubbling fish tank, the swinging pendulum of a clock, or similar attractions. One of our babies stopped fussing and settled in her infant seat while watching me exercise on a cross-country-ski machine. When you've exhausted all the in-house entertainment, try a car ride.

A walk for two. "Oh, how I look forward to our daily walk!" revealed a mother who learned how to survive and thrive with her high-need baby. Secure baby in a sling and take a long walk. Not only will the exercise relax you, but the motion, closeness to a

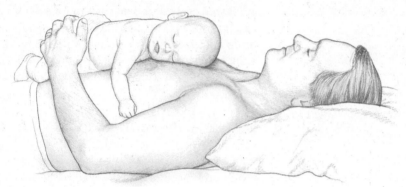

The warm fuzzy is a fuss-buster dads can employ.

The warm fuzzy. Mothers do not have the only "womb" in the house. This fuss preventer really makes dads shine. Lie on the bed, floor, or grass. Drape your bare-skinned but diapered baby flat, tummy to tummy, over your bare chest. Place baby's ear over your heart. Feel the tension release. The rhythm of your heartbeat plus the up-and-down motion of your breathing can make even the most upset baby forget to fuss. Note: This touch technique works best in the first three months. Older babies often squirm too much to lie still on daddy's chest.

Another warm fuzzy. Once baby reaches a squirming stage, or you wish to sneak away from your sleeping baby, try this variation of the tummy-to-chest touch. Nestle with baby side by side, with baby's head in your armpit and baby's ear against the left side of your chest (where baby can hear your heartbeat). Once baby is deeply asleep, lift your arm and creep away.

A warm bath for two. This one's for mom. First, comfortably immerse yourself in a half-full tub. Have dad or someone else hand your baby to you. Let baby nestle against your breast, or breastfeed (your breast being just a couple inches above the water line). The combination of warm water, a free-floating feeling, and mom should untense baby. An additional tub tip: Leave the drain partially open and a warm-water faucet running slightly. This provides the soothing sound of running water and keeps the water comfortably warm.

THE COLICKY BABY, ALIAS THE HURTING BABY

You're holding your two-week-old happy baby — the model of a thriving infant, apparently without a care in the world. Suddenly and unexpectedly he stiffens his limbs, arches his back, clenches his fists, and lets out ear-piercing shrieks. Like a person who hurts and is angry at the hurting, he draws up his flailing limbs against a bloated, tense abdomen and continues the unrelenting, agonizing screams. Even his face cries "ouch": wide-open mouth, almost a perfect circle, with furrowed brow and tightly closed or widely opened eyes, as if yelling, "I hurt and I'm mad." As baby's tension mounts, your frustration escalates, and you are driven to the edge by feeling as helpless as baby in determining the cause and alleviating the pain. He's inconsolable, and you are both in tears. You hurt together.

Stretched to the limits, he shuts down his agonizing screams and withdraws into a spent sleep, retreating from system overload and giving a momentary reprieve to his puzzled parents. A friend enters during the calm before the next storm and exclaims, "What a healthy-looking baby. You're so lucky!" You reply, "You should have seen us a few hours ago when we were both a wreck." Your friend leaves, naturally feeling that you are imagining things. Surely there couldn't be anything wrong with such a cherubic-looking baby. Then as though someone turned on a start-screaming switch, the violent outbursts resume, this time lasting more than an hour. Round two of baby's fight with himself begins. You try to cuddle, baby stiffens in protest; you try to nurse, baby arches and pulls away; you rock, sing, ride. The soothing techniques that worked yesterday aren't working today. And you replay the familiar worry, "What's wrong with my baby; what's wrong with me?" as you excuse yourself from the company of the perfect mothers with their perfect babies.

"How could such a good baby two hours ago be in such a snit now?" you wonder. He's like Dr. Jekyll and Mr. Hyde. By some strange quirk of justice your baby is worse toward the end of the day, when you are least able to cope. Your sweet morning baby turns sour in the evening.

Enter the cure-alls from the unending stream of well-meaning friends. Baby still screams, and you feel, more and more, it's a

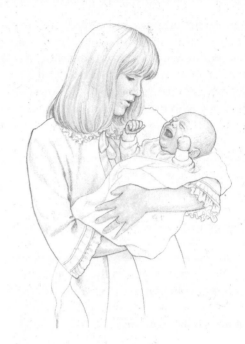

A colicky baby in full voice.

reflection of your mothering, yet somehow you know it's not. He hurts; he's mad; you don't know why, and probably neither does baby.

By the time you go through all of Aunt Nancy's herbal teas, the doctor-advised feeding changes, and every conceivable holding pattern, as mysteriously as the fight began, around three to four months of age it stops, and life goes on. Baby seems none the worse for wear, and you close one of the most difficult chapters in life with your new baby.

That's colic!

Is Your Baby Colicky? How to Tell

If you wonder whether or not you have a colicky baby — you don't! The violent, agonizing outbursts of prolonged incon-solable crying leave no doubt about colic. Sometimes when parents think they have a colicky baby, we'll send them to visit a few members of the "colic club" — parents in our practice who truly have colicky babies. They often return relieved, saying, "We don't have a colicky baby after all." Around 20 percent of all babies have some daily outbursts of crying during the early months.

What Is Colic?

"Colic" is a description, not a diagnosis. While no one agrees on the cause or the defi-nition of colic, physicians regard a baby as colicky if sudden and unexplained outbursts of inconsolable crying

- last at least *three* hours a day, occur *three* days per week, and continue for at least *three* weeks
- begin within the first *three* weeks of life
- seldom last longer than *three* months
- occur in an otherwise healthy, thriving baby

We sometimes refer to this as "the rule of threes."

Over the past thirty years, I have grown to realize that most colicky babies fit into one of two categories: the evening-only colicky baby and the all-day colicky baby.

Evening-only colic. Also known as the "P.M. fusser," this baby is generally happy during the day. Friends would never know that baby has colic unless they come over after dinner. She will smile, make eye contact, and coo and gurgle like any other baby during the day.

Then comes the evening blast! As if some internal alarm clock goes off, baby suddenly begins to fuss. Fussiness escalates into more intense screaming, and then into full-blown colic, as previously described. It lasts any-where from one to four hours. Often baby screams nonstop, with only a few brief inter-ludes of quiet. Baby finally falls asleep, exhausted, as do the parents. This may occur four to seven nights each week for the first few months. The good news about this type of colic is that baby generally sleeps well, and mom and dad get to enjoy the rewards of par-enting a happy baby during the day. Another bit of good news is that, unlike with all-day colic, there is rarely an underlying medical cause for evening-only colic. (See "Un-Happy Hour!," page 386.)

All-day colic. This baby is rarely happy. He spends most of the day fussing, squirming, or screaming. He may have several hours, usually in the evening, when the crying is more intense and continuous. Most babies with this type of colic will also be restless sleepers, with frequent night wakings. A few, luckily, may be so exhausted that they sleep well at night. In this situation, I ask parents, "Is your baby *ever* happy?" The answer is often no! This baby has very little happy, quiet time. He is always busy, either eating, sleeping, or fussing. There is little opportu-nity for parents to bond with baby, make intimate eye contact as baby gazes peace-fully at their faces, or enjoy the rewards of parenting. Besides being the most severe type of colic and the most difficult for par-ents to cope with, this intense type of colic merits the term "hurting baby," and it is the type for which parents and doctor are likely to detect an underlying cause.

Why Colic?

The most frustrating feature of colic is not knowing why baby screams and why what worked one day doesn't work the next. If you have a colicky baby, it's normal to go through the mental torture of "Why me, what am I doing wrong?" And because your baby hurts, you hurt. You are vulnerable to all the well-meaning friends offering their own personal diagnosis: "It must be your milk." "He's spoiled." "You're holding him too much" — or not enough. Let's turn a critical eye toward exposing the most popular myths about colic.

The Tense Mother–Tense Baby Myth

Fussy and colicky behaviors come more from the temperament of the baby than the nurturing abilities of the parents. Research has taken the pressure off mothers. There seems to be no proof that tense mothering causes tense babies. But mothers who are tense during pregnancy have a slightly increased chance of producing colicky babies. Also, some studies suggest that having a colicky baby is a self-fulfilling prophecy. Mothers who expect to have colicky babies often do. In our experience, the mood of the mother influences how she *handles* her colicky baby rather than being the *cause* of the colic. A tense baby doesn't settle well in tense arms.

If parents caused fussy babies, you would expect firstborns to win the Most Fussy Baby title. Not true. Fussy and colicky babies show no respect for birth order. Our fourth baby was the fussiest, and she was born following one of our most relaxed pregnancies and least hectic family situations. Nor is colic a social disease. We cannot blame baby's behavior on hurried life-styles. Anthropologists report that babies born into cultures that hold their babies almost constantly and give prompt nurturing responses to babies' cries are less fussy than those in other cultures, but all cultures are blessed with colicky babies. The Chinese refer to this behavior as "the hundred days' crying."

Deflating the Gas Myth

"But he's so full of gas!" a mother reports. Many babies are gassy during the early months. Put your hand on the bloated tummy of a recently fed, happy one-month-old, and you are likely to feel rumblings that pass just in time for the next feeding. However, X-ray studies cast doubt on gas as the culprit of colic. Abdominal X rays of most babies, whether colicky or not, frequently reveal a lot of gas. X rays taken of colicky babies reveal no gas during the bout but gas after the fit. Researchers believe that babies gulp air *during* the crying, and gas is the *result* rather than the *cause* of colic. Although gas may be conducive to discomfort in some babies, this research takes the wind out of the gas theory of colic.

What does this research mean to comforting parents? Aborting a crying fit or promptly intervening on the opening note of the scream may lessen the amount of air baby swallows. Colic cries promote air swallowing. Watch a baby during one of these angry spells. Notice how baby holds his breath during a prolonged crying jag, sometimes even turning blue around the mouth, causing parents to join baby's panic. Then after holding this note seemingly forever, baby takes a sudden, forceful catch-up breath (and so do you); some of that air gets gulped into the stomach. This excess air bloats the intestines, perhaps prolonging the colicky episode.

UN-HAPPY HOUR!

Plan ahead for the P.M. fusser. One of our babies fussed predictably around five o'clock most afternoons, an exhausting time we dubbed "happy hour." We figured that she was just releasing pent-up tension, but we feared that she was getting conditioned to regard the end of the day as a painful time. So we decided to plan ahead with a before-colic ritual to condition her to expect an hour of comfort rather than an hour of pain.

At least an hour before expected blast-off, either lie down with your baby and take a nap for two or enjoy an infant massage, preferably on the floor with baby warmed by a ray of sunlight coming through the window. Immediately after the nap or massage, nestle baby in a baby sling and take a walk. As you stroll past moving cars, moving people, and up and down hills, baby often gets so interested in her environment that she forgets to fuss. And if your baby is still going to fuss, she might as well fuss outside in an environment that's therapeutic for both of you.

TRACKING DOWN HIDDEN CAUSES OF COLIC

My perspective on colic changed one day when a mother consulted me about her inconsolably crying baby. After I diagnosed colic, she challenged me, "Do you call it colic when you don't know why a baby is hurt-

ing?" This mother was right. Professionals and parents tend to lump all outbursts of crying into "colic." When an adult hurts, we play detective and track down the cause of the hurt and fix it. What has been frustrating about colic is that we seldom know the cause, nor do we know how to fix it. At least until now! To determine what's bothering your baby, consider three general possible causes: medical, dietary, and emotional. Here is a three-step approach to tracking down hidden reasons for a baby to be hurting and suggestions for treatment.

Step One: Seek Help from Your Doctor

In our pediatric experience, the two most common hidden medical causes of colic are:

1. gastroesophageal reflux disease
2. food or formula sensitivities

If you find the cause, you're likely to find a cure. Suspect that your baby has an underlying medical cause for the pain if any of the following is true:

- Baby's crying pattern *suddenly* changes to more painful outbursts.

- Baby frequently *awakens* in pain.

- The crying occurs in frequent, long, inconsolable bouts and is not limited to evening time.

- Your parent's intuition tells you, "My baby hurts somewhere."

If you have determined that a visit to the doctor is in order, there are a number of

GETTING THE WIND OUT OF GASSY BABIES

Swallowing air and passing gas is a normal part of growing up. But excessive intestinal gas can make a young baby miserable. A mother of one of my gassy little patients describes these bloated episodes: "When my daughter is trying to pass gas, it is like a mother going through a difficult labor." Try these ways of getting the air out.

Letting Less Air In

- If breastfeeding, be sure baby's lips form a good seal far back on the areola.
- If bottlefeeding, be sure baby's lips are positioned on the wide base of the nipple, not just on the tip.
- Tilt the bottle at a thirty-to-forty-five-degree angle while feeding so that air rises to the bottom of the bottle; or try collapsible formula bags.
- Eliminate fuss foods from your diet if breastfeeding (see page 152).
- Feed baby smaller amounts more frequently.
- Keep baby upright (at about a forty-five-degree angle) during and a half-hour after feeding.

- Avoid prolonged sucking on pacifiers or empty bottle nipples.
- Respond promptly to a baby's cries.

Getting More Air Out

First and foremost, be sure to burp baby during and after feedings (see burping tips on page 213). You can also try the following techniques and remedies (see "Comforting Colic," on page 400, for more about these):

- abdominal massage
- baby bends
- simethicone drops
- glycerin suppositories

---

measures you can take to ensure that you get the most out of it.

Make a Fuss List

Before your appointment make a list addressing the following items:

- Is the baby in enough pain to be distressed and to distress you? Or is he just fussing?
- When did the episodes start, how long do they last, and how often do they occur?

- What triggers the colic episodes, and what turns them off? Do they occur at night?

- Describe the cry.

- Where do you feel the pain is coming from? What do your baby's face, abdomen, and extremities look like during the episode?

- Is the crying related to feeding? Give the details about feeding: breast or bottle, frequency, air swallowing. What changes of feeding techniques or formulas have you tried? What worked? Do you hear your baby gulping air?

- Does your baby pass a lot of gas?

- What are your baby's bowel movements like — easy, soft, or hard — and how frequent are they?

- Does your baby spit up? How often, how soon after feeding, and with how much force?

- Does your baby have a persistent diaper rash, and what does it took like? Is there a red, inflamed, ringlike rash around baby's anus? (This suggests a food sensitivity.)

- Elaborate on your home remedies. What has worked and what hasn't?

- Volunteer your diagnosis.

Keep a Colic Diary

Record in your fuss book, in vivid detail, as much information as you can about your baby's painful episodes, using the preceding list as a guide. You might be surprised at what correlations you uncover. One mother noticed, "On days I wear him most of the time, he forgets to fuss come evening."

Make a Distress Tape

To help your doctor appreciate how devastating these colicky episodes are, record one of your baby's crying jags. Because there is so much body language that accompanies the screaming, if you want to get your point across make a videotape of you and your baby during a colicky episode so that your counselor can truly witness a mother-infant pair in distress. I have found it very therapeutic for the parents to view their own tape periodically to appreciate their baby's distress and to see how they are coping.

Tell It Like It Is

Don't hold back how much your baby's crying bothers you. Both mother and father should attend the doctor's visit. Fathers keep mothers honest, preventing them from downplaying how much their baby's crying upsets them. Perhaps they fear that such a revelation will shatter their perfect-mother image in the eyes of their pediatrician. Fathers usually tell it like it is. During one case of colic counseling I didn't appreciate the magnitude of the problem until the father volunteered, "I had a vasectomy last week. We'll never go through this again!" I got the picture. (Dad was subsequently reconnected and fathered two more babies.)

Don't lose faith in your doctor if he or she cannot determine why your baby is hurting or cannot cure your baby's colic. When I see parents and their colicky baby, I hurt for them, I hurt for their baby, and I also feel like a failure when I cannot pinpoint the cause and prescribe instant treatment. Oftentimes the best your doctor can do is take a detailed history, administer a thorough physical exam, and, unless an underlying medical problem is uncovered, prescribe trial-and-error dietary elimination and detective work along with the tincture of time. (But we believe it is important to first approach colic as a medical problem in the general category of *the hurting baby;* otherwise treatable painful problems may be missed.)

Step Two: Investigate the Possibility of Gastroesophageal Reflux

In our pediatric experience, the most common medical cause of the "hurting baby" or colic is gastroesophageal reflux, also called GERD (gastroesophageal reflux disease), acid reflux, heartburn, acid indigestion, and just plain "reflux." In this painful medical condition, the acid-containing stomach contents regurgitate back into the esophagus. Normally, once swallowing is over and all the food has entered the stomach, a circular band of muscle called the lower esophageal sphincter (LES), where the esophagus joins the stomach, contracts like a door that closes to keep stomach contents and stomach acids from regurgitating, or refluxing, back into the esophagus. Reflux is basically an immaturity of the LES. If, instead of closing, the LES remains open, stomach acids reflux back into the esophagus and irritate, or "burn," the sensitive lining of the esophagus, causing pain. Not all babies with reflux spit up. Babies may spit up a little or a lot. If the stomach contents reflux just partway up the esophagus, baby may hurt but may not spit up or vomit. This is called silent reflux. Sometimes the refluxed gastric contents enter the back of the throat, causing a sore throat, choking, gagging, coughing, and erosion of dental enamel, and can even be aspirated into the lungs, causing respiratory infections, wheezing, and asthma-like symptoms.

Usually infants associate feeding with comfort, but the baby with reflux may associate feeding with pain, and so refuse to feed and show poor weight gain. Or, because breast milk and formula neutralize the stomach acids, the infant may want to "feed constantly" and may gain weight well or even overgain. Because gravity holds the stomach contents down and lessens reflux, babies are often more comfortable when upright but shriek in pain when put down or during sleep.

Not only does reflux hurt babies, it hurts parents, who may be led to believe that their baby cries a lot because she is just a "fussy baby" or that something is wrong with their parenting, which is not true. Undiagnosed and untreated reflux often results in the "hurting family."

In the early months, two-thirds of all babies have some degree of reflux, which accounts for the frequent spitting up that most babies do. Spitting up does not usually bother these babies, dubbed "happy spitters." It is not painful, does not slow weight gain, and is more of a laundry problem than a medical one. Reflux becomes a problem when it causes painful irritation or damage to the esophagus, interferes with growth and development, interferes with feeding and sleeping, or contributes to respiratory problems.

Reflux usually starts in the newborn period, peaks around four months, and begins to subside around seven months of age, when babies begin spending most of their days upright and start eating solid foods, and by the law of gravity, food stays down better. Most infants outgrow reflux by one year of age (I call this "walking away from reflux"). Yet in some children reflux continues throughout childhood and sometimes into adulthood, where it is manifested more by "heartburn" and "wheezing" episodes. Don't always assume the reflux is gone when the spitting up stops.

Clues That Baby Suffers from Reflux

A baby with reflux may have many or only a few of the following signs. Sometimes baby may regurgitate only partway up the esophagus and thereby not visibly spit up. The best clue is your gut feeling telling you that your baby "hurts somewhere."

- frequent blasts of inconsolable, painful crying — "unlike the usual baby cries"
- frequent episodes of spitting up, which may include forceful regurgitation through the nose

- frequent inconsolable bouts of abdominal pain, day and night
- painful bursts of night waking
- fussiness after eating; drawing up legs, knees to chest
- arching or writhing as if in pain
- diminishing fussiness when carried upright, sleeping prone (on the stomach), or propped up at least thirty degrees
- frequent unexplained colds, wheezing, and chest infections
- stop-breathing episodes
- frequent "wet" or "sour" burps, throaty or swallowing noises, gagging, or hiccupping
- excessive drooling

Detecting Reflux

Your doctor may suspect reflux based upon your observations. Parents need to be keen observers and accurate reporters. Go through the above list of clues and write down which of these your baby has and how often. Be clear about the severity of these symptoms. (To measure how much your baby spits up spill a tablespoon of milk on a plate as a gauge of the amount of spit-up.) Does baby suffer only an occasional spitting up or the odd restless night? Or is it a daily, even hourly, occurrence, enough to interfere with your infant's well-being — and yours? To describe how much your baby truly is hurting, show your doctor a videotape. Let your doctor know how much of a problem this is for your family. One patient said to me, "I am camping out in your office until you find out what's wrong with my baby."

Oftentimes a doctor will diagnose the problem as GERD and begin treatment based upon a parent's history alone and not do any tests. If the diagnosis is in doubt, however, a doctor may order one or more of the following tests:

Barium swallow X ray (fluoroscopy). In this test, also known as an "upper GI series," baby swallows some barium, which outlines the esophagus, stomach, and upper intestines. The main reason for this upper GI study is not to diagnose reflux, but rather to exclude other causes of vomiting, such as anatomical abnormalities of the stomach or intestines that could contribute to or cause a partial obstruction.

pH probe. A thin, flexible tube is placed through your baby's mouth or nose into the esophagus and down to just above the entrance to the stomach. The tip of the tube measures stomach acid that is regurgitated up into the esophagus. The pH probe is the most sensitive test for measuring the frequency and degree of acid reflux. The probe is left in for twelve to twenty-four hours. The insertion can be done either overnight in the hospital or in your own home. A technician skilled in probe placement comes to your home (or to the hospital or doctor's office), places the probe in baby's esophagus, and attaches it to a small recording machine. The recording is then monitored for twelve to twenty-four hours.

Dr. Bill suggests: A useful diagnostic tool I have found is to have parents record the severity, frequency, and timing of their baby's hurting episodes while the pH probe is in place. I then see if there is a correlation with the probe readings of acid reflux. If there is, this suggests acid reflux is indeed the cause of baby's hurting. Newer probes have buttons that parents push to signal crying, vomiting, and so on.

Scintography. Baby is fed a bottle of breast milk or formula that contains a radioactive substance. A computerized scan of baby's abdomen reveals if the stomach takes a long time to empty (called "delayed gastric emptying"), which contributes to reflux. This scanning technique is not considered reliable for showing the presence or degree of reflux; it merely shows if delayed gastric emptying is contributing to reflux. It can also show aspiration of reflux material into the lungs.

Endoscopy (esophagoscopy). This procedure is done on an outpatient basis while baby is under light general anesthesia. A pediatric gastroenterologist inserts a flexible tube with a fiber-optic camera at the tip into baby's esophagus, stomach, and upper intestine. The doctor then examines these areas for abnormalities and especially looks at the lining of the esophagus for inflammation, called esophagitis. The presence and degree of reflux esophagitis give a clue to the severity of the reflux and guide the doctor in deciding how aggressive the treatment regimen should be.

Dr. Bill notes: I recently saw a nine-month-old baby for fussy-baby counseling. His mother had been advised to let him cry it out. She was told she was anxious and overreacting, and that he was just manipulating her. Mother's instincts said, "I know something is wrong with him." After listening to her, I suspected severe GERD and referred the infant for an endoscopy. The endoscopy showed severe erosion and ulcerations of the lower end of the child's esophagus. The damage from the reflux was so severe that baby needed surgical correction. Mother knows best! Lose points for the let-him-cry-it-out crowd!

When Is Testing for Reflux Necessary?

A hurting baby who frequently spits up probably has reflux and may not need any tests to confirm this. The above tests are, however, useful in the following situations:

- *To diagnose "silent" reflux.* With this type of reflux, baby has many of the above signs but does not spit up.

- *In complications from reflux.* If baby is suffering from any complication of acid regurgitation, such as failure to thrive or respiratory problems, testing may be appropriate.

- *When reflux does not improve* with positional and feeding strategies (see below) or increasing doses of medication. Tests may reveal an anatomical problem in the gastrointestinal system that needs additional treatment.

Consider Surgery for GERD

Surgical correction of GERD is now being performed more frequently for two reasons: the debilitating nature of GERD has become more widely appreciated, so that doctors are now becoming more knowledgeable and aggressive about its treatment; and surgical procedures have become safer and more refined, and now can often be done through laparoscopy, sparing the child from a large abdominal incision and prolonged postoperative recovery. The general term for GERD surgery is *fundoplication,* in which a band of upper stomach muscle is wrapped totally or partially around the lower esophagus, in effect tightening the valve and lessening reflux. In the Nissen procedure a total 360-degree wrap is performed, whereas in the Thal procedure a partial wrap is performed. Because with the total wrap a child can lose the protective ability to vomit or burp, the partial wrap is often the preferred choice. Surgery is considered particularly beneficial for infants with GERD who are neurologically impaired.

The main criteria that doctors use in deciding when and if to perform fundoplication surgery are how much the GERD is bothering the child, whether the GERD is increasing in severity and frequency, how much esophageal damage is seen on the endoscopy, and whether the more conservative treatment regimens are working. Ideally, fundoplication is performed before severe esophageal damage occurs, which if untreated can lead to lifelong debilitating narrowing of the lower esophagus (called "esophageal stricture").

Eighteen Ways to Comfort the Baby with Reflux

How long and how aggressively reflux is treated depends upon the severity of the reflux and how much it is interfering with an infant's growth and well-being. The doctor will supervise and prescribe medications, but parents are responsible for a lot of the treatment. Babies with reflux require parental intensive care, as you will soon learn. Treatment for reflux is aimed at keeping baby comfortable and thriving and minimizing possible esophageal damage until the natural intestinal maturity enables baby to outgrow this condition. The basis of reflux treatment is:

• *Developing a feeding pattern* and choosing foods that keep the stomach emptying rapidly and the food going down instead of up.

• *Positioning your infant* — day and night — in a way that allows gravity to help keep the food down.

• *Developing a parenting style* that lessens crying, since crying puts pressure on the stomach, which worsens the reflux.

Here are ways you can comfort your baby with reflux:

1. Practice attachment parenting. This high-touch style of parenting decreases baby's need to cry (remember, crying increases reflux) and increases parents' ability to cope. Less crying and more coping is the basic recipe for living with reflux. Attachment parenting (especially the three baby B's of breastfeeding, babywearing, and belief in the signal value of baby's cries) not only comforts the hurting baby, but helps parents more intuitively read their baby's pre-cry, or about-to-reflux body language, and intervene appropriately. Attachment parenting also increases the maternal hormones prolactin and oxytocin, which have a calming and relaxing effect on mother. Above all, shun the cry-it-out crowd. Babies with reflux cry because they hurt. Consider your nurturing response to your baby's cry as baby's best medicine. (See Chapter 1 for detailed information on how this style of parenting helps parents and babies thrive.)

Dr. Bill notes: *Don't take it personally that your baby cries a lot. A baby knows that his parents are there and care, even if they can't always relieve his pain.*

2. Keep baby semi-upright, especially during feedings. Gravity helps minimize reflux by helping the food stay down instead of go up. Wear your infant in a baby sling most of the day (see page 285 for instructions). Don't leave a baby with reflux sitting for long periods in a car seat or infant seat. Sitting positions bend baby in the middle, put pressure on the stomach, and increase reflux in some infants. (See also "Colic Carries," page 401.)

3. Keep baby quiet after feedings. Cuddle with your baby or wear your baby in a sling for at least thirty minutes after a feeding. Sway, don't bounce. Above all, don't jostle or vigorously play with baby after feedings. This can cause stomach contents to splash around and increase reflux.

4. Offer smaller feedings more frequently. Follow Dr. Bill's rule of reflux feeding: *Feed half as much twice as often.* Less food in the stomach at one time lessens reflux. Feeding frequently stimulates more saliva production. Saliva contains a healing substance called epidermal growth factor, which helps repair the damaged tissues in the esophagus. It also neutralizes stomach acid and lubricates the irritated lining of the esophagus.

5. Burp baby efficiently. Excess swallowed air aggravates reflux. If breastfeeding, burp baby when switching breasts. If bottlefeeding, burp baby after every few ounces of formula. Some newer feeding systems reduce air bubbles collecting in the bottle.

6. Breastfeed your baby. Breast milk is appropriately dubbed *the "easy-in, easy-out" meal.* Reflux is typically much less severe in the breastfed baby, and a breastfeeding mother is able to cope better for the following reasons:

- Breast milk empties from the stomach much faster than formula.

- Breast milk is more intestine friendly than formula.

- Breastfed babies naturally feed more frequently, and breast milk is a natural antacid.

- Breastfed babies have softer and easier-to-pass stools.

- Mothers enjoy the relaxing effect of maternal hormones while breastfeeding.

A parent notes: At age five months and four pediatricians later, Jacob was diagnosed with gastroesophageal reflux. I am forever grateful I did not give up in my search to find out why he was hurting! The goal of one of Jacob's reflux meds was to help digestion, so he would not reflux. I figured, what could be better for him than the most easily digested food for babies? . . . mom's milk! When the specialist to whom our doctor referred us first met Jacob, he was shocked to see him looking so happy. He told me that most babies with Jacob's degree of reflux failed to thrive and were very sickly. I am convinced that Jacob thrived because he was breastfed.

7. Don't bottle-prop or leave baby unsupervised during feedings. Babies with reflux can gag, choke, and have stop-breathing episodes during a feeding.

Dr. Bill advises: The stress of mothering a colicky baby can itself decrease your milk supply, which then may contribute further to baby's fussiness and cause you to give up breastfeeding. Remember our Parenting 101 advice: Baby needs a happy, rested mother. Get help from a lactation consultant to keep up your milk supply, get help at home, and carve out de-stress time just for yourself.

8. Try a pacifier. While the most effective pacifiers will be your breast and your holding, some infants with reflux are helped by the frequent use of pacifiers. Nonnutritive sucking can often ease reflux. This is why breastfeeding mothers often find that their babies with reflux want to "nurse" constantly. (On the other hand, some babies with severe GERD refuse to feed often because they associate feeding with pain.) Frequent sucking stimulates saliva production, which, as mentioned above, eases the irritation of reflux. Be aware, though, that in some cases vigorously sucking on pacifiers can aggravate reflux by increasing air swallowing. So, learn to read your baby for what style of sucking works.

9. Minimize air swallowing and gas. If breastfeeding, be sure baby has formed a tight seal (see "Positioning and Latch-on Skills," page 128). If bottlefeeding, try bottles and nipples that minimize air swallowing. Simethicone drops are marginally effective. This substance breaks large stomach bubbles into smaller stomach bubbles, which are easier to pass. Excess air in the stomach and intestines acts as a pneumatic pump, so when a stomach full of bubbles contracts, it can cause stomach contents to reflux. (See "Getting the Wind Out of Gassy Babies," page 387, and "Baby Bends," page 402.)

10. Avoid constipation. By increasing abdominal pressure while straining, constipation can aggravate reflux. Also, food that can't move down into overly full intestines can bounce back up. (See "Treating Constipation," page 696.)

11. Thicken feedings. If your baby is bottle-feeding and ready for solids (around six months of age), and if recommended by your doctor, thicken baby's feedings with two or more tablespoons of rice cereal in each eight-ounce bottle. Heavier food tends to stay down more easily. Thickened feedings help some infants with reflux but may aggravate reflux in others. I'm not convinced thickened feedings help, and too much rice cereal can be constipating.

Dr. Bill advises: Since many infants with GERD are also allergic to milk-based formulas, if bottlefeeding try a hypoallergenic formula (see page 202), which empties from the stomach faster than standard formulas.

12. Work out a reflux-friendly sleeping position. While it is always safest to put infants under six months of age to sleep on their backs to reduce the risk of SIDS, babies with severe reflux often sleep more comfortably on their left side. (The gastric inlet on the left side of the body is higher than the outlet, which helps gravity keep the food down.) Discuss with your doctor whether the reflux is severe enough to warrant side or tummy sleeping. Otherwise put your baby to sleep on her back. Try these other reflux-lowering helpers during sleep:

• Use a box or chair to elevate the head of baby's crib at least thirty degrees.

• Try The Tucker Sling. This sling fits around the upper part of the crib mattress like a contour sheet. A diaper-shaped part goes between baby's legs and fastens around the waist with Velcro. The sling, designed by a mother whose infant, Tucker, suffered from severe GERD, keeps baby from sliding down to the foot of the mattress when the mattress is elevated.

- If baby sleeps in your bed, try placing baby on a *reflux wedge,* available at infant product stores.

For information on reflux wedges and slings, see www.tuckerdesigns.com.

13. Don't smoke around baby. Nicotine stimulates gastric acid production and opens the lower esophageal sphincter.

14. Don't dress baby in clothing that is tight around the waist.

15. Try medications for GERD: While the following medications can certainly help ease the discomfort of reflux and minimize esophageal damage, they should always be used *in addition to,* not instead of, most of the above parenting, positioning, and feeding suggestions.

- *Antacids.* These over-the-counter medicines neutralize stomach acids. Given three or four times a day with a feeding (product and dosage to be determined by your child's doctor), they start working rapidly, but the neutralizing effect lasts only a couple of hours or less. For older children, chewables work better because they stimulate and mix with the saliva to help the antacid stick to the lining of the esophagus where it can better neutralize stomach acids. Long-term use of some antacids can contribute to constipation or diarrhea.

- *Acid suppressors or reducers.* These medicines (e.g., Prevacid, Zantac) block varying degrees of stomach acid production. They can take anywhere from thirty minutes to a couple of hours to take effect, but they may last for eight hours. They are usually given twice a day. If reflux tends to wake your child, give a dose one hour before bedtime.

- *Motility medicines.* These remedies work by increasing muscle tone and therefore tighten the lower esophageal sphincter muscle or increase the movement of the muscles of the stomach and upper intestines, thereby speeding up gastric emptying. They are sometimes referred to as prokinetics. Whereas antacids and acid blockers do not decrease reflux but rather just make it less painful and lessen the damage to the esophagus, motility medicines do decrease the amount of reflux but may have more side effects.

Be sure to work closely with your infant's doctor and/or pediatric gastroenterologist to develop the reflux management regimen that works best and is safest for your child. Be sure not to exceed the dosage recommended by your doctor or even use over-the-counter antacids without your doctor's advice. All medicines have a risk-benefit ratio, and medicines that neutralize stomach acid or interfere with its production should be used only if the reflux is severe enough that it truly bothers baby and/or could damage the lining of the infant's esophagus. Yet, untreated reflux may have serious long-term consequences, such as esophageal damage or asthma. One reason for antacid caution, for example, is that stomach acids have a beneficial effect. They help digest proteins and aid in the digestion of many vitamins and minerals. Stomach acids also kill harmful bacteria and help keep the normal bacteria of the gut in balance. Finally, the right amount of stomach acids balance the hormones that promote stomach emptying. Consider using an antacid only if your baby's GERD has not responded to the suggestions above.

16. Keep a diary. You need to be a keen observer and accurate reporter of your child's symptoms, since the doctor will often gauge the aggressiveness of the treatment regimen based upon your reporting. The doctor also relies upon your recording and reporting to modify treatment, such as changing medications or adjusting dosages. In a reflux diary list the main symptoms your child has, the treatment regimen, and the progress (better, worse, no change).

17. Get support. Ask your doctor for the names of parents whom you can consult who have children with reflux. Join a support group for parents of children with reflux, such as the Pediatric/Adolescent Gastroesophageal Reflux Association (PAGER), at www.reflux.org. Because reflux is being increasingly recognized as an underlying cause of infant illnesses such as colic, frequent respiratory infections, and asthma, both the understanding of this condition and its treatment are enjoying rapid advances. For current updates, consult our website, www.AskDrSears.com.

Advice from a parent: Never stop searching for answers to why your baby hurts. Be persistent in getting proper medical help.

18. Additional reflux tips for toddlers and older children. While most babies outgrow reflux by about one year of age, some children continue to suffer throughout childhood. Try these tips for toddlers and older children:

- *Chew-chew-chew.* Teaching your child how to take small bites, chew food well, and eat slowly results in less air swallowing. Also, food chewed into smaller particles empties from the stomach faster.

- *Let your child graze.* Small, frequent minimeals are easier to digest than fewer large ones. (See "Getting Your Toddler to Eat," page 253, for tips on offering your child a nibble tray.)

- *Sit and stand still and eat.* Jostling causes stomach acids to splash up into the esophagus. Encourage your child to sit or stand still for thirty minutes after eating.

FOODS THAT MAY AGGRAVATE REFLUX

- acidic foods: citrus fruits and juices (orange, grapefruit, and lemon), tomatoes, peppers, onions
- alcohol
- caffeine: coffee, tea, soft drinks (caffeine increases gastric stomach acid production)
- carbonated beverages
- chilies
- chocolate
- fatty foods
- fried foods
- high-sorbitol fruit juices (prune, pear, and apple)
- meats with a lot of gristle
- peppermint and spearmint
- spices
- stringy foods: seeds, skins, stringy fruits and vegetables

- *Lessen before-bedtime eating.* Eat dinner earlier in the evening and serve low-fat, mushy rapid-transit foods for the evening meal and bedtime snack. Adults with reflux often remind themselves, "Don't dine after nine."

- *Get friendly with your blender.* Fruit-and-yogurt smoothies and blended vegetables pass through the stomach quickly and are therefore less likely to cause reflux. (See our family's smoothie recipe on page 257.)

- *Keep your child lean.* Obesity aggravates reflux.

- *Avoid foods that linger in the stomach* or increase acid production and may aggravate reflux.

Step Three: Track Down Fuss Foods

Do gassy foods cause gassy babies? Every experienced breastfeeding mother has a fuss-food list — foods that she eats that may cause colicky behavior in her baby. Suspicious foods include gassy vegetables, dairy products, caffeine-containing foods, certain grains and nuts, among others. (See "Upsetting Foods in Breast Milk," page 152, for a discussion of colic-promoting foods in the breastfeeding mother and ways to identify them.)

Not only can what's in mother's milk upset baby, but how it's delivered can cause a bloated abdomen. Overfeeding is an uncommon but subtle cause of excessive intestinal gas. Feeding too much milk too fast may produce lactose overload and increased intestinal gas from the breakdown of the excessive lactose. Offering *smaller volumes* of formula *more frequently* or offering *one* breast at a feeding may be easier on baby's digestion (providing, of course, baby gets adequate nutrition in this change of feeding pattern).

The Colic–Cow's Milk Connection

New research supports what old wives have long suspected. Some babies show coliclike symptoms if their breastfeeding mothers drink cow's milk. Researchers found that the potentially allergenic beta-lactoglobulin in cow's milk is transferred into baby through the breast milk. This allergen causes intestinal upset just as if the baby had directly ingested the cow's milk. One study showed that eliminating cow's milk products from a breastfeeding mother's diet lessened colicky symptoms in around a third of the babies. Another study showed no relationship between cow's milk that mothers drank and the colic that those babies had. Many mothers in our practice report their baby's fussiness and colic remarkably subside when they eliminate dairy products from their diet, and the colicky symptoms reappear after they reintroduce cow's milk into their diet. If your baby's colicky behavior is due to dairy or other food products in your diet, the colicky symptoms usually appear within a few hours of your eating the suspected food and disappear within a day or two after you discontinue it.

Some mothers need to eliminate all dairy products totally, including ice cream, butter, or margarine made with whey (check labels for dairy contents: casein, whey, and sodium caseinate). Others can simply reduce the quantity of milk they drink, yet still eat yogurt and cheese without causing colicky behavior in their baby. Perhaps one of the reasons that colic disappears around four months is that this is the time when a baby's intestines mature enough to keep many of the food allergens from entering the bloodstream. (For an alternative to drinking cow's milk, see the almond milk recipe on page 153, or use a rice or soy beverage or goat's milk.)

Be Objective

In your eagerness to pin the cause of colic on something, along with everyone else's zeal to find the magic cure, it is easy to cloud your objectivity in labeling dairy products or other foods as the culprit. In our experience, if a baby is allergic enough to dairy products to cause colic, baby will often show other signs of allergy — for example, rashes, diarrhea, runny nose, night waking — signs that persist after the "colic" is gone.

Here's another fuss-foods clue. Sensitivities to food or dairy products in a breastfeeding mother's diet or sensitivities to formula usually are reflected in baby's stools. Frequent green, mucousy stools (or the opposite — constipation) accompanied by a red allergy ring around baby's anus suggest a food sensitivity. When you eliminate the offending food or dairy product, baby's stools become more normal, and the sore rash around the anus disappears.

Formula Allergies and Colic

Infants fed a cow's milk–based formula may become colicky if sensitive to cow's milk as an allergen. The American Academy of Pediatrics Committee on Nutrition recommends that soy formula *not* be used routinely in colicky infants because of the likelihood that infants who are allergic to cow's milk proteins are also likely to be allergic to soy. A predigested formula recommended by your baby's doctor (Alimentum, Nutramigen or Neocate) should be tried if you suspect a formula allergy. Use the elimination-and-challenge approach described on page 152 to uncover formula allergies.

No Smoking, Please

Colic occurs more often in babies whose mothers or fathers smoke or if a breastfeeding mother smokes. Researchers believe that not only does the nicotine transferred into mother's milk upset baby but the passive smoke in the home acts as an irritant. Babies of smoking parents fuss more, and mothers who smoke may be less able to cope with a colicky baby. Recent studies show that mothers who smoke have lower levels of prolactin, the hormone that increases a mother's sensitivity and allows her to persevere during those trying times.

Step Four: Consider Emotional Causes of Colic

After years of hurting with colicky babies and their parents and reviewing the research, we have concluded that colic has many causes: physical, medical, dietary, and emotional.

Colic Is Not Just a Disease

Could colic be a neurodevelopmental problem, not always an intestinal problem? Do we attribute colic to the wrong end of the baby? In some babies colic is a behavior, not a disease, and certainly not an incurable one. It's something a baby does, not something he has. Colic is one chapter in the whole book of fussy or high-need babies who have a supersensitive, intense, disorganized, slow-to-adapt temperament that we term a *colic tendency.* Whether or not this tendency escalates into colicky behavior depends, to

FUSS FOODS

Your baby's colic could be due to something in your diet that is passing through your breast milk. Oftentimes, baby's food intolerance is dose related. Perhaps you can drink a small amount, such as one glass of milk a day, without it bothering baby, yet two or three glasses are more than baby can comfortably tolerate. You can eliminate all potential offending foods at once or just a few at a time, depending on how severe the colic is. Be patient, it sometimes takes a week or two for the offending food to get out of your system. Dairy products are the most common offender. Here's a list of foods that may be the culprit.

beef	cabbage
caffeine: coffee, tea, soda	onions
chicken	green peppers
chocolate (sorry!)	nuts
citrus fruits	peanuts and peanut butter
corn	shellfish
dairy products	soy products
egg whites	tomatoes
gassy vegetables:	wheat
broccoli	
cauliflower	

some extent, on the caregiving environment baby meets.

Is Colic Due to Upset Biorhythms?

To ensure well-being, everyone has biorhythms — internal master clocks that automatically secrete regulating hormones and govern our daily changes of body temperature and sleep-wake cycles. When our biorhythms are *organized,* we feel right and act right. When our biorhythms are upset — for example from jet lag — we become "fussy."

Some babies enter the world with disorganized biorhythms. We say they are unsettled. Other babies enter the world organized and expect the caregiving environment to keep them organized. Failure to become organized or stay organized results in a behavioral change we call colic. Perhaps there is a group of organizing hormones that cause babies to settle. If these organizers are missing, babies become internally unsettled. Instead of fussing all the time, they let loose with periodic outbursts of colicky behavior or store up a day's worth of tension and release it in one long evening blast.

Could colic be a deficiency of calming hormones or an excess of upsetting hormones? There is some experimental support for the disturbance-in-biorhythm theory of colic. Newborn experimental animals separated

---

PLANNING FOR UN-HAPPY HOUR

To survive evening colic, prepare the evening meal in advance. Frozen pre-cooked casseroles and colicky babies mix well. Giving baby (and yourself) a late-afternoon nap sometimes settles the evening blow and recharges your coping system in case baby erupts. Wearing your baby for an hour or two in the late afternoon may relax baby enough to eliminate the evening outburst.

---

from their mothers have disturbed secretions of adrenal hormones, the body's regulating hormones.

Progesterone is a hormone known to have calming and sleep-inducing influences. Baby receives progesterone from the placenta at birth. Could the calming effect of maternal progesterone wear off around two weeks (when colic typically begins) and cause colic if the infant does not begin producing enough of his own progesterone? Some studies have shown low progesterone in colicky babies and improvement in the colicky behavior when these babies were given a progesteronelike drug. Other studies have shown mixed results. Breastfed babies in one study had higher levels of progesterone.

Prostaglandins, hormones that cause strong contractions of intestinal muscles, are newcomers to the disturbed-biorhythms theory. Coincidentally, when researchers injected prostaglandins into two babies to treat their heart disease, the two infants became colicky. Observations that babies who were the product of stressful births were more likely to become fussy lend support to these hormonal theories.

A final bit of icing on the biorhythm cake: Colic magically subsides around three to four months of age, at the time when baby's sleep patterns become organized into more predictable biorhythms. Any relationship? Our personal belief is that fussiness and colic in some, but not all, babies are the behavioral and physical manifestations of the internal regulating systems gone haywire. Much research is needed to identify the relationship between internal regulating hormones and baby's behavior and the effect of parenting styles on these substances. Until this research is available, we simply have to rely on common sense — that holding and nurturing calm a baby.

COMFORTING COLIC

Traditionally, colic has been "treated" by laying a reassuring hand on the tummy of the baby and the shoulders of the parents and temporizing, "Oh, he'll grow out of it!" Most approaches to colic are aimed more at helping parents cope than at relieving baby's hurt. By maintaining the mind-set "the hurting baby" rather than "the colicky baby," you and your doctor form a partnership to persevere in finding the cause and the remedy for your baby's pain.

Even though no one completely understands colic, let's make two assumptions: The whole baby is upset, and baby has pain in the gut (the term "colic" comes from the Greek *kōlikos,* meaning "suffering in the colon"). Treatment, therefore, is aimed at relaxing the whole baby and particularly baby's abdomen. Review the soothing suggestions we describe for calming the fussy baby, beginning on page 378. Here are additional tips to relax tense tummies.

The Colic Dance

Want to make a best-selling dance video? Put ten veteran parents with their colicky babies on a dance floor and watch the different steps. While each dance movement is as unique as a fingerprint, the choreography that works the best contains movement in all three planes: up and down, side to side, forward and backward — as in the womb. Here's your first dance lesson.

The right hold. Place baby in the neck nestle position or football hold (described below). Hold baby firmly, but relax. Convey an "I'm in charge" impression. Snuggle closely with a lot of skin-to-skin contact or use a baby sling.

The right dance step. Move in three planes (up and down, side to side, back and forth), and alternate these three motions. The up-and-down motion, the most colic-soothing dance step (the "elevator step"), is best performed by springing up and down as you walk — heel-toe-heel-toe.

The right rhythm. Moving in a rhythm of sixty to seventy beats per minute soothes babies best. (Count one–one thousand, two–one thousand. . . .) Interestingly, this rhythm corresponds to the uterine bloodflow pulse rate that baby was used to. Continue dancing until either the dancer or the fusser wears out.

Change partners. Some babies prefer mother's dance routine, probably because they are used to her style after nine months. But a change of partners is sometimes needed. Babies appreciate a new set of calm arms when mothers are tense from a whole day of baby holding. Dads have their own unique dance steps, too. When dad wears out, call in an experienced grandmother. She has time, patience, and experience.

Colic Carries (Mostly for Fathers)

Like dance routines, try all variations of baby holding until you find one that works. Here are some time-tested favorite colic carries that fathers of high-need babies refer to as "fussbusters."

The football hold. (See the illustration on the next page.) Drape baby stomach down along your forearm. Place baby's head near the crook of your elbow and his legs straddling your hand. Grasp the diaper area firmly and press your forearm into baby's tense abdomen. You will know you have found the right hold when you feel baby's tense abdomen relax and his previously tight limbs loosen and limply dangle. Or try reversing baby so that his cheek lies in the palm of your hand, his abdomen along your forearm, and his crotch area snuggled in the crook of your elbow.

The neck nestle. Snuggle baby's head into the groove between your chin and chest, in the neck nestle position. Croon a low, slow, repetitive tune. As baby quiets and falls asleep while dancing or being carried in the neck nestle position, ease baby into the warm fuzzy position (see page 382.)

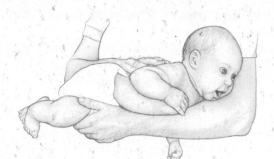

The football hold, a time-tested colic carry.

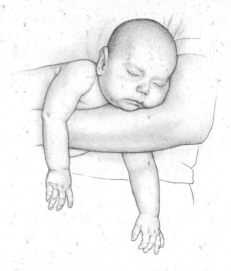

The limp-limb sign is a sure indication that baby is deeply asleep.

Bouncing baby. Hold baby close enough to engage in an eye-to-eye gaze, with one hand firmly under his bottom and the other on his upper back and neck. (Be sure to support the wobbly head of a newborn.) Bounce baby by moving your hands up and down rhythmically at sixty to seventy beats per minute. For an added touch, pat baby's bottom.

Bounce while you dance. One father in our practice scheduled his daily exercise routine during his baby's predictable evening fussy times. He bounced on a small trampoline while holding baby. It worked to take the tension out of baby and pounds off daddy.

Baby Bends

Besides creative rocking, baby bends are great for untensing baby, especially for a baby with pain in the gut. Here are some time-tested favorites, most of which are not effective when baby is at the peak of an attack. Do what you can to calm baby somewhat first, then he'll be more able to receive the physical benefits of bending.

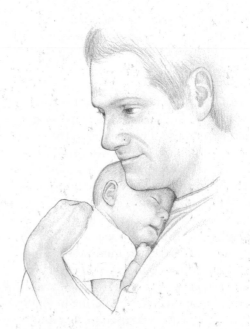

A comfortable neck nestle.

The gas pump. Grasp both lower calves and pump baby's legs, knees to tummy. Occasionally alternate the pumping actions with bicycling motions.

The colic curl. This is a favorite of tense babies who stiffen and arch their backs and have difficulty relaxing and molding into any holding position. Cradle baby with him sitting in your arms facing forward, resting his back against your chest. Bending baby relaxes the abdominal and back muscles, which often relaxes the whole baby. If your arms give out, try the kangaroo carry in the baby sling (see page 289). Or if you and baby like eye contact and like to play facial-gesture games, reverse the bend. Hold baby's back away from you and bend his legs up against your chest.

Roll out the pain. Drape baby tummy down over a large beach ball and roll him back and forth in a circular motion. Lay a securing hand on baby's back while rolling.

Press out the pain. Drape the awake baby stomach down on a cushion, with his legs dangling over the edge, to apply some soothing pressure to his belly.

Soft Touches

The big hand. Dads, place the palm of your hand over baby's navel and your fingers and thumbs circling baby's abdomen. Let baby lean his tense abdomen against your warm hand.

The "I Love U" touch. Picture an upside-down *U* over the surface of your baby's abdomen. Underneath are your baby's tense intestines, which need relaxing, and the colon, out of which you try to massage the gas. Rub some warm oil onto your hands and knead baby's tense abdomen with your flattened fingers in a circular motion. Start with a downward stroke for the *I* on baby's left side

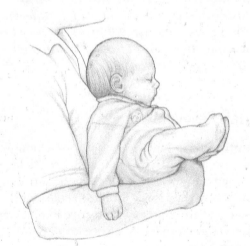
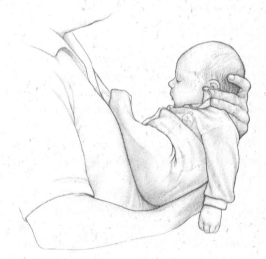

Two variations of the colic curl.

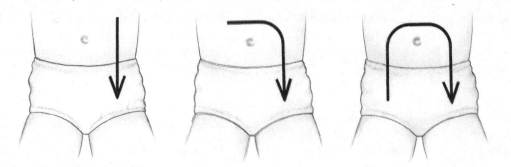

The "I Love U" touch helps move gas along baby's intestinal tract.

(your right, see illustration). This stroke moves gas down and out of your baby's descending colon. Then massage along the upside-down *L*, moving the gas along the transverse portion of the colon and down the descending colon again. Then massage along the upside-down *U*, stroking upward along the ascending colon, across the transverse, and down the descending colon. Abdominal massage works best with baby on your lap, feet facing you, or in a warm bath, or both.

A Mother's Story

"I tried warm baths with my baby. This helped, but only as long as he was immersed in the warm water, and realistically, you can't spend your life in a bath! I also massaged his tummy while he was in the water. With his feet toward me, I would place my left hand across his middle and knead rather deeply with my fingers, concentrating on his left side close to the rib cage. This helped, but he only liked it when he was in the water. After his bath I would rub him with lotion, starting with his precious little feet and working up each leg. I found when I reached his thigh his wails immediately turned into cackles of laughter. I began to concentrate on massaging his thighs when colicky periods began, and even without the bath, the reaction was always the same.

"The thigh massage I found most helpful went like this. I would lay Eric in my lap on his back with his head on my knees and his feet at my stomach. I would place a hand on each thigh, thumb in the groin area and fingers on the outside of the leg. Then I would use a rather firm, deep kneading motion with equal pressure on both the inside and the outside of the leg, squeezing, rolling, then releasing. It worked every time, turning those pitiful wails into laughter — at least for a while!"

Gas Relievers

Antiflatulent (simethicone) drops, a nonprescription digestive aid given before feedings, lessens the formation of gas in the intestines. At this writing these drops are considered safe and are sometimes effective in relieving excess gas formation. Bloated babies are often relieved by the doctor inserting a lubricated pinkie into baby's tight rectum.

RX FOR FUSSING

Why Babies Fuss (or Hurt)

- [ ] Missing the womb
- [ ] Separation from mother
- [ ] High-need baby
- [ ] Formula allergy
- [ ] Allergy to foods in breastfeeding mother's diet
- [ ] Gastroesophageal reflux

- [ ] Ear infection
- [ ] Urinary tract infection
- [ ] Constipation
- [ ] Diaper rash
- [ ] Broken bone from recent fall
- [ ] Drug withdrawal (newborn)
- [ ] They're just being babies

What to Do

- [ ] Babywearing
- [ ] Frequent feedings
- [ ] Prompt responses to cries
- [ ] Colic carries and dances
- [ ] Soothing lullabies and music
- [ ] Baby swings
- [ ] Moving attractions: fish tank, grandfather clock, videos, exercise machines
- [ ] Car rides: freeway fathering
- [ ] Feeding while carried in a sling
- [ ] Infant massage, especially abdominal

- [ ] Warm fuzzies: dad's chest
- [ ] Warm baths
- [ ] Looking at self in mirror
- [ ] Elimination diet if breastfeeding
- [ ] Hypoallergenic formulas
- [ ] Smaller, more frequent feedings to avoid overfeeding
- [ ] Upright position, especially after feeding
- [ ] Tense-tummy exercises
- [ ] Medicinal gas relievers
- [ ] A visit to the doctor

Sometimes stool will shoot out and the "colic" stops.

If your infant is constipated, nonprescription glycerin rectal suppositories for babies may help expel some stool and relieve the backed-up gas. Insert the suppository about an inch into the rectum and hold baby's buttocks together a few minutes to allow the suppository to dissolve. (See treatment of constipation, page 696.)

A Home Remedy

Parents have reported that some herbal teas are successful in relieving the pain in their colicky babies. Try chamomile and fennel teas. Put one-half teaspoon of the herb in one cup of boiling water. Cover and steep for five to ten minutes, then strain. Cool and give baby a few teaspoons of the tepid tea.

►*A WORD OF CAUTION ABOUT COLIC REMEDIES: From time to time new research shows that colic remedies thought to be harmless to a baby may not be safe. Always be sure to check with your doctor before giving your baby any prescription or nonprescription remedies. Also see our website, www.AskDrSears.com, for updated information.*

Should Baby Cry It Out?

We put the cry-it-out approach to sleep in the chapter on nighttime parenting. We want to keep it asleep as a "treatment" for the colicky baby. This severe method of dealing with colic is a no-win situation for baby and for parents. In a study comparing two groups of colicky babies, one group was given an immediate nurturant response to crying, while the other group was left to cry it out. The group whose cries were properly attended to cried 70 percent less. The babies in the cry-it-out group, however, showed no decrease in colicky crying. Besides not helping the baby, the cry-it-out approach desensitizes parents, who may already be struggling with ambivalent feelings toward their baby. The last thing they need is any advice that creates even more distance between parents and their baby.

Parents, as we've said before, it is not your fault your baby cries, nor must you always stop baby from crying. There may be times when baby needs a good relief cry. But baby doesn't need to cry alone. Your role is neither to ignore nor frantically hush baby's cry, but to do all you can to help if there is pain. Then if baby still cries, stay relaxed yourself and allow him to release and express what can only come out through crying. We all know how therapeutic a good cry can be, and even more so in someone's supporting arms. Babies have feelings just as intense as ours, and it helps them to be able to get it out so they can get back to feeling balanced and happier, and maybe even sleep better.

Parents need to know how stress causes them to react to their baby's crying. Many remember only too well the feelings of despair because of fatigue and lack of sleep — visions of throwing baby out the window do not mean parents would actually do it! Stress can push new parents to the extreme edge, and they can picture themselves losing control, shaking the baby, screaming at the baby to shut up. Stress management becomes an important tool in dealing with a crying baby. If you have thoughts like these, seek help immediately from a professional counselor or a sympathetic friend.

IS COLIC PREVENTABLE?

Mike and Lori were parents of a previously colicky baby who was now a happy and calm

> ### DON'T SHAKE THE BABY
>
> Colicky cries not only pierce tender hearts; they may also push anger buttons. If baby's escalating cries are getting to you, hand baby over to another person or put baby safely down and walk out of the room until your scary feelings subside. Angrily shaking a baby may damage his fragile brain structures, sometimes fatally.

two-year-old. Expecting their second baby, they came in for prenatal counseling and began, "Is there anything we can do to increase our chances of having a calmer baby? We don't want to go through that again."

A Colic-Prevention Experiment

I counseled these parents that, while there is no magic preventive medicine for colic, there are ways to lower your chances. Over a three-year period we tried a colic-prevention experiment in our office. This is what we advised and what we observed.

Strive for a peaceful pregnancy. While a stress-free pregnancy is as rare as a never-fuss baby, studies have suggested that mothers who go through pregnancy with a lot of unresolved stress have a greater risk of having colicky babies.

Try a drug-free pregnancy and birth. Studies have shown that mothers who had a drug-free birth were less likely to have colicky babies. Also, mothers who took addicting drugs or drank alcohol heavily during pregnancy were more likely to have fussy babies.

Practice the seven Baby B's of attachment parenting. Of all these concepts we found babywearing to be the most useful fuss preventer. Every couple in our experiment left the hospital with a baby sling, and a brief course in babywearing by our office staff followed. Both mom and dad were instructed to wear their baby most of the day.

Identify the "colic candidate" early and intervene. Some babies give a clue in the first day or two of life. They show a few sparks that warn the real explosion is soon to follow.

When I was working as director of a university hospital newborn nursery, I was astonished at how disturbing are the cries of some newborns. I would open the door of the nursery and hear one of those ear-piercing cries and want to shut the door and run. Babies' cries are something I definitely have a low tolerance for. So in addition to studying the sound qualities of the cry, I wondered if we could identify babies with particularly disturbing cries in the newborn nursery and mellow out these cries during the first few weeks. Most babies have the good manners to start out with attachment-promoting cries, which if promptly attended to don't escalate into detachment-promoting cries. A few click immediately into the ear-piercing, shrill detachment cry, which makes all within earshot want to run from the baby. These cries sometimes invoke anger rather than sympathy toward the baby. Nursery nurses identify these babies early on, often saying, "This one's going to be a handful." In most of these "crybabies" I have studied, babywearing early in the newborn period not only lessens the frequency of crying but mellows the nature of the cry into more tolerable and attachment-promoting cries. The following is an example that actually occurred during the writing of this book.

Jeffrey, the secondborn of a very attached and committed mother, was the product of a stressful labor and birth. Jeffrey's cry was shattering. Even in the delivery room his cry almost cleared the room of all personnel. Susan, Jeffrey's mother, even admitted that his cry was disturbing their bonding relationship. As an experiment, I advised the parents to wear Jeffrey in a sling for at least four hours every day, more if possible. Also, they were instructed to tape-record his cries over a period of two weeks. Within a week, Jeffrey's cry mellowed considerably, enabling the mother to "finally enjoy being with him; he cries much nicer now." Susan and her husband created a caregiving environment in which Jeffrey had no need to be angry and certainly no need to cry angrily.

Attachment Parenting Can Help

It is customary for medical professionals to advise parents to wear their babies and use other comforting techniques *after* fussy or colicky behavior has already begun. Indeed, I used to do this. I then realized the importance of preventive medicine for colic. I started advising new parents to begin wearing their babies right after birth, especially those babies who had already been labeled "fussy" in the hospital. As I expected, the incidence of colic and fussy behavior dramatically decreased in my practice.

I have noticed, and research has confirmed, that parents who employ the attachment style of parenting have fewer fussy babies. I have observed, however, that even parents who practice all the concepts of attachment parenting may be blessed with a colicky baby. Even babies whom I call right-from-the-start babies get colic. (But in these babies suspect a medical cause.) There's something fundamentally distressing about not being able to comfort a crying baby. But attachment parents who have colicky babies are better able to cope with the colic, are more likely to seek out the cause, and are generally more sensitive to baby's crying. In these families, even if they cannot cure the

colic, it does not promote a distance between the parents and baby, but they use this passing trial as just another factor that cements the already strong parent-infant bond.

I find it very interesting that colic usually does not begin until after the second week of life. Could it be that the infant is giving us a two-week grace period to help her get organized and adjust to life outside the womb? If her expected parenting style is not fulfilled, her system goes from neutral equilibrium to disequilibrium, from unorganized to disorganized, resulting in the total behavioral decompensation we call colic.

Even with babies whose colic is due to a medical rather than a behavioral cause, parents who wear their babies are better able to cope with the colicky behavior. The closeness they achieve creates a *sensitivity* in these parents, causing them to be especially responsive to their infant's needs. Babywearing parents also learn to anticipate the triggers of colicky behavior and avoid these triggers before they occur.

Babywearing is especially valuable in preventing evening colic. It could be that baby has spent most of his day trying to compensate and fit into his environment using his own semisuccessful self-soothing techniques. By the end of the day he is so exhausted from trying to fit that he bitterly decompensates into colicky behavior. Babywearing during the day, in effect, compensates and helps baby organize the day and thereby relieves evening colic. The tenseness that would have built up during the day and would need to be released at night in colic is not there because babywearing has done its part to help the baby fit. (See "Babywearing Reduces Crying and Colic," page 303.)

ENTERING THE PROMISED TIME

When will it stop? Colic begins around two weeks of age and reaches peak severity around six to eight weeks. Seldom do the violent outbursts continue longer than four months of age (unless it's due to an undetected medical cause), but fussy behavior may last throughout the first year and mellow between one to two years of age. In one study of fifty colicky babies, the evening colic disappeared by four months in all of the babies studied. What's magic about three to four months? Around that time babies develop more internal organization of their sleeping patterns. Exciting developmental changes occur that lead babies to the promised land of fuss-free living. They can see clearly across the room. Babies are so delighted by the visual attractions that they forget to fuss. Next, they can play with their hands and engage in self-soothing finger sucking. Babies can enjoy more freedom to wave their limbs freestyle and blow off steam. Also, during the second half of the first year baby's intestine is more mature, and perhaps milk allergies subside. Or by this time the cause has been found or comforting techniques perfected. Like pregnancy and labor, colic too will pass.

17

Working and Parenting

One morning Martha and I were guests on a TV show. I was asked to comment on "the working mother," which tops my dreaded-question list. While I was trying to be pediatrician turned politician and muster up an unoffending answer, Martha piped up, "If I hadn't worked while you were an intern, we wouldn't be sitting here right now."

THE REAL ISSUE: ATTACHMENT

The issue is not the working mother, the issue is *attachment* with your baby. The solution is to combine earning and parenting. Separating mothers into two camps does nothing but provide judgmental material for magazines and devalues one side or the other. The approach we take is to present the facts and then offer, instead of guilt-laden judgment, support for attachment and thoroughly researched advice for incorporating working and attachment. To write that full-time attachment mothering makes no difference would be dishonest, ignoring what both research and experience have shown and trading truth for popularity. Likewise, to pontificate that a baby will be absolutely disadvantaged if mother works is equally shortsighted. We have worked out a practical approach based upon our own career juggling, and our experience in counseling hundreds of working and caring parents.

For Mothers Who Are Undecided

Your baby is due in a few weeks, and you have begun your maternity leave. As you clean out your desk, you wonder, "Will I ever return? Should I return? Do I have to? Do I want to?" For the many women in this quandary who have the luxury of choice, here are answers to some questions often asked by mothers about to face the decision whether to work, stay home, or both.

Does the amount of time I'm with my baby really make any difference to my child's outcome?

What you are really asking is "How important am I?" Reread Chapter 1, "Getting Attached," and read the first few pages of Chapter 19, "Growing Together," on the meaning of mother-infant attachment, how it affects your child, and what's in it for you. Especially consider the concepts of mutual giving, mutual shaping, and mutual sensitivity. Notice that your presence influences not only what you give to baby, but what baby *gives to you*, how interacting with your baby shapes your mothering skills. What baby does for mother is an important but underappreciated fact. Your presence is important to your baby's development, and your baby's presence is important to your development.

Are there studies showing that full-time mothering makes a difference?

Yes, but not the studies that make headlines in magazines. Again, the issue is not full- or part-time mothering, but attachment. Even the artificial divisions "full-time" and "part-time" are misleading. You can be full-time at-home but only part-time interacting with your baby, or part-time at work and full-time interacting with your baby when at home. In a nutshell, the studies conclude: *The most important contributor to a baby's physical, emotional, and intellectual development is the responsiveness of the mother to the cues of her infant.*

It's the attachment with your baby that counts, not just the time you spend. A baby has an intense need to be with her mother that is as basic as her need for food. But the need for food is not continuous, nor is the requirement for mother. The baby needs to be held, carried, talked to (attached), but not necessarily always by mother. Mother's availability, like feeding, is on an as-needed basis to be delivered as much as possible by mother herself. "Responsiveness" is the current buzzword among infant development specialists. Another is "reciprocity." These infant-stimulation terms boil down to a more understandable concept — *harmony*. Your baby has a need and gives you a cue. Because you are present and tuned in to baby, you pick up on the cue and respond. Because baby trusts that she will receive a consistent and predictable response, she is motivated to keep cueing. The more you and baby practice this cue-response interplay, the better baby learns to cue and the better you learn to respond. The mother-baby relationship is in harmony. Baby and mother bring out the best in each other.

WHO WILL MOTHER YOUR BABY?

When considering a return to work, ask yourself these questions: What are my options for substitute care? Is my husband willing and able to share the parenting and provide a nurturing alternative? Do I have a substitute caregiver who is basically a nurturing and responsive person? If yes, then easing back into work may be an option. If not, consider full-time mothering.

Don't sell yourself short. One reason some mothers turn their babies over to someone else is they truly believe their baby will be better off. They have such a poor self-image or such poor mother-daughter modeling from their own childhood that they cannot picture themselves as good for their babies. Your baby does not shop around; he doesn't know any "better." You are his only mother, and *you are good enough.* You need your baby to open you up to learning how to be a mother.

And don't forget the mothering hormones (see page 307); studies have shown it's the frequency of mother-baby interaction that is the most potent stimulator of these mothering boosters.

What about quality time?

The concept of quality time was marketed by the child-care industry to lessen guilt during the you-can-have-it-all style of the eighties. Initially meant for working fathers, quality time made its way into the guilt-easing package for working mothers.

There is a certain value to the quality time concept. In certain situations, quality time may be the only option. One sincere, caring mother told us, "I have to work all day, so quality time is all I can afford. I give up a lot of time I would ordinarily spend on entertainment to be with my child, so that when I am not working I am fully devoted to my infant. Besides quality time, I probably give him more quantity time than some nonworking mothers who spend a lot of time each day pursuing their own forms of entertainment." This mother is truly doing the best she can do. While quality time is important, so is the quantity of time. Here are some advantages of simply being there.

Baby's spontaneity. Babies are spontaneous. Their play is mood dependent. One of the fallacies of baby care is that we must always be stimulating our babies. Most babies, however, have a *prime time of receptivity* each day, a period during which they learn best from their social interactions. Most babies have their best time in the morning. Evening times are often a baby's worst. The "happy hour" from 6:00 to 8:00 P.M. is often a cranky, fussy time of the day that is enough to drive mothers back to work. To rush home from a full day's work and feel you then have to stimulate your baby is not in the parent-infant contract. A more realistic approach is simply being available and approachable when baby needs to play or be comforted.

Missed milestones. Precious things happen when a parent is not around, shooting another arrow at the quality time target. Everyone loses when the first crawl, the first step, the first word, occur and baby's favorite guests are not at the party.

Teachable moments. Another fact of baby care that dilutes the quality time concept is the well-researched observation that baby-initiated play has more educational value than parent-initiated interactions. Baby looks up into the sky and sees his first bird. That's an opener. Is there someone there to share his discovery and expand on it by talking to baby about birds flying in the sky?

What are the effects of mother-baby separation?

Basically, they are a lessening of the benefits of mother-infant attachment. In recent years there has been a flurry of research validating, almost down to the cellular level, the importance of mother's presence. Fascinating findings (for example, infant animals separated from their mothers have higher levels of stress hormones and lower levels of growth hormones) are beginning to open a lot of eyes toward realizing the value of attachment. How long and how often baby can tolerate separation from mother depends much upon the strength of the mother-baby attachment, the quality of substitute attachment caregiving, and the temperament of the baby.

Of course, no matter how much weighing of advantages and disadvantages you do in advance, baby will ultimately have a voice in the decision too. If you are blessed with a high-need baby (see the preceding chapter for a profile of this little person), full-time mothering for a longer time may be your only real option.

A mother notes: I left a promising career to stay home when my baby was born, feeling my career as a mother was even more promising.

"I Have to Work — We Need the Income"

If your preference is to be at home with your baby, but for financial reasons you have to work, consider these alternatives.

What does it cost to work? By the time you deduct from your paycheck the costs of convenience food, transportation, clothing, child care, increased taxes, and medical bills (infants in day-care centers get sick more often), you may be surprised by how little you have left.

Evaluate your priorities. Are you working to pay the utility bills and to feed your family? Or are there desired luxuries that can be temporarily put off? No material possessions are more valuable to your infant than you are. Consider whether you can afford not to give your child your full-time self, at least for two or three years.

Economize. Take a long, hard look at your family's spending habits. Some people are better at penny-pinching than others, and to some it is a consideration that makes them angry. (Why should they have to discipline themselves?) Yet if they can truly understand the worth of having mother with her small children full-time, the effort and delay of gratification will be worth it. With serious economizing, it is possible for some to raise a family on one income and even make a few dreams come true along the way.

Consider borrowing the extra income. The high-touch stage of infant care does not last forever. Have you considered borrowing the extra income while your child is an infant and returning to work later to repay it? Grandparents are often a willing lending source if they realize that this is one of the most valuable investments they can make in their grandchild's future.

Plan ahead. During your early years of marriage and during pregnancy, economize to save as much money as you can. Let the savings from your second income help your family while you are a full-time mother. Many couples become accustomed to a standard of living that depends upon two incomes. Early in your marriage consider living on one income and saving the other, lest you become trapped in the two-income standard of living after baby arrives.

Start a home business. We feel for some couples this may be a realistic answer to the second-income dilemma. Home businesses are most successful when you do the type of work you *want* to do. Any work that you dislike will wear thin after a while. Examples of successful home businesses that we have seen work are mail-order distributing, bookkeeping, typing and word processing, selling, working with arts and crafts, giving piano lessons, working as a sales distributor, or starting your own home day care. We have professional women in our practice who bring their businesses into their homes and turn a spare room into an office. Telecommuting is a technological boon that has enabled many mothers to stay connected to their office while staying home with their baby. For example, one mother is an editor who works at her own portable home computer that is tied into the main office. She goes to her office without leaving her nest. The exciting part of home businesses is that many of them become so successful that it not only helps mother and baby stay attached, it helps husband and wife stay attached, and as the child gets older he or she can become involved in the family business. We know two mothers who wanted to stay home with their new babies but needed the second income. They started a garage business making car seat covers. This company subsequently mushroomed into a multimillion-dollar corporation.

Consider different working-time options. Besides the usual full-time or part-time employment, consider two other novel options:

- Flextime work. Work with flexible hours allows a parent to adjust the hours to be at home when the child is sick or has a special need, and it best allows spouses to share the child care.

- A shared job. In this type of arrangement two parents share the work of one full-time job. This situation allows parents to cover for each other when the children have special needs or are sick. It benefits employers because they get two minds for the price of one. For any arrangement less than full-time, you may have to bargain with employers for benefit packages.

KEYS TO WORKING AND ATTACHING

We begin this section with two real stories.

What Not to Do

Jan is a career woman about to deliver her first baby. Her professional voice tells her that she has studied long years to get her degree, that she feels fulfilled by her job and wants to return to it. Her maternal voice tells her, because she has researched this baby well, that a strong mother attachment is important. She fears that she may not be able to return to work easily if she gets hooked on motherhood. Subconsciously she keeps herself from getting too attached to her baby and is preoccupied with the day she has to return to work. She spends a lot of time interviewing substitute caregivers, buying things for baby, and planning her dual-career juggling act. Before she realizes it, her month at home is over, and the office scene now consumes her day. She dismisses frequent baby pangs as a side effect of mothering that soon will pass — and it does. Baby seems to be thriving in the hands of a nurturant caregiver, and Jan has entered the ranks of master jugglers.

In time a *distance* develops between mother and baby — and between father and baby, too. The signs are subtle at first, then obvious. Come the toddler years, she and her child are locking horns. Discipline becomes a list of methods desperately snatched from the nearest book. She finds herself seeking more and more help from counselors about how to handle her unruly daughter. The attachment was not developed at a time when both mother and baby needed it, and they are now playing the difficult game of catch-up.

A Story About Healthy Working and Attaching

Mary and Tom are about to become first-time parents. The couple, both with interesting careers, realistically evaluates the family situation and concludes that Mary needs to work (even wants to), at least part-time. During "their" pregnancy Mary and Tom read a lot about the importance of mother-infant attachment and father-infant attachment. They vow not to let working and parenting be an either/or decision. They both will work outside the home, but they will also work at building a strong attachment to baby, and this is how they do it.

First, Mary puts out of her mind the day she plans to return to work lest she be preoccupied with "what happens when." She doesn't let economic pressures rob her of the joy of becoming attached. She chooses her birthing scene wisely, keeps baby with her after birth, breastfeeds on cue, and wears baby James most of the day — the entire attachment-parenting package. Tom shares every aspect of parenting except the breastfeeding. The attachment strengthens.

After a month of being an attached mother, Mary feels connected with her baby and at peace with herself. Feeling connected to their baby elevates Tom and Mary's whole decision-making process to a higher level. Mary still realizes she must work, but she is even more committed to mothering because she realizes how important it is to maintain the attachment. She realizes she can't rewind the parenting tape of the early, formative months, but she can always catch up on income. She decides to *ease* into working, first very part-time, then maybe more — using baby as a barometer of separation.

In some ways her strong mother-infant attachment makes it tougher to leave James; in other ways it is easier because she knows in her heart (confirmed by research) that strong early attachment makes later separation healthier. A secure mother-infant attachment allows baby to better tolerate substitute care and helps mother to feel less guilty about leaving.

The attached couple thoughtfully selects a substitute caregiver, one who is naturally nurturing and sensitively responsive. Mary spends time showing her how she wants her baby mothered.

While at work, Mary periodically clicks her mind onto images of her baby. After all, working people let their minds wander a bit; she might as well let it wander to her baby. Every few hours her breasts tingle and leak as a reminder that though professionally she is at the office, biologically she is a breastfeeding mother. She pumps and stores milk, glad for this connection with James. The connection continues — because Mary orchestrates it.

Sometimes the couple is able to juggle work schedules so that dad parents while mom works. After all, if mom shares earning, dad can share baby care.

At night James sleeps next to mom and dad, for some catch-up closeness from missed time during the day. The attachment continues at night. As Mary and Tom take inventory of their "home baby-raising business" they make adjustments, considering the needs of all *three* persons.

They realize the need to put a part of their previously busy life-style on hold for a while, because James will be a baby for a relatively short time, and their current financial situation is likely to improve. They even include James in their social life, gravitating toward like-minded friends and learning from veteran career jugglers.

What is the secret of their success? Because they were convinced attachment parenting makes a difference, they found a way. And they see the payoff. Years later, after Mary's office closes, Tom's company relocates, and their professional lives change, James will display the dividends of a long-term attachment investment.

Connecting and Staying Connected

Central to our approach to the working-parent issue is not whether or how much a mother works, but *how close the attachment is between baby and mother.* Even though the focus is on employed mothers, a broader issue is how *both* mother and father can be employed and parent. Here are tips for keeping connected to baby.

Make the most of maternity leave. Don't dwell upon the day you will return to work, lest the preoccupation rob you of those precious weeks of connecting with your baby. During the weeks or months at home with baby, practice as many of the attachment concepts as you can. Get hooked on your baby. Let your baby develop your nurturing skills. Enjoy the time spent with your baby as you let mutual giving bring out the best in both of you.

Realize your importance. Ponder the whole concept of attachment as discussed in the questions and answers earlier in this chapter. Be aware of the importance of parent-infant attachment. Especially consider the concepts of mutual giving, shaping, and sensitivity. Once the magnitude of what it means to nurture another life hits you, you will be more motivated to make attachment a priority.

Reconnect with baby. Let quality time be nurturing time, a time to reconnect with your baby after work. Continue breastfeeding after returning to work if you enjoyed this feeding style while you were a full-time mommy (see page 165 for tips on breastfeeding and working). Wear baby as much as possible while working around the house, shopping, and running errands. Incorporate baby into your away-from-the-workplace life. Indulging baby in *things* to make up for relationships is not part of the attachment style of parenting. Catch-up nurturing is.

While at work keep the attachment going. New technologies can be helpful. You and your baby may be able to look at each

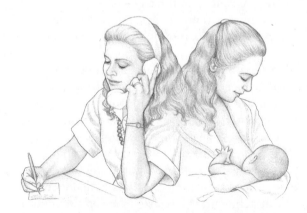

Attachment parenting helps the working mother reconnect with her baby after work.

other through a Web camera set up on a computer. Baby's pictures, pumping milk, and telephone calls to caregivers make long-distance connecting easier. Sometimes you may find all these baby reminders upsetting. Take these feelings as a sign of your continued sensitivity to your dual career. Completely shutting off baby thoughts eight hours a day is a desensitization process that leads to the most common infection of employed mothers — *distancing between mother and child.*

Blend jobs. If possible, choose employment that allows you the maximum time to mother. Here are some suggestions:

- Telecommunicate as much as possible.

- Start a home business.

- Find nearby employment that enables you to come home for reconnecting times or enables the caregiver to bring baby to your workplace.

- Work a flextime schedule, in which you have a certain amount of work to do but can choose your hours to accommodate baby-care times.

- Use on-site child care that allows you to stay in close and frequent touch with baby while at work.

- Work and wear. Bringing your baby to your job depends on the baby and the job. A fussy baby and a librarian mommy couldn't peacefully coexist in the same workplace. But there are plenty of jobs that enable you to wear your baby in a baby sling while working. Some examples are clerking in a baby shop — a natural shopper-stopper — selling real estate, even office work in a setting where baby sounds are socially acceptable. The cradle or playpen in the office corner can be an option. A patient of ours is a substitute teacher who wears her baby to class. Can you imagine the attachment message she gives these impressionable future parents? (See the discussion of working and wearing baby, page 298, for more baby-at-the-workplace tips.)

Know yourself — know your baby. No career, even mothering, works if you push yourself beyond job satisfaction. A mother in our practice summed up her realistic appraisal of herself and her baby: "Full-time mothering was too much for me; full-time working was too much for my baby." She reached a compromise. Besides working part-time, she got involved with a mothering support group at our suggestion so she could learn to broaden her enjoyment of her mothering profession.

Martha notes: When asked that inevitable question "And what do you do?," I respond, "I'm a specialist in early childhood education." And with no trouble at all, I could sit down and write out a detailed job description to go with that lofty title.

Share baby care. If you are bringing home part of the bacon, honor your husband with his share of the household duties, especially taking over for the sitter whenever possible. One of the better by-products of employed mothers is more-involved fathers.

Shortening the Distance

Over the years we have noticed that expectant mothers planning to return to their jobs a few weeks after birth subconsciously may not let themselves become closely attached to their baby "because it will be so hard to go back to work." Many of these babies and mothers who get a short start become victims of the dual-career juggler's disease — *distancing*.

We tried an experiment in our practice. Prenatally or around the time of birth, when mothers told me they would be returning to work, I asked them to put "W-day" completely out of their mind. "Enjoy full-time mothering while you can. Get hooked on your baby. In a couple of weeks before your return to work, we'll discuss preparations." Amazing changes occurred in these mothers.

• They procrastinated and asked for a medical release to extend maternity leave. I was happy to oblige and prescribed Dr. Bill's standard mother-needs-to-stay-home-with-baby-awhile-longer remedy: *"Because Mrs. Smith's baby is allergic to any milk other than her breast milk, it is medically necessary to extend her maternity leave so that she can safely meet her baby's nutritional needs."* (This statement is technically correct. At least in the early months, infant intestines show allergic reactions, albeit sometimes microscopic, to any food other than human milk. Therefore, mother's milk can be considered a preventive-medicine prescription.)

• The concept of leaving baby at one place and working in another became foreign to them — as if having to leave parts of themselves in two places. The baby had become part of mother's life.

• These mothers had various outcomes. Some made drastic changes in their lifestyles and took a year or two off to be full-time moms. The rest went back to work,

but all had come to the same conclusion. *They would work but still meet the needs of their babies.*

• The mothers who returned to work sought jobs that gave them the maximum flexibility. These mothers settled only for substitute caregiving that offered a high level of sensitive nurturing. Some mothers even negotiated improved child-care policies at their workplace, such as sick-child leave and flextime.

What had happened to these mothers? A month or two of attachment parenting began a relationship that was too valuable to dilute, and whatever it took to maintain this connection they did. These babies did for their mothers more than all of the advice in the world could have done — they showed mother her importance.

CHOOSING SUBSTITUTE CAREGIVERS

After many mothers come to grips with the agonizing reality of dual-career juggling, next comes the search for their substitutes.

Options for Care

The first step for most mothers in this position is to consider the care options that are feasible in their circumstances.

In-home care. Having your baby cared for in your own home is preferable. The advantages of home care are familiar surroundings, familiar toys, the germs that baby has already learned to live with, no transportation hassles, and your familiarity with the home. Shared care by your spouse is usually best; next comes grandparents or close relatives. Though more costly, a trained nanny, an au pair girl, and live-in help are other options. But once you go beyond the inner circle of family, relatives, or intimate friends, a seemingly endless search begins.

Shared home care. An option for part-timers is sharing child care with a friend — "I'll mother yours and you mother mine two and a half days a week," or whatever schedule you work out. This deal brings you the advantage of having a like-minded caregiver, and, as in a profit-sharing partnership, each is motivated to give the other person's child the level of care they expect for their own. Friends with the same due date and back-to-work schedule as yours, and mates in your childbirth class, are ready sources for this arrangement.

Home day care (family day care). In this arrangement baby is cared for in another mother's home. Mothers often do home day care to supplement their family's income and to be home with their own children. The same nurturing priorities that prompted this mother to set up this arrangement may carry over into her care of your baby. You can only be sure of this if you know this person well or have carefully checked out her references. But this is not so ideal if the care provider piles in kids to the maximum allowable limit, has weak sick-child policies, and is not an attentive person. An ideal rule of thumb is that one caregiver can usually care for one one-year-old, two two-year-olds, three three-year-olds, and so on, which is modified by the number and ages of her own children. These houses should be licensed, and you should be able to see the license. Remember, licensing deals with safety and medical issues; it does not guarantee a nurturing environment. That is your job to determine.

Parent co-ops. Four or five mothers of similar values get together and agree to care for one another's babies in their own homes in rotation. Since one caregiver cannot manage more than two babies under a year, the co-op hires a full-time caregiver as a parent's assistant. Or several like-minded parents chip in and hire one or two highly qualified and highly paid caregivers to come to one of the houses to look after the babies.

On-site day care. Corporations that value keeping their employed mothers satisfied offer day care at the workplace. Check it out. If your corporation doesn't have this setup, lobby for it.

Commercial day care. In general, day-care centers are not advisable for infants under one year because of too many kids, too few staff members, and the increased chances of contagious illness at a child's most infection-vulnerable time.

Finding the Right Caregiver

Before you start the search for a specific caregiver, formulate the qualities you want — keeping in mind the realistic fact that your clone doesn't exist. As a starter, consider that you want *one substitute parent.* Consistency of care is the least you can offer your baby. The same caregiver with the same mind-set as you is idealistic, yes; but it's a place to begin. Next, try the following sources for possible leads.

Friends. Spread the word around your like-minded friends. They may know of available caregivers, and the fact that they know your mothering style gives you a bit of a preselection.

Baby's doctor. Pediatricians often have bulletin boards of child-care positions; be sure your doctor knows and recommends the caregiver (although this does not replace your thoroughly checking this person out yourself). The doctor is likely to know mothers who run a mini-day-care center in their own homes, rather than those who will come to yours. Consider putting up your own help-wanted notice on the doctor's bulletin board.

Resource and referral agencies. Training in how to find quality care is provided by these agencies. They also maintain a referral list of licensed day-care houses and facilities in your community. If no agency is available in your area, contact your local social service agency.

Also consider these sources:

• your church or synagogue
• senior-citizen organizations
• hospital auxiliaries
• your local La Leche League group
• newspaper ads — best to write your own
• nanny, au pair, and baby-sitting agencies

Interviewing Candidates

For those of you who have to sift through resumes and conduct interviews trying to decide to whom you will entrust your precious baby, here's how to make the decision process less overwhelming and the selected caregiver less of a stranger.

Make a list. Before starting the selection process, make a list of questions you need to ask (see list below). Put the most important questions at the top so if the answers aren't satisfactory you don't waste time covering your whole list.

Screen first. To save time and fruitless interviewing, ask applicants to send you resumes and references. Select from these whom to telephone interview. Begin at the top of your question list and, as you get a phone feel for the person, either complete the list or gracefully terminate the conversation. If uncertain, by all means get a personal interview. Don't let a good person get away. Phone interviews, while timesaving and helpful, can be misleading. Beware the person reluctant to provide references. The right caregiver expects to be asked for references.

Your first impressions. First by phone, then face-to-face, impress upon the prospective caregiver how you value substitute care and the importance of her nurturing your baby the way you want your baby mothered. But don't get too specific, since you want to find out her own nurturing values before you reveal yours, lest she simply parrot what you want to hear. Besides the usual name, age, address, phone number, and so on, try these probing questions:

• What will you do when my baby cries? How will you comfort him? In your experience what comforting techniques work best for you? What do you feel about spoiling? (In these openers, try to get the person to talk about baby care — while you listen and see if you match mind-sets. Is she basically a nurturing, sensitive, and responsive person?)

- What would you like to know about my baby? (Get a feel for her flexibility. If you have a high-need baby, can she match her giving with baby's needs? You may need to offer more pay for this kind of baby care.)

- How do you feel about holding a baby a lot?

- What do you feel a baby this age needs most? (As you are getting a feel for her nurturing abilities and her flexibility, you're also getting a sense of whether you can work with this person and trust your baby with this person. Also, watch how she interacts with your baby during the interview. Is it forced or natural? And how does your baby interact with her?)

Now it's time to get down to the specifics:

- Why do you want to look after babies?

- Tell me about your last job. Why did you leave it?

- How will you play with my baby during the day?

- How will you handle feeding my baby? (If you are breastfeeding, does she understand the importance of offering your pumped breast milk?)

- How will you put my baby to sleep?

- If my baby throws a tantrum, how will you handle it? How will you discipline him if he seems defiant?

- What are the most common accidents that you feel he is likely to have? What precautions will you take? Have you taken a CPR course? (If yes, ask to see the certificate. If no, would she be willing to take a course on her own time?)

- What would you do if my baby was choking on a toy? (Ask this to test her knowledge; see page 719 for answer.)

- What factors may interfere with your being on time? Do you travel a long distance? By car or by public transportation? (Was she on time for your appointment? — a question to ask her references also.)

- Do you drive? (Ask this only if driving is a requirement for your caregiver.)

- Tell me about your previous child-care experience.

- Do you have children of your own? What are their ages? (Determine if the care of her own children may compromise her availability for the care of yours. If she has school-age children, what alternate care does she have if her children are sick? If she has a baby or preschool child and wants to bring her child along, discuss this option. Meet mother and child together to see how they interrelate and get a feel for the temperament of her child. Do you want your child also to spend the day with this child? Realize that there will always be a "her child — my child" compromise, and if her child is going through a high-need stage at the same time as yours, guess who will get the attention.)

- How long do you plan to do child care? (Consistency is important for your child to build up an attachment.)

- Are you willing to do some housework? (Ideally have the caregiver do some household chores while baby is sleeping, which gives you more time with baby after work. But a person who will keep both your baby nurtured and your house immaculate is a rare find.)

• How is your health? What is your physician's name, and could I check on the date of your last examination? Are you a smoker? (Smoking and babies don't mix.) Do you drink? How much and how often? Do you use other drugs? (While you are unlikely to hear a yes answer, get a sense of her level of comfort or agitation at answering the question.)

Ask yourself if she is a physical match for your baby. While frail grandmothers, so soft and patient, may wonderfully rock a three-month-old all day, they may not have the stamina to keep up with a busy toddler. During your interview get a feel for this person's mannerisms, and consider your feeling for the overall person. Is she kind, patient, flexible, nurturing, with an overall presence and mannerisms that are contagious in a healthy way? *Basically, is she a person you want your baby to form an attachment to?*

If with the first interview you don't succeed, keep trying, remembering the importance of making the right match. Be prepared, however, to make some compromises. You will quickly realize the person you want may not exist, and the demand for quality caregivers far exceeds the supply. Keep this in mind when you begin negotiating fees.

Giving Your Substitute a Trial

After you've made your choice, agree beforehand on a trial period of a few weeks to see if she, baby, and you fit. Here's how to tell.

Use baby as a barometer. Expect an initial change in baby's behavior for two reasons. Not only is he getting used to different care,

but you are, too. Sometimes it's more the difference in mother (tired, preoccupied, stressed from work) that accounts for baby's behavior changes. But after a week or two baby should settle down into his previous behavior. If he becomes clingy, aggressive, angry, wakeful, or mopey and that spark has diminished, something is amiss. Either it's a baby-caregiver mismatch or you need to reassess the timing of your return to work.

Use the caregiver as a barometer. Is she enjoying your baby? Or do you come home to a frazzled, irritable, tense person who can't wait to relieve herself of this burden? That's a red flag. (Accept some days' wear and tear as normal baby-tending effects.) If, on the other hand, she and baby show signs of a match, you can sleep better.

Look for good-care signs. Besides baby's emotional state, is there evidence of good maintenance? For example, are diapers changed often enough? Does baby's bottom have a rash and odor not present presitter? In all fairness it could be coincidental to teething, change of diet, or diarrhea.

Make spot checks. Periodically arrive unannounced early or on a lunch break. If you have a high-need baby who needs a lot of holding, how much has he been left to cry it out? Short of a hidden video camera or audio recording, spot checks tell you a lot. Without your having to be either paranoid or lax, in time a caregiver will earn your trust, making such regular surveillance less necessary. But some continued monitoring reinforces the fact that you expect her to take her job conscientiously.

Ask for neighbors' and friends' observations. Tell your friends and neighbors about your situation and ask them to kindly report any concerns. If your sub takes baby to the park for group play, ask the other mothers to comment.

Introducing Your Sub

It's not fair to caregiver or baby to throw the two together without a proper introduction. Before the day of departure, have the caregiver spend some time with you and your baby. This gradual acquaintance serves several purposes: It helps baby get acquainted with her, it helps her get acquainted with baby, and it allows you to model for your sub how you want your baby cared for. Especially if baby is in the stranger-anxiety stage, a gradual warm-up is best (see page 514 for tips on introducing baby to strangers). Remember to put on your friendly face when greeting this new friend. If she's OK to you, she's OK to baby. This is also a good time to see your sub in action. You can always change your decision. If the initial impressions are good, ease the caregiver into baby care as you ease into your work.

It's best not to start right off with eight-hour days and forty-hour weeks. Begin leaving baby for short intervals, ideally between feedings, and *gradually* lengthen the time away. Begin back to work on a Wednesday or Thursday to ease the separation.

THE COMMERCIAL DAY-CARE OPTION

Although group day care is not recommended for infants, there are times when this really is the only reasonable alternative for working parents. Here are some ways to make the best of this situation.

Selecting a Day-Care Center

Child-care providers deserve the respect and compensation given to teachers. They are more than pigtail-and-bubble-gum babysitters. These persons are substitute parents. Learn what quality day care should be and seek it out, rather than settling for mediocrity. Your child will benefit. Here are some tips to help you in making the selection.

- Check out the center, or preferably several of them, spending some time watching the caregivers and children relate. Find out which person will be primarily looking after your baby. Watch how she relates to the children in her charge. How does she discipline them? When they cry, how does she comfort them? Is she sensitive? Does she give the children eye-to-eye contact? Does she touch and hold them? Does she engage in lively conversation? Does she appear to enjoy handling babies? Is she able to adapt to the ever-changing moods of some toddlers? Does she have a sense of humor? Also, above all, watch how the children relate to the caregivers. By observing staff and children interacting, you will get a feel if there is a genuine connection there.

- Ask about the ratio of caregivers to children. The rule of thumb we mentioned earlier for home day care (one one-year-old child, two two-year-olds, and so on) would be unaffordable in commercial day care. The maximum should be no more than four children for one caregiver.

- Examine the licensing to be sure that it is current.

- Inquire about the credentials of the staff.

- Ask what the philosophy of the center is. Use leading questions, like "What will you do when my baby is crying? What do you feel about spoiling?"

- Browse around the facilities. Are they clean? Is the equipment safe? Are the toys age appropriate?

- Are the children generally happy? Does the staff appear caring, connected, and attentive, or more distant and detached from the kids?

- Ask about their sick-child policy, whom they admit, whom they don't. Watch their sanitation procedures. Do they wash hands after changing diapers, maintain separate diapering and food-serving areas, sanitize the toys when necessary, and discourage sharing of bottles, pacifiers, and other personal items?

- Is all the staff trained in CPR? Ask to see their certificates. Do they have a policy for handling disasters and emergencies such as fires?

- Visit the center at a time when other parents are dropping off or picking up their children. Ask for references.

- Finally, is this a place you enjoy being?

Don't feel you are imposing on the day-care center by asking probing questions. The industry to which we are entrusting the future of our country should have high standards and be willing to demonstrate them. If the only available day-care center fails the test questions, seriously consider getting welfare assistance so you can stay with your baby until appropriate care can be located.

Too Sick to Attend Day Care? How to Tell

It's seven o'clock in the morning and family rush hour begins. The teakettle is whistling,

---

A DAY-CARE TIP

Establish routines for day-care drop off and pickup to make transition times easier for small children. A special "hug and kiss refuel" on departure and on reunion eases the separation anxiety. Remember, too, that it is hard for a child who is engrossed in play to drop everything the minute the parent walks in. Briefly join in your child's activity, show interest in what he is doing, and gradually close out the activity. (See page 535 for departure tips in closing out play.)

---

the toaster's popping, and the traffic report is the usual bad news. Enter a whine that will turn your already overbooked day upside down. By reflex you lay hands on your baby's head. "Oh, no, a fever!" To day care or not to day care, that is the question. Suddenly you realize that it is not so easy to change jobs at the touch of a forehead.

How sick is sick enough to miss day care? This decision affects three parties: Does your baby feel too sick to attend day care? Is she contagious to the other children? How convenient is it for you to take a day off from work? Here are some practical guidelines on what germs are the most catchy.

Diarrhea Illnesses

Here is one set of germs that all doctors agree are very contagious. Frequent, watery, mucousy, and sometimes bloody diarrhea is a sure indication to stay home, both for your baby's sake and to prevent an outbreak in the center. Add vomiting — parents call this a double ender — and your baby is certainly too weak and too upset to leave home. As soon as the vomiting is over, the stools are no longer explosive and watery, and your baby feels better, she may return to day care. Be prepared for the bowel movements to remain loose and frequent for weeks, as the intestines are notoriously slow to recover. During this convalescent stage of diarrhea, your baby is not contagious.

Colds and Fevers

While diarrhea illnesses merit quarantine, respiratory and febrile illnesses are a different bag of germs. Most cold germs do not threaten an outbreak in the day-care center as much as diarrhea germs do. In fact, studies in school-age children have shown that excluding children from school does not diminish the spread of colds; admitting kids with colds to school does not increase their spread (the contagious period is variable, and babies are most contagious a day or two before they act sick). When you send your two-year-old to day care with a cold, this is one time to teach her not to share. Show her how to cover her nose and mouth with a tissue when she sneezes or coughs and to turn her head away from others. Two-year-olds may be able to learn this sanitation gesture but are likely to forget. If your baby has a fever (persistent temperature of at least 101°F/38.03°C) it is prudent to keep her out of day care until you ask your doctor whether she is contagious.

Sore Throats

Sore throats, especially those associated with fever and throat sores (for example, hand, foot, and mouth disease, see page 710), are very contagious and are a red light for day-care attendance until the fever and the throat sores are gone — usually around five days.

WHEN TO STAY HOME WITH A COLD

If your baby's nasal secretions are clear and watery, and your baby is happy and playful, pain free, and has only a low-grade fever (100°F/37.8°C) there is no need to keep your baby home from day care. If the nasal secretions become more thick, yellow, and green, especially if accompanied by a fever, an earache, frequent night waking, or a peaked look — in mother jargon, a sick-looking face — this is a stay-home-and-call-the-doctor cold. Your baby may have an ear or sinus infection. In reality, a cold can be contagious for two or more weeks, yet it is unrealistic to expect to miss work for that long. When to send only a mildly sick baby to day care depends a lot on the ability of the day care to separate potentially contagious children.

Before you jump to change your whole day, here's a nasal secretions tip: The goop from the nose is always thicker upon awakening in the morning, since it has had a chance to stagnate during the night. To help assess the situation, squirt a few saline nose drops into each of your baby's stuffy nostrils and encourage a gentle nose blow, or remove the secretions with a nasal aspirator (see page 665). If the remaining secretions are clear and your baby breathes better, you can breathe easier, and it's off to day care.

Eye Drainage

The nose is not the only thing that runs when baby gets a cold. Eye drainage is often associated with an underlying cold, especially a sinus infection. These eyes are not contagious, and usually neither is the rest of the baby. This type of goopy eye drainage does, however, merit a doctor visit.

Some runny eyes are due to conjunctivitis (often called pinkeye), a contagious infection that will send day-care providers rushing to make a come-get-your-baby call. If the eyes are bloodshot in addition to draining, this is contagious pinkeye, which is quickly treated and made noncontagious by an antibiotic eye ointment or drops. The baby may attend day care as long as treatment has begun. If the eyes are not bloodshot, this is seldom contagious conjunctivitis, and your child may still attend day care.

Colds Versus Allergies

Day-care centers often reject a coughing, sneezing child because of a cold when it's really an allergy that is not contagious to playmates and is no more than a nuisance to the child. How to tell a cold from an allergy? Back to the telltale nasal secretions. Allergic noses run and drip, are clear and watery, and are accompanied by other allergic signs: watery eyes, sneezing, wheezing, a past history of allergies, and the fact that it's hay fever season. The nasal drainage from a cold is too thick to run. It dangles. Also, with a cold there are other signs of infection, such as fever. In general, allergic children are noisy (sneezy and wheezy), but don't act sick. They may attend day care and are not contagious. Children with colds act sluggish, mopey, or cranky and may be contagious.

Coughs

Most colds end but the coughs of some linger, keeping babies out of day care and parents out of work. But all coughs are not automatically stay-home illnesses. A dry, hacking cough that neither awakens the baby nor is associated with fever, pain, difficult breathing, or other cold signs is not a reason for quarantine. These nuisance-type coughs linger on for weeks, are rarely contagious, and seldom bother the child or her mates, who themselves may also be coughing. Then there's the baby who coughs a lot at night but seems well during the day except for annoying throat-clearing sounds and may have several similar episodes during allergy season. This child suffers from postnasal drip, she is noncontagious, and this seldom is a reason to stay home from day care.

Of course, any cough accompanied by fever, chills, and the coughing up of green or yellow mucus warrants medical attention and absence from day care. Your baby can return to day care when the fever subsides and she feels better (usually in a few days), though the cough itself may linger for a week or two.

Rashes

The problem with rashes is that the day-care provider sees them and sends your baby home. But not all rashes are contagious or uncomfortable enough for a baby to miss day care.

Impetigo. A bacterial infection in the skin, impetigo begins as tiny red spots resembling picked-at pimples that enlarge to coin-sized blisters which rupture and produce an oozy, sticky, honey-colored crust. These circular spots may be as small as a pimple or as large as a quarter. They tend to occur in patches where babies scratch, such as beneath the nose and on the diaper area, but may occur anywhere on the skin. Scratching spreads these eruptions. You can cover the infected areas with the prescribed antibiotic ointment and a square bandage and send your baby back to day care. More severe cases may require oral antibiotics and a longer stay-at-home break.

Ringworm. A circular rash with red, raised borders, ringworm is caused by a fungus and is even less contagious than impetigo. Cover the area with an over-the-counter antifungal cream (or a prescription cream if necessary) and pack your baby off to day care.

Chicken pox. Unlike the rashes just mentioned, chicken pox is one of the most contagious of all childhood infections and a sure prescription to stay home. It begins as a flu-like illness (low-grade fever and tiredness), and the spots usually appear a day later. Initially, they resemble tiny bites over the back, chest, abdomen, and face. I'll frequently have patients waiting at my office door at 9:00 A.M. wondering if "these spots" could be early chicken pox. I pronounce them prickly heat or flea bites and dispatch the spotted baby to day care.

If you're uncertain about your baby's spots, circle a few with a felt-tipped pen; in a day they'll change from pimples to blisters if they're chicken pox, and new crops will appear. After several days, the early spots will crust. Baby can return to day care once all the spots are scabbed over, about a week after they first appear. (See also page 708.)

Head Lice

Where there are lots of children in a crowded place, expect little parasites to tag along. A typical scene: You get a call at your office or your baby is sent home from day care with a note informing you that she has head lice. Your first reaction is embarrassment ("But my house is so clean!") followed by incredulity ("She has to miss day care and I have to miss work because of a lousy louse?").

What's wrong with this picture? First, head lice are no reflection on your housekeeping. They live in warm, crowded environments like classrooms and day care, where they can easily pass from head to head as babies snuggle together. Lice don't carry disease and are more of a nuisance than a medical problem. They reside deep in the hair, most commonly around the nape of the neck and around the ears. In return for a warm, fuzzy place to live, they often don't bother the host, except for an irritating itch and unnecessary quarantine by the day-care provider.

Lice themselves are difficult to see (they're tiny, light brown, and may sometimes be seen with a magnifying glass), but you may find the whitish nits (egg sacs) attached to the base of individual hairs. You can distinguish nits from dandruff because nits are round and adhere to the hair shaft, unlike the flat flakes of dandruff that slide off easily.

If you see nits, you don't have to immediately share your discovery with your doctor. An over-the-counter lice shampoo (follow directions on package) and a specially designed nit-removal comb will suffice for an evening at-home treatment. Your baby may return to day care the next morning, but be prepared for the day-care provider to scan every hair looking for nits — hence the term "nit picker" — and to call for pickup if even one egg is found.

Who Plays Nurse When Baby Is Sick?

For dual-income families, who stays home when baby can't go to day care, mom or dad? Who can most afford to stay home? Who is most needed at work? Do you and your spouse split the shift or bring in the reserves? (Sick babies should have their mothers if at all possible — mother preference intensifies when baby is sick.)

While there is no better nurse than a caring parent in a child's own home, this ideal may not be possible, especially for financially strapped and single parents. Consider these alternatives.

Try shift work. Mom is nurse in the morning, dad in the afternoon. Your child gets special TLC from both parents and both sharpen their sick-child-care skills.

Take your baby to work. If your baby is not sick enough to stay home but is not permitted in day care, prepare a "sickroom" at work if circumstances permit. If you have your own office, set up camp in the corner, including her favorite books, toys, and blankets. This scene is also a prime chance for your child to learn about your work. If the older patient is willing and able, give her some time-occupying task to "help" you at work. Your child will feel important and get her mind off being sick.

Have grandmother on call. If blessed with a nearby extended family, ask grandma to pinch-hit. Grandmothers have time, unlimited patience, and the price is right.

Use a sick-child-care center. Explore what facilities for sick children are available in your community. Some day-care centers and hospital pediatric wards have get-well rooms, staffed with sensitive caregivers trained to care for sick children. However, they are expensive.

Plan ahead. Before your baby gets sick — and she will — devise a family game plan rather than scrambling for on-the-spot decisions with the first fever. Decide with your spouse who will stay home. Have backup caregivers on call. Find out your day-care center's sick-child admission policies. Are there home-care agencies available, and what is their cost? Find out what's available, affordable, and above all what's best for your child.

Sick-Leave Benefits

Taking a baby out of day care may mean paycheck deductions for working parents, but a day at home with your sick child can have its compensations. Being at home with your sick baby is a chance to rebond. Especially if you have recently locked horns with your child or she is going through an independence streak, a day at home may do wonders for your relationship. Babies go from independent to dependent when sick, as if clicking into a memory of what "mother" and "father" really mean. Making chicken soup and popsicles, giving back rubs and reading stories — a day at home with your baby is a chance for your nursing, and parenting, skills to shine.

18

Special Situations

Over the years of counseling families, we have come to recognize the phenomenon we call the need-level concept: Given the right advice and support, parents can adjust their level of caring to meet the need level of their baby. Special family circumstances and special-needs babies have a way of bringing out special qualities in parents. In the following challenges, we will show you how this happens.

PARENTING THE ADOPTED BABY

The long-awaited phone call comes. You're going to be parents, without the customary nine months of biological preparation. While there are a wide variety of circumstances, here are some general ways to ease into adoptive parenting.

Consider open adoption. During the writing of the first edition of this book, our eighth child, Lauren, came into our family by adoption. It was then that we realized that in most circumstances it's healthy to lift the veil of secrecy surrounding adoption. Open adoption means keeping lines of communication open between birth mother (or birth parents) and adopting parents. This permits prearranging a plan that is best for all parties. Many adopting parents and birth mothers are choosing open adoption because this arrangement benefits everyone, especially the child.

Open adoption benefits adopting parents by removing the surprises. They learn more about the genetic background of their child, and they don't have to live in fear that the birth mother will suddenly invade their lives. The birth mother, for her part, is continually reassured that the child is loved and well cared for. Removing the mystery about what happened to her child helps the birth mother reaffirm that she made the right choice. As a birth mother who chose open adoption once said, "Instead of having an abortion, I made four people happy — including myself."

Later on, letters of contact answer questions the child may have that can only be answered by the birth mother, avoiding imaginings that threaten self-worth. Statements such as "I gave you to your parents because I could not at that time give you the life I wanted you to have" are not from a person

429

who didn't care, and it's important for the adoptee to feel that.

Yet another value of open adoption came to us when we realized a biological mother could not sweep her birth memories under a rug and uncaringly get on with her life. This mature type of adoption exposes the myth that birth memories disappear. They won't! Open adoption encourages coming to grips with the fact that the baby has and always will have two sets of parents. In essence, open adoption allows all parties to tell the truth — and truth is therapeutic.

Get all the facts. Be certain to learn as much as you can about the biological parents: family history of inherited disease, prenatal care of the mother, possible drug use during pregnancy, and any other necessary medical or social information.

Be involved in the pregnancy. If you have the ideal adoptive situation — knowing the birth mother during her pregnancy — do what you can to ensure good prenatal care. Be sure she understands the importance of a drug-free, smoking-free pregnancy. Help her choose the right childbirth class and birth attendants, especially a labor support person. And be sure to assist her in receiving professional counseling before (and after) the birth.

Be involved in the birth plan. If possible (and if the birth mother is comfortable with the idea) be present at the birth. After the birth attendants ensure that baby is healthy, have baby "delivered" into your arms. Bond with *your* baby. Some adopting parents in our practice have even checked into a hospital room. They have fed and cared for their baby from birth to discharge from the hospi-

tal, taking part in the baby-care classes that the hospital offers.

Part of your birth plan that you both have previously worked out is what contact the birth mother will have with the baby immediately after delivery. In the movies, a baby is snatched from visual or skin contact with the mother and rushed out of the delivery room. The theory of this inhumane practice is out of sight, out of mind. Supposedly, this helps the mother forget the birth and get on with her life. Nonsense! The birth mother needs to be able to say good-bye.

While long-distance adoptions may delay an early bonding, try to assume the care of your baby as soon as possible after birth. Baby needs to know to whom he or she belongs. Granted, the legal formalities are important, but you are not simply transferring ownership of a package. You are assuming care of a person. Adopting parents often worry, If we miss the early bonding period, will baby and we be eternally deprived? No! Bonding is a lifelong process. Early bonding just gives you a head start. (See discussion of delayed bonding, page 44.)

Try attachment parenting. Adopting mothers often wonder if they will be adequate mothers. What are they missing by not having the biological boost of the hormones of pregnancy and birth? In my experience adopting mothers are so thrilled to finally have a baby that they are able to make up for these biological helps. For some parents it's love at first sight; for others it's a gradual process. The style of parenting you practice will affect the way your relationship progresses. The attachment style we advocate is particularly helpful for adopting parents. Try to practice as many of the attachment concepts as you can.

Adopting parents, both mothers and fathers, can also experience postpartum depression. This is most likely due to a combination of being fatigued and overwhelmed by so many changes so fast. Seek the support of other adopting parents and learn from their experience. For example, a special custom in some adopting families is to celebrate two birthdays: baby's biological birthday and the day baby legally became theirs.

Think about when to tell, how to tell. At this writing Lauren is ten years old. Here is how we told her she came into our family by adoption. First, we have never referred to her as our "adopted daughter." She is our daughter. This presentation conveys to inquirers that to us how she entered our home is of secondary importance to the fact that she's ours. Also, we have not kept the A-word a secret from Lauren. During the first couple of years Lauren heard the word "adoption" frequently, and when she was around the age of two, with the aid of storybooks about adoption, we eased Lauren into associating herself with the word. In order not to devalue her, we *minimized the difference* of adoption, since children equate being different with being less. Yet, we do celebrate two birthdays, her biological one and the day her adoption was finalized. Likewise, we thought it unwise to make a big deal of her "specialness" or that she was "chosen" since, as adoption counselors have discovered, this status may burden the child with the feeling that she has to measure up. By letting Lauren become familiar with the word "adoption," we helped her become comfortable with the term long before she understood its full meaning. Finally, as Lauren got older, we filled in — and will continue to fill in — the blanks according to her interest and understanding.

(For more information see "Adoption Resources," page 745.)

PARENTING TWINS

With twins, parenting means double the fatigue, double the fun. While most parents find the first year of life with twins a bit of a blur, here's how to make caring for multiples easier.

Doubly prepared. With ultrasound now routine during prenatal care, twins seldom come as a surprise. And remember, multiples usually come two or three weeks early. Waiting until the last minute may find you with an unfeathered nest. Read Chapter 3, "Preparing for Baby," and do most of your baby buying and nursery designing before your final months of pregnancy. In the last trimester, join the Mothers of Twins Club in your community. Attend their meetings before the birth of your babies and continue throughout at least the first year or two. There is no better resource than experienced parents sharing time- and energy-saving tips.

Double team. With singletons father involvement is a choice. With multiples it's a must. In caring for twins the mother-father roles are not clear-cut. Except for breastfeeding (and even here dad has duties), all the high-maintenance tasks of infant care can be shared by father. Yes, attachment parenting multiples takes more time and effort, but you get double the rewards. You may not be able to do the whole attachment parenting package all of the time. Do the best you can with the resources you have.

Dinner for two. Try to get both babies on a simultaneous feeding schedule. If dad is home, and you are bottlefeeding, each parent can feed a baby at the same time. If you are breastfeeding use the holding positions illustrated in the discussion of breastfeeding twins, page 193.

Double duties. As with simultaneous feedings, try to get babies on a similar sleep schedule. Having two set times during the day when all three of you lie down together helps establish a consistent nap routine. In the early months, double bathing will be impossible without four hands. If you find two in the tub too cumbersome, bathe one while the other one plays. Realize that babies don't need daily baths. Bathe one baby one day, the second the next, and yourself the third. Daily sponging of the face and diaper area during the out-of-tub days should suffice.

Doubly organized. With the birth of your twins comes an honorary degree in time management. Do what you have to do and *delegate the rest*. Give dad, grandma, or a trusted friend your shopping list. Let wait what can wait. Ask your equally tired friends at Mothers of Twins for shortcuts, for example, with preparing food. Diaper service is a real asset if you're using cloth diapers.

Double up in bed. Instead of putting babies in separate bassinets in the hospital, most twins calm more quickly and settle better if placed side-by-side or face-to-face in the same bassinet. After all, they have been womb-mates for nine months. As they get older, juggle sleep areas depending on whether they sleep better snuggled next to each other or separately. (See co-sleeper arrangement, page 333.)

Get help. Hire household help, at least in the early months. For parents of twins this is not a luxury; it's a necessity. If your friends ask what you need or what they can give you, ask for housekeeping help and solicit brought-in meals.

Carrying double. Carried babies cry less. Veteran parents have learned that this style of parenting calms babies. Double this for twins. One crying baby can set off the other, and the cumulative effects of double wailing can be nerve-racking. Get two baby slings, one for mom and one for dad, and frequently wear your babies out for a walk. The great outdoors can be a mind saver when you are feeling housebound.

Seeing double. If you have trouble telling your identical babies apart, try these labels: a bracelet on one, painting toenails different colors, cutting one's hair differently, and identifying clothing. Even for identicals, if you give each a total body scan you usually notice an identifying birthmark, dimple, or other feature that belongs only to one. Trying to match four look-alike shoes is the worst case of mistaken identity. Either buy different-looking pairs or use different shoelaces. As twins get older, even the most identical-looking ones develop unique features.

Name that twin. Keep in mind you are parenting individuals, not twins. Call them by their names, rather than "the twins."

Alike but different. As these little mates grow older, be prepared for them to play both ends. They like the specialness of being twins but also want to be individuals. One day they may want to dress alike; the next they may want to dress differently. Ride with the flow, treating them alike when they want to be twins and differently when they want to be individuals.

There's an extra dimension to watching twin development — babies relating to each other. Doubling the humor balances doubling the work load. The arrival of the sitting and crawling age is a major relief milestone for parents, as the duo can entertain each other, giving you much-needed baby breaks. Then comes the surveillance stage, as your eyes wander Ping-Pong-like, keeping both babies under your watchful gaze. The high-maintenance stage of twin raising soon lessens but never passes. Such are the joys of parenting a baby — and another baby. (For more information about parenting multiples see "Twins and Multiples," in "Resources," page 747.)

SINGLE PARENTING

Our hearts go out to mothers who by choice or by circumstance begin their parenting careers without a mate. While there are a variety of single-parenting circumstances for mothers and fathers, our discussion is limited to single mothers. Here are a few tips on being a nurturing mom to your baby while leaving some time to nurture yourself.

Choose the parenting style best for you. In our experience the style of parenting that works for most single parents most of the time is attachment parenting. You may not be able to do all of the elements of attachment parenting all of the time, but try to do as many as you can as often as you can. This way of parenting is more difficult when solo, but it's also more important. Without the help of

another parent to bounce decisions off of, you will need extra sensitivity toward your baby's behavior and extra knowledge of your baby's needs. Attachment parenting gives you the self-confidence to make decisions and the wisdom to carry them through. Consider the advantages of attachment parenting as discussed in Chapter 1 and you will see how this way of caring for your baby will improve the behavior of your child and make parenting life easier for you.

Don't do it alone. Single parenting is a misnomer. You may be a single parent, but you're not a superparent — nor should you have to be. Even two-parent households need help. Connect with support groups, other single parents, relatives, anyone who can lend an experienced and nurturing set of arms.

Reserve time for adult company. Realize you are set up for burn-out. To make up for baby not having an involved father, you may be tempted to immerse yourself in motherhood and slip into the trap of "My baby needs me so much I don't have time for anything or anyone else." Your baby needs a happy mother.

Solve custody squabbles sensitively. While the child is still an infant, divorcing parents would be wise to adopt the motto of juvenile courts: *Do what is in the best interest of the child.* A common situation is the baby who is not yet weaned but father demands overnight visitations. If you face this situation, a valuable resource is the "Custody or Visitation" pamphlet available from La Leche League. Visit www.lalecheleague.org or call (800) 435-8316 or (847) 519-7730.

Single moms often feel guilty, wondering if they are doing enough for their child, and cheated, wondering if they are getting enough out of life for themselves. Remember, parenting is a guilt-laden profession and even in the best of home circumstances, you will never feel that you are always the best mom you can be. Martha and I were both children of single parents, having lost our dads in early childhood. I remember as a child resenting the fact that my mother had to work long hours to support us, when that wasn't the case with the other kids on the block. Yet as a child, and to this day, not only did I feel loved but I sincerely believed that my mother was doing the best she could in less-than-ideal circumstances. If you can leave your child with these messages, you can feel you have done your best as a single parent.

THE DOWN SYNDROME BABY — A SPECIAL KIND OF PARENTING

As Martha gave her final push and I eased the precious head out of the birth canal, out popped a pudgy little hand with a curved little finger. In a flash I realized that we were parents of a baby with Down syndrome. The baby we expected was not the baby we got.

As we parent Stephen, we continue to realize that a child with special needs exacts from us a special kind of parenting. For special-needs children the principle of mutual giving really shines. As Stephen develops special skills, we develop special skills. He continues to stretch us while also bringing out the best in us. Here are the most common concerns parents have about the most common chromosomal abnormality.

How Frequent

Down syndrome (formerly called mongolism), named after Dr. Langdon Down, who described these children in 1866, occurs in one out of seven hundred births. The chance of having a Down syndrome baby increases with the age of the mother:

- women under age 25 — 1 in 2,000 births
- women at age 30 — 1 in 1,300 births
- women at age 35 — 1 in 400 births
- women at age 40 — 1 in 90 births
- women at age 45 — 1 in 32 births
- women at age 50 — 1 in 8 births

Depending on how they are presented, these figures can be scary. If a doctor says to a mother, "At age thirty-five you have five times the chance of having a Down syndrome baby that you did at age twenty," that would scare many senior mothers from conceiving. Here's how I present the risk factors to my patients who ask. At age twenty you had a 99.95 percent chance of *not* delivering a baby with Down syndrome; at age thirty-five your chances are 99.75 percent. Doesn't that figure sound more reassuring? This is why in my opinion the "thirty-five-year-old scare" is too young; forty-five perhaps? Even at age forty-five you have a 97 percent chance of delivering a baby *without* Down syndrome. So for mothers of later childbearing age, these figures are looking up.

Because of these risk factors, we believe that it is unwarranted to scare a thirty-five-year-old mother into prenatal diagnostic tests (either amniocentesis or chorionic villi sampling). Weigh these facts: At age thirty-five your statistical chance of delivering a Down syndrome baby is 0.25 percent. However, the risk of damage to a normal preborn baby during the tests may be around 1 percent. Whether or not you have prenatal diagnostic testing is an individual judgment call between you and your doctor.

Why Down Syndrome Occurs

Normally a sperm and an egg each contain twenty-three chromosomes. At fertilization they combine to form a cell with forty-six chromosomes. Sperm and egg cells undergo normal divisions, called meiosis, producing exact copies of the original cell. Sometimes, by chance, during meiosis the division is unequal. One cell gets one less chromosome and dies. The other cell gets one extra chromosome and lives. If this cell joins with a sperm (or egg), the resulting fertilized egg contains forty-seven chromosomes. In the case of Down syndrome the extra chromosome is number 21, so the genetic name for this syndrome is trisomy 21, that is, the cells have three number-21 chromosomes. There are other trisomies, which usually end in miscarriage or early infant death. Why an extra chromosome causes the features of Down syndrome is unknown. This unequal division of cells is called *nondisjunction.* It occurs by chance and accounts for 95 percent of the chromosome abnormalities in Down syndrome.

A rare genetic form of this syndrome (occurring in around 2–3 percent of these babies) happens by the mechanism of *translocation.* In this situation one of the number-21 chromosomes parts company with its mate and attaches to another chromosome, giving the appearance of the cell's having only forty-five chromosomes. However, the person is normal because he or she has all the genetic material of forty-six chromosomes. But when a sperm or an egg from this normal person containing the translocated number-21 chromosome joins with another sperm or egg, the resulting fertilized egg appears to have forty-six chromosomes but actually has three number-21 chromosomes. To confirm which type of chromosome abnormality your baby has, a geneticist analyzes your baby's chromosomes in a blood sample. The type of chromosomal abnormality, either nondisjunction or translocation, can be ascertained by looking at the chromosome alignment in your baby's blood cells. While most translocation abnormalities occur by chance, occasionally one parent is a *carrier* of cells that may contain a translocated number-21 chromosome and therefore has an increased risk of having more Down syndrome babies. If analysis of baby's blood reveals a translocation type of abnormality, analysis of the parents' blood will reveal whether this happened by chance or whether a parent is a carrier and therefore has a risk of future babies inheriting this abnormality.

Another type of Down syndrome is called *mosaicism,* meaning some of the baby's cells contain the normal number of chromosomes, and others have an extra number 21. This is why many cells of your baby's blood are analyzed. Sometimes, but not always, a baby with mosaic Down syndrome is less affected.

Why Us?

Chromosomal abnormalities happen by chance. You did not cause this by anything you did or did not do during pregnancy. A woman is born with a certain number of eggs and does not produce new ones during her life. The longer an egg lives, like any tissue, the more likely something is to go wrong. Why this happens in sperm is more of a mystery. New sperm cells are continuously being made. There is no such little creature as an old sperm. For some unknown reason the risk of nondisjunction occurring in sperm increases in men over fifty.

Possible Medical Problems

Down syndrome babies are prone to a number of potential medical difficulties. Among them are these.

- **Heart defects:** Around 40 percent of Down syndrome babies are born with an abnormally developed heart. Most of these conditions are now surgically correctable.

- **Intestinal defects:** Around 4 percent of these babies are born with a blockage in the upper intestine, called duodenal atresia. This must be surgically corrected to allow food to pass.

- **Hypothyroidism:** This occurs in around 10 percent of children with Down syndrome. Because the chance of this condition increases with age and may not be apparent on examination, it is wise to check your baby's thyroid function at least every two years.

- **Vision problems:** Many children with Down syndrome develop a variety of eye problems, such as crossed eyes, nearsightedness, farsightedness, and cataracts.

- **Hearing problems:** Around 50 percent of these children have varying degrees of hearing problems. Their increased susceptibility to middle ear infections contributes to this.

- **Instability of the vertebrae:** In approximately 10 percent of these babies the first two vertebrae, where the spinal column joins the neck, are unstable (called atlanto-occipital instability). Babies with this condition are prone to spinal cord injuries from a jolt during contact sports. All Down syndrome children should have X rays of the upper spine before being allowed to participate in contact sports.

- **More colds:** Down syndrome babies have reduced immunity, which together with small nasal passages makes them more prone to sinus and ear infections.

How Smart Are These Babies?

Children with Down syndrome have less-than average intellectual functioning; some are more impaired than others. With early intervention and special education many of these children join mainstream classes in school. Language lags are the most noticeable of the impairments. Because they do not go through motor milestones so quickly, it's like watching the remarkable unfolding of development in slow motion. Because parents cannot take milestones for granted, infant development takes on an added element of anticipation and excitement.

What they may lack academically, these babies make up for socially. Like all children, babies with Down syndrome have good and bad days. But, in general, these babies are affectionate and just plain happy. Many share constant hugs and kisses and radiate a generally carefree attitude. Their giving and caring attitudes are so contagious that those around these babies wonder who is really normal. There is indeed an up side to babies with Down syndrome.

Parenting These Special Babies

With these babies the attachment style of parenting really shines. It gives you the ability to read the special needs of your baby, almost like having a sixth sense. You will need a deeper sense of intuition and observation because your baby's cues may initially not be so easy to read. (See breastfeeding the baby with Down syndrome, page 188, for practical attachment suggestions.)

Weighing how your baby looks and acts in relation to other babies will tear you apart. As I was coming to terms with parenting a special-needs baby, every time I examined a baby in my office I would think, "Our baby doesn't look like that or feel like that." In reality, I was filling my mind with the gut-wrenching feelings that our baby was less valuable than other babies. The real breakthrough came when I was able to focus on the special qualities of our baby rather than on what he is missing compared with other babies.

Find out what resources, such as early intervention programs, are available within your community. Consider joining a Down syndrome support group if there is one in your area. You will be amazed at the practical suggestions and insights from parents who have gone through situations similar to yours and have coped and thrived and are able to share their experiences. One mother wrote to us: "Stephen will bring flashes of color to your life that you never knew existed." Some parents plunge right into as many support groups and community resources as they can and feel comfortable immersing themselves in learning as much as possible about parenting their child with special needs. Other parents feel more comfortable choosing only a few support resources, deciding it is better for their own family situation if they do not focus their entire lives on Down syndrome but, rather, incorporate their special-needs baby into the mainstream of family life. They feel this approach emphasizes more of the individuality of their special baby. For example, when baby Stephen rubbed his palm across my cheek, the caress of his soft touchy hand was unlike any touch I have ever felt. Special-needs babies can bring special gifts to the family. In my experience parents who practice attachment parenting get in harmony with their special-needs baby and develop an incredible sensitivity toward him. This sensitivity carries over into their social, marital, and professional lives. This sensitivity is also contagious to siblings. Parenting special babies is a family affair. I have noticed that when siblings pitch in and care for their special-needs brother or sister, it mellows out their usual egocentric and selfish natures, enabling them to become giving, nurturing, and sensitive children. In general, a special-needs baby can elevate the sensitivity level of the whole family.

On the other hand, parenting a special-needs baby can cause marital stress. It is necessary to keep some balance in your baby care. Some mothers focus totally on the special needs of the baby and withdraw from the needs of other members of the family. It is natural for a mother of a special-needs baby to feel, "My baby needs me so much; my husband is a big boy and can take care of himself." Each spouse needs to care for the other so that they can better care for their baby.

A word of advice for friends and relatives: The worst thing you can do is shower *sympathy* on the parents of a baby with Down syndrome. Statements like "I'm sorry for you . . ." devalue the baby — and the parents. After all, mother delivered a baby, perhaps not "normal" by our standards, but a unique person who will make his or her own contribution to that family and to society. After the birth of our baby, when the parade of friends began, the most uplifting statement I remember is from an experienced grandmother who offered, "My wish is for you to become excited about your special baby." (For more information about babies with Down syndrome, see "Down Syndrome" in "Resources," page 746.)

MIXING BABIES AND PETS

If you have raised a dog through puppyhood, bringing up a baby should be a breeze — but not without some planning.

Have Pet — Add Baby

Introducing a new baby to a pampered pet may bring out problems as intense as sibling rivalry. Here's how pet and baby can safely and peacefully get along.

Before Baby Arrives

If your pet has been the baby in a childless house, get it used to being around babies before yours arrives. Invite over friends with babies. Let your pet sniff (under supervision, of course) and get used to the scent of babies. Remember, the attention you lavished on Fido will now go to baby, so a bit of prepartum weaning is wise. When your pet demands attention, sit in a rocking chair and "mother" a baby doll, meanwhile letting your pet learn an ability that few humans have — delaying gratification. Like life with a new sibling, after an initial decrease of attention, sharing the house with the baby will eventually mean more attention for the pet.

Veterinarians recommend bringing home from the hospital an unwashed blanket or sleeper of baby's so that your pet can get used to baby's scent before the real person arrives.

And, of course, if dog or cat has been a member of the family bed, get it used to sleeping outside your bedroom before your new bedroommate arrives.

If your pet is proven not to be baby friendly, tough and heartless as it may be, find a new home for it before baby arrives. It's not worth the risk.

When Baby and Pet First Meet

When mom, dad, and baby bundle return to the pet's home, be prepared for frisky jumps into your arms. Pet misses you. Sit down on the floor or couch at pet level for a get-acquainted sniff. After pet and baby have met, let dog or cat snuggle next to you during baby feeding and holding time — like you would a sibling.

Postpartum with Pet

The first two weeks at home with baby and pet are a get-acquainted period. Never leave them together alone. Snappy dogs are unpredictable, and cats like to jump into bassinets and snuggle next to babies.

Have Baby — Add Pet

Do you really want a pet? Before choosing another family member consider the time, energy, and expense involved in caring for another set of legs — four at that. If a friend offers you a pet, remember there's no such thing as a free pet. While visions of your toddler romping through the yard with a dog seem appealing, during the high-maintenance stage of babyhood do you have time and energy to take care of two babies?

Beware of this parent trap: Stray dogs or cats wander into your yard, and your older children pounce to adopt the stray. Clutching their homeless furry friend, your child pleads, "Please, mommy, can we keep her?" The combination of a begging child and hungry pet is hard to snub. As charter members of the can't-say-no club, our home has provided shelter — and more than overnight — to many a stray. And sometimes at a cost we weren't prepared for. Here's a pet-bargaining tip: When your older child wants a pet, be sure he or she agrees to care for the animal — and get it in writing.

Choosing a Pet

Certain pets and babies don't mix. Kittens and cats are usually kind to babies. Certain breeds of dogs are more baby friendly than others. Avoid unpredictable breeds, such as Doberman pinschers. Shun breeds that have high-strung personalities, such as little "yappers" who often compensate for their size with unpredictable and unpleasant behaviors. Try a gentle breed, such as a Labrador retriever. Purebred is less risky, but a healthy pound dog with a gentle nature may be brought home on trial. Before purchasing or bringing home a pet, be sure the previous pet owner agrees on a two-week trial. If the pet's temperament and the baby don't mix, keep baby and return pet.

Keeping a Healthy Pet

While it's true pets bring more joy than germs to children, keeping your pet well is part of the total family health package. Before selecting a pet (gift or purchase) have your vet check the animal. Periodically, have the vet deworm and deflea your pet. A flea-bitten baby and a flea-ridden pet make an uncomfortable combination. Keep your pet's immunizations current. Free or lowcost immunization clinics are available in most communities.

If Dog Bites Baby

Seek proof from the owner that the dog has been fully immunized and the shots are current. Dog-bite cuts become easily infected. Clean the wound with antiseptic soap, and cover with an antibiotic ointment until the wound is healed. If the bite inflicts a severe wound, your doctor may prescribe an antibiotic. If the dog is a stray and immunizations are unknown, call the dog shelter or local dogcatching agency to quarantine the dog for signs of rabies. Check the outcome with these agencies and notify your doctor if rabies is suspected. Make note of the circumstances surrounding the bite. Was it provoked or unprovoked? Was the dog acting strange?

Safety Around Pets

By two years of age your child can understand how to behave safely around pets. Remember, babies treat animals like toys. They pull ears, tails, jump on dogs, and throw cats. Let sleeping and feeding pets lie. Teach your child not to grab the dog's bone or dish while the pet is eating. Put feeding dishes out of reach of the curious toddler. The most common cause for biting is a dog defending his food.

Teach your child how to approach a strange dog, and be especially vigilant when visiting the home of someone with a pet. Let the animal approach the child. Have your child stand still as the pet circles and sniffs. Teach your child not to stare at the animal, provoke the pet with jerky movements, or run from the dog. Speak to the dog in a high-pitched, soothing voice like you would talk to a baby. Children tend to provoke dogs, and some dogs are more easily provoked than others.

Pets and babies do mix, but only with care.

IV

Infant Development and Behavior

What changes can we expect from month to month? What can we do to help our baby be bright and happy? How will each stage affect our lives? Can we really make a difference in how our child turns out? These are common questions new parents ask concerning the growth and development of their babies. The most exciting new discovery is the profound effect that the style of parenting has. How a baby grows used to be viewed as a sort of developmental elevator. From month to month baby went up a floor, the door opened, and baby got off to encounter new skills. Given a reasonable amount of nurturing, nutrition, and health care, baby would graduate from one developmental stage to another at a pace determined primarily by genes and temperament.

This simplistic view is partially true, but there's more. Each baby enters the world with his or her own potentials, like a capabilities cup. Some babies have larger cups than others. How close baby comes to fulfilling his or her potential depends to a large extent on the nurturing and responsiveness of the caregivers. You can influence how full your baby's capability cup becomes. In the following pages, we'll show you.

19

Growing Together: Enjoying Your Baby's Developmental Stages

L et's look again at that developmental elevator. A baby reaches each developmental floor equipped with certain competencies. How these competencies flower into skills depends upon *interaction* with the caregiving environment baby finds on that floor. If the interaction is responsive and enriching, baby gets back on the elevator with more skills, and the ride up to the next floor is much smoother. Because baby reaches the next floor with more skills, the interaction on the next level of development is even more rewarding.

GROWING TOGETHER

Our approach in the following chapters is to focus not only on the growth of the baby but also on that of the parents — the growth of a relationship. *Infant development* and the modern cliché *infant stimulation* mean not only what the infant does and what parents do for the infant, but what baby and parents do for one another. They grow together as a family. Here's how it happens.

Mutual sensitivity. As you travel through the first two years of development together, something good happens to both of you. You become more sensitive to each other.

Mutual shaping. As you and your baby become mutually sensitive to each other, you begin to shape each other's behavior. Mutual shaping of behavior is well illustrated by the ways parents and baby shape one another's language. On the surface parents appear to undergo a regression to the level of the baby. They act, talk, and think down at the baby's level. The parents first become like the baby in order that the baby can more easily become like the parents — all developing communication skills that none had before. This concept of mutual shaping is one of the most important ways parents and baby learn how to fit together.

Mutual competence. As you and your baby become more sensitive to one another and shape one another's behavior, you develop competence. Your baby gives a cue. You watch, listen, learn, and respond. Because of your keen perception and quick response, baby is more motivated to continue giving cues.

Take, for example, the way baby develops social competence. In the first days, even hours, of life baby cries to get fed or comforted. Parents respond. In time baby refines these "Pick me up" cues to facial or body language gestures. Parents perceive this new language and respond. Because of this responsive social setting, baby learns better social language, and parents develop better cue-reading abilities.

Baby is not, as previously thought, a passive player in the parenting game. She takes an active part in shaping behavior and building the competence of parents, providing they develop a parenting style that lets it happen.

ATTACHMENT PARENTING: HOW IT BUILDS BETTER BABIES — AND PARENTS

Over our many years in pediatric practice we have noticed a remarkable correlation between certain parenting styles, and their lack, and the development of babies. The style of parenting that works for most families most of the time is attachment parenting. In Chapter 1 we listed the seven tools of attachment parenting (see page 6), and in subsequent chapters we have discussed how this style of nurturing benefits a baby's growth and development. Let's briefly review the most important points.

Attachment Parenting Helps Babies (and Parents) Thrive

All babies grow, but not all babies thrive. Thriving takes growth a step further, to baby's fullest potential. Helping babies thrive is what attachment parenting is all about. Research has proven what parents have long known — that something good happens to parents and babies when they're attached. For example:

- Infants of parents who practice attachment parenting show more advanced developmental skills compared with infants given more restrained and distant styles of parenting.

- Infants who are breastfed on cue and have a timely weaning, are worn in slings during the day, sleep beside their mother at night, and are given an immediate nurturant response to crying eventually become more independent. These styles do not, as previously believed, create overly dependent children.

- Infants whose cues are sensitively attended to later develop more competent social skills.

- Attachment parenting enriches brain growth. In studies, sensitively nurtured infants scored higher on mental development and IQ tests.

- Infant animals who stay closer to their mothers have a higher level of growth hormones and enzymes essential for brain growth. Separating from or not interacting with their mothers causes the levels of these growth-promoting substances to fall.

Fascinating results from these attachment studies. Here is what we believe happens when parents and baby connect.

Attachment Parenting Organizes Babies

By organizing behavior, attachment parenting helps babies conserve energy.

WRITING YOUR BABY'S STORY

Want to make a memory that lasts a lifetime? Create your baby's own book. Beginning with your birth story, journalize your baby's development.

Recording tips. Your recording system can range from a minimum-effort simple scratch pad, and a stick-on-sticker baby calendar, to authoring your baby's full story on a computer. We found it easiest to keep a pocket-sized tape recorder handy on the most accessible kitchen counter. Dictate those memorable events when they occur, sometimes as they are occurring, baby's first steps, for example. Periodically type these notes or hire a friend to type them for you. (The "Martha notes" excerpts throughout this book are drawn from her journals of Matthew and Stephen.)

What to record. Too much verbiage obscures the main event. Start each topic with an opener, a highlighted minititle similar to the format we use in this book. This makes it easier to scan and retrieve information later. Record high points of your baby's development: first sit, first step, and first words. Also highlight humorous events and cute scenes — we call them the catch of the day: "Today I caught Johnny unrolling the toilet paper across the room!" And don't forget special occasions, like birthdays. Note special clips of *your* development. Oftentimes you will respond to a baby's cues in a way that amazes you: "I did that?" or "It worked!" Don't let your wisdom go unrecorded.

In the early months or years you will probably make daily or weekly entries because baby does so many new things so fast. As baby grows or the reporter tires, you may record only the headlines of special events or make once-a-month entries. It's fun later to pick up your baby's story and reflect on the person he was and the person he is now. It also helps you reconnect with your growing child during phases in your life when the fleeting features of childhood have faded from your memory. You might even want to give a copy of your diary (easier to duplicate if it is typed) to your "baby" as a wedding gift, or when he or she becomes a parent. By referring to the fussy moments and sleepless nights recorded in mother's journal, your grown child will gain insight into how he or she was parented.

Because their behavior is better organized, attachment-parented babies cry less than other babies. If they cry less, what do they do with their free time? They spend more time in quiet alertness and divert the energy conserved from not crying into growing. During quiet alertness babies interact and learn the most from their environ-ment, and their physiologic systems work better.

Attachment Parenting Is Good Brain Food

The brain grows more during infancy than at any other time, doubling its volume and reaching approximately 60 percent of its adult size by one year. As the brain grows, nerve cells called neurons, which resemble miles of tangled electrical wires, rapidly proliferate. The infant is born with much of this wiring unconnected. During the first year, these neurons learn to work better and connect up with each other to make circuits that enable baby to think and do more things. The more baby interacts with the caregiving environment, the more nerve connections she makes, and the better the brain develops. Attachment parenting helps the developing brain make the right connections.

The Shutdown Syndrome

One day, first-time parents Norm and Linda came to me for consultation, along with their four-month-old high-need baby, Heather. The family had been practicing the attachment style of parenting and, though often exhausting, it had worked for them. Heather had been a happy, thriving baby. Then well-meaning friends (aka baby trainers) persuaded Norm and Linda that they were spoiling Heather, that she was running their lives and manipulating them, and she would be forever dependent.

Somehow they lost confidence in their intuitive style of parenting and yielded to these pressures of a more restrained and distant style of parenting. Heather was scheduled, left to cry herself to sleep, and was not carried as much. Over the next two months Heather's weight leveled off. She went from happy and interactive to withdrawn. Her sparkle left, and she was no longer thriving — neither were the parents. Heather was about to undergo an extensive medical evaluation for failure to thrive. After listening to the parents' story and examining Heather, I diagnosed the shutdown syndrome and explained: Heather had a high need to connect with her parents. Because of their responsive style of parenting she was an organized baby and trusted that her needs would be met. And it was working. When the attachment plug was pulled, her connection was lost, as was her trust. A sort of baby depression resulted, and her physiologic systems slowed down. I advised the parents to return to their previous parenting style, carrying her a lot, breastfeeding on cue, responding sensitively to her cries by day and night and, above all, adopting a style of parenting that worked for them, not someone else's parenting advice. They did, and Heather thrived once more.

HOW BABIES GROW

Before we begin our journey through infant development from birth to two years, here are some basic principles that will help you understand and enjoy the individual variations of your baby.

Getting-Bigger Charts

At each well-baby checkup your doctor will plot your baby's height, weight, and head circumference on a growth chart. In the most commonly used charts, each line represents a percentile, which means that's where your baby is, compared with a hundred other babies. For example, the fiftieth percentile, or average, means that one half of babies plot above the line, the other half below. If your baby plots in the seventy-fifth percentile, he is larger than average. Twenty-five babies plot above your baby, and seventy-five below. Note that these charts are not infallible. They represent averages of thousands of babies. Average growth is not necessarily normal growth. Your baby has his or her individual normal growth. These charts are simply handy references to alert the doctor to any unhealthy trends. (See the growth charts in the appendix.)

Getting-Smarter Charts

Your baby gets bigger not only in size but also in competence. Developmental charts show the average age at which infants perform the most easily identifiable skills, such as sitting or walking, called *developmental milestones*. The developmental chart used most by pediatricians, the Denver Developmental Screening Test (DDST), shows that 50 percent of children walk at one year of age, but the normal range for beginning to walk is ten to fifteen months of age. Expect your baby to show uneven development in many of the developmental milestones. He may plot "ahead" in one milestone and "behind" in another.

Progression Is More Important Than Timing

When a child does what is not as important as moving through a progressive sequence of developmental milestones. Your baby will progress from sitting to pulling up to standing to walking. He may accomplish these motor milestones at different ages than the baby next door. But they both will follow a similar progression. Compare your baby only with himself as he was a month ago.

Infants spend different amounts of time at each stage before moving on to the next higher stage. Some infants seem to make a quick stop at one level and then quickly progress to the next. Some may skip a level entirely. Avoid the neighborhood race to see whose baby walks first. Milestone races are neither an indication of baby's smartness nor a badge of good parenting.

Why Infants Grow Differently

Not only do babies look and act differently from one another, they grow differently. That's what makes them unique. It helps parents to understand the wide variation in normal growth patterns and the way that many of life's little setbacks may affect growth and development.

Baby's body type. Your baby is endowed with tall and slim genes, short and wide genes, or in-between genes. Ectomorphs (tall and slim "bananas") often put more calories into their height than weight, so that they normally plot above average in height and below in weight, or they may start out hovering around the average line and eventually begin a stretching-out phase, soaring up the chart in height but leveling off in weight. Mesomorphs ("apples") show a stocky squared-off appearance. They usually center around the same percentile in both height and weight. Endomorphs ("pears") plot in the reverse of ectomorphs, often charting in a higher percentile for weight than height. All of these variations are normal and indicate the importance of looking at your baby (and his family tree) while looking at the chart, and putting the two together.

Growth spurts. While the chart implies a smooth, steady progression, many babies don't grow that way. Some babies grow in bursts and pauses, and when you plot them on the growth chart, you notice periodic growth spurts followed by periods of leveling off. Other babies show a consistent, steady increase in height and weight over the first year.

Health and nutrition. Sick babies temporarily divert their energy into healing rather than growing. During prolonged colds your baby's growth may level off. With diarrheal illnesses your baby may even lose weight. Expect catch-up spurts after the illness is over. Breastfed and bottlefed babies may show different growth patterns, and the growth charts currently in use do not differentiate. Some breastfed babies, especially high-need babies and frequent feeders, may plot high on the weight chart and be unfairly dubbed "overweight." Nearly all of these "overweight" breastfed babies begin a natural slimming process around six months to a year, when breast milk fat naturally lowers. Both breastfed and bottlefed infants who plot on the overweight side in the first six months normally begin a slimming process that we call "leaning out" between six months and a year as their increasing motor milestones help them burn off the chubby rolls. (See page 139 for weight differences of breastfed and formula-fed infants.)

THE FIVE FEATURES OF INFANT DEVELOPMENT

As we travel through infant development from birth to two years, we will group baby's developmental skills into five general areas: gross motor skills, fine motor skills, language skills, social and play skills, and cognitive skills.

Gross motor skills. How your infant uses the larger muscles of his body — trunk, limb, and neck muscles — is determined by his gross motor skills. They include such milestones as head control, sitting, crawling, and walking. The progression of gross motor skills from birth to two years means getting more and more of his body off the ground, moving from head to toe.

Fine motor skills. Finger and hand skills that baby uses to manipulate toys rely on fine motor skills. Like gross motor skills, fine motor skills develop in an orderly progression, from imprecise punchlike reaching to pinpoint pickup with the thumb and index finger.

Language skills. Here is where your skills as a baby communicator really shine. Parent input can affect language development more than any other of your baby's skills. You may think that babies don't talk much until one and a half to two years. Baby "talk" begins at birth. The cry of a newborn that causes nurses to come running, that causes mother to drip milk and embrace her baby, and causes a parent to bump into furniture during a nighttime sprint toward the 3:00 A.M. summons — that's language! To a tiny baby, language is any sound or gesture that makes a caregiver respond. During the first year, called the prelinguistic stage of language development, baby learns to communicate before she is able to say words. Early in the newborn period a baby learns that her language, the cry, is a tool for social interchange that she can use to get attention and satisfy needs. By sensitively responding to your baby's early cries, you help her refine these somewhat demanding signals into more polite body language requests that are easier on the nerves.

Mothers are naturals at talking with their babies. Language researchers who have studied mothers all over the world notice a sort of universal mother language, called motherese. Mothers are intuitively able to speak down to the baby's level, yet they're able to shift to a higher level of communication when their infants are ready.

Social and play skills. The ways a baby interacts with caregivers and plays with toys make up her social skills. Like language development, interaction with caregivers can profoundly affect social development. In the fun-things-to-do-with-your-baby suggestions for each stage of development, we give time-tested play tips to help you and your baby have more fun.

Cognitive skills. We have frequently watched our babies' facial expressions and said, "I wonder what he's thinking." While you will never be certain what goes on in your baby's developing mind, it is fun to deduce what your infant is thinking by his expressions and the way he is acting. Cognitive skills include the ability to think, to reason, to make adjustments to different play situations, and to solve problems such as how to crawl over obstacles. We will point out what signs to watch for to give you a clue to what your baby is thinking.

Make Your Own Chart

A valuable exercise during the first two years is to make your own growth and development chart like the one shown in this chapter. Using a large poster board, list the areas of development down the left-hand side and monthly stages of development across the top. Divide the sheet into blocks and plot your baby's skills. Concerning cognitive development, fill in what you think is going on in baby's mind. For simplicity, you may wish to combine social and language milestones, as we have done on our chart and throughout these chapters. Charting your baby's development not only improves your skills as a baby watcher, it adds to your overall enjoyment of growing together. (See the growth charts in the appendix.)

SEVEN WAYS TO BUILD A BRIGHTER BABY

You can make a difference in your baby's brain development. New insights into how a baby's brain grows show that parents can have a profound effect on how smart their child later becomes. The brain grows more during infancy than at any other time, tripling its weight and reaching approximately 60 percent of its adult size by one year. As the brain grows, nerve cells called neurons proliferate, resembling miles of tangled electrical wires. The infant is born with much of this wiring unconnected. During the first year, these neurons grow larger, learn to work better, and connect up with one another to make circuits that enable baby to think and do more things.

Here's how these circuits work. The tips of each neuron resemble fingerlike feelers attempting to make connections with other nerves. During development two important

(text continues on page 454)

INFANT DEVELOPMENT AT A GLANCE: BIRTH TO TWO YEARS

First Month	Second Month	Third Month
Master Skill		
Exhibits attachment-promoting behaviors, cries, cuddles, coos	Visually connects to parents	Hand play
Gross Motor Skills		
Lies flexed as in utero Springlike feel to muscles Lifts head barely to clear surface Occasional muscle twitches Bears no weight on legs	Limbs relax, stretch partway out Lifts head 45 degrees Head wobbly while held sitting Muscle twitches lessen	Stretches limbs all the way out; cycles and makes freestyle movements Holds head higher than bottom, searches Briefly bears weight on legs Holds head steady when held Rolls from back to side
Hand Skills and Self-help		
Hands tightly fisted Can't hold rattle	Hands partially unfold Swipes aimlessly Briefly holds rattle	Hands open and inviting Makes swiping reaches, more misses than hits, karate chops Holds and shakes rattle longer Grabs clothing and hair of others Sucks fingers and fists Plays with hands, midline
Language and Social Skills		
Demanding cries Grunting, throaty sounds Fleeting smiles Sleep grins Tells parents' voices from strangers' Sees best 8–10 inches, blurred vision Sleeps, wakes, feeds erratically	Coos, squeals, gurgles Wet noises, chest rattles Smiles responsively Shows emotions: delight, distress Catches moods: upset when parent is Quiets self with thumb Holds eye contact, studies face Vaguely mimics facial gestures Tracks moving persons Cries when put down	Draws out vowel sounds: "aaah," "eeeh," "eeee," "oooh" Makes louder sounds, screeches Cries differently for different needs, anticipating pauses between cries Begins to laugh
Cognitive (Thinking) Skills		
Inborn attachment-promoting behaviors: cries for comfort or feeding Behavior mostly reflexive (automatic) rather than thought out Anticipates distress will be followed by comfort Begins to learn trust	Shows engaging behaviors: communicates moods, protests if anticipated needs not met Gives cue, expects response, trusts both Makes associations: cries — gets held or fed	Learns cause and effect: hit mobile, it moves! Learns competence: can cause persons to react by smiles, cries, body language
What Babies Like		
Skin-to-skin cuddling Being carried in arms or sling Feeding on cue, not on schedule Eye-to-eye contact Hearing parents' voices Womblike sounds	Being worn in sling Looking at mobiles Black-and-white patterns Music box: prefers classical music Animated talk and gestures Infant massage Lying on dad's chest	Standing on your lap, leaning on your chest and peering over your shoulder Playing with own hands Playing sitting semiupright better than lying on back Swiping at mobiles Manipulating grab rings and shaker toys Freestyle floor play, "flapping wings"

ourth Month	Fifth Month	Sixth Month
Displays accurate visual tracking	Reaches accurately	Sits
Stands supported Sits propped on arms Lifts head 90 degrees, scans 180 degrees Rests on elbows Rolls from tummy to side	Sits propped on floor and with pillow in high chair Stands, holds on only for balance Rolls from tummy to back Rocks on tummy: airplanes Assumes push-up position: chest and part of tummy off floor Wiggles a few feet forward Cranes neck forward to see Possibly grabs toes	Sits briefly by self, uses arms for balance and to break falls, may slump forward Sits in high chair Stands briefly while leaning on furniture Rolls over both ways Digs in with toes and hands to move toward toy
Two-handed embracing reach Accurately gathers in dangled toy Explores clothing, pats mother's breast Uses mittenlike grasp	Reaches with one hand— good aim Transfers toys purposely hand to hand and mouth Begins block play	Reaches precisely Points at toys Manipulates blocks Uses whole hand to rake in and pick up small objects with thumb and fingers
Shapes mouth to change sounds: "ah-oh" Blows bubbles, sputters loudly Laughs hilariously when tickled Social gesturing: flaps arms to signal "Pick me up" Develops binocular vision: better depth perception, gazes intently, tracks accurately	Babbles "ba-ba-ba" to get attention Turns head toward speaker Attempts to mimic sounds, inflection, and gestures Watches mouth movements Vocalizes different sounds for different needs May show beginning interest in solid foods Shows interest in colors	Strings out longer and more varied sounds Experiments with pitch and volume of new sounds, notices reactions they produce Reflects moods by sound and body language; shouts, belly laughs, clapping arms, grunts, growls, droopy face Mimics facial gestures better
Forms mental images of what to expect when gives a cue (e.g., nursing) Is aware that persons and things have labels (e.g., "cat")	Learns which sounds and gestures get a response Shows decision-making expressions during hand play Figures out objects and changes hand shape to accommodate shape of objects before making contact Uses hand to push away your arm when you're giving medicine	Shows more "intentionality" during play: tries to figure out how to pick up third block with a block in each hand Spends longer studying toys and what to do with them
Greeting caregivers and inviting play Amusing self with fingers Playing with bracelets, rattles Rolling on beach ball Changing to forward position in sling	Pushing off with feet Grabbing your nose, pulling hair Squeeze and squeak toys High-chair and lap play Playing peekaboo	Playing with blocks Banging toys Swinging, bouncing Floor play, propped up Playing wheelbarrow, rolling on foam cylinders Changing to hip carry in sling

6 to 9 Months	9 to 12 Months	12 to 15 Months
Master Skill		
Crawls, uses pincer grasp	Cross-crawls, cruises	Walks
Gross Motor Skills		
Sits erect unsupported	Masters cross-crawling	Walks alone: officially a toddler
Lunges forward to grab toy	Goes from crawling to sitting	Tries various walking styles
Crawls on hands and knees	Scales and climbs furniture	Climbs up stairs, backs down
Pivots in circle	Crawls up stairs, not down	Tries to climb out of high chair
Pulls self up to standing	Cruises around furniture	Get-up-and-go movements: crawls,
Stands leaning on furniture	Stands without holding on	squats, stands, walks
	Walks with assistance	
	First solo steps, stiff, unsteady, wide based, frequent falls	
Hand Skills and Self-help		
Picks up tiny objects with thumb and forefinger	Well-developed pincer grasp	Uses tools: utensils, toothbrush, hairbrush, telephone
Feeds self (messy)	Points and pokes with index finger	Opens cabinets, removes contents
Pounces on moving toys, drops toys, watches them fall	Changes hand to accommodate shape of objects	Fits graduated cylinders
Drinks from cup	Stacks and drops blocks	Tosses ball with hands
	Shows hand dominance	Cooperates in dressing
		Feeds self, holds bottle
Language and Social Skills		
Babbles random consonant-and-vowel combinations ("ah, da, ba, ma, di, mu") and jabbers these sounds together	Two-syllable sounds ("ma-ma," "da-da"), associates sounds with right person	Says 4–6 intelligible words
Adds tongue movement to change sound: "ah-da"	Understands "no"	Uses *b, c, d, g* words: "ball," "cat," "dog," "go"
Consistently responds to own name	Imitates sounds: cough, tongue clicks	Utters partial words: "ba" for "ball"
Social directing: uses arms to invite caregivers to play, raises arms to signal "Pick me up"	Understands gestures: waves bye-bye	Says and gestures "no" ("na-na-na") and shakes head
		Asks for help by pointing and gesturing, some sounds
		Recognizes names and points to familiar persons
		Understands and follows one-step directions: "Throw ball to daddy"
		Laughs at funny scenes
Cognitive (Thinking) Skills		
Labels: associates mental images with words and pictures (e.g., "cat")	Shows memory of recent events	Growing vocabulary and growing mind make memory easier
Develops concept of "in" and "out" — notices how smaller containers fit into larger ones	Cue words trigger mental pictures of action to expect: "go . . ." — looks toward door	Associates familiar persons and things with word for them
Shows stranger anxiety	Remembers where toy is when hidden under one of two covers	Gives impression that your words and gestures trigger thoughts
	"Mama's coming" triggers mental picture of mama, stops fussing	Begins learning how things fit: tries to match lids, stack blocks
	Shows separation anxiety	
What Babies Like		
Bouncing to music	Container play: pouring, filling, dumping	Pushing and pulling toys while walking
Peekaboo, pat-a-cake	"Pickpocketing" dad's shirt	Throwing balls, flinging toys
Words and rhyming games	Flirting with self in mirror	Touching games: this-little-piggy and where's-daddy's-nose
Following and grabbing bubbles	Banging and matching lids on pots and pans	Emptying cabinets, sorting containers
Rolling balls	Stacking 2 or 3 large blocks	Riding on daddy's shoulders
Small object fascination		Talking to toys
		Mimicking animal sounds, "woof-woof"

15 to 18 Months	18 to 24 Months
Understands simple language	Figures out before acting, understands most daily language
Walks in circles, backward, pivots Walks faster, trots, prances Walks up stairs — needs help Stops and stoops to pick up toy Climbs onto furniture, tries to climb out of crib Rides on four-wheeled toy Tries to kick balls, many misses Positions self in a chair	Runs, tries to escape from caregiver Looks down to dodge obstacles Jumps in place and off step Pedals first tricycle Kicks ball without stumbling May climb out of crib Walks up stairs without help, both feet on each step, may need help coming down Opens doors
Scribbles random lines and semicircles Opens drawers Cooperates in dressing Throws ball with whole arm Dips morsels of food	Unwraps packages Removes clothing, washes hands Fits lid on shoe box Builds tower of 6 blocks Folds paper, fits simple puzzle Throws ball overhand Seats self at table
Says 10–20 intelligible words Uses complete words: "ba" becomes "ball" Puts two short words together: "bye-bye," "all done," "no-no" Makes first sentences: "Go bye-bye" Responds to verbal requests without accompanying gestures Chatters and parrots Understands "up," "down," "off," "hot" Uses feeding words: "num-num," "ba-ba" Understands "other" Gesticulates: "shhh" for "hush"	Says 20–50 intelligible words Attempts multisyllable words: "Ben-ben-ben" for Benjamin Answers "What does dog say?" Makes three-word sentences, telegram style: "Me want more" Normal to "say little, understand all" Likes challenge words ("helicopter," "dinosaur"), with cute mess-ups, of course! May give first and last name Hums and sings Normal behaviors: tantrums, whining, biting, screaming
Sorts shapes, graduated rings Learns by exploring all over house Identifies familiar picures in book: "find the cat" Matches round peg in round hole Separation anxiety lessens: Can retain mental pictures of persons when they're out of sight	Figures things out in head before rushing into task Copies circles, makes line drawings Aligns simple inset puzzles Shows mind-set: peanut butter *must* be on top of jelly Understands and remembers two-step request: "Go to kitchen and bring daddy a pretzel"
Pushing toy lawn mowers, buggies Pounding toys: rubber hammer Stacking 4 or 5 large blocks Playing body-part games: "Where's nose?" Dancing to music Turning knobs, pressing buttons Playing peekaboo and chase	Pulling wagons Helping around house Gymnastics: somersaults Standing on stools, "helping" at sink Using own play shelves, table and chairs Rearranging furniture "Reading" picture books, turning pages one at a time

improvements are made on this beginning nervous system. First, the number of connections between neurons increases, and second, each neuron acquires a coating called myelin, which helps messages move faster and insulates the nerve, preventing short circuits. The new and exciting field of neurobiology tells us that the more connections the nerve cells make, the smarter the child's brain. Smart-start parenting means helping your baby's brain make the right connections.

1. A Smart Womb Start

At the moment sperm meets egg, your baby's brain growth takes off. In fact, a baby's brain develops faster during the nine months in mother's womb than at any other time in the child's life. The development of the fetal nervous system is affected — for better or worse — by what's in mother's blood during the nine months of pregnancy. Inhaling or ingesting substances called neurotoxins, such as cigarette smoke, excessive alcohol, and many kinds of drugs, has been shown to harm the baby's brain development and increase the risk of having learning and behavior problems later on.

Besides the "don'ts" of drugs, alcohol, and nicotine during pregnancy, there are some "do's" that affect the developing fetal brain in a healthy way. A maternal diet rich in brain-building omega-3 fats (see page 150 and www.dhadoc.com) is smart nutrition. While it takes very poor maternal nutrition to harm a baby's developing brain, in general, the better you nourish your body, the better you nourish your baby's growing brain.

2. A Smart Milk Start

As discussed on page 119, research has shown that breastfed babies enjoy an intellectual advantage over bottlefed babies. Even more exciting, breastfeeding research suggests a dose-response relationship: The more frequently and longer a mother breastfeeds, the smarter her kids are likely to be. Here are two reasons that breastfed babies enjoy a brighter beginning:

- *Smarter fats.* Mother's milk is rich in brain-building omega-3 fats, such as DHA (docosahexaenoic acid), ARA (arachidonic acid), and cholesterol. Dubbed "smart fats," these nutrients contribute to the growth of the baby's brain tissue, especially myelin, the fatty coating that insulates each nerve fiber, enabling messages to travel faster and more efficiently between brain circuits.

- *Smarter communication.* As discussed on page 5, the responsiveness of caregivers to the cues of the infant is a powerful builder of brighter babies. Breastfeeding is an exercise in baby-reading. A breastfeeding mother learns to read her baby's cues of hunger and satisfaction since, unlike the bottle-feeding mom, she can't count the number of ounces of milk she is giving. The perk of extra intuition hormones that a breastfeeding mother enjoys helps her be more sensitive, tuned in, and more appropriately responsive to the cues of her infant. Since breast milk is digested faster than formula, breastfed babies feed more often and therefore enjoy more interaction and touch time, which are also powerful influencers of an infant's emotional and intellectual development.

3. Smart Moves

Why does babywearing build brighter babies? Answer: Their brains grow better. Babies learn a lot in the arms of busy caregivers. Carried babies cry less. What do they do with this extra time and energy? They learn. Carried babies show an increase in awake-contentment time, also called "quiet alertness" or "attentive stillness" — the behavioral state in which an infant learns most by being able to best connect and interact with his environment. And the more babies interact with their environment, the more meaningful are their neurological connections. Babies divert the energy they would have spent on fussing into thinking. During babywearing, mom gives her baby a 180-degree view of his environment and allows him to more easily scan his world. Babies who are carried learn to choose — picking out what they wish to look at and shutting out what they don't. This ability to make choices enhances learning.

To appreciate how babywearing helps infants learn, let's use a principle from Parenting 101: Get behind the eyes of your baby and imagine the world from her viewpoint. First get into a stationary infant seat or crib and imagine the world you see. You lie unattended, flailing your arms, arching your back, and wasting a lot of energy in purposeless motion. You don't learn much lying motionless gazing passively at a meaningless sky or ceiling.

Now imagine being worn in a sling. You are now what we call a "slingbaby." With mom you travel down the aisles of the supermarket. You see the same variety of shopping attractions that mom sees. You're being carried through the park, where you watch kids play. You're with mom when she's poking around the house or talking on the phone. You go where your mom goes, see whatever she sees, and hear whatever she hears.

Because we believe that babywearing is valuable for a baby's intellectual development, every new parent who comes into our practice gets a demonstration on how to wear their baby in a sling. Later these parents often tell us, "When I pick up the sling and put it on, my baby lights up and raises her arms. She knows that soon she'll be in my arms and in my world." Whenever I mentioned the cue word "go" to nine-month-old Matthew, he would crawl toward the wall where we hung the baby sling. Matthew's connection between the word "go" and the tool for going, the baby sling, is known in infant development jargon as *a pattern of association.* Like thousands of short-run movies filed in the infant's growing neurological library, patterns of association are rerun whenever baby is exposed to a situation that reminds him of the original "movie."

Slingbabies fuss less, learn more, and are just plain easier and more fun to be with. (For more about the benefits of babywearing, see Chapter 14.)

4. Smart Play

Babies learn about their world through play, and parents can learn about their babies' preferences and capabilities at each stage of development by watching them play. By observing and sharing in baby's play, parents can begin to get a faint idea of all the decision-making and problem-solving processes going on in baby's developing mind. In the following chapters, as you read and grow with your baby, you will learn age- and stage-appropriate brainy baby games, toy tips, and the concept of "toys for two" — toys that help you interact more meaningfully with your baby. (See www.AskDrSears.com for more developmental toys and play tips.)

5. Smart Talk

How you talk to your baby has a profound effect on your baby's brain development, and here's where parents, especially mothers, can really shine. As you ride the developmental elevator with your baby through the following chapters, you will learn many brain-building tips for talking with your baby. (See "Tips for Talking to Your Baby," page 472.)

6. Smart Listening

It's not only how you talk to your infant but also how you listen that helps build a brainy baby. As we discussed on page 5, the responsiveness of caregivers to the cues of their infant is a powerful enhancer of brain development. When it comes to learning to be a good listener, here is where attachment parenting really shines.

Once upon a time, the "fear of spoiling and being manipulated" mind-set gave rise to a philosophy of infant care we call "baby training" (see page 9). This lower-touch, cookbook style of parenting promises to help babies fit more conveniently into their parents' life-styles. New insights into infant development have shown how detrimental this approach can be. The current buzzword among infant development specialists is *responsiveness,* which means tuning in to the cues of the infant and responding sensitively.

As you take a course in infant development in the following chapters, you will learn listening tips, the most important of which is responding *appropriately,* knowing when to say yes and when to say no, and how to tell the difference between a need and a want. Infants whose language is listened to and whose needs are responded to appropriately learn to trust their environment, and trust is one of the earliest and most valuable brain-building blocks. (See "The Shutdown Syndrome," page 446, for a story about how lack of trust slowed an infant's development.)

7. Smart Foods

New research is confirming what parents have long observed: What children eat affects — for better or worse — how they act, think, and learn. Since a baby's rapidly growing brain uses 60 percent of the total nutritional energy consumed by the infant, it stands to reason that the healthier the food, the healthier the brain. The food baby eats affects not only how well the brain grows, but also how well the nerves send messages to one another via biological bridges called neurotransmitters. Best foods for growing brains are:

- *Smart fats.* The best fats come from breast milk, with its omega-3 fatty acids, including the smart fat DHA. Low-fat diets are not smart for babies. Nature is smart. Around 50 percent of the calories in mother's milk comes from healthy fat. Since a baby's brain is 60 percent fat, and since fats are the major structural components of the brain cell membrane and the insulating sheath around each nerve, getting enough fat and the right kinds of fat can help build a better brain. (See "Smart Fats for Baby, Healthy Fats for Mom," page 150, and "Feed Your Baby Smart Fats," page 238.)

- *Smart carbs.* Also known as "mood foods," carbohydrates (sugars) help growing brains in two ways: Carbs are the primary energy source for the nervous system; and carbs regulate neurohormones and neurotransmitter function. A steady supply of "smart carbs" (such as complex carbohydrates or fiber-filled carbs) improves alertness and concentration. (See "Feed Your Baby the Best Carbs," page 240, and "Grazing," page 223.)

- *Other smart nutrients.* An adequate supply of vitamins, namely vitamin C, folic acid, and the other B-vitamins are important for optimal brain growth. Minerals, namely calcium and iron, are also important nutritional brain-building blocks. (See "Value Your Vitamins," page 244, "Mind Your Minerals," page 245, and "Pump Up Baby's Iron," page 245.)

The parenting style you practice, the way you play with your baby, and the food you feed your infant, all stack up to be important blocks for building your baby's brain.

20

The First Six Months: Big Changes

More changes occur in the first six months than during any other growth period. Baby doubles his birth weight; posture progresses from barely a one-inch head lift to a full sit-up; hand skills progress from tight-fisted, aimless swiping to precise reaches. Baby's thought process matures, too; primarily reflexive responses give way to the beginning of thought-out actions and the initially uninterpretable cries develop into understandable cues. Parents also grow at an amazing rate at this stage, progressing from "I have no idea what he wants" to "I finally understand his signals." Let's now take a journey through one of the most exciting stages of a child's life: the first six months.

THE FIRST MONTH: BIG NEEDS

"What should we be doing with our new baby?" is a question that concerns new parents. Hold him a lot and love him a lot is the answer. The first month is a stage of adjustment for parents and organization for baby. Hold the toys for later. Babies do not show great strides in motor development during this stage, nor do they need a lot of things — except the arms of loving parents.

Opening Moves

Watch your tiny bundle curled up in the bassinet. So peaceful, so quiet. It's hard to imagine this is the same baby who turned roly-polies in your uterus. When he awakens, gaze at him face to face. His arms and legs dart out as if stretching after a deep sleep. Those were the punches and kicks you felt during the final months inside. Now you can watch what you felt.

When playing with your newborn, notice the springlike feel to the muscles. If you pull his arms or legs away from his body or try to open his hands, they quickly spring back to their original flexed position. Enjoy this tight, springlike appearance and feel while they last, as baby's whole body will loosen up over the next few months. When unflexing baby's leg or arm, you will often hear and feel crackling sounds around the knee and elbow joints. These are normal joint noises coming from the rubberlike ligaments and loose bones. These sounds, too, will disappear.

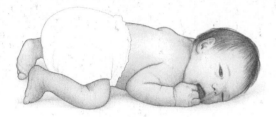

A newborn in the fetal position.

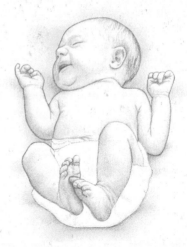

Newborns' muscles have a springlike feel, and their limbs tend to return to a flexed position.

The behavioral state your newborn is in often determines how he moves. While most of the time baby's wiggles seem random and jerky, recent studies have shown that when newborns are relaxed and in the quiet alert state their movements take on a more organized pattern of periodic bursts and pauses. The more time baby spends in the quiet alert state, the more these jerky muscle movements organize into more rhythmic patterns. This is one reason we emphasize parenting styles that promote the state of quiet alertness.

If your baby startles easily, his chin quivers a lot, and his arms and legs seem trembly, wear your baby in a sling or wrap your newborn in a blanket, which contains and helps to organize these jerky muscle movements. These normal newborn shakes usually subside by the end of the first month.

What Newborns Can See

Dim the lights; a newborn is coming. As though emerging from a dark to a light room, a newly born baby squints. Add to this light-sensitive squinting the puffy eyelids from the birth squeeze, and the world may not look so clear for the first few hours. As a further light shield, newborn pupils are often somewhat

smaller than normal for the first week or two. Within minutes to an hour after birth most newborns show a wide-open, interested-in-the-world look.

During the early days except for fleeting eye-opening moments, newborns keep their eyes closed. This can be frustrating to parents trying to connect visually. Try this eye-opener: Hold your baby in front of you with one hand supporting his head and the other under his bottom, between eight and ten inches (twenty and twenty-five centimeters) from your eyes. Turning from the waist, swing him gently to an arc of about 120 degrees and come to a slightly abrupt stop. This rotating motion prompts baby to open his eyes reflexively. Another method is to support your baby's head and raise him gently from a lying to a sitting position.

Newborns see; they just don't see far. They see most clearly at a distance of eight to ten inches, which, amazingly, is the usual eye-to-eye distance during breastfeeding. Catch your baby in a bright-eyed state of quiet alertness. Hold him in front of your face, making eye-to-eye connection around eight to ten inches away. As you move baby closer and farther from this *intimate space* — the distance that best holds baby's attention — notice that baby breaks the visual connection and loses interest because your visual image becomes more hazy.

What Newborns Like to See

Here's a clue: It has round curves, contrasting light and dark patterns, and sharp outlines. No, it is not a breast, but you're close. Another clue. It moves, blinks, and smiles. Newborns love to look at faces, especially a familiar one. Give him yours. There's something uniquely appealing about the order of features in the face. Researchers showed four different diagrams to forty newborns at a mean age of nine minutes. The babies turned their heads and eyes and displayed interest in the diagram that showed the facial parts in the right configuration. They showed less interest in diagrams in which the facial parts were scrambled. If you play the face-preference game, dad may win. Because of their preference for light-dark contrast, babies often pay more attention to the *male* face, especially if it has a beard or mustache. While a parent's face will always be baby's best eye-catcher, next in order of preference are black-and-white drawings or photos of a face, and black-and-white contrasting patterns such as checkerboards, stripes, and bull's-eyes.

Newborns are very discerning about what they choose to look at. If you don't wear glasses and suddenly put on a pair, or if your baby gets used to seeing you with glasses on and you take them off, he may look puzzled and turn away, as if thinking, "What's wrong with this picture?" This visual perception indicates that even a newborn can store

---

TIPS FOR HOLDING BABY'S VISUAL ATTENTION

- Sit or hold baby upright.
- Wait for baby to be in the quiet alert state.
- Keep object or face around ten inches (twenty-five centimeters) from baby's face.
- Use animated facial gestures (wide-open mouth and eyes) while speaking in a slow, rhythmic, exaggerated tone.

---

familiar patterns in his visual memory bank. The newborn is programmed to pay attention to the human face even from birth.

Fixating

"Sometimes he's cross-eyed, sometimes he's not," parents often observe. Periodic crossed eyes are normal. *Constant* crossed eyes need medical attention. Eyes may not be constantly straight until six months of age. Because newborns do not use both eyes together, images do not fall at the same point on the retina in each eye. This results in poor depth perception. As baby learns to hold her head and eyes still, images become clearer, depth perception improves, and baby holds a longer fix on your eyes. This *binocular vision* starts to develop around six weeks and is well established by four months.

How to Tell If Your Baby's Eyes Are Crossed

Because some babies have wide nasal bridges, you may not see much of the whites of the eyes. Consequently the eyes may appear crossed, but really aren't. Here's how to tell. Shine a penlight into your baby's eyes (or take a flash photo). Notice the location of the light reflex, the white dot on baby's eyes. It should be in the same place in each eye. If the dot is in the center of the pupil in one eye but off center in the other, one or both eyes have lazy muscles. Report your findings to your doctor. During well-baby exams, this is how your doctor checks baby's eyes.

Gazing

During the first few weeks your baby's eyes scan your face but seldom are still and fixed directly onto your eyes for more than a fleeting second or two, despite your pleading, "Look at me." Even though your baby starts focusing better around two weeks, expect her eyes to continue to move most of the time. Holding a fix on either a still or moving object does not click in until around four months.

Sometimes if a newborn is in a relaxed, interested, and quiet alert state, a face or an object may hold her attention for several minutes. Try this gazing game: Hold your baby within her own clear-vision distance (which you can determine by slowly telescoping your baby toward and away from your face until you reach a distance that best holds her attention — this is usually somewhere between eight and thirteen inches/twenty and thirty-three centimeters).

Babies are more likely to become bored with visual games when lying on their back but become more attentive when placed in the *upright* position.

What Newborns Can Hear

Newborns prefer mother's high-pitched voice to father's and prefer sounds with a womb-like beat. That's the music they're used to. They calm best to soothing sounds with a slowly rising and falling rhythm, like classical music. Loud rock music that has a disorderly rhythm disturbs their peace.

Newborns appear to recognize the sounds they heard repeatedly while in the womb, such as a favorite piano piece that mother played often during her pregnancy. Babies and children are also more attentive to stories that mother frequently read out loud during her pregnancy.

You don't have to tiptoe and whisper around a sleeping newborn. Babies have a remarkable ability to block out disturbing noises. This stimulus barrier operates even when baby is awake. Sometimes you may call your baby's name, and he doesn't even notice, and you wonder if he hears you. Babies are selective about what they give their attention to. If baby is interested in a dangling mobile and you call to him, his visual pursuits override other senses, and he tunes you out. Try again when he is not so focused on something else. (Expect the same behavior when your newborn becomes a two-year-old.)

Newborns also protect themselves against sensory overload. During a loud, disturbing commotion some babies become upset; others fade into a deep sleep, as if saying, "Too much going on here. I'm tuning out."

Amazingly, newborns can associate the sound with the direction of its source — which is called *orienting.* Call your baby from the right side, and she may turn to the right. Now try the left side. Not all newborns orient to all voices all the time, and don't be alarmed if it takes another month or two for your baby to turn toward your voice. Mother's voice is special. Newborns can pick out mother's voice from the sounds of strangers.

When hearing the same sounds newborns become *habituated,* infant-stimulator jargon for becoming bored. If you're not able to make sound connections with your baby, try varying the tone of your voice. Also, babies become confused if they cannot see who's talking to them. They like to look at who's talking. To hold your baby's attention to your voice, first get an eye-to-eye visual fix and then begin talking. (For tips on checking your baby's hearing, see page 681.)

►*SOUND ADVICE: Exposure to loud noises — a rock concert, for example — may damage hearing. As a practical guide, music you can carry on a conversation over is safe. If you have to shout over the noise, it's too loud.*

PICKING UP EACH OTHER'S SCENT

The sense of smell is acutely developed in newborns, and in their mothers. Not only can a newborn distinguish mother's voice from a stranger's, he can also pick out her individual scent. An interesting study of six-day-old newborns showed that when mother's breast pad (with or without her milk) was placed alongside her newborn's face, baby turned toward it, though he ignored breast pads from other mothers. This special scent recognition also holds true for mothers. Blindfolded mothers can identify their own babies by smell.

A Mind of Their Own

Much of what a newborn does is by reflex. When hungry or upset he automatically cries. He acts before he thinks.

Mental Pictures

Most of a newborn's early learning is directed toward comfort and satisfaction. He wants to be fed, held, and comforted, and he has the same language for all these — the cry. Put yourself in the mind of your newborn. "I cry, I get picked up. I keep crying, I get fed. I cry again when I'm lonesome, and I get held more." After repeating these cue-response scenes hundreds of times, a newborn develops a mental picture of what to expect following a cry. It is as if each time baby gives a cue, a flash card appears in his mind, and he previews what's going to happen. Infant development specialists call these mental pictures a *schema.* The more mental pictures, the better the mind develops. So the initial reflex, crying, matures into a thinking or cognitive process as the baby calls up a flash card reflecting the solution to his need and musters up the language to get it.

Mothers go through the reverse of this mental process. Initially, as you are learning to read your newborn's cues, you think before you act. "Is he hungry? But I just fed him. Is he wet? Is he manipulating me? Probably!" As you overcome these worrisome mental gymnastics, you learn to respond more intuitively, almost by reflex. You act before you think. As you and baby practice this cue-response connection, you both settle into a state of harmony. You and your baby are learning to fit — baby with a mind full of beautiful attachment pictures, and you with a new comfort level of reading your baby.

A newborn who is used to this cue-response network learns to *trust* her caregiving environment. She learns how to get her needs met through the help of others. The nine-month-old, for example, raises her arms in anticipation that daddy will pick her up and recalls the mental pick-up-and-play flash card that she expects.

A Mutual Mind-set Develops

As baby is developing mental pictures of mother's (and father's) responses, mother also imagines what baby is thinking and needing. Baby gets into the mother's mind, and mother gets into the baby's mind.

What about the baby whose cues are not responded to, usually because of the parents' unwarranted fear of spoiling or of being manipulated? The mind of a baby whose cues are not given a nurturant response is not so rich. She doesn't know what response to expect and doesn't develop a mental picture of what to anticipate. Her mind is full of blank flash cards. Mother also is left empty. Because baby has not learned to trust that cues will be read, she does not learn to cue better. Mother becomes less comfortable reading her baby's cues. Baby and mother share less of each other's thoughts, and a distance develops between them.

One day I was explaining to a new mother how she and her baby could get into each other's mind. She understood, but seemed worried, exclaiming, "This sounds exciting, but what if I goof and don't give our baby the right response? What if he's wet and I think he's hungry?" I reassured her, "You can't goof when you pick up and nurture a baby. When your baby cries and you pick him up and he continues crying, you simply go through a trial-and-error checklist until you click into

---

BABY'S BEHAVIORAL STATES

- **Crying.** Loud, fretful complaints are accompanied by flailing, uncoordinated limb movements. Baby is only minimally attentive. This behavior is upsetting to baby and to his caregivers.

- **Active alertness.** A state similar to quiet alertness, but here baby's limbs and head are moving, and baby is less visually attentive. Baby seems distracted by his own motions.

- **Quiet alertness.** Eyes are bright, open, attentive; limbs are relatively quiet. Baby appears to be contemplating the environment. This state is most conducive to interaction and learning.

- **Drowsy.** Eyes are open and fluttering or starting to close; baby is slightly attentive, with stirring body movements and sleep grins. Baby is either waking up or falling asleep.

- **Light sleep.** Baby startles easily and shows facial and limb twitches, irregular breathing, spurts of movement. Limbs are flexed toward the body.

- **Deep sleep.** Baby shows minimal movement, expressionless face, regular breathing, and limp, dangling limbs.

the need that needs filling. The important message you give your baby is the anticipation of being listened to and responded to."

Enjoying Your Newborn's Smile

With baby's first smile, you swoon and forget the sleepless nights and constant holding. You are thrilled, and you feel, "My baby really loves me." Enter the spoilers: "Oh, it's just gas." After years of watching newborns smile, we wish to deflate the gas bubble. Newborns do smile, and not because of gas (unless after passing it).

As veteran smile watchers we divide smiles into two types: inside smiles and outside smiles. Inside smiles, occurring in the first few weeks, are a beautiful reflection of an inner feeling of rightness. Some are *sleep grins;* some are only a happy twitch in the corner of the mouth. Relief smiles occur after being rescued from a colicky period, after a satisfying feeding, or after being picked up and rocked. During face-to-face games is another time to catch a smile. Baby's early smiles convey an "I feel good inside" message

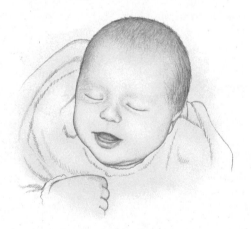

Sleep grins are among baby's first smiles.

and leave you feeling good inside. Be prepared to wait until next month for the true outside (or social) smiles, which you can initiate and which will absolutely captivate all adoring smile watchers. Whatever their cause, enjoy these fleeting grins as glimpses of the whole happy-face smiles that are soon to come.

NEWBORN REFLEXES

Newborns and adults show two types of action: *cognitive,* meaning you think before you act, and *reflexive,* meaning your reaction is automatic. When you show your baby a rattle, his brain thinks, "I'll use my hand to get the rattle." And the brain sends the message to the muscles, instructing them to grab the rattle. If you tap your baby's knee with the rattle at just the right place, baby's knee jerks automatically, or by reflex. Much of a newborn's early behavior is reflexive, but as his nervous system matures he puts more thought into his actions. There are around seventy-five primitive reflexes in the newborn period. Most are curiosities, some are protective, and a few serve some additional purpose. Here are some interesting and useful reflexes.

Mouthing reflexes. These reflexes help a baby find the source of food and ingest it. Of these, the *sucking* and *swallowing reflexes* are the most important for survival. Notice that your baby automatically sucks when you stimulate (in order of decreasing sensitivity) the soft palate, the interior of the mouth and lips, and the cheek and chin. A relative to the suck reflex is the *rooting* (or search) *reflex.* Using your nipple, tickle your baby's face and watch him turn his head toward your nipple as if searching for food. The rooting reflex subsides around four months as reaching skills begin and the infant's search for food becomes more voluntary.

Startle reflex (Moro reflex). If baby is exposed to a sudden loud noise or you withdraw support of baby's head and back while holding him, he reacts to the sensation of falling by quickly extending his arms out from his body and cupping his hands as if trying to cling to and embrace someone. Especially if there is no one to grab on to for comfort, the reflex may be accompanied by anxious grimacing or crying. This protective reflex is a clinging response in which baby is giving the message, "I need a person between these embracing little arms." The startle reflex is most noticeable during the first month and gradually disappears by three or four months. Anthropologists speculate that the startle and grasp reflexes are primitive

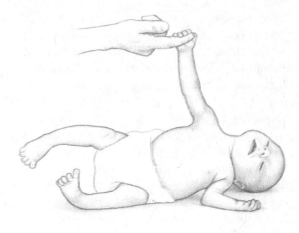

The grasp reflex.

attachment behaviors that infants used to hold on to their mothers.

Grasp reflex. Stroke the palm of your baby's hand with your fingertip or place your finger into the palm from the pinkie finger side and notice how your baby's fingers wrap tenaciously around yours. Sometimes baby's grasp is so strong that you can partially lift him off the surface he's lying on before he lets go. (Try this only on a soft surface, like a bed, as baby has no control of when he will let go.) For another demonstration of the grasp reflex, place a rattle in your baby's hands; notice how difficult it is to pry the rattle away from little Hercules. The grasp reflex is strongest in the first two months; it begins disappearing by the third month and is usually gone by six.

Righting reflexes. Survival behaviors called righting reflexes help baby learn to keep her trunk, head, arms, and legs in proper alignment for breathing and development. Place your baby facedown and notice she lifts her head just enough to clear the surface and

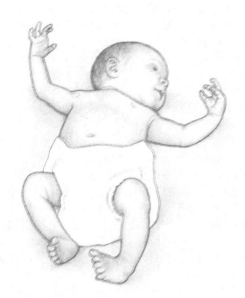

The startle reflex (Moro reflex).

turn her head to one side. If a blanket or pillow falls over baby's head, she may mouth it initially and then twist her head vigorously from side to side and flail her arms to push away the blanket to breathe and see.

Gag reflex. To protect baby from choking while learning to feed and swallow, the gag reflex automatically expels an object from baby's throat. If a finger or an object stimulates the back of the throat, the jaw lowers and the tongue thrusts forward and downward to push the object out. The gag reflex persists throughout life, but the tongue-thrusting part of the reflex disappears around six months. These reflexes explain why babies have difficulty handling early solids.

Tonic neck reflex (fencer's reflex). While your baby is lying on his back, turn his head to one side and notice his arm and leg thrusting outward while the opposite arm and leg flex, resembling the *en garde* position of a

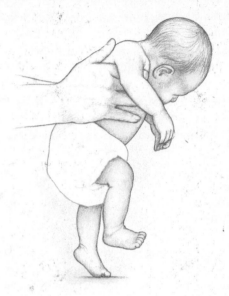

The stepping reflex.

fencer. This reflex both helps and hinders baby's muscle development. It encourages baby to look at the hand extended in front of him and keep his attention on a toy in that hand. But it inhibits baby from using his arms, hands, and head in midline play in front of his body. Around three to four months this reflex begins to subside, allowing your baby to hold toys in front of him and engage in hand-to-eye and hand-to-mouth play.

Stepping reflex. Hold your baby over the table or floor so that the sole of one foot presses on the surface. The weight-bearing foot will lift up, and the other foot will lower, as if baby were taking a step. If you "stub her toe" on the edge of the table, she will lift her foot as if stepping up on the table. This reflex, which disappears around two months, is an amusing curiosity with an unclear purpose.

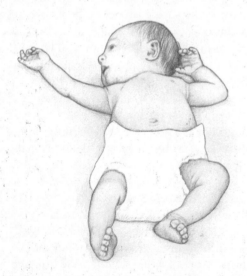

The tonic neck reflex (fencer's reflex).

Withdrawal reflex. Baby is protected against pain by the withdrawal reflex. If baby's heel is pricked to obtain blood, as during routine hospital tests, the leg and foot flex and withdraw to avoid the pain. At the same time, the other leg thrusts outward as if pushing the offender away.

THE SECOND MONTH: BIG SMILES

During the first month babies seldom make enough major changes to write grandmother about. It is a stage of becoming organized, discovering to whom she belongs, and learning to fit into her new home. It is a time for parents to recover from birth, survive on less sleep, and adjust to life with a new baby. In the second month you are, in the words of surviving parents, "over the hump."

The second month is baby's social debut — the coming out of herself. She opens up her hands to greet people. She opens her vision to widen her world and her mouth to smile and make more noise. The feeling of rightness and trust developed during the first month opens the door for baby's real personality to step out.

The Great Imitator

Baby's intense interest in your facial gestures prompts her to mimic your changing facial expressions. Like a dance — you lead, baby follows. Nothing can entertain a baby like a face. Walt Disney capitalized on this observation by creating cartoon characters with big and exaggeratedly round eyes, nose, cheeks,

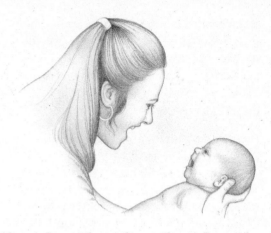

In the second month, baby will mimic your facial expressions.

and ears. The best of these, Mickey Mouse, has survived the longest.

When your baby is in the quiet alert state, try this face-to-face game: Hold your baby within best focusing distance (around eight to ten inches/twenty to twenty-five centimeters) and slowly stick out your tongue as far as you can. Give baby time to process your antics, then repeat two to three times a minute. When baby begins to move her tongue, sometimes even protrude it, you know you've registered a hit. Try the same game with opening your mouth wide or changing the contour of your lips. Facial expressions are contagious. You may catch your baby mimicking your yawn, or vice versa.

Mom, the mirror. In playing face-imitation games you mirror your newborn's expressions back to him. When a newborn frowns, opens his eyes or mouth wide, or grimaces, mother instinctively mimics her newborn's expressions and *exaggerates* them. Baby sees his face in his mother's. Infant development specialists regard mirroring as a powerful enforcer of baby's self-awareness.

Visual Development

The fleeting glances of the first month evolve into ten or more seconds of engaging eye-to-eye contact that captivates caregivers and mesmerizes babies. These penetrating stares and facial-welcoming gestures seem to say, "Hi, mom and dad!" In the first month baby mostly scanned your face; now she studies your face in more detail.

Martha notes:* When Matthew is looking at me, he scans my face very methodically and systematically. He seems to be studying my face. He will start out looking at my eyes and from there he will look up to my hairline and follow the hairline all the way around, then come back to the eyes, down to the mouth, up to the hairline and back to the eyes. He will study my face like this for long periods of time.

Eyes and head move together. As you begin to walk away, notice baby's eyes can now follow you for a few moments. Unlike the asynchronous eye and head movements of a newborn, baby's eyes now move more smoothly, and her head finally catches up with her eyes to move together. She's more able to track your face or a toy moving from side to side, perhaps even a full 180 degrees.

---

*As you journey through this section on infant development, you will read passages entitled "Martha notes." These are based on entries in Martha's daily journals written when our son Matthew was a baby.

Sees farther. Last month baby showed little interest in the world beyond her reach. She could not see it clearly. This month brings about an increase in her intimate space, and more of her ever-widening world is now in focus.

As if given a better camera at two months, baby becomes interested in many of the goings-on elsewhere in the room. She studies your face for a while, shifts her gaze to focus on something in the background, scans the room, pausing momentarily as if to snap the pictures she likes, and then shifts back to peer at your face — still her favorite picture.

Eye-catchers. To spark the interest of a curious two-month-old, here are the sights that most delight. During the early months babies like black and white better than a rainbow of colors. They prefer patterns that contrast with

---

WHAT BABIES LIKE TO LOOK AT

- your face — always the favorite
- contrasts (mainly black and white)
- black-and-white photos: glossy eight-by-tens of mom's and dad's faces
- broad stripes, approximately two inches (five centimeters) wide
- black dots, one inch in diameter, on a white background (the younger the baby, the wider the stripes and the larger the dots)
- checkerboards and bull's-eyes
- silhouettes (for example, plants in front of a window)
- mobiles, especially with black-and-white contrasting designs
- ceiling fans and ceiling beams
- fires in fireplaces

each other rather than soft colors that blend together. Even two-month-olds have selective visual tastes. Rather than synthetic patterns and pastel designer wallpaper, they prefer the colors of nature: bright flowers in the garden, reds and yellows of changing autumn leaves, and bare tree branches silhouetted against a winter sky. Babies often get bored indoors. Take her outside where the rhythmical movements of trees, clouds, flowers, and even automobiles open the eyes of everyone.

Sit me up to see my world. Want to see more of those bright sparkly eyes? Get baby off her back. Babies seem to be less interested in using their visual or motor skills to relate to their environment when lying on their backs. Perhaps the reclining position reminds them too much of sleep. Instead of letting your baby lie in a crib staring at a mobile, sit her upright in an infant seat or in your lap or carry her over your shoulder.

Become an eye watcher. Your baby's eyes are the window to her feelings. Wide-open sparkly eyes are invitations to play. Slowly drooping eyelids signal that sleep is coming. An intense look reflects interest, while a blank expression indicates boredom. Glazed may mean sick. If your baby turns away from eye-to-eye contact, she is telling you that she is losing interest and it's time for a change. Raising and frowning eyebrows add another clue to baby's early eye language. Eyes do mirror moods.

Baby's First Smile Makes It All Worthwhile

Here it is, the sight you've been longing for — real smiles. A baby's smile develops through two stages. The smiles of last month were reflex smiles, automatic reactions to an inner feeling of rightness. They were fleeting,

---

GUESSING YOUR BABY'S EYE COLOR

Place your bets on future eye color now, but all the pigment of the iris may not cross the finish line until a year or two of age. During their baby's two-month check-up, parents invariably ask me, "Doctor, what do you think her eye color will be?" In my early years of the eye-color guessing game, I usually lost. Now I know how to play the odds, and here they are.

Darker eyes, brown or dark green, usually stay dark, especially in darker-skinned races: African American, Indian, and Asian. Lighter eyes (blue, gray) are less predictable, often going through many color changes in the first three months before settling on a color

direction by three months and darkening to their final color by six to twelve months. When in doubt, I look at the parents. If both parents have brown eyes, guess brown (75 percent chance of being right); if one has brown eyes, still guess brown (50 percent right); if both blue, guess blue (but baby may still turn out brown-eyed). Though parents' genes primarily determine eye color, even Great-grandma Lily may leave her mark. Curious brown triangular or round specks on the iris are often a distantly inherited trait. Add eye color to the many fleeting changes of the early months. Photo capture it while you can.

limited to the muscles of the mouth, and usually appeared only for a few seconds as baby drifted off to sleep or after a feeding. Those were the "I think they're smiles but I'm not sure" grimaces. Now there is no doubt. These are returned social smiles in response to your smiles and facial gestures. The whole face lights up. Baby's eyes are wide open and, if she is really into it, crinkled up at the corners. Dimples appear in baby's chubby cheeks as she flashes her pearly gums and toothless grins. These facial smiles often escalate into total body smiles as baby wiggles with pleasure during a smiling game.

Remember, smiling is a two-way communication between smiler and smilee. Reinforce your baby's smiles by smiling back. Jazz up your smile to intensify baby's smile. Sometimes this smiling game will escalate into a chorus of mutual total body language: Parents exaggerate their facial gestures and babble a barrage of baby talk while baby wiggles with delight and spurts out her first coos and squeals, sounding like her first laugh. After you have both come down from the high of your first laugh together, you melt into a comforting cuddle. This first smile is such a powerful enforcer of parenting behavior that you momentarily forget the sleep you are losing and the rest of your social and professional life that is now on hold.

Engaging Behaviors

Remember those helpless feelings when you didn't know what baby needed, and how frustrated you were when you couldn't stop her cries? In the previous month, except for a cry and a few decodable "Pick me up" signals, you often didn't know where you stood. Now the two-month-old is easier to read. The smiles are an opener to relate and play. The cries take on a more purposeful pattern. Around two months, babies show a set of interesting cues we call *engaging behaviors* — social signals that show you how they feel and what they need.

Martha notes: Matthew lets me know when he's hungry, and he knows that I usually hold him cradled in my arms for feeding. He knows that I fiddle with my blouse and unhook my bra to get ready, so already during this ritual he is letting me know that he anticipates a feeding. He starts to nibble a bit, to rev up his breathing patterns, and to turn toward me in an expectant sort of way. He has already told me that he is hungry, and now he is telling me that he expects to be fed.

Anticipation and protest behaviors. By two months of age your baby may begin showing trust-in-parent signs; the earliest of these is *anticipation*. After rehearsing the cue-response script of "I cry — I get picked up and nursed" (meaning breast, bottle, or comfort) for two months, baby is now ready to show the audience that she understands her lines. Likewise, if her opening lines are misread, she shows *protest behaviors.*

Martha notes: If I miss Matthew's early cues, he protests. He pounds my chest with his tiny little fists in a desperate kind of way and bobs his head back and forth. One day as I was preparing to feed him, I decided to hand him over to dad so I could get one more thing done before I actually sat down for a prolonged feeding. He immediately started to howl. This was the opposite of what he was expecting and wanting. He was angry and very upset and wouldn't settle down until I satisfied his anticipation and fed him.

I have found it much more pleasant for both Matthew and me if I respect his anticipatory behaviors. When he has given me a cue that he is hungry and I respond immediately he is a wonderful sight. If I miss his hunger cues or try to delay a feeding, he may cry for a period of time and his mouth will be very tight and his lips pursed. During the feeding he will continue to be upset. His sucking movements will be tense and his face will be quivering. Disappointing his expectations produces feelings of mistrust which are reflected in his sucking patterns and are not good for either of us. Because of this, I find that my response time is consistently getting shorter.

Catching your moods. Moods are contagious to attached babies and their mothers, and around this stage a mutual mood sensitivity begins. When mother is upset, baby is upset. We have noticed that babies who are most sensitive to their parents' feelings are the ones who have the most trust in their parents. Naturally, a mutual sensitivity develops when two people grow close to each other.

Feeding Behaviors

Scratch the schedule. By two months of age, if not sooner, you will realize that feeding schedules are an illusion of writers outside of the inner circle of baby feeders, especially with breastfeeding babies. Some breastfed babies, for example, like to cluster-feed, bunching several feedings into an hour or two, then going three to four hours without feeding. Shun the rigid term "schedule" and think in terms of feeding *harmony:* reading your baby's cues and not the clock's and being more flexible in response to your baby's individual temperament and your life-style. We prefer the more flexible term "cue feeding" to the "demand feeding" label attached to the hungry little field general.

Now that baby can see clearly for a distance of eight to ten feet (two to three meters), she looks beyond your face and body while nursing and is distracted by other guests in her restaurant. Your baby may suck a little, then stop and look at an interesting scene or passerby, then resume sucking. Going on and off the breast, and even the bottle, is a time-consuming yet passing nuisance. (See page 178 for how to handle this nuisance.)

Two-Month Talk

Your baby's sounds give you a clue to what mood she is in. Cooing sounds are baby's earliest attempts to communicate delight. Remember, language is made up of both sounds and gestures. Notice the amusing sounds that accompany your baby's smile. The initial part of the smile (the mouth opening) is often accompanied by a brief "ah" or "uh," followed by a long, sighing, cooing sound as the smile widens and grows. During the second month baby's vocalizations range from brief one-syllable squeaks and squeals to prolonged expressive sounds: "eh, ah, oh!" Toward the end of the second month baby's throaty, grunting sounds become higher pitched, more vowel-like and musical, including coos, squeaks, and gurgles. Sounds produced during sleep both amuse and worry parents. Baby's breathing may sound rattled as the air moves through puddles of saliva in the back of the throat — the same sound that produces the normal chest rattle that you may now feel.

How Mothers Talk to Babies

Many times during the early months you will wonder how much of what you are saying really gets through to your baby. Research confirms what parents have long suspected — when mother talks, baby listens.

Let's try a home video experiment. When your baby is in the quiet alert state, capture an eye-to-eye fix and begin your natural mother talk while your husband tapes the scene. When you play back the tape, you will see baby's and mother's body language are in synchrony. If you play the videotape in slow motion, you will notice that the listening baby's head and body movements seem to dance in time to the rhythm of mother's voice. You really are getting through to your baby, although imperceptibly.

Natural baby talk. You don't have to learn how to talk to your baby. You're a natural. Mothers instinctively use motherese — upbeat tones and facial gestures — to talk to their baby. They raise the pitch, s-l-o-w the rate, and E-X-A-G-G-E-R-A-T-E the main syllables. Notice that you put your whole face into the act by over-widening your mouth and eyes while talking. The quality of mother's speech is tailored to the baby's listening abilities, slowing down and speeding up according to baby's attention. To make sure baby gets the message, mothers instinctively draw out their vowels — "Gooood baaaby." How mother talks is more important to a baby than what she says.

Taking turns. Mothers talk in slowly rising crescendos and decrescendos with bursts and pauses, allowing baby some time to process each short vocal package before the next message arrives. Though you may feel that talking to your baby is a monologue, you naturally speak to your baby as if you're imagining a dialogue. Video analysis of the fine art of mother-baby communication shows that mother behaves as if she imagines baby talks back. She naturally shortens her messages and elongates her pauses to the exact length of time that coincides with the length of the imagined response from the baby, especially when she is talking to the baby in the form of a question. This is baby's earliest speech lesson, in which mother is shaping baby's ability to listen. The infant stores these early abilities away and later recalls them when beginning to speak.

Tips for Talking to Your Baby

The preceding research findings on speech analysis show that every mother naturally receives an honorary degree as her baby's speech teacher. Following are some more tips to help your early communication get off to an even better start.

Look at the listener. Capture baby's eyes before beginning your conversation, and you will be able to hold her attention longer and are more likely to get an appreciative response.

Address baby by name. While baby may not associate the name with herself for a few more months, hearing it frequently triggers a mental association that this is a special sound she has heard before and signals that more fun sounds will follow — much as an adult perks up to a familiar tune.

Keep it simple. Use short two- or three-word sentences and one- or two-syllable words with lots of drawn-out, exaggerated vowels: "Preeetty baaaby." As when composing a telegram, avoid cluttering your dialogue with "the" and "a." Drop the pronouns "I" and "me." They have no meaning to baby. Refer to yourselves as "mommy" and "daddy."

Keep it lively. Say "Wave bye-bye cat" as you direct your waving bye-bye at the cat. Babies are more likely to recall words that are associated with *animated gestures*. Give your speech some spark with inflections at the end of the sentence. Exaggerate cue words. File away which sounds get the best audience reaction. Babies become bored easily, especially with the same old sound.

Ask questions. "Matthew want to nurse?" "Go bye-bye?" Talking in questions will naturally amplify the sound at the end of the sentence as you anticipate baby's response.

Talk about what you are doing. As you go through your daily maintenance tasks of dressing, bathing, and changing baby, narrate what you are doing, much like a sportscaster describing a game: "Now daddy takes off the diaper . . . now we put a new one on . . ." It's normal to feel a bit foolish initially, but you are not talking to a stone wall. There is a little person with big ears processing every word she hears, storing it on an endless memory record.

Watch for go signs and stop signs. Wait for your baby to show engagement cues (smiling, sustaining eye contact, and hands-out gesturing) as if to say, "I like it, keep on talking." Also, observe stop signs of disengagement (vacant staring and turning eyes and head away from your face) that say, "I've had enough of this chatter, let's change gears."

Give baby a turn. When asking a question, give baby time to answer. As when you talk to another person, pause frequently to give baby a chance to get in a little coo or squeak. Baby is likely to tune out a steady commentary.

Give baby feedback. If baby responds or when baby opens the conversation with a smiling total body wiggle or a charming coo, imitate her vocalization and replay it back. Mimicking her language adds value to it and reinforces baby's attempts to continue to get her point across.

Read to baby. Babies love nursery rhymes and poems with an up-and-down singsong cadence. Reading aloud can help you satisfy two persons with the same story. Reading to a toddler while holding and sometimes breast-feeding your new baby may hold both busy babies' attention. There will be days when your adult mind needs more than Mother Goose. Read your favorite magazine or book aloud to baby, pepping up the story for a baby's ear.

Say it with music. Infant researchers believe that singing affects more of the brain centers for language than do words without music. Even if you are not an opera star you will at least have an admiring audience of one. Babies at all ages love familiar songs, either self-composed or borrowed. File away baby's top ten favorites and replay them frequently. A desire for parents to repeat their entertainment is a forerunner of the incessant encores to come: "Again . . . again, Mom [or Dad]."

Two-Month Moves

Loosening hands and arms. The tight fist and body-clenched arms of the first month loosen a bit during the second month, as if the reflexes that kept baby's muscles flexed tightly inward were overruled by the maturing brain's saying, "Loosen up and enjoy the world." Baby's tightly clenched fingers unfold one by one to fan out into an open hand. When you place a rattle in the palm of baby's hand she will tightly grasp the toy and hold on to it awhile. But don't expect her to voluntarily reach for the rattle until next month. Baby's tightly clenched fist doesn't eagerly release its treasured toy. Stroking the back of a baby's hand may persuade the tight fist to loosen its grip.

First reaches. Baby's first attempt to reach out and touch her world seems totally aimless, but there is a bit of directionality in her punches. The short little jabs in the general direction of a dangling toy score more misses than hits. But practice makes perfect.

➤*SAFETY TIP: Always stay with your baby while there is a mobile within reach. Even though her waving hands seem aimless,*

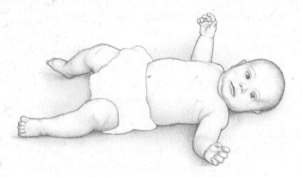

The flexed-limb posture of the first month unfolds into a more relaxed position in the second.

baby's finger, or worse, her neck, can get caught in the dangling strings — which should be no longer than eight inches (twenty centimeters).

The opening of eyes, voice, and hands during this second month is a prelude to the social person to emerge during the next month.

THE THIRD MONTH: BIG HANDS

"My three-month-old is so inviting," exclaimed one mother. "Mine seems so responsive," said another. "I just love the way he waves his arms at me," added another mother. The third month is a fun period for both baby and parents. Your baby is more alert, active, organized, and responsive. Communication is better by the third month because both parents and baby have become comfortable with each other's cues. For these reasons, parents often describe the third month as easier.

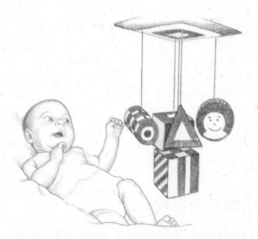

Baby begins to use her hands as tools in the second month.

Handy Hands

Those adorable little hands. How often you've played with them, prying open tightly curled fingers and rubbing the soft palms over your face. Now baby can play with his own hands. The beginning of hand play is the most noteworthy feature of the third month. The previously clenched fists unfold, and the hands remain half-open most of the time.

At this stage babies realize their hands are familiar and easily accessible toys and, most important, part of themselves. Watch baby play with his hands in front of his face. He may explore one hand with the other, sometimes holding the whole fist, other times grabbing just one or two fingers. Of course, these curious hands find their way to their familiar target, the mouth, as baby delights in fist and finger sucking. These are baby's first tools, and now he begins to use them.

Reach out and grab someone. Watch out, hair and clothing, here come the hands. Everything in grabbing distance is fair game. Babies love to pull hair, grab glasses, grab daddy's tie, and, a favorite, pull on mommy's blouse during nursing. These first grabs are powerful and not very polite. Once baby gets

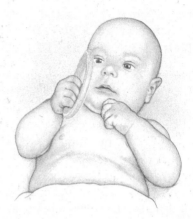

Toy of the month: A rubber or plastic ring or bracelet is the most educational toy for the three-month-old. Watch as baby uses hand and mouth to explore this simple toy.

hold of a fistful of hair, he doesn't easily let go.

The first reaches are not very defined either. When trying to reach and grab a dangling toy, the arm movements are still short, boxerlike karate chops, swiping and still often missing. Next month he'll be more on target.

Holding power. Baby shows increasing power in holding on to toys. Now instead of dropping a rattle immediately (as he did a few weeks ago), if you place a rattle or ring into baby's half-open hands, his fingers curl around it, and he holds on to and even studies it momentarily until he drops it because he is tired or bored. Here are a few tips for choosing a rattle for your baby:

- The lighter the rattle and the easier it is to grip, the longer your baby will hold it.

- Black and white or contrasting colors best hold baby's attention.

A POSTURE TIP FOR STIMULATING HAND PLAY

The position of baby's body influences hand skills. The horizontal position hinders hand play; the upright posture stimulates it. When lying flat on the floor, baby will be more interested in freestyle cycling her hands and feet and stretching them out from her body. Also, when baby is lying on her back, the tonic neck reflex causes her head to turn to one side and her arm to dart out on that side and her hands to stay closed. Instead of lying flat, baby should be in a semiupright position in your arms or in an infant seat. As you raise your baby to a semiupright position, notice that her head faces forward and she looks toward a person or toy instead of to one side, and her hands and arms stay open and inviting as if she is flirting with you or the toy. Semi-upright posture encourages the arms and hands to come together, stimulating baby to play with her hands or with toys in front of her.

- Babies prefer the feel of fabric to plastic rattles.
- A safe rattle that won't cause choking has dimensions of no less than one and one-half by two inches (four by five centimeters) and no sharp or detachable parts.

Baby's Visual Development Shines

Watch your baby's eyes fix on an interesting floral pattern on the furniture or wallpaper, or on the ever-favorite face. Notice how she now studies these patterns longer, paying more attention to the detail instead of momentarily scanning them, as in the previous month.

Tracking also matures. Observe your baby holding a visual fix, tracking you, radarlike, as you walk by her and leave the room. She may cry as you depart. Besides seeing better at this stage, babies see farther. When in the quiet alert state, baby may gaze at ceiling fans, light and dark contrasting ceiling beams, shadows on the wall, or plants on a ledge fifteen to twenty feet (five to six meters) away. Dark contrasting objects on light walls are the most appealing.

Martha notes: I can keep Matthew's attention by holding a black-and-white six-faced cube about two feet in front of his eyes. He is riveted to the "moving picture" for at least five minutes. He studies each side as it slowly rotates and appears to discern the design difference on each side. Sometimes as Matthew starts to fuss I pop out the cube and he stops fussing.

Three-Month Talk

Here's when the real conversations begin. One reason you may find this stage easier is that you are able to read your three-month-old. Watch your baby's facial and body language and try to guess what he is thinking by the way he is acting. By reading baby's mouth and facial language you can often tell what emotion is soon to follow — is he going to cry or smile? By quickly intervening with "Hi, baby [name]!" you can often divert a cry to a smile. Seeing your happy face makes baby forget to fuss.

Communicative cries. Not only is baby's body language easier to read but his cries, too, are more revealing. Different cries reflect different needs — and require different responses. The red-alert cries warrant an instant pick-baby-up. The fuss cries, however, may merit a longer-distance response from another room. Notice the *anticipatory pauses* in your baby's cries. He is telling you he expects a response and is likely to protest if misread.

Vocalizing increases. Baby begins to "talk" more. Sounds become louder, more vowel-like, and baby begins to draw out the vowel sounds longer: "aaah," "eeeh," "eee," "oooh." Listen to those long strings of gurgles, goos, growls, screeches, hollers, and sighs as baby experiments with the way different tongue and mouth movements produce various sounds. Baby becomes amazed at how loudly he can screech — and the instant attention his howls bring from his caregivers. Very early baby learns that his sounds have shock value. But this loudspeaker may need some fine-tuning. Even at this stage baby can adjust his tone to yours. If you greet baby's ear-piercing screeches with a whisper, he is likely to modulate his voice.

Three-Month Moves

Since it is safest for babies to sleep on their backs, provide baby with some daily tummy time and tummy talk to help strengthen his head-lifting muscles. Place your baby tummy down on a padded surface on the table or the floor. Get down to his level. Lock in the eye-to-eye fix and begin talking. Baby may raise his head forty-five degrees or more and carry on a head-to-head visual conversation. Instead of quickly plopping his head down as he did last month, baby may hold his head up for a while and begin *searching* by rotating his head from side to side.

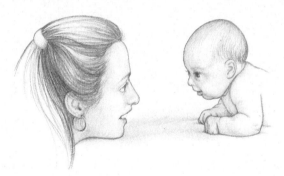

Tummy talk. Your three-month-old will raise his head to make eye contact.

Next game. Roll baby over on his back (most babies cannot yet roll over themselves), hold both hands, and gradually pull baby to a sitting position. Head and trunk lift together. Notice how much less now than last month baby's head lags behind his body. When held sitting, baby begins to hold his previously wobbly head steady. The unsupported head may still tire and quickly sag, but baby can now regain control of the droopy head and resume holding it erect.

Stand and lean. Place your hands under baby's arms and hold him standing up. Last month he probably would have quickly crumpled down on his wobbly legs. This month he may bear most of his weight for a few moments, being supported only for balance. Now hold baby standing on your hands and lean his chest against yours. Notice how much stronger baby's legs are this month.

Floor play. The *up-down game* begins. While most three-month-olds still like to be held a lot, baby may like to be placed on his back on the floor to enjoy freestyle play. The restrictive tonic neck reflex begins to diminish, allowing baby's stretched-out limbs to swing and cycle freely — called "flapping his

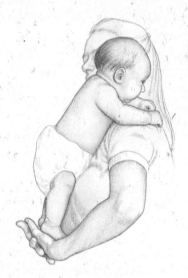

At three months, baby loses some of his wobbliness.

wings." Naturally, his admiring audience cheers on his performance from above. Better yet, get down with him so he'll have company.

Learning cause and effect. By three months baby discovers that he can make things happen. A certain play action causes a certain reaction — called *contingency play:* "I swipe or kick the mobile — it moves." "I shake the rattle — it makes noise."

As baby stores these cause-and-effect patterns of behavior in his developing brain, he begins to make adjustments in these patterns to improve their outcome. For example, by this time your baby has learned to suck in such a way that he gets the milk most efficiently.

Martha notes: I notice that Matthew will latch on to my breast, give a few sucks, and then wait for the milk-ejection reflex to start

the milk flowing. Only then does he start actively sucking and swallowing. He learned that this was the easy way to get a feeding started.

As baby becomes brighter and you become more observant, you both are well on your way to growing together.

A THREE-MONTH REVIEW

The first three months were the fitting-in period. You and your baby were getting used to each other. Your regular sleep and feeding patterns were organized into whatever routine worked for your family life-style and the needs of your baby. By trial and error you developed a parenting style that worked. And whatever career juggling needed to be done, you did.

By the end of this first stage, baby has learned two fundamental lessons: *organiza-*

SAFETY TIPS

- By three months babies can scoot, wiggle, and roll. Never leave a baby unattended on a changing table or in an infant seat on a countertop, even for a second. Use the safety belt in the infant seat and place the seat only on a carpeted floor.

- Use a guardrail or cushions alongside baby if she is in your bed (see illustration on page 319). Never leave baby unattended on a couch or any other piece of furniture that she can roll off.

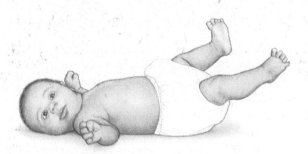

Baby "flaps his wings."

tion and *trust.* The fussy period of learning to fit into life outside the womb has subsided (somewhat), and baby knows to whom he belongs. Because his needs have been consistently responded to, he has developed the most powerful infant development stimulator: trust. Based upon an inner feeling of rightness, baby wastes less energy fussing and now diverts this energy into developing skills — called baby competence. Because his cues have been read, he values himself — the beginning of baby's self-esteem.

You have graduated from novice to veteran at reading and responding to your baby's cues. You understand your baby's language, primitive though it may be. Perhaps life with a new baby has not been all rosy — it never is. But at least by this stage you feel more comfortable in the two *R*'s of parenting: *reading* your baby's cues and *responding* in a way that works — at least most of the time. It is normal for you to feel a bit shaky in these two skills. But if you and your baby are still

---

FLAT HEAD

During the second or third month of life, some babies begin to develop a flat area on the back of the head. This is called *positional plagiocephaly,* and it typically occurs either on one side or directly in the middle of the back of the head when a baby spends too much time sleeping with the head in one position. You can easily see this asymmetry by viewing your baby's head from the top. As baby develops a flat spot, it becomes more comfortable for him to continue sleeping with his head resting on the flat area. This preference only makes the problem worse. You can prevent this by rotating your baby's sleep position (always keeping baby on his back or side). If your baby develops a flat spot, use a wedge or rolled-up blanket to prop baby on his side so that the nonflat part of his head rests on the bed. For example, if the left side of baby's head gets flat, prop him on his side facing to his right. During the day when you put baby down to play, place him so all the action is on the side opposite his flat spot. A few months of this position change should straighten out the problem. Do not worry. This flat area is purely a cosmetic issue and has no effect on the baby's brain growth. There is an extremely rare condition in which the skull bones don't expand as baby's brain grows, creating an asymmetric skull. Be sure your doctor examines baby's skull carefully to make sure this is not the case. Severe cases of positional plagiocephaly can be treated using a pressure helmet, which slowly molds baby's head back into shape. These are expensive and rarely necessary.

strangers, it's time to take inventory of your parenting style. Reread Chapter 1. Is your nest too busy or cluttered with nonbaby things? Consult parents who seem to be in harmony with their babies. The earlier you and your baby begin growing together, the more you'll enjoy parenting during the next stage.

THE FOURTH MONTH: BIG LOOKS

Now the real fun begins. The social, motor, and language skills that started in the previous stage really blossom during the next three months, which we call the interactive stage.

The Master Skill — Binocular Vision

As you become a veteran baby watcher, you will notice that each stage has one important skill that, once mastered, has a snowball effect in helping baby better develop other skills. Binocular vision is the master skill of the fourth month. Baby can now use both eyes together, giving him better depth perception — the ability to judge accurately the distance between his eyes and the things he sees. Imagine what baby had to put up with in the previous month. After swiping at and missing targets for three months, baby can finally get a consistent fix on a toy *and* grab it accurately.

When your baby develops binocular vision, here's what he can do with it. First, he tracks better. Watch him hold a visual fix on a toy or person moving from side to side, a full

> ### "MY BABY'S NOT DOING THAT!"
>
> There will be times when you feel, "My baby's not doing that yet!" Don't worry. Nearly all babies go through the milestones we discuss, but they may not always be "on time." The month-to-month progression is more important than the timing. Enjoy the *sequence* of development and don't focus on which month you are reading about.

180 degrees. And, while tracking, his head begins to catch up with his eyes so that both begin to move together.

Gazing begins. Gazing is more than seeing. It includes the sense of sight plus the ability to move the head and eyes to keep a visual fix on a moving target. To see if your baby has mastered this skill, try the *mutual gazing game:* When baby is in the quiet alert state capture his attention with a visual fix. Then slowly tilt your head. Watch him tilt his. Rotate his body and notice he turns his head to keep his favorite face in view. This is gazing — a powerful visual skill that captures all who lock into baby's eyes.

Martha notes: One of the most exciting things about our four-month-old's development is the way he reaches for me with his eyes. He expresses thanks with his eyes. He turns his face and eyes toward me. They are so expressive and adoring. He appears to be fully aware of me as his source of love, nourishment, and well-being. He craves my presence and totally enjoys our togetherness. It's a love affair, full-blown. I recognize the love in his eyes as one more emotion that he's capable of expressing.

Favorite colors. Besides being able to see more clearly, babies widen their color preference. While black and white were the favorites — and may remain so for a while — your baby may begin to show an increasing interest in colors. Babies prefer natural colors, like the reds and yellows of flowers, and they still shun pastels. To encourage baby's interest in color, continue to contrast light and dark colors — alternating red and yellow stripes, for example.

Martha notes: When I'm reading books to the older children, Matthew is very interested in looking at pages that are white or yellow and have large, dark printed letters. He studies the letters intently and makes cooing noises. It almost looks as though he's trying to read what he's looking at.

Reach Out and Touch Someone — Accurately

The development of binocular vision is a prelude to an important hand-eye skill — *visually directed reaching,* meaning the eyes lead the hands to grab the desired object or person accurately. Watch your baby's eyes follow his hands as he reaches for a toy. It seems as if hands and eyes are finally saying, "Let's move together to improve our aim."

Hand play. One of the most intriguing developments of this stage is increased interest in hand play. Now that baby's eyes have clear depth perception, he may constantly play with his favorite and ever-present toys — his hands. Sucking on fingers and fists now

becomes a treasured pastime. To relieve gum soreness, the beginning teether gnaws on his hands as readily available teething objects.

Martha notes: Matthew's favorite hand toy is a red rubber ring around three to four inches in diameter. We watch all the things he can do with this simple inexpensive toy. He can grab it, squeeze it, bring it toward the midline in front of his face, study it, grab it with the other hand, pull it with both hands, release it with one hand while holding it with the other, transfer the ring to the other hand again, and gum the ring as it inevitably finds its way to its final destination, his mouth. He seems amazed at his complete control of this simple toy.

Gathering in. Most babies do not yet reach accurately with one hand. Dangle an interesting toy in front of your baby's face within reaching distance. Rather than reach out with one hand with pinpoint accuracy, he will most likely embrace the toy with both hands as if gathering it in toward himself. Sometimes he'll miss the toy entirely, and his embracing hands will meet and continue on to the mouth. Now move the toy while he is reaching for it, and he'll probably miss it or turn away because you have violated his rules of the reaching game. Hold the toy still. At this stage most babies cannot yet make in-flight corrections to grab moving toys accurately.

▶*SAFETY TIP: Beware of the reaching and grabbing tendencies of the four-month-old. Keep baby beyond the reach of harmful objects, such as hot beverages or sharp and fragile items. Never hold a hot beverage while holding a baby, no matter how careful you plan to be. Babies have lightning-fast reaches.*

Moves of the Month

Rolling over. When your baby rolls over depends more on baby's temperament than motor maturity. Very active babies, who enjoy stiffening and back arching, are apt to roll over sooner. When lying on his tummy, the active baby may practice push-ups and torque his head to one side, surprising himself when he flips over. Mellow babies are content to lie and gaze at visual delights. They flip around less and are likely not to roll over until five to six months. Most babies at this stage roll from tummy to side or from side to side, and they usually first roll from tummy to back before rolling from back to tummy.

Preteething Signs

Though you may not see those pearly whites for several more months, your baby may now begin to feel them. Here are the usual signs that baby senses teething discomfort:

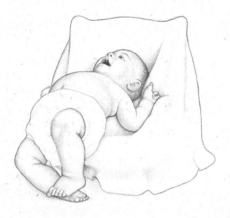

Active babies are likely to roll over at an earlier age than mellow babies. Keep a watchful eye on your little squirmer.

- Drooling begins, accompanied by a pink raised rash around the lips and chin (drool rash) and often looser bowel movements (drool stools) and a similar rash around the anus. For the next few months expect a constant case of wet mouth.

- Baby may massage his gums with his tongue and suck on his favorite teethers — fingers and fist.

- Baby may chomp on your nipples or slide his sore gums over your nipple to massage his gums. (See page 179 for taming the nipple chomper and page 495 for teething tips.)

Fun and Games with a Four-month-old

Grab-and-shake games. Offer baby rattles, four-inch (ten-centimeter) rings, rag dolls, and small cuddly blankets.

Sit-and-hit games. Dangle an interesting toy or mobile within baby's reach. Watch him punch at it or try to gather it into his arms.

Kick toys. Pom-poms, a helium balloon on a short string, rattles, and pleasant noisemakers can be attached to baby's ankles for him to activate with his kicking. He can also kick at mobiles or balls within range — all under supervision, of course.

Finger games. Under supervision, give your baby piles of yarn to explore with his fingers. Change the texture by using different kinds of yarn. Tying six-inch strips of yarn loosely to baby's fingers helps him realize that he can move each of these interesting appendages

THREE FAVORITE FOUR-MONTH-BABY POSES

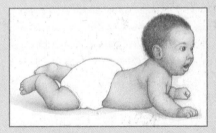

Head up — chest up. Get out the cameras. The classic four-month-baby pose is here: head up ninety degrees, upper body propped up resting on elbows with chest completely off the floor, and eyes searching from side to side for admiring photographers.

Sitting all propped up. Sit your baby on the floor, and he may momentarily prop himself up with both arms before falling forward on his nose or toppling sideways — be there to catch. At four months of age baby's lower back muscles are usually still too weak for baby to sit erect. To determine if your baby is developing a sense of balance yet, hold him in the sitting position by his hips and momentarily let go. Baby may thrust out his hand to catch his fall as he leans sideways, indicating he is developing a sense of balance.

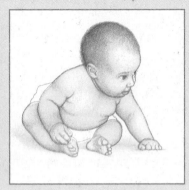

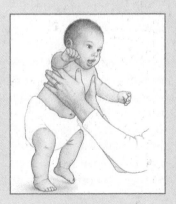

First stands. Hold baby in the standing position. By four months most babies can bear all their weight for a few seconds before collapsing. Continue holding his hands, and baby will often pull back up to a standing position. Watch baby's face showing delight in his newly found standing skill; arms will also flap in delight. (Early standing does not cause bowed legs, despite grandmother's warnings. Babies only stand for a few seconds. It's lying in the curled-up fetal position all night that contributes to curled legs.)

separately. Later, lightweight puppet figures can be attached to the dangling yarn.

➤ *SAFETY TIP: Never leave a baby unattended with a piece of string or yarn or a balloon. Keep string or yarn shorter than* *eight inches (twenty centimeters). Make a safe "yarn pile" by tying a dozen six-inch strips together at their centers.*

Sofa sitting. Sit baby in the bend of a sofa pillow. He may spend five to ten minutes looking around and enjoying this new posture and vantage point.

Rolling games. Drape baby over a large beach ball and roll it slowly back and forth. This helps him develop balance.

Peekaboo. This old favorite can be played by hiding behind a piece of cloth or cardboard or popping up from behind a couch. Be sure to talk to your baby and make exaggerated faces: "Where's mommy? Here I am!"

Pull-up games. Hold a thin bar, such as a golf club or baton, in front of baby's chest. He will grab on, tighten his grip, and gradually pull himself up.

Mirror play. Babies love to sit or be held in front of mirrors, enjoying their own movements. (See "Magic Mirror," page 380.)

Gitchee-gitchee-goo. Tickling games that use tactile and vocal gestures get you both laughing.

LANGUAGE DEVELOPMENT, FOUR TO SIX MONTHS

Baby's language in the early months was hard to decode. Now baby becomes a better communicator. During this stage baby learns that language is fun, and she also learns how to use sound and body language to affect caregivers.

New Sounds

Watch baby's wide-open mouth. Here comes the "ah," then the mouth circle closes a bit, and "ah" changes to an "oh." Once baby realizes her sound-changing power is affected by simply altering the contour of her mouth, she doesn't want to quit. Baby stretches out these sounds into long strings of "ah-oh-ah-oh" and long, drawn-out vowels, "eeeeeee," especially during exciting play or in anticipation of the pleasurable event of nursing. Notice baby's short catchup breaths between these long strings of sounds.

Cue sounds. Try to associate certain sounds with specific needs. If "ah-ah-ah" and "eeeeeee" means "I want to feed," listen and respond. Baby will soon learn the sound value of various vocalizations and be more motivated to keep talking.

Loud sounds. Not only does baby realize she can make different sounds and longer sounds, now she can make *louder* sounds by pushing more air through her voice box. Watch baby take a deep breath, and out come the hollers. Soon baby learns which sounds have shock value. Attention-getting yells and protests seem to trigger a more rapid response from listeners. Baby is not being deliberately annoying. She is just trying on new sounds to see which one she likes best and is testing which ones shake up her audience. She will soon learn that pleasant sounds get a pleasant listening response. You can help baby modulate her hollers by answering a yell with a whisper. Baby will get the message.

Laughing sounds. When excited during play, baby pushes air through those quivering little vocal cords so fast that laughter is full of squeals. Want baby to laugh more? Playful tickles, gitchee-gitchee-goos, and silly sounds are likely to invoke laughter. You are your baby's favorite comedian. You're playing to an audience of one, and you can count on lots of laughs. Remember, as silly as baby's silly sounds sound to you, your silly sounds sound just as silly to baby. Laugh together.

Raspberries. First on the top-ten baby sounds between four and six months is a variety of bubble-blowing sputters affectionately known as raspberries. These delightful baby sounds occur when baby blows air through the saliva-filled mouth against pursed lips. As baby approaches teething time, expect many of the sounds to take on a wet and sputtering quality.

First babbles. Sometime between four and six months babies start to make the earliest of true language sounds — *babbling,* the sounds produced when baby combines a vowel sound with a consonant and repeats it over and over ("ba-ba-ba-ba"). Babbling will be most noticeable in the next stage of language development, from six to nine months.

Help Your Baby to Be a Good Communicator

Enjoying language not only helps baby learn to communicate better, it also helps you to communicate better with your baby. Try these early language lessons.

Familiar openers. Open the dialogue with familiar words, such as your baby's name, and repeat them frequently with a musical quality in your voice. By four months, most babies respond consistently to their names. At this age baby will also notice words that obviously refer only to him, such as "cutie" or "sweetie." Baby recognizes the unique tone of voice that you reserve for him. If you want to know how important baby's name is to him, try this test: Talk to your baby from behind without using his name; then speak

---

PRECIOUS RECORDINGS

Want to have some fun with precious baby sounds? Tape-record baby's sounds at each stage of development. When listening to these recordings, even in the early months you will be able to pick out certain repetitive patterns, such as the comforting sounds of "ah" or the excitement of "eeeeee!" We keep a tape recorder at the bedside. You will usually get the best of baby's vocalizations when he first wakes up. These delightful wake-up sounds announce to the world that today's play is about to begin. Audio capture the sounds and video capture the body language while you can, as these dialects and infant mannerisms pass all too quickly.

---

the same sentence beginning with his name. Baby will turn toward the speaker more consistently if addressed by name.

Attention holders. Babies tune in to conversations and can tune them out as well. Use opening words such as "hi" and "hello" to engage baby's attention and hold it through the conversation. When you notice your baby's gaze begin to wander, repeat these opening cue words to reengage baby.

Matching. Engage your baby in a face-to-face dialogue. Start with a very open-mouthed, wide-eyed, expressive "ah." Wait for your baby to open his mouth and perhaps mimic the sound. Then slowly circle your lips down into the "oh" sound and see if baby matches the sound. The ability to match your sounds indicates that speech is an intelligent activity that your baby recognizes and voluntarily attempts to reproduce.

Labeling. Give names to familiar toys, persons, or household pets. Start with one-syllable words such as "mom," "dad," "ball," "cat." When your baby's gaze indicates that he is interested in the cat, teach him the name for it. First use an opening phrase — "Hi, baby!" — to engage baby's attention. Once baby turns to you and locks in on your gaze, slowly turn your gaze toward the cat, allowing baby to follow your eyes. When both of you are looking at the cat, point and exclaim, "Cat!" in a very excited tone. During this stage of development baby may associate the label "cat" with the whole sequence of events — your steering his gaze toward the cat, your pointing at the cat, and your saying the word "cat." He probably will not turn toward the cat if you give him only the label without the accompanying directing gestures. In the next development stage, from six to nine months, baby may turn and point toward the cat as it walks by with no cues other than your saying the word "cat."

Expansion of baby-initiated language. Expansion carries labeling one step further. When baby initiates interest in a familiar object, gazing at the cat walking by, for example, expand on his interest by exclaiming, "There's cat!" Expansion capitalizes on a well-known principle of education: *Learning that is initiated by the baby is more likely to be remembered.* Follow through on other baby-initiated cues. When baby sneezes, quickly exclaim, "Bless you!" After many repetitions of this response, baby will turn toward you after a sneeze, anticipating your "Bless you." Expansion and following through reinforce baby's emerging sense of competency, making him feel that his primitive language has value. Therefore, he has value.

Echoing. Another way to capitalize on baby-initiated language is to echo the sound back to baby. Mimicking the sounds that baby produces further reinforces that you hear what he says and are interested in his sounds — therefore you are interested in him.

Taking turns. Remember that dialogue has a rhythm of listening and responding. Try to develop a rhythm in your conversation with your baby. Encouraging him to listen is an important part of language development. Taking turns in conversation fosters attentive stillness, an important quality in learning language and the state in which baby is most receptive to learning how to communicate. Taking an active part in helping your baby enjoy language not only helps baby to learn to communicate better, it also helps you communicate with your baby. Learning about your baby helps you learn from your baby.

Mutual gazing. Watch your baby orient his head toward yours, smile, wiggle, vocalize, and with these cues invite a social exchange. Baby is now able to initiate, maintain, or stop a social interaction by simply moving his head.

Mutual gazing is a potent interpersonal magnet. Adults seldom hold a mutual gaze for more than a few seconds, except perhaps when falling in love. Parents and babies, however, can remain interlocked in a mutual gaze for much longer. I have seen babies gaze at their caregivers, trancelike, for up to thirty seconds. Babies nearly always outlast their caregivers at the blinking game, holding their eyes focused and motionless much longer than the adult.

Social Signals

The ability to engage and disengage a caregiver or to direct caregivers toward meeting his needs is one of the most fascinating social interactions of the four-to-six-month stage. Now baby can tell you what he needs, not with words but with body language that requires careful listening.

Martha notes: *When Matthew wants to nurse he has a definite signal of nuzzling, and when that signal isn't picked up he goes into a vocalization that is peculiar to wanting to nurse: a string of breathy vowel sounds — "a-a-a-a" — during short bursts of inhaling and exhaling, all the while orienting toward my breast.*

One day Matthew was fussing a bit and squirming in my arms, and none of my comforting measures worked. He would look over toward the rocking chair and squirm his body in that direction. It took me a while to understand what he wanted. When I finally got around to giving him the rocking chair it was an instant success.

DECODING SOCIAL SIGNALS

Here's an exercise to help you learn to interpret your baby's early signals. List your favorite social signals in one column, your interpretation of these signals in another, and how baby reacts to your response in the third column. After a few months of practicing this exercise, you will be well on your way to becoming a keen baby watcher. For example:

Social Signals	What Baby's Trying to Tell Me	How Baby Responded
• Leans toward me, eyes wide open, waving arms in embracing motion	• "Let's play!"	• We "talked" nonstop for three minutes.
• Makes short, breathy, staccato cries	• "I'm going to cry unless you pick me up right away."	• He quieted as soon as I picked him up.
• Smacks lips and clutches at my blouse	• "I want to nurse."	• He chowed down.
• Fusses and arches back when held	• "I want to be put down on the rug to kick and play."	• He just wanted to be put down on the floor to kick.
• Fusses when put down on rug	• "I want to be walked around and held in a baby carrier."	• He quieted when I put him in the sling.

Social Gesturing Begins

Gesturing is another exciting body-language behavior that begins during this stage. At this point baby's gesturing cues may be very subtle, such as nodding his head toward a desired object or turning his body toward the bed when you approach it. In a later stage of development baby will gesture better with his hands and arms.

The better you listen and respond, the better baby learns to "talk." The feeling "I'm understood" is a powerful builder of baby's self-esteem.

But What About Spoiling?

"Is baby manipulating me?" you may ask. Once upon a time there was a school of misguided baby-care "experts" who taught vulnerable new parents that responding so quickly to baby's needs would spoil their babies, that babies would be clingy, dependent, and manipulative. That school is now closed. Volumes of research have disproved the spoiling theory. Responsive parenting turns out secure, independent, less whiny children. Put the fear of spoiling out of your mind.

THE FIFTH MONTH: BIG REACHES

Reaching one-handed is an exciting developmental accomplishment at this stage. To appreciate the serial development of baby's ability to reach, let's review the sequence of reaching from birth to five months. Even in the first couple of months a finger may momentarily flit or dart out in the direction of the object of interest. This subtle, almost imperceptible gesture is the beginning of reaching.

Around three months of age baby discovers that her hands are easily reachable objects, and, even more amazing, they are a part of herself. Baby begins pointing, swiping, and batting at close objects. Her misses usually outnumber the direct hits. There is very little directionality in the early swiping movements. From three to four months the beginning of midline play (using the hands in front of the body) is another important milestone in the development of reaching. One hand serves as a target for the other. The development of binocular vision enables baby to begin gathering-in motions in the fourth month, and baby develops some direction to his reaching.

Reach Out and Touch Someone — With One Hand

Around the fifth month, the two-handed embracing type of reaching progresses into

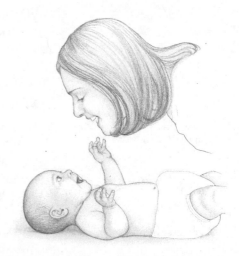

Developing babies enjoy floor play with mom or dad.

an accurate one-handed reach. In baby's first touch-grasp motions, she uses her whole hand in a mittenlike grasp to trap the object between all of her fingers and the palm of her hand. Also around the fifth month, baby reaches out with one hand for objects that are nearly an arm's length away. Watch your baby grasp the intended toy precisely in her hand, examine it, and then transfer it to the other hand or to her mouth.

Martha notes: Matthew is now more of an interactive person. He will take the toy I give him and is able to appreciate and use the toy.

When Matthew gets tired during a game it is often because I have been handing him the same toy over and over. If I start handing him different toys, then his interest in the game is renewed.

When Matthew is playing with an object he does primarily three things with it. He explores it with his hands, he brings it to his mouth to explore it, and he looks at it with his eyes. As he draws the toy closer to his face in order to bring it to his mouth, his eyes try to stay on the object, but when it's right in front of his face it has probably gone out of focus, so in order to see the toy again he will stretch his arms out to bring the object to a comfortable seeing distance from his face. This is why Matthew seems to be telescoping the toy back and forth in front of his face.

Maintain Voice Contact

Baby's developing ability to associate the voice with the person adds a new dimension to keeping in touch with your baby. Use this ability of voice recognition and localization to calm your baby. When your baby is fussing in the other room, call out, "Mama's coming." Baby will often quiet down and will be waving his arms and kicking his legs in anticipation when you enter the room.

Not until around a year of age can you expect baby to keep an image of you in his mind when he can't see you. Voice contact ("Mama's here") will help lessen baby's worry, but expect baby to fuss during your disappearing acts for many months.

Favorite Five-Month Activities

Playing airplane. Place your five-month-old on his tummy and notice how he flaps his arms, pedals his legs, rocks on his tummy, arches his neck for the takeoff, and plays airplane.

Pushing off. Here's how you help him "take off." Push your hand against the soles of his feet while he is on his runway and watch him propel himself forward by pushing off on your hand. Digging in and pushing off is why you may discover that your baby has squirmed all the way across the crib.

Pushing up. Last month baby was content to lift his head and chest up and rest on his elbows. Now he can do a complete push-up, lifting his chest off the floor with his arms extended as props.

Playing with the feet. Reclining in your lap, baby may now be able to crane his neck forward to grab and play with his flying feet.

Pulling to sit and stand. Now pull your baby up by the hands to a sitting position and notice how he assists you by lifting his head

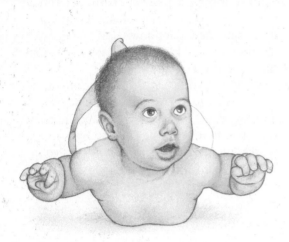

The "airplane" pose.

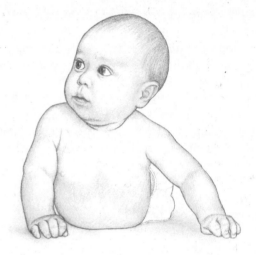

By five months, baby can do a complete push-up.

forward and flexing his elbows, making it easy to pull him to sitting and standing positions.

First sitting. One of my favorite five-month poses is baby sitting without support, leaning forward propped up on both outstretched arms. In the previous stage he might have immediately toppled over, but now he can spend a few minutes enjoying these first sits and may even let go with one arm and start playing with his toes or reaching for a toy while maintaining his balance with the other arm. The ability to sit up with support gets baby his first high chair, and the five-month-old may be ready to join the family table.

Rolling over. The push-up position allows baby to roll easily from tummy to back. Watch your baby's rolling-over sequence: As baby pushes himself up, he pushes higher with one arm and then leans his head and shoulders backward and torques like a flywheel, increasing his twisting momentum. Besides torquing himself all the way over from the complete push-up position, baby discovers the follow-

ing shortcut to rolling over: Place a favorite toy alongside baby. He'll notice the toy and try to roll toward it. He tucks one elbow underneath him and pushes himself over with the other arm, letting the elbow on the tucked-in arm act as a sort of roll bar. Most babies roll from tummy to back before rolling from back to tummy because they can muster up more leverage with their arms and roll better on their rounded abdomen.

Standing better. Previously, baby could stand only if you supported his trunk under his arms. Now he can bear almost all of his weight himself, his outstretched hands holding on to you only for balance.

Playing with a Five-month-old

Here are some good ways for you and baby to enjoy his expanding skills.

Grab and pull. Any part of your body is fair game for reaching. As our babies would grab a fistful of my chest hair, I would yell "Ouch," and they would squeal with delight at their achievement. Baby can now reach for and hold on to the bottle or the breast during feeding.

Martha notes: Matthew is now grabbing on to different parts of my face, such as my nose, chin, and lips. He also grabs my face with a hand on either side of my chin and pulls my chin toward his face, grabs on to my chin with his mouth, and then begins to suck on my chin. He really enjoys these reach and suck patterns.

Block play. There is no better toy than the simple block. Try these starter blocks:

- small enough (one-and-a-half-inch/four-centimeter sides) to be easily picked up with one hand
- contrasting colors: red, yellow, blue
- wooden blocks

Set your baby in a high chair, propping him up with pillows until he's old enough to sit steadily in the chair unsupported. Place the starter blocks on the tray or table in front of baby and observe the amazing play skills of the five-month-old. Watch your baby grab a block in a mittenlike grasp, fondle it, study it, transfer it from hand to hand or from hand to lips. Soon he will learn to bang the blocks, drop them, and stack them. Watch your baby turn the block over and over from hand to hand.

Start with one block and let your baby get used to it. Then place a second block before him and notice how he holds one block with one hand and grabs the second block with the other. Now he looks at both hands full of blocks and wonders what to do. Probably

---

TOY TIPS FOR THE FIVE-MONTH-OLD

- squeeze toys and squeak toys
- toys of different shapes and textures that baby can really sink his hands into, such as several short pieces of yarn tied together at the center
- blocks — a favorite at any age
- grab-and-transfer toys such as rings

▶ *SAFETY TIP: Toys such as blocks and balls should have a diameter of at least one and one-half inches (four centimeters) so that baby can't swallow them.*

---

he'll start banging them together. Within a month or two he will learn to put one block down to grab another. Manipulating blocks is a valuable play and learning exercise for baby. He has complete control of this toy, and it helps encourage thumb-and-forefinger grasping that will develop over the next few months.

Table fun. Sit baby on your lap at the dinner table and allow him to play with paper or cloth napkins and spoons.

▶ *SAFETY TIP: At the table be careful to keep dangerous utensils, such as knives and forks, and hot food and beverages far away from baby. If baby does accidentally grab a sharp utensil, avoid trying to grab it from his hand, which may cause baby to hold on more tightly and result in a cut. Instead, squeeze the back of his hand and his wrist. This prevents baby from clutching the knife tightly and waving it around. With the other hand slowly pry the fingers off the knife until it falls out of his clenched fist.*

Cushion play. Beginning around five months we have had the most fun playing with homemade cylindrical and wedge-shaped cushions. You can buy leftover pieces of foam at an upholstery shop. If you are really hip on being an infant stimulator, cover the foam with patterned material, such as black-and-white stripes.

Cylindrical shapes (called bolsters), seven to ten inches (eighteen to twenty-five centimeters) in diameter and approximately two feet (sixty centimeters) long, make practical rolling cushions for baby to practice trunk, head, and reaching exercises. For example, you can hold your baby by the feet and play wheelbarrow or drape your baby over the cylindrical cushion and notice how he enjoys the mobility that these floor cushions allow. He may push himself forward by digging his

toes into the carpet and learning to rock himself back and forth on the cushion using his own foot power.

Wedge-shaped cushions can support baby's chest, allowing him to dangle his head over the edge of the wedge and play with toys within his grasp. Use a wedge three to four inches (eight to ten centimeters) high for this age.

Martha notes: *Matthew is still very frustrated when he is on his tummy and realizes that he could make tracks if he could only get his tummy off the ground. He flaps his arms and kicks his legs, but it gets him nowhere. This is one reason that I think he likes his foam wedges and rolls, because these at least get his tummy off the ground and give him the sensation of moving forward.*

THE SIXTH MONTH: SITTING BIG

From five to six months is a transition stage in baby's development. Before this period, baby is stuck. He can't move around or sit and play by himself. In the next stage, six to nine months, he becomes able to do both. In the sixth month, then, baby begins learning to sit and move about, and it is these major milestones that we focus on in the next few pages.

The Sitting Sequence

Learning to sit is the master skill of the sixth month. The sequence of learning to sit from four to six months is one of the most fascinating steps in baby's development. In the first

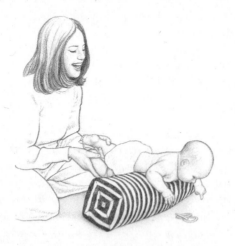

Cylindrical or wedge-shape cushions are great props for floor play.

few months (Figure A) baby seems to have little strength in his lower back muscles. When put in the sitting position he flops forward on his nose. Around three to four months baby shows some lower-back-muscle strength by easing forward, but again goes flop. Between four and five months (Figure B) baby still slumps or topples sideways but begins using his outstretched arms as forward and sideways props. Between five and six months baby may let go. His back muscles are now strong enough to support sitting erect, but usually still with the hands as props. Now sitting is just a matter of learning balance.

Watch how your clever beginning sitter learns balance. When baby starts to let go, first with one hand, then the other, he holds his straight back forward at a forty-five-degree angle. As balance and back-muscle strength improve, he sits erect at ninety degrees to the floor (Figure C). The novice sitter teeters and wobbles on his rounded bottom while thrusting out his arms like sideways balance beams.

Once he masters sitting balanced, baby no longer needs his head and arms for balance props but can use them for communication and play. When the skillful sitter begins turning his head to follow you and lifting his arms to gesture or to play, usually between six and seven months, baby is truly sitting alone.

Helping the Beginning Sitter

Because baby does not yet have the strength to right himself from a topple, backward and sideways falls are the price to pay for a good sit. Your baby will learn to sit well if you leave him alone. But if you help your baby enjoy the early sitting experiences, he will realize the interesting views he has in this position and will better enjoy developing his skill. Here's how to help:

- Cushion the inevitable backward and sideways falls by surrounding baby with pillows. There's nothing like a fall on a hard surface to scare baby and dampen his motivation to sit.

- To steady the wobbly beginning sitter, place baby in a homemade horseshoe-shaped piece of foam rubber. (We used a Nurse Mate pillow purchased as a

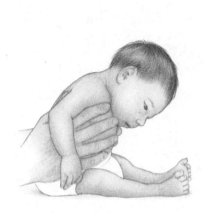

Figure A.

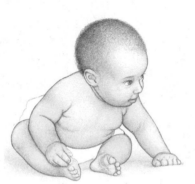

Figure B.

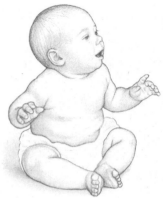

Figure C.

breastfeeding aid for the early months — a good example of extending the usefulness of an item!)

- For the summer sitter, hollow out an area in the sand. (Cover the sand with a blanket if you don't want sand in the eyes, mouth, and diaper.)

- When enjoying floor play together, sit baby between your outstretched legs so he can use them as grab rails.

- Use toy interactions to help baby learn balance. When enticed to use his hands to reach for a toy, the sitting baby "forgets" to use his hands as balance props and learns to rely solely on his trunk muscles for balance.

- If baby continues to rest on his hands as forward props, place blocks in front of him to motivate him to lift his hands off the floor by grabbing the blocks.

- To encourage hand play, dangle a favorite toy, eye level, in front of baby. Then move the toy to each side, encouraging baby to move his arms toward the toy while sitting.

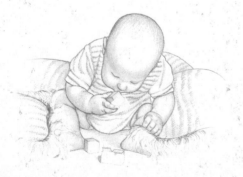

The sitting baby becomes more adept at playing alone.

During these balance-training exercises, notice how baby uses his arms to maintain balance. At first, baby reaches with one hand toward a toy while thrusting out the other for balance. As balance improves, watch baby reach for a toy to one side with both hands and reach behind himself without tumbling over.

A Relief for Parents

When baby can sit alone better, parents can sit alone longer. Sitting skillfully alone and playing is a major relief milestone for parents. Once he masters sitting, a six-month-old becomes less of a lap baby and carried baby and more of a high-chair and floor baby.

Pushing Up and Moving Around

The sixth month is literally a turning point for baby. Each month baby has been raising more of her torso off the floor. Now she can push her tummy off the ground almost as far as her belly button. Watch what baby can do from the push-up position. She can let go with her hands, raise her feet, and rock on her belly — playing teeter-totter. Or she can keep her hands and feet touching the ground and pivot around in a semicircle in pursuit of a favorite toy. As a finale, the rocker can pivot on her weighty abdomen by the sheer momentum of her wiggling legs and waving arms — playing airplane.

Next comes *pivoting*. Using her arms to steer, baby tries to turn a circle by pivoting on her abdomen, which still seems stuck to the floor. While baby is in the middle of pivot practice, place a favorite toy to one side just beyond her reach. Watch baby pivot around to get nearer the toy. If she is really in a hurry, she may turn a quick flip and roll toward the toy.

PLAYPENS: DON'T FENCE ME IN

Babies don't learn much in pens. In the sit-and-play stage some babies may temporarily enjoy their own little "playroom" with lots of stuff within easy grabbing distance. But in later months, as the beginning explorer peers through the net at the whole big room out there, he is likely to protest confinement.

Pens do have their place. A portable pen and a mobile baby may, of necessity, belong together at your place of work. Plopping baby in a pen while you answer the phone or remove dinner from the oven is often a safety saver for the busy parent. But keep the sentence short; put pen and baby within easy relating distance while finishing your work, making sure to frequently acknowledge the inmate.

If you need baby to be in the pen, keep it safe. Beginning sitters and crawlers flop around a lot on the pen floor. Keep hard toys out. Soft, cuddly toys make good pen-mates and are safer to fall against. (See page 601 for a checklist of playpen safety.)

As baby progresses from the sit-and-play stage to the move-and-explore stage, pack up the pen and put it in its rightful place (perhaps even next to the crib) at your next garage sale and babyproof the whole house.

Here's how you can participate in baby's developing skills.

Chest rest. While a baby likes to play on his tummy, frequent push-ups can tire the young athlete. Also, he may be frustrated by having to use his arms and hands for support and not for play. Place a three-inch foam-rubber wedge under baby's chest. This prop frees his hands to play with toys in front of him more comfortably and for longer periods without getting tired. He can also roll off onto the carpet without hurting himself.

First scoots. Place an enticing toy just beyond the floor-baby's reach. Watch baby dig in with toes and fingers and squirm, scoot, or combat crawl toward his target. Some babies can move a foot or two at this stage as they practice their first crawls.

Martha notes: Matthew now fusses less when the toy rolls beyond his reach when he is lying on his tummy. He knows he can propel himself forward and therefore does not start crying for help because he knows he doesn't need it. He can simply scoot himself forward enough on his tummy to grab the toy. So he is combining both awareness of distance and the awareness of his body's ability to close that distance. He therefore has no need to fuss.

RAISING HEALTHY TEETH

Going are those adorable toothless grins. Coming is a novel smile each month. Around five to six months, parents become interested in teething. Here are the most common concerns parents have about caring for those precious pearly whites.

When should we expect our baby's teeth to appear?

When teeth first appear is as variable as the timing of baby's first steps, but in general expect the first sharp nubbin around six months; some babies teethe earlier, some later. And heredity plays a part. If you check your own baby book, if grandmother was a tooth-record keeper, your baby's teething schedule may resemble yours.

Actually, babies are born with a full set of twenty primary teeth. They are just buried in the gums, waiting in line for their time to sprout. Teeth push through in upper and lower pairs, usually the lower appear before their upper gum mates, and girls teethe slightly earlier than boys. The "rule of fours" is how teeth usually appear. Beginning around six months expect four new teeth every four months until complete, usually by two and a half years. Teeth come through gums at unusual angles. Some come out straight, others first appear crooked but straighten as they twist their way through. Don't fret about spaces. It's easier to clean between spaced teeth, and the spacing of the baby teeth does not necessarily reflect how the permanent teeth will appear.

How much should we expect teething to bother our baby?

As you wonder why your sleeping angel turns night waker, you hear the telltale ping against the spoon or feel the cutting edge. Actually babies don't "cut teeth," nor do teeth "erupt." Teeth slowly slide and twist their way through gum tissue. But sharp teeth pushing through sensitive gums do hurt, and babies protest. Here are the nuisances to expect and suggestions to comfort the budding teether.

Drooling. During teething time expect the saliva faucet to be on. In addition, listen for the young announcer's voice to sputter. Many of the following aggravations stem from this excessive drool.

Drool rash. Sensitive skin and excessive saliva don't sit well together, especially when the skin is rubbing against a drool-soaked bed sheet. Expect a red, raised, irritating rash around lips and chin. Place a drool-absorbing cotton diaper under baby's chin or a towel under the sheet while baby sleeps. Gently wipe excess drool off the skin with luke-

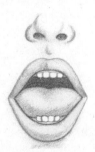

6-12 months: incisors

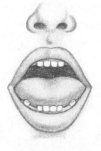

12-18 months: first molars

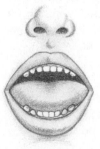

18-24 months: canine teeth

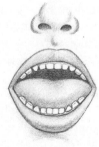

24-30 months: two-year molars

warm water and pat (don't rub) dry. Lubricate with a mild emollient such as Nature's Second Skin or cold-pressed coconut, almond, or safflower oil.

Drool cough. Besides drooling out the mouth, the excess saliva escapes through the back door, dripping down baby's throat, causing gagging and an irritating cough.

Drool diarrhea. Not only does the face react to excess saliva, but so does the bottom. Expect loose stools and a mild diaper rash during peak teething time. This temporary nuisance self-clears as each teething burst subsides.

Fever and irritability. The inflammation caused by hard teeth pushing through soft tissue may produce a low fever (101°F/38.3°C) and the disposition of someone who hurts. Give baby acetaminophen (see page 657 for appropriate dosage) as needed.

Biting. The budding teether longs for something or some person to gnaw on. Teeth marks on crib rails and clicking gums on silver spoons are telltale signs of sore gums needing relief. Expect these hard gums to clench your knuckles, arm, finger, and sometimes the breast that feeds baby (for survival tips, see discussion of biting and breastfeeding, page 147). Offer something cool and hard. Gum-soothing favorites are a cool spoon, popsicle, frozen bagel, teething ring, and, a favorite Sears family teether, a chicken leg bone stripped of the tiny bone slivers. Try cold teething biscuits for another melt-in-the-mouth teether. We are hesitant to recommend commercial numbing substances because it is difficult to learn their exact contents and find research that validates their safety.

Night waking. Growing teeth don't rest at night; neither do teething babies and their parents. A previously steady sleeper may frequently awaken during peak teething times and may have difficulty resettling into the preteething sleep schedule. Offer a dose of acetaminophen before bedtime, or, if baby is in severe pain, a one-time double dose. Repeat the dose four hours later if needed.

Refusing to feed. This is the most variable of all teething concerns. Some teethers never miss a meal, some avid breastfeeders accelerate their nursing for comfort, but a few may pass up even their most trusted human pacifier. Offer cool, mushy foods — for example, applesauce and frozen fruit-juice slush. Put these on a cool spoon to make a real hit.

Doctor, could it be her teeth?

You may feel that your doctor doesn't share your degree of concern about your baby's teething problems. Your doctor is being cautious and has the best interest of your baby at heart. Some medical studies, at odds with mother's observations, claim teething discomforts are overrated. Another reason for your doctor's ambivalence about possible teething-related symptoms is the worry that you will attribute a symptom to teething and miss a serious underlying illness. Many a doctor has agreed with the mother and considered teething over the phone but diagnosed an ear infection when examining the baby in person.

How can I tell if my baby is teething?

Besides the trademark drool and other related signs, try the gum-massage test. (Babies are more likely to accept a finger probing into their mouth than to allow a look.) Run your finger along the front edges of the gums, and you will feel swollen ridges of preteething gums.

It is sometimes difficult to tell if a baby is teething because the amount of teething discomfort varies considerably among babies. Some are steady, once-a-month teethers; many teethe in bursts and pauses, where suddenly baby has a miserable week and you feel four swollen ridges along the gum line. Expect the most discomfort when many teeth come through at once. Some babies experience exquisite pain and swelling during molar teething. If allowed to look, you may notice a mound of swollen tissue around a budding tooth. Don't be alarmed if you notice a mushy blue blister above an erupting tooth. This is actually a collection of blood beneath the superficial layer of gum tissue. These painful swellings are best treated by cool compresses (for example, popsicles), which soothe the swelling.

I've taken our baby to the doctor several times for what turned out to be false alarms. I thought he had a cold, but it turned out to be teething. How can I tell?

You are right to let your doctor make the decision. When in doubt, don't attribute baby's behavior to teething. But here are some general ways to tell the difference between teething and an illness such as an ear infection:

- Teething mucus is clear saliva and *doesn't run out the nose.* Cold mucus is thick and yellow. A nasal discharge usually means an allergy or an infection, especially if accompanied by eye drainage.

- Teething rarely causes a fever higher than 101°F (38.3°C).

- Teething may be confused with an earache. Babies pull at their ears during teething, probably because of referred pain from the teeth to the ears. Ear pulling in babies is usually an unreliable sign. With an ear infection babies usually hurt more lying down and have accompanying signs of a cold.

- Babies don't act progressively sicker with teething. As a general rule, when in doubt, check it out with the doctor.

When should we first take our baby to a dentist?

Sometime between baby's first tooth and third birthday, schedule baby's first dental checkup. Better early than late. Getting your baby used to painless dental checkups long before the first cavity drilling makes it easier on baby, parents, and dentists. Ask to hold your child during any dental procedures or at least to be present during the exam. Some pediatric dentists ask parents to assist by sitting knee to knee (see the illustration on page 499) with the child's head resting on the dentist's lap. Well-teeth checkups, like well-baby exams with your pediatrician, give the dentist an opportunity to teach you some preventive care, such as proper teeth brushing, avoiding night feedings, and correct fluoride dosage.

When should I start brushing baby's teeth?

Dentists now recommend cleaning gums with gauze to remove plaque beginning around the time that teeth first appear, usually six to seven months. Try the following brushing tactics.

Model good dental hygiene. Let baby watch you brush. Show excitement, capitaliz-

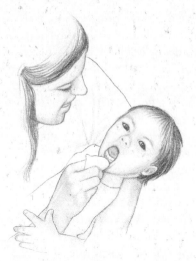

A gauze-wrapped finger makes a good first "toothbrush."

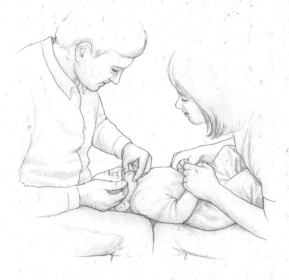

The two-person toothbrushing position.

ing on "Brush off the sugar bugs, just like mommy and daddy." Around his first birthday, get baby his own toothbrush and enjoy side-by-side brushing just for play. If you first get baby to enjoy imitating toothbrushing, it will be easier for you to get down to the business of getting germs off little teeth.

First toothbrushing. The best chances for a cooperative baby and clean teeth is to use your moistened gauze-wrapped fingertip as a toothbrush. Gauze also works well in the older baby who refuses to let you invade his mouth with a toothbrush.

Toothbrushing positions. Placing baby on your lap with his head facing you is a good position for a wide-open-mouth entry. Sitting or standing behind baby with him looking up also gives you a good view. An older baby can be held cradled in your arms to one side. Or try the two-person knee-to-knee position as shown in the illustration

above or sit on the floor with baby's head between your legs.

Toothbrushing and toddlers. Once baby gets a mouth full of teeth, especially molars, a toothbrush works better than a mommy-made, gauze-on-finger brush to get in the crevices between teeth. Don't forget to take a few gentle swipes over the surface of the tongue, which harbors the same bacteria as the gums. Letting your toddler hold the brush while you clean helps his acceptance. Children mostly protest brushing their back teeth for fear of choking, so begin with the front teeth and ease toward the molars.

Which toothpaste? Toothpaste isn't necessary for starter brushing, but if desired, a half-pea-sized dab will do. Dentists caution against letting baby swallow too much fluoride-containing toothpaste. (See the question about fluoride on page 501.) Toddlers enjoy the ritual of putting on the toothpaste, but then they object to the sharp taste. Use a mild-flavored children's paste if necessary.

Which toothbrush? Choose a short brush with two rows of soft bristles on a small head. Store a spare brush. They get lost, get dirty, and wear out quickly. Change brushes when the bristles get bent.

Why all the fuss about first teeth? Baby will lose all of them anyway.

It's important to care for the baby teeth. These primary teeth hold the right spaces for the secondary, or permanent, teeth. Healthy first teeth also contribute to proper alignment of the jawbones and eventual bite. And don't discount the healthy vanity of a smiling preschooler. No one likes to show off a row of rotten teeth.

Besides brushing, what else can we do to help our baby's teeth?

Here are suggestions for your own home-dental program for cavity-free kids.

Breastfeed. Pediatric dentists who study the effects of breastfeeding on oral development believe that one of the most beneficial contributors to healthy teeth and healthy jaw alignment is a breast in the mouth for as long as mother and baby are willing and able. Apparently the unique sucking action of breastfeeding helps prevent malocclusion. A saying we have heard in dental circles goes, "Your infant's breastfeeding efforts will be later reflected in his face."

Avoid sticky stuff. Keep your baby off a steady diet of highly sugared junk foods, especially tacky lollipops, caramel, and hard candy that stick and lodge between teeth and have a long-enough contact time for germs and enamel to get well acquainted. Tooth decay begins with the formation of *plaque* — a sticky film that forms on the teeth and provides a residence for decay-promoting germs. The bacteria and the plaque react with the sugar in the food, creating a decay-producing acid. The more plaque, the more decay. The goal of dental hygiene, therefore, is to keep the plaque from forming in the first place, by frequent brushing, and keep the sugar off the plaque, by a healthy diet. When our toddlers would protest toothbrushing, we'd tell them it was to wipe off the "sugar bugs."

Don't let baby sleep with a bottle of milk or juice. Bottles are not friendly to a sleeping baby's teeth. Especially blacklist honey-dipped pacifiers. When baby falls asleep, saliva flow decreases, diminishing its natural rinsing action on the teeth. The sugary stuff bathes the teeth. Plaque and bacteria have an enamel feast, resulting in severe tooth decay called bottle mouth. If a baby is hooked on the nap or nighttime bottle, try watering down the juice or milk, each night diluting it a bit more until it's all water. If baby clings to his nighttime bottle and won't settle for any diluted substitute, be sure to brush the teeth well on the first morning trip to the bathroom.

Check out advice on night nursing. "Nursing caries" does happen to breastfed babies, but buffers in human milk allow it to be tolerated in the mouth, so that tooth decay is much less likely than with bottles of juice or formula. They are most likely to be found in those all-night snackers who feel night nursing tops the list of baby's bill of rights. We consulted pediatric dentists who have thoroughly researched the night-nursing concern. Many believe that nighttime breast-feeding only slightly contributes to tooth decay. In many cases the tooth decay would have occurred with or without the night nursing.

If you are still night nursing and it's working for you, consult a pediatric dentist knowledgeable about the benefits of breastfeeding and oral development. Have baby's teeth periodically checked to see if they have any beginning decay or enamel weakness that would prompt you to curb night nursing. If you get your dentist's OK to continue night nursing, it would be wise, besides your routine before-bed brushing, to start the teeth off each day with a thorough cleaning.

To stop breastfeeding or even night nursing when the teeth come in, as an occasional dentist may advise, is like throwing out the baby with the bathwater. Considering the overall medical and dental health-promoting benefits and the emotional and developmental advantages of long-term breastfeeding, a more prudent approach would be frequent dental checkups and after-nursing brushing.

What about fluoride? How can I tell if my baby is getting enough?

Here's what every parent should know about fluoride:

- Fluoride helps teeth in two ways: The fluoride that baby ingests (in food or water) enters the bloodstream and gets into the teeth, strengthening the developing enamel, making it more resistant to decay. Fluoride applied topically (through toothpaste or fluoride applications by your dentist) helps strengthen the new enamel that is being formed as teeth repair themselves

(called remineralization) from the normal wear and tear.

- While still inside the gums, the permanent teeth begin mineralizing and developing enamel even before birth. Fluoride administered after birth is incorporated into the developing teeth, making them stronger.

- Nature's own experiment: People living in areas where the fluoride is naturally present in the water supply have 50 percent fewer dental caries.

- Fluoride, unlike many vitamins and minerals, has a narrow range of efficacy-toxicity, meaning the right amount helps, and too much harms the teeth by making them brittle — a condition called fluorosis. This is why fluoride is available only by prescription and must be given to a baby in the exact dosage prescribed.

- Formulas are not made with fluoride-supplemented water.

- A pea-size dab of fluoride-containing toothpaste is all that baby needs. Do not use both a fluoride-containing toothpaste and fluoride supplements, as this would be too much.

- The amount of fluoride naturally present in drinking water varies in different areas of the country. Check with your dentist or local water company, inquiring how many parts per million. If your tap water contains at least 0.3 parts per million, your baby doesn't need, and probably shouldn't have, fluoride supplements.

- The Committee on Nutrition of the American Academy of Pediatrics recommends that if the water baby drinks contains less than 0.3 parts per million of fluoride, baby should be given a daily supplement of 0.25 milligrams of fluoride beginning at age six months and continued (with increased dosage) until adolescence.

- Even though your local tap water may be fluoridated, some infants drink little water, and some are always quenching their thirst. Also, if you drink bottled water, it will not be fluoridated unless you specifically request it.

- Many foods, such as grains and vegetables, naturally contain fluoride. Babies can get fluoride from the following dental sources: fluoride supplements prescribed by your doctor (often combined with vitamin drops or chewable tablets), fluoride applied topically in toothpaste or in dental treatments, and a fluoridated water supply.

- The jury is still out on whether predominantly breastfed babies need fluoride supplements. At this writing the evidence suggests they do not, although little fluoride enters the baby through mother's milk and this amount is not altered significantly by a change in her diet.

21

The Second Six Months: Moving Up

During the first six months parents and trusted subs are the center of baby's universe. While this remains true during all stages of development, from six to twelve months baby develops the skills to extend his world of interest. He becomes less an arms and lap baby and more an exploring floor baby. During this stage, growth accelerates. Baby's weight increases by a third, first words appear, and true thumb-and-forefinger pickups emerge, as well as first crawls and steps. These skills also bring about parents' development as safety patrol officers. Baby's motor development allows him to get more and more of his body off the ground. By six months he is halfway there, sitting; by twelve months he's on his own two feet, and the baby chase begins.

SIX TO NINE MONTHS: EXPLORING BIG

Two important skills form the next steps up the ladder of infant development: progressing from *sitting to crawling* and learning to *pick up objects* with thumb and forefinger. At each stage of development baby masters one primary skill that then triggers a series of accomplishments. In this stage, *sitting without support* is the master skill. This, in turn, opens a wide new world for baby to explore. He now sees his environment straight on, an entirely different perspective from the one he gets lying on his back. By six or seven months, most babies can sit unsupported. Since he no longer needs his arms to prop himself up, baby is able to use them more fully for socializing and play.

The Crawling Sequence

Line up ten beginning crawlers at the starting gate and watch them make their individual ways around the track. They all reach the finish line, but with different styles and different speeds. Each is normal. While no two babies crawl the same, most follow a similar sequence of development.

Lunging Forward

Intense curiosity coupled with increasing strength in trunk, arm, and leg muscles seem to plant an idea in baby's mind: "I have the capability to handle my toys. Now how do I get to them?" Here's how one skill leads to another. The ability to sit unsupported encourages baby to try lunging forward in pursuit of a desired toy. Place your baby's toys just beyond his reach and you will notice that he lunges to lengthen his reach, extending his hands and arms to rake the toy in pawlike fashion until it is comfortably within reach.

Baby translates a stationary skill (sitting) into a moving skill (lunging). This is the precursor to crawling. As you place the toy farther beyond baby's reach, notice what happens. He lunges his trunk forward as much as possible, stretching his arms toward the toy. Next he learns to fold his outstretched legs in toward his body. This tucked-in position shortens the rocking axis, allowing baby to roll forward over his feet. As he begins to lunge forward on his little rocker bottom, he builds up momentum until the forward-lunging movements of his body gradually overcome the weight of his bottom, and he falls, usually on his tummy, just short of his intended goal.

➤ *SAFETY TIP: When a baby is practicing these forward-lunging skills, choose soft toys for him to go for in case he falls splat on top of his goal. Such an encounter with a hard wooden, metal, or plastic object could be very uncomfortable.*

First Crawls

Baby's first crawls are frustrating. As with many developmental skills, intent precedes ability. Like a stuck turtle's, baby's propelling arms and legs kick, but her heavy abdomen won't budge off the ground.

The styles of beginning crawlers are variable. Some babies inchworm along the floor. This early style progresses toward a commando-type crawl, with baby squirming forward on her tucked-in elbows, her head scanning from side to side searching for objects to capture. Some babies begin moving more backward than forward in a type of crab crawl as they push instead of pull with their arms. Others prefer the thrusting motions of their legs as they dig in with their feet, making a sort of bridge with their extended legs and arms and then thrusting forward in leapfrog fashion, propelling themselves ahead a foot or two at a time.

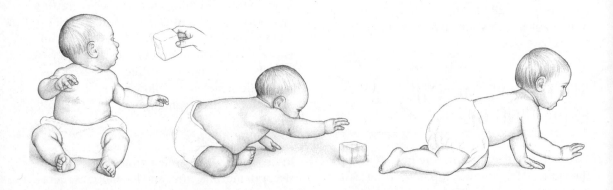

By age six or seven months, baby is able to sit without support, setting the stage for lunging and then crawling, as he moves out to explore a wider world.

Making a Bridge

Until baby can get her pelvis and abdomen off the ground, her crawling is inefficient. Once her heavy middle is raised — "making a bridge" — she's off. Baby first rocks back and forth on hands and knees. Now she's up on four wheels and ready to explore ways of rolling on them.

Cross-crawling

A major turning point in crawling skills is mastered when baby learns to alternate arms and legs, getting the arm on one side and the leg on the opposite side to move forward together and strike the floor at the same time. This refinement in baby's ground transportation is called cross-crawling. This stance allows baby to balance steadily on the hand and knee that remain in contact with the floor while elevating the opposite ones. This is the most efficient and speedy of the crawling styles and takes baby in the straightest line. Cross-crawling is a locomotor skill that teaches a baby to use one side of his body to balance the other.

Want to really appreciate the efficiency of cross-crawling and have some fun? Along with your friends, get down on the floor and start crawling. Notice that most adults crawl "wrong." They move the arm and leg on the same side of the body together, which is off balance, instead of moving the opposite arm and leg ahead and maintaining their balance. How smart this nine-month-old engineer is to have developed such a balanced suspension!

The Mental Side of Crawling

Imagine the learning power that a baby derives from learning to crawl. He experiments with various styles and then "chooses"

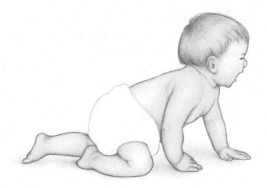

Cross-crawling: Each arm moves in conjunction with the opposite leg.

the one that works best. Baby learns problem solving and cause-and-effect relationships — "I push with my feet one way and I move faster than if I push another way." Baby also learns self-reinforcement: The more he moves and reaches the pursued toys, the more motivated he is to improve his locomotor skills.

You can tell that baby is thinking about how best to crawl by watching how he accommodates his crawling style to different textures. Place baby on a deep-pile carpet and notice that he uses his feet and toes to dig in, thrusting forward leapfrog style. Now place him on a smooth kitchen floor, and he is likely to inchworm his way and slide along the smooth surface. Some babies like to bear crawl on hands and feet on tiled surfaces because the soles and palms stick instead of slide. Watch how your baby learns to navigate using different styles on different "roads."

During this stage of development it is not so important *how* baby moves in pursuit of a toy. The important milestone is that he realizes his capabilities to move from place to place and experiments with various methods. Sometimes he may dig in and scoot; other times he may twist and roll toward the toy; sometimes he may crawl. During the next stage of development baby refines these various modes of transportation and selects the one that is most efficient.

Advanced Maneuvers

Babies like to crawl up and over obstacles. For fun and games, place a foam-rubber roll or wedge between baby and an interesting toy. Also, make yourself an obstacle. Lie down on the floor and place the toy on one side of you and the baby on the other, and feel your baby crawl over you.

From Crawl to Sit

Besides developing new locomotor skills, baby enjoys combining skills. Around seven months a baby can go from sitting to lunging to crawling forward. Baby next learns how to maneuver his body in the opposite sequence, going from the crawling position back to a full sit. To master this maneuver, baby uses the foot tuck. Watch baby crawl along and then quickly stop, tuck one foot underneath, and swing sideways, vaulting over the tucked-in foot while digging in and pushing with the other foot and hand. Presto, he's sitting upright! Baby's ability to achieve a sitting position by himself is another relief milestone for parents. Previously he would fuss because he couldn't right himself back to the sitting position. He needed a nearby helper. Now he doesn't.

Reinforcing the Little Mover

I remember how each time our son Matthew showed a new skill, he seemed to do best amid the encouraging cheers of his siblings. For example, when baby crawls up the step, rolls over, or goes from crawling to sitting, watch how she beams afterward. When you notice she is pleased with herself, praise her. By acknowledging her performance, you share her joy, and she may give an encore.

Pulling Up and Moving Around

The desire to ascend from a horizontal to a vertical position stimulates baby to grab hold of furniture, railings, or parent's clothing and pull himself upright. Watch the delight on your baby's face at the thrill of his first pull-up.

Taking a Stand

Once baby has mustered all the skill and energy needed to pull up to a standing position, he wants to stay there awhile and enjoy the view. At this stage baby may stand briefly while holding on to your hand only for balance, not for support. An eight-month-old may be able to lean against a sofa for five to ten minutes. Many babies at this stage still do not plant their whole foot on the floor, preferring to stand on tiptoe with their feet turned in, a position that greatly compromises their balance. The tiptoe tendency is probably due to the baby's tensing his whole body to get into this exciting new position.

Help baby take the right stand. If he is hanging on to a sofa and his feet are turned in and overlapping, gently turn them out and plant them flat, teaching baby to use his feet as a firm base of support. If baby still crumples easily when standing, support his bending legs with your hands around the back of his knees. By taking some of the frustrations out of failed attempts, you can help baby enjoy a new skill and reinforce its development.

WAIVE THE WALKER

We strongly discourage you from exposing your infant to a walker for both safety and developmental reasons. Providing exercise for baby, keeping the pre-walking baby occupied, and as a baby-sitting aid to keep the mobile baby happy are not good enough reasons to justify the safety and developmental risks that walkers pose for babies.

The number of walker accidents steadily increases each year, prompting the American Academy of Pediatrics to propose a law banning the sale and use of infant walkers. Studies show that as many as 40 percent of infants placed in walkers suffer a variety of injuries, such as skull fractures, neck injuries, lacerations, knocked-out teeth, and burns. Some of the most common injuries occur from falls, such as when a baby gets up enough speed to crash through a safety gate and falls downstairs, tips over when rolling over throw rugs or thresholds, or bends over to pick up toys on the floor. Baby's fingers can get caught in collapsible walkers, especially the older models with exposed springs and coils.

Walkers give babies wheels to navigate into dangerous places.

The second reason we strongly discourage walkers is that they reverse the normal sequence of motor development. Infants develop from head to toe, with their upper-body skills progressing ahead of their lower-body skills. In typical motor development from birth to one year, baby gets more and more of his body off the ground. He begins by raising his head, then his chest, then his tummy, then his hips, then raises himself on hands and knees, then stands with support, then takes a few steps while holding on, and then walks solo. In relying on the walker to do the work, baby loses the ability to keep experimenting with his own body in order to develop crawling and walking skills. In fact, studies have shown that babies who spend a lot of time in walkers are more likely to be slower in developing a normal gait. These studies showed that "walker-trained" infants demonstrated a stiffer-legged gait.

If you absolutely must have a gadget that entertains the pre-walking baby, never leave the baby unattended.

First Cruises

Around eight or nine months babies lean against furniture only for balance, not for support. Next baby cruises around furniture using the couch or coffee-table top as his balancer. Finally, baby tries letting go with both hands and may even stand momentarily by himself before grabbing on to the nearby couch or table or crumpling to the floor from lack of balance.

Pick Up and Play: Hand Skills

Baby may act like a little carpet sweeper, picking up even the tiniest pellets that are lying around on the floor.

➤ *SAFETY TIP: The combination of a fascination for small objects and the ability to move toward them makes mouthing objects that can cause choking a prime safety concern at this stage. Be especially vigilant*

about what you leave around for these curi-
ous little fingers to find. Any object smaller
than an inch and a half (four centimeters)
in diameter can lodge in baby's airway.

Development of the Pincer Grasp

One of the most interesting examples of how
two skills develop simultaneously and complement each other is the way a baby's fascination for small objects develops at the same
time as the hand and finger capability of
exploring these objects — the evolution of
thumb-and-forefinger pickup, or pincer grasp.

Watch your baby go for a pile of O-shaped
cereal. She first rakes tidbits toward herself,
pawlike, and tries to grab them, mittenlike,
with her fingers and palm. She frustratingly
loses the food bits in her pudgy little hands.
Pointing with index finger alone is the earliest sign that baby is about to master the pincer grasp. She touches the object with a
pointed finger, tucking the remaining fingers
into her palm. Soon the thumb follows the
lead of the index finger, and baby picks up
objects between the pads of thumb and forefinger. As baby's picking-up ability matures to
the tips of thumb and forefinger, you will
notice a less pawlike action and more direct
thumb-and-forefinger pickups.

Learning to Release

An important part of baby's reach-grasp
learning is developing the ability to release
the grasped object. Babies become fascinated with holding something, such as a
piece of paper, and then opening their hand
and allowing the object to drop to the floor.
Learning to release toys leads to one of
baby's favorite games at this age, "I drop —
you pick up." She soon associates the action
of dropping with your reaction of picking

up the toy. Thus, she learns to associate cause
and effect.

Transferring Objects

Releasing helps a baby learn to transfer
objects. Put a ring toy into baby's hands and
watch what happens. He first pulls on the
toy, playing a sort of tug-of-war. If one hand
lets go first, the other gets the ring, and
baby's eyes go from the empty hand to the
hand that holds the ring. He transfers the toy
from hand to hand, at first accidentally, then
intentionally. The ability to transfer a toy
extends baby's playtime. Now he can sit and
entertain himself for ten to twenty minutes,
shuffling a toy back and forth from one hand
to the other.

Developing a Stronger Grip on Things

Around six months a baby's reach-and-grasp
sequences become more one-handed, purposeful, and tenacious. Baby can now consistently and quickly grab a toy handed to him.
Put a toy in front of the sitting baby and see
how steadily and accurately baby reaches his
mark. Now try to take away the toy. Notice
how baby protests your pull. He tenaciously
holds on to the toy with a strong grasp. When
you manage to extract the prized toy from
baby's clasp, put it on the floor in front of
him and observe the way he immediately
pounces and recaptures the toy in his grasp.

If you really want to appreciate how baby
puts his mind into his reach, videotape him
reaching for a toy block. In the previous
stage, baby would strike and palm the toy,
and his whole hand would encompass it,
adjusting to its shape only after he touched it.
Now, watch baby begin to change the shape
of his hand to fit the shape of the toy before
he actually reaches it. He is developing a

visual "feel" for the object, which helps him determine its shape before he touches it. He is now making in-flight corrections as his hands approach the target.

Parents, if you are wondering why we go into such detail in describing infant development, it's because we want you to appreciate the big capabilities in your little person. Also, remember you are *growing together.* As your baby refines his developmental skills, you refine your skills as a baby watcher — a valuable exercise in learning to read your baby.

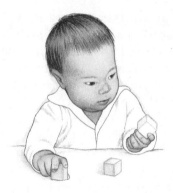

Babies start engaging in block play at about five months.

Fun for Little Hands

Block games. Sit baby in a high chair and put two blocks in front of him. After baby is engrossed, with a block in each hand, place a third block in front of him. Watch the decisive look on his face as he figures out how to get the third block.

Next put the blocks on a place mat just beyond his reach. After lunging toward the blocks and realizing they are out of his grasp, he may pull the place mat toward himself and voilà! the blocks come, too. This may be baby's first experience in learning how to use one object to get another.

Now play the pounce-on-the-moving-block game. Put the blocks on a place mat in front of baby. Slowly pull the place mat across his path. Watch baby sit with his hands open, starlike, ready to pounce on anything within his reach.

Playing with body parts. Being able to reach for things stimulates baby to explore his body parts. He cranes his neck forward and bends his legs upward, bringing his toes within reach of his outstretched hands. As with so many other objects, once baby has a firm grasp on his toes he often brings them to

his mouth. Notice that baby frequently points his big toe upward, making it an easier target to grab.

Not only does baby like to grab and suck on his own body parts, he also frequently grabs the parts of you within his reach, such as your nose, hair, or glasses. Within reason, try not to turn off this grabbing and pulling at your person. It's part of being a baby.

Martha notes: Matthew likes to practice his one-handed reaching while eating. While nursing he waves his arms, pats his head, pats my face or breast, and begins to explore my clothing. Often I enjoy this; sometimes it's a distracting nuisance during feeding.

Picking grass. Nature provides fun targets for inquisitive little fingers. Sit baby down in the grass. At first he grabs a whole clump of grass with his entire hand. Then baby becomes fascinated with the blades of grass extending upward, and he tries to grab individual pieces of grass with the thumb and fingers. He soon refines his grass-grabbing techniques by picking up one blade of grass at a time with the thumb and forefinger.

Playing pickpocket. Capitalize on baby's fascination for small objects, especially pens in shirt pockets. Dads, wear a shirt with a vest pocket and an obvious pen. Hold your baby and watch the pickpocket strike. Baby may precisely grab the pen, hold it very possessively, and you will have difficulty getting it back; he is not likely to put it back in your pocket at this stage. Babies love the pickpocket game and learn to associate dad's wearing a shirt with pockets and pens to grab. One time I came home from work and picked Matthew up. He reached toward my pocket, but to his amazement it was empty. He looked surprised and very disappointed. He had stored in his memory that pens belong in shirt pockets that belong on dads. Babies easily become confused when expected patterns of association are not fulfilled.

Spaghetti play. Place a plate of cooked and cooled spaghetti in front of baby — hold the sauce, please — and watch the little fingers pick.

Hand Dominance

While baby may not reveal a definite hand dominance for several more months, sometime between six and nine months you may get a clue as to which is baby's dominant hand. Put a toy in the midline in front of baby and watch which hand consistently goes for the toy. Now put the toy to the left side. If baby is right-handed, he may reach across his body with the right hand, his left hand standing in readiness to assist the right. Now try the same exercise with the toy on the right side of baby to see which hand consistently reaches for the toy. Over the next three months most babies will reveal their dominant hand.

In Search of Baby Handcuffs

When babies master a skill, they have an insatiable appetite to use this skill over and over. This is fun, but also a nuisance. Babies are especially attracted to strings, buttons, or bows. Buttons are potentially dangerous because they can be pulled off and mouthed. So intense is baby's desire to grab that it is wise not to show him or expose him to anything that he is not allowed to touch.

At the dinner table, for example, all the reachable delights may set off a grabbing frenzy as baby's hands dart out and snatch plates, newspapers, utensils, napkins, anything else that gets in the way of the windshield-wiper arms. As you clean up your baby's handiwork, remember this stage will soon pass. If your lap baby is becoming increasingly a handful at the dinner table, you can diffuse a grabbing frenzy by placing him

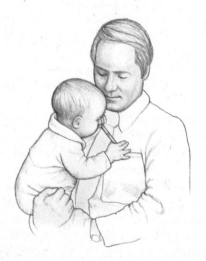

Pickpocket.

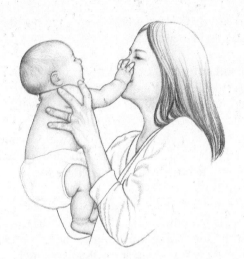

Reach out and grab someone. Anything within grabbing distance is enticing to a six-to-nine-month-old.

on the floor with some plastic cartons and let him grab to his hands' delight.

Language Development

In addition to crawling and the pincer grasp, baby's first language is another highlight of this stage. Babies cry less, talk more, and begin to combine sound and body language to get their point across. A major breakthrough in speech development occurs around five months of age when babies learn they can change the sounds they make by changing the shape of their tongue and mouth. By six months babies begin to babble, which consists of long, repetitive strings of syllables containing a vowel and a consonant. Between six and nine months baby learns to change "ba-ba," sounds made with the lips, to "da-da," sounds made with the tongue. After going through the consonant alphabet with all sorts of combinations — "ah-ba-di-da-ga-ma" — baby begins to sort these first "words" together — "ba-ba-ba-ba" — and razzes up these sounds with the wet noises of teething mucus. By nine months many babies are saying "mama" and "dada," but may not yet consistently match the right word with the right person.

Gesturing and Social Directing

Gestures are one of the most important forerunners of verbal language, because they are later replaced by their equivalent in words. Instead of crying to be picked up, baby often extends his arms and raises his big eyes toward you in a "Please pick me up" gesture. Also, because of the ability to use her hands for play and movement, a baby at this stage often becomes less interested in being held and will give you a "Put me down" sign, darting her hands toward the floor and squirming in your arms until you put her down to pursue her target. Respond to baby's hand signals as you did to her cries. This reinforces the use of body language instead of crying as a way of communicating. Besides using her own hands to signal needs, baby directs your hands to move with hers. Watch her grasp your finger and make your hand and arm move where she wants them to be. This hand-on-hand directing is most noticeable during feeding.

Martha notes: Matthew shows different "Pick me up" signals when he is upset and when he wants to play. When he wants to play, his arms are wide open, extending completely outward from his body in an embracing fashion. When he is upset, he doesn't hold his arms outstretched but rather holds his arms tightly to his side at the elbows with the forearms raised, his little hands and fingers open, but in a pinched-together gesture which further communicates his discomfort while also saying, "Please help me."

Reading Baby's Language

By nine months most babies have developed a true language (sounds plus gestures) that parents understand but strangers seldom do. Reading these gestures is where your previous exercises in baby reading really pay off. And watch for specific sounds to signal specific needs. Our baby Matthew vocalized "mum-mum-mum-mum" when he wanted to be held. Here are some favorite gestures and sounds.

Pointing fingers. Babies begin pointing and touching in a way similar to how new mothers have been observed touching their babies for the first time, first with their fingertips and then with their fully opened hands. Baby also begins to understand *your* pointing.

Martha notes: Around six months Matthew began pointing at the family cat. He approached the unsuspecting cat for the first time with his open hand and his fingers extended, starlike. He first touched the cat's head with just the tip of his index finger. He explored the cat for a while with the tips of all his fingers before resting his whole hand upon the cat and clutching the fur with his clenched fist.

Entry greetings. Look and listen to your baby's special gestures to initiate special play. When daddy enters the room, for example, baby comes to life. His face lights up and lets out a big smile, his arms wave, and he turns toward dad with a whole body language that says, "Let's play!"

Mood sounds. Listen and watch your baby vocalize pleasure and displeasure. When happy, baby brightens with uplifting facial gestures: bright eyes, facial muscles drawn upward, and cheeks bulged out with a smile. He giggles, squeals, belly laughs, and bounces his whole body while muttering joyful sounds like "ba-ba-ba-ba."

When sad, baby utters the grunts and growls of complaints. At this stage the universal "n" sound emerges to signal negative feelings. Baby may protest medicine taking by a string of "na-na-na-na." Baby puts on his unhappy face: mouth twisted into a grimace and facial muscles drooping. And, if you don't quickly get the point, these sounds and body language escalate into a cry.

Helping Language Development

Language, like a sense of humor, is caught, not taught. You don't directly teach your baby to speak. You fill her ears with the right sounds, and baby catches the spirit that talking is fun. Speaking is more natural that way. Here are some ways to foster language development.

Play word games. Word games teach baby that language is fun and stimulate baby's developing memory. One of our favorites is:

Round and round the garden goes the
   teddy bear,
*(draw a circle around baby's tummy
   with your finger)*
one step, two steps,
*(walk your finger from his belly button to
   his neck)*
tickle you under there!
(tickle baby under the chin)

Give cues. Cue words are words or phrases that trigger a response from baby because of a pattern of sounds he has heard before. One of our favorites is the bump-heads game. When Matthew was in this stage of development, I would say, "Bump heads!" and Matthew and I would gently bump foreheads. After repeating this game a number of times, Matthew took the cue and actually started moving his head toward mine as I said, "Bump," even before I started moving toward him. What was going on in Matthew's mind? I believe that he had stored this game in a series of "records" in his memory. Upon hearing the cue word "bump," he dropped the needle into the right groove and set the whole record playing. Playing word games and watching your baby's response to certain cue words lets you know how your baby's memory is developing.

Associate words with objects. During this stage, watch your baby begin to associate words with the most important objects in his environment. When reading to your baby, connect persons and objects in the book with those in his environment — saying, for example, "See *cat*" as you point toward the cat in the book.

Table talk. Place baby at a table full of kids and adults and watch him join in the conversation. Notice how baby follows the discussion, turning his head from speaker to speaker and learning a valuable language art — listening.

Fun and Games for the Six-to-Nine-month-old

The best activities are those that hold baby's attention and stimulate the two master skills

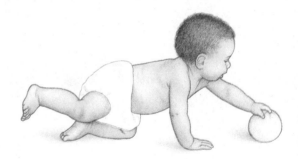

Your six-month-old will enjoy grabbing and holding a soft ball.

of this stage, crawling and thumb-and-forefinger pickup.

Play ball! Balls rank next to blocks as the best baby toys. Don't expect your minor leaguer to field or return your throws just yet. But baby can grab and hold a ball. Use balls that are large enough to be held with both hands, preferably made of soft foam or cloth that baby can get his fingers into and hold on to with one hand. Sit on the floor facing baby with your legs stretched out in front of you and roll the ball toward him. This pregame warm-up sets the stage for opening day of the real ball game in a few months.

Mirror play. Sit baby within touching distance of a mirror (floor-to-ceiling mirrors are the best). Watch your baby try to match her hands and face to the image in the mirror. Now you appear alongside, and baby becomes fascinated at your image next to hers in the reflection.

Roll games. Playing on foam bolsters, which began in the previous stage, becomes even more fun at this stage, because baby can crawl up and over these cushions and

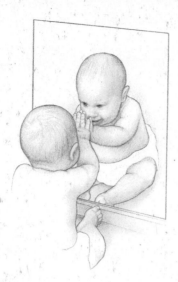

Babies of this age become fascinated with mirror images.

entertain himself. Drape baby over the bolster cushion and place a toy just beyond his reach. Notice how baby digs his feet in, pushing and rolling himself forward on the foam cylinder in hot pursuit of the toy.

NEW FEARS AND CONCERNS IN THE SECOND SIX MONTHS

A friend of yours, but a stranger to baby, wishes to greet you and your baby-in-arms. You open your arms to your friend, but your baby doesn't open hers. Instead she fearfully clings to you, periodically peering over her shoulder to check out the intruder. The harder you work at making a proper introduction, the tighter baby clings.

Your baby is experiencing what is commonly called stranger anxiety. This — and its close relative, separation anxiety — is normal among children in the second six months; it seems to be a protective behavior that keeps babies close to home base at a developmental stage when their motor skills entice them away.

Stranger Anxiety

Stranger anxiety normally occurs between six and twelve months, when your onetime social butterfly turns shy. While she formerly enjoyed the game of going from arms to arms, now she settles only for yours. Your baby may reject even her closest significant others previously dear to her. This social behavior is a normal and passing phase, no reflection on your parenting, nor an indication of child insecurity. In fact, some of the most securely attached babies may go through periods of stranger anxiety before eagerly embracing unfamiliar persons.

Your baby regards you as the standard by which she measures everyone else, and she rates everyone else by your reaction. She sees strangers through your eyes. If your baby needs a social chairman, here's how to help.

Easing into strangers. Quickly greet the advancing person with a welcoming smile and begin a joyful dialogue, but still keep a distance. Give your baby time and space to size up the stranger and read your happy face. Based on your reaction to the stranger, baby forms a concept about the unfamiliar person. If she's OK to you, she's OK to baby. Then you take the lead. Make the proper third-party introduction: "See Aunt Nancy, she's nice." Meanwhile Aunt Nancy makes no advances. Then you *gradually* close the distance. When Aunt Nancy is within baby's intimate space, take baby's hand and pat Aunt

Nancy's face, all the while reading baby's body language for when to advance and when to retreat. Brief Aunt Nancy about your strategy so she knows not to rush at baby. Grandparents, especially, need to understand how important it is to let baby approach them. This avoids hurt feelings or lectures on how you are spoiling that baby. This method also helps babies approach "strange doctors."

For more difficult cases. If your baby is very stranger anxious, set the stage for a more subtle introduction. Warn your friend about what your baby is experiencing. This is a matter of normal infant development; don't be apologetic ("But she really is a good baby"), trying to cover up for these first impressions. Suggest the stranger begin by warming up to one of baby's favorite toys; for example, cuddling T. Bear or pulling out a special toy so that baby will want to approach the stranger to get the toy.

If all your social strategies fail to release the clinging vine, sit baby securely on your lap while you enthusiastically relate to the stranger and let baby join the fun at her own pace.

Martha notes: When a familiar person approaches, Matthew initiates play by smiling and gesturing. When a stranger approaches, he gets a look of concern on his face as though he is measuring this person and measuring his ability to respond. Sometimes he will respond to the stranger's game and start to smile brightly and babble and activate his limbs. Sometimes he waits until he's sure of what the game is. When he sees someone he is familiar with, such as mother, father, or siblings, he automatically goes into animated socializing. The way he expresses caution with a stranger is his eyes widen and a sort of vulnerable expression crosses his face with just a momentary pause, as though he is checking things out before he proceeds with play. Sometimes he needs prompting from me to encourage him to go ahead and take part in the game with the stranger. I watch and see at what point he no longer tolerates being placed in the arms of a stranger and walked away with. He tolerates this quite well as long as I ease the transition by gesturing and smiling that it's OK, as long as the person he's being handed to is relaxed and comfortable with him. If he senses in any way that he is not safe with that person, he fusses. A few months ago he showed all-out beaming angelic smiles that were just so cute that he was able to charm any stranger. Now he doles out his smiles with much more discretion. This tells me that he is reasoning about why he should be smiling. He is becoming a more discerning person. When responding to a stranger his smile will be very slow in coming and it will be studied. He will look from the stranger back to me and then back again as though checking in with me to see if it's all right if he smiles. Sometimes he gives a tentative smile then turns away from the person and hides his face in my shoulder. He will then continue to socialize with that person only if I support and encourage him.

Separation Anxiety

Separation anxiety usually begins around six months with the crawling phase and may even intensify from twelve to eighteen months when baby begins walking. A wise parent will respect the normal phase of separation anxiety and, if possible, plan necessary separations from baby outside of this sensitive period. Because this phenomenon is of such concern to parents, let's take a closer look.

IS BABY TOO DEPENDENT?

Our eight-month-old baby cries every time I put her down and walk into the next room. I can't seem to leave her without her getting upset. We're very close, but could I have made her too dependent on me?

No! You have made her secure, not dependent. Your baby is experiencing separation anxiety, a normal and healthy behavior that is not caused by your making her too dependent.

One day as we watched eight-month-old Matthew playing, we developed a theory as to why separation anxiety occurs and why it's healthy. While Matthew crawled around the room, every few minutes he would look back to see if we were watching. He would get upset if he saw us walking out of the room or couldn't keep a fix on us.

Why this curious behavior? As experienced baby watchers, we have learned that babies do what they do for a good reason. Separation anxiety seems to peak at the time when baby begins experiencing locomotor skills. Could separation anxiety be a safety check that clicks on when baby has the motor abilities to move away from the parents but does not yet have the mental capabilities to handle separation? *Baby's body says go — his mind says no.* Otherwise, he would just keep on going.

Giving "It's OK" signals. Don't feel you have made your baby too dependent on you and that he will remain clingy and not develop a healthy independence. On the contrary, separation anxiety is often a measure of how secure a baby's attachment is and how securely he will ease into independence. Here's why. Suppose baby is playing in a room full of strange toys and strange babies. Baby begins to cling to you. Instead of reinforcing his fears of the strange and unfamiliar, you give baby "It's OK" cues. Baby releases from you and becomes familiar with the strange environment, periodically checking back into home base for reassurance that it's OK to proceed into more unfamiliar situations. The presence of a strong attachment figure, usually the parent or a familiar, trusted caregiver, acts as a coach to give baby the go-ahead to explore further. During a strange situation the attachment figure interjects a reassuring "It's OK" as baby begins to explore another level. As soon as baby becomes familiar with one level, he goes on to another level. As baby climbs the ladder of independence, he checks in to be sure someone's holding the ladder.

Easing baby into separation. If baby can't see you, he does not yet have the mental capacity to figure out that you are just around the corner or will soon return. Making voice contact sometimes reassures a baby who can't see you, and it stimulates baby's ability to associate your voice with a mental image of you, quelling an attack of separation anxiety before it happens. Not until the second year do most babies develop *object and person permanence,* the memory ability to make and retrieve mental images of a person or thing he cannot see. This ability to retain a mental picture of a trusted caregiver will enable baby to move more easily from the familiar to the unfamiliar. (See page 525 for more discussion of object permanence.)

Close Parent-Infant Attachment Fosters Independence

As we mentioned earlier in a different context, we think it helps to understand mental development if we compare the developing of baby's mind to the process of making a phonograph record; this is our deep-groove theory. The stronger the parent-infant attachment, the deeper the attachment groove in baby's record and the easier baby can click into this groove when needed. Earlier theories about spoiling claimed that an infant who is strongly attached to his mother would never get out of the groove, become independent, and explore on his own. Our experience and the experiments of others have shown the opposite. In a classic study, called the strange-situations experiment, researchers studied two groups of infants (labeled "securely attached" and "insecurely attached") during an unfamiliar play situation. The most securely attached infants, the ones with the deepest grooves, actually showed less anxiety when separated from their mothers to explore toys in the same room. They periodically checked in with the mother for reassurance that it was OK to explore. The mother seemed to add energy to the infant's explorations. Since the infant did not need to waste effort worrying about whether she was there, he could use that energy for exploring.

When going from oneness to separateness, the securely attached baby establishes a balance between his desire to explore and his continued need for the feeling of security provided by a trusted caregiver. When a novel toy or a stranger upsets the balance, or mother leaves and thus reduces baby's sense of security, baby feels compelled to reestablish the original equilibrium. The consistent availability of a trusted caregiver provides needed reassurance and promotes independence, confidence, and trust, leading to an important milestone by the end of the first year — the ability to play alone.

NINE TO TWELVE MONTHS: BIG MOVES

Progressing up the developmental ladder from crawling to scaling to cruising and finally walking is one of the most exciting motor sequences in infant development. Get your video camera ready. This budding choreographer will show you a parade of interesting moves as he climbs the ladder of developmental success.

Locomotor Development

By nine months most babies have mastered the style of crawling that is most efficient, comfortable, and speedy. For most babies this means cross-crawling, which allows better balance by keeping one limb on each side of the body on the floor at all times. Cross-crawling teaches baby to coordinate the use of one side of his body with the other and prepares baby for other physical skills.

Once baby masters a developmental skill such as crawling, she wants to experiment with variations on that skill. Baby may get a bit cocky in her crawling style, wiggling her bottom, wobbling her head, and getting her whole body into the crawling act.

Crawling opens up a new social avenue for baby. Now she can come to you and doesn't have to wait for you to come to her. Like a puppy eager to greet her owner, baby crawls right up your pant leg, pulling herself to a

WHAT ABOUT SAFETY GATES?

Putting a gate at the top of the stairs is like waving a red flag in front of a baby bull. The impulsive explorer scales right up the gate and rattles it back and forth until sometimes baby and gate come sliding down the stairs. Whether to rely on a gate or teach your baby how to crawl safely down stairs is a matter of baby's temperament and crawling abilities. Watch your baby crawl toward the top step. Around ten to eleven months most babies develop some caution about heights (see page 526). Some crawl toward the edge, stop, look, and feel over the edge with their hands. These are the babies who can be trained to back down the stairs safely. Impulsive babies, however, do not take time to slow down and feel for the edge; they are likely to hurl themselves down the steps. These babies and those who show quickly progressing motor and climbing skills (early walkers) are ones who need watchful monitoring and a secure safety gate.

standing position and giving you "Let's play" overtures.

Bypassing the Crawling Stage

Some infant development specialists feel that a baby who misses the crawling stage is at risk for coordination problems later on because crawling is a prelude to learning balance. While this may be true for some babies, there are many perfectly normal, well-coordinated children who quickly bypass the crawling stage to move on to other forms of locomotion. One of our babies "walked" on her knees instead of crawling. Another scooted on his bottom with one leg straight out and the other leg bent under. Some babies scoot so well that they quickly lose interest in crawling. And perhaps the enjoyment of these cute styles of locomotion by baby's cheerleaders reinforces them.

From Crawling to Scaling to Climbing

Watch baby crawl over to the bed or sofa. He grabs the bedspread or upholstery and pulls himself up as far as he can go, a skill called *scaling*. Climbing and scaling are simply crawling upward rather than forward, an example of how baby expands one skill into another. Because neurologically baby develops from head to toe, his arms are stronger and more coordinated than his legs and feet. Baby first pulls up with both hands while his weaker legs bow and his feet curl inward. Finally, baby learns to push up with his legs while pulling with his hands. After baby scales the side of the sofa or high chair, he looks around in amazement that he got there all by himself and enjoys his new view. Then, for a moment, he appears stuck in the standing position. Eventually his legs give out and he crumples quickly to the floor.

Now the fun begins. After baby has mastered crawling and scaling, here comes the climber. Baby will enjoy climbing over a pile of cushions and especially the climbing-over-pop game while dad lies on the floor. Then baby discovers the ultimate climbing activity. You'll catch him looking up at his staircase to the "sky." Your baby may be able to climb a whole flight of stairs by the end of the first year, especially when encouraged by a cheering squad of proud parents and siblings. But

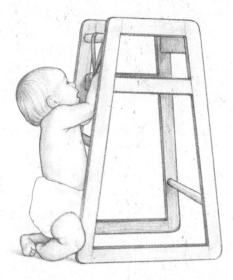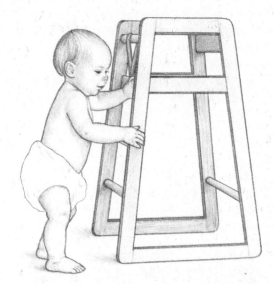

As locomotor development progresses, baby will advance from crawling to scaling, using his arms to pull himself up.

notice your baby's confused body language when he is stuck at the top of the stairs. Babies don't know intuitively that the safest way to get down stairs is backward. They are likely to turn around and propel themselves recklessly forward. While babies do not need any help climbing up, they are likely to need help getting down. Teach your baby to back down steps by turning his body around. Show him how to dangle one foot over the edge of the step to touch the step below. Baby will then use his feet as feelers to test the distance for climbing down steps (or off the sofa). You know that your baby can comfortably handle stairs when he swings his body around at the top of the staircase and approaches the second step feet first.

Standing Supported

Once baby has learned to scale a piece of furniture, he likes his newly found skill and the view from up there and decides to stay there

awhile, developing the skill of standing supported. But the first efforts are off balance as he tries to unfold his wobbly feet and get off his tiptoes. Once baby learns to stand like a little ballerina, feet flat and turned out, he can balance better.

Let the beginning climber scale your pant leg, and you can feel the progress that baby makes in learning to stand. Initially you feel a lot of weight as baby grips your pants for both balance and support. Gradually you feel less and less of baby's weight as he holds on only for balance.

Cruising Along

Once baby can stand leaning against a sofa or low table, don't expect him to stay put. When first cruising, baby is likely to get his sidestepping feet entangled. He soon learns that cruising sideways is uncomfortable. Watch how baby compensates. He turns his legs, then his feet, so they can walk

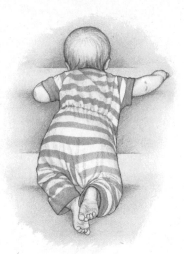

Crawling becomes climbing by the end of the first year.

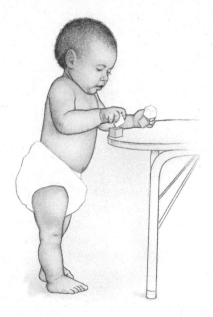

To help baby enjoy standing, place some favorite toys on a waist-high table and let baby stand and play.

frontward instead of sideways, and then turns the upper half of his body to align with the lower half. Now he learns to get one foot in front of the other, and around the table he goes, holding on first with both hands, then one hand.

Now that baby can stand and cruise, he wants to stand and play. Put toys on a low table and watch him entertain himself for five or ten minutes.

➤*SAFETY TIP: Cruising gives baby a motor skill not only to enjoy but also to use to get into trouble. Now that baby has a fascination with tabletop play, he will want to grab and bang anything within reaching distance on his cruise pad. Remove sharp breakable and mouthable objects from your coffee table or any low-lying table that the cruiser is likely to explore. Babies love cruising along desks and reaching for dangling phone cords or any object they can grab.*

➤*SAFETY TIP: Falling against the sharp corners of coffee tables or climbing on them and falling off are common accidents for beginning cruisers. Either store the coffee table for a year or place protective covers on the edges.*

From Cruising to Freestanding to First Steps

As the cruiser sidesteps along furniture, he periodically lets go. Amazed at his courage, baby looks up for a cheering audience. His legs quickly give way and he goes boom. Here's an exercise to put him on cruise control. Arrange furniture (sectional sofas work best) in a circle and watch baby cruise around the inner circle, holding on with one hand for support. Then put increasingly wider gaps between the sections. This setup motivates baby to close the gap by toddling across the open spaces. This show may lead to baby's first freestanding and first steps.

Standing free. During one of baby's around-the-living-room cruises, watch him let go and freestand. Baby is surprised and puzzled. Now that he's left standing alone, he's faced with two decisions: how to get back down and how to move forward. He will plop down on his well-padded bottom, crawl over to the sofa, and pull back up to a standing position and try again, this time standing longer.

First steps. Once baby begins cruising, she is ready to walk in front of you being supported by your hands. Stand baby between your legs, hold both hands, and take steps together. Then, as baby learns to freestand

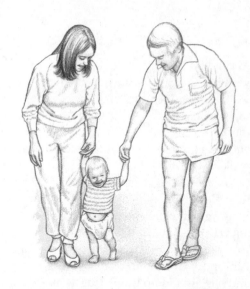

A cruising baby is ready to try walking supported by your hands.

longer, she's ready to take her first solo steps. Watch the balancing act as she figures out that moving forward from a standing position is just a matter of learning to balance on one foot while the other foot shuffles ahead. (Notice how your baby's ankles roll inward, exaggerating her knock-knees and flatfeet. The rubberlike ligaments supporting the ankles do not strengthen for several years, so enjoy these flatfeet for a few more birthdays.)

To start out, baby widens her stance, opens her arms sideways, and keeps her head pointed forward — all positions that achieve better balance. Her first steps are quick, staccato, and stiff legged — like a wooden soldier's. Her face has a mixed expression of wonder and caution, but after a few days of stepping better, she consistently has an "I can do it" look.

Helping the beginning walker. To reinforce baby's walking skills, take her hands

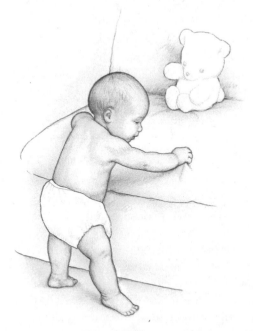

A standing baby soon becomes a cruising baby, supporting himself on whatever furniture is within reach.

EARLY WALKERS — LATE WALKERS?

Around 50 percent of babies walk by one year, but there is a wide normal range for walking, from ten to fifteen months. Walking is a matter of coordinating three factors: muscle strength, balance, and temperament, and the latter seems to influence the age of walking the most. Babies with easier temperaments often approach major developmental milestones more cautiously. Since, early on, crawling is speedier than walking anyway, the confirmed crawlers are content to zip around the floor like miniature race cars and show no interest in joining the tall and busy world up there. Late walkers are more likely to be content to entertain themselves with seeing and fingering fun than with motor accomplishments. A late walker goes through the crawl-cruise-stand-walk sequence slowly and cautiously, calculating each step and progressing at his own comfortable rate. When he does finally walk, he walks well.

The early walker, on the contrary, may be the impulsive, motor-driven baby who has raced through each motor milestone before parents could get their camera ready. While there is no definite profile of early walkers, they tend to be high-need babies who early on left the lap stage and squirmed out of infant seats. Body type may also affect the age of walking. Lean babies tend to walk earlier. Early and impulsive walkers are often more accident-prone than their more cautious walking mates.

Parents who carry their babies a lot often ask, "Will I delay her walking by carrying her around so much?" The answer is no. In fact in our experience and in the studies of others, babies who are the product of the attachment style of parenting (for example, worn in a baby sling for many hours a day) often show more advanced motor skills. No matter which baby in the neighborhood walks first or wins the speed race, the age of walking has nothing to do with eventual intelligence or motor skills. Baby walking, both the timing and the style, is as unique as personality.

and walk with her between your legs or alongside you, gradually letting go with one hand, then the other. And as baby practices her first solo steps, stand a few feet away, holding out your encouraging arms and giving baby a "Come on."

From Crawl to Squat to Stand

Even though baby may be taking a few steps, when he zeros in on a desired toy across the room, the rookie walker usually plops down from standing and clicks into a faster mode of ground transportation — often cross-crawling or scooting. The next decision for the beginning walker is how to get back to the walking position. Initially baby needs a crutch, and he crawls over to the wall or a piece of furniture, scales it to a standing position, lets go, and takes a few steps, falls, and begins the same cycle all over.

"If only I could short-circuit the couch and go directly to standing," baby might imagine.

And in the next stage that's just what he does (see page 533).

Hand Skills

In the previous stage, when you placed a tiny morsel of food within baby's grasp, baby would rake it toward himself and maneuver it into the ends of his thumb and finger, eventually picking it up with thumb and forefinger. In this stage, after dozens of pickup practices, baby develops a neat pincer grasp. Put a tiny O-shaped cereal pellet in front of him and watch him unerringly grab it with a clean thumb-and-forefinger pickup, without first raking it in or resting his hand on the table. Baby puts the tip of the index finger on it and curls the finger toward the thumb and, snatch! he's got it.

Baby Accommodates Hands to Objects

Place a new pencil (unsharpened) on a table and watch baby grab it. Now turn the pencil

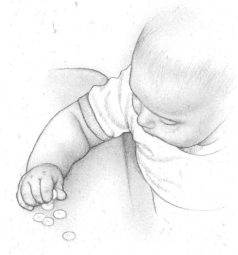

The pincer grasp enables baby to pick up small objects.

at a different angle, and watch baby turn his hands parallel to the long axis of the pencil, making in-flight corrections on the way to the target. Before, baby impulsively grabbed a toy whole-handedly without first figuring out how best to pick it up. Now baby makes decisions about how to manipulate the toy before grabbing it.

Container Play

The master curiosity of this stage is the relationship between toys: how a big toy is related to a little one and how a little object fits into a bigger one. Improved manipulating skills enable baby to figure out play combinations of objects — banging toys together, stacking, and the ever-favorite fill-and-dump. Being able to manipulate two toys together opens endless play possibilities for these curious little hands, and near the end of the first year baby discovers containers and the concept of emptiness. Here are some activities that will help baby enjoy his new skills.

- Give baby a large plastic glass or a shoe box and watch the curious hands poke around inside the container. Now give baby a block and observe how he introduces the block and the container. Hand and mind work together to figure out how to put block into box and, of course, how to dump it out. After mastering put-in-and-dump-out, baby shakes the container and listens to the block flopping around inside. Notice the figuring-out expressions on baby's face as he goes through the many play combinations with a simple block and a simple cup.

- Put cotton in your ears and bring out pots and pans! Baby delights in putting little pots into bigger pots and, of course, the noise of banging and dropping.

- Bathtub and sink play (always supervise) gives the master dumper an exercise in *filling and pouring.* Scooping up a cup of water and pouring it out makes a big splash on baby's list of favorite games.

- Place baby in a large laundry basket half full of small clothes, preferably socks and baby clothes. After baby takes the clothes out of the basket, put your little helper outside the basket and show her how to "put it in," picking up a sock and putting it back into the basket for her.

Getting Into Your Baby's Mind

If only you could get into that little mind and find out what your baby is thinking. Well, you can — sort of. You can learn what baby thinks by observing how she plays. You can deduce what mental processes baby is capable of by giving her an opening cue and noticing how she responds. We call this the fill-in-the-blanks approach. A guess, yes, but until your child can tell you what she is thinking, it's the best you can do. While baby can't yet talk, she can use body language to tell you her thoughts.

Signs of Developing Memory

Mental pictures. One day I was reading to nine-month-old Matthew. I pointed to a picture of a cat and said, "Cat." Watching his face, I saw a light of recognition go on. He looked toward the door because the family cat resides outside. Then he began patting the cat in the picture. The picture of the cat triggered a *mental association.* Matthew had stored in his memory the image of a cat and remembered that he usually pets the cat. Also, I observed that he now had the mental capability to recognize the similarity between the cat in the book and the cat in his life.

Name that tune. At this stage babies do remember recent events. One day we took nine-month-old Matthew to an exhibit at Disneyland called "It's a Small World." The theme song and the accompanying visuals made quite an impression upon him. The next day when we sang the melody of "It's a Small World," Matthew's excited eyes and smile showed that he was remembering what he had seen and heard the day before.

Martha notes: Matthew is becoming very set in what he wants to do and where he wants to be and is beginning to remember activities when we're interrupted. He seems more aware of places. If he is anticipating being taken in one direction and we go the opposite direction, he will protest with intensity depending on how badly he was hoping for his own direction.

Cue words. We believe babies store bits of information, and if they hear a cue word it's just like pressing a button in a baby's mental jukebox and a whole memory record comes down. For example, Matthew and I would enjoy daily walks to the ocean. When he was nine months I would say "Go" and Matthew would crawl over to the door because the word "go" triggered visions of playing outside, going for a car ride, or any other activity associated with going out the door. He didn't react any differently no matter what I added to "go." By one year, however, his mind was capable of more complete memory. Now when I said, "Go ocean," he anticipated not only being carried out the door but also going for our usual walk to the ocean. If I turned in a direction away from the ocean, he would protest. He could associate definite words and actions with definite events to follow. Anything that didn't fit his mental expectations merited a squawk. This illustrates the value of talking with your baby, explaining things step-by-step so he won't be taken by surprise or unnecessarily disappointed, a setup for tantrum behavior.

What's behind the door? Baby's vivid memory now enables him to remember what is behind closed doors. At eleven months Matthew sat in front of an open kitchen-cabinet door and noticed the enticing pots and pans, which he grabbed, pulled off the shelf, and rattled in a way only a parent could love. (Fortunately for human ears, baby's playtimes are short.) When Matthew finished his sound effects, we took away the pots and pans and closed the door. From then on Matthew remembered the noisy toys behind the closed door and daily crawled toward the cabinet, scaled up the door, and tried to open it.

Games to Play

Find the missing toy. A mental skill that may begin to mature at this age is the concept of object permanence — the ability to remember where a toy is hidden. Previously, out of sight was out of mind. If you hid a toy under a blanket, baby showed little interest in finding the toy. Try this experiment. Let baby see you place a favorite toy under one of two cloth diapers lying in front of him. Watch baby momentarily study the diapers as if trying to figure out which diaper is covering the toy. By the "I'm thinking" expressions on his face, you get the feeling that he is trying to recall in his memory under which diaper the

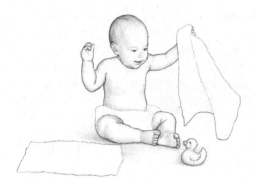

Near the end of the first year, baby may show interest in finding a toy he has seen you hide under a diaper. This is the beginning of awareness of object permanence.

toy is hidden. He makes his decision, pulls off the diaper covering the toy, and shows great delight in making the right choice. Try this several times, always putting the toy under the first diaper, then let him watch you put the toy under the second diaper. If you have consistently hidden the toy under the first diaper, even when baby sees you put the toy under the second diaper, most of the time he initially searches under the first diaper because that scene is still fixed in his memory. Sometime between twelve and eighteen months, as baby's reasoning abilities mature, he may consistently remember that you switched the toy under the second diaper or see the bulge under the second diaper and realize the toy must be under there.

Hide-and-seek. Baby's new ability to remember the place where a parent's bobbing head was last seen makes this game a favorite. Let baby chase you around the couch. When she loses you, peer around the edge of the couch and call her name. Baby will crawl to where she saw you peering. Eventually she will imitate you by hiding and peeking around the couch herself.

Next, add the game of *sounding*. Instead of letting baby see where you are hiding, stay hidden but call her name. Watch her crawl, and later toddle, around the house in search of the voice she mentally matches with the missing person. Keep sounding to hold the searching baby's interest.

Mental Protections

Babies become more mentally discerning at this stage and begin to have a feel for harmful objects or situations. But this is an extremely valuable skill, so don't rely on it.

Awareness of heights. Usually by one year of age babies develop a mental awareness of heights, as demonstrated in the classical visual cliff experiment. Crawling babies were placed upon a long glass-top table. Immediately beneath the glass of half the table was a checkerboard pattern. The same checkerboard pattern was placed beneath the other half of the glass table but on the floor four feet below. The babies were positioned on the checkerboard half of the table and encouraged to crawl across it toward their mothers. When babies reached the end of the first checkerboard pattern their hands still touched glass, but their eyes told them there was a drop-off, and the babies stopped crawling when they reached the apparent cliff. This experiment demonstrated that babies at this stage do have the mental capabilities to determine edges and heights and are able to decide not to go over the edge. But don't leave your baby playing on a tabletop! For particularly impulsive babies, called hurdlers, their tempera-

ment overrides their mental awareness of danger, and they may crawl right over the edge.

Mother gives the go-ahead. As an interesting twist to the visual cliff experiment, when the babies crawled toward their mothers and their mothers projected a happy, nothing-to-fear attitude, most babies crawled across the visual cliff. When mothers projected an expression of fear, the babies stayed put. The conclusion: Mother acts as an emotional regulator of the infant, who is able to read her facial signals or bounce his own signals off her and react to a situation according to the feedback he receives.

Babies read our faces about everything, especially as it relates to them. If you tend to be chronically anxious or depressed, your baby applies what he sees on your face to himself and to life in general. A face that radiates genuine joy toward life is a wonderful legacy to give your child (and yourself).

Mastering the World of Words

As baby masters the wonderful world of words, you may finally feel you are getting your point across. At last, baby understands you, though he still does not consistently comply. Simple and familiar questions usually trigger an understandable response: "Do you want to nurse?" "Do you want to go outside?" No "yes" or "no" words yet, but baby's body language is crystal clear. Unless, of course, he doesn't know himself what he wants.

Under one year of age babies still say very little with words, understand a lot with their mind, and have very powerful body language.

A baby's receptive speech (the ability to understand) is always several months ahead of expressive speech. Just because a baby says very little does not mean she does not understand what you are saying. In fact, if you double what you actually imagine your baby understands, you will probably accurately assess her language comprehension at all ages.

Baby Words

As well as understanding your verbal and body language, baby now increases his own repertoire. Though still mostly jabbering, baby surprises you by periodically changing inflections and intonations in his talking, giving you the feeling that *he* knows what he is saying even if you don't.

The term "word" means a sound used consistently to refer to an action or object, even if the sound is not intelligibly articulated. This is true of most baby words, which are not always intelligibly articulated, thus not understood — except perhaps by parents. Most babies at this stage have familiar words ("dada," "mama," "cat"). Babies love to imitate your speech sounds, including coughing and tongue noises such as hisses and clicks.

Baby not only has more language at this stage than the last, but it's definitely louder. The shouting stage begins, followed by the screaming stage. Plug your ears. This soon will pass. Baby is just trying out his voice and is amazed at the intensity of sounds he can generate and the response of those within earshot. If you feel you must do something to teach your baby to use his "quiet voice" in the house or car, *show him how* by whispering. This "secret voice" gets his attention and gives him something else to imitate.

"NO-NO-NO!"

By the end of the first year most babies understand "no" to mean "stop." How quickly baby complies depends on the gestures and tone of voice that accompany "no." When a baby is about to pull on a lamp cord, gently grab his little hand, look in his big eyes, and point to the cord while saying, "No, don't touch — hurt baby!" Then redirect his curiosity to a safer and yet equally interesting activity. At this stage baby may even shake his own head to mimic your gestures, as though this helps him understand. Avoid saying no in a rude, punitive way. Maintain respect for your baby when you speak to him. Your goal is to teach, not to frighten. And, of course, expect your baby to come back at you with frequent noes. Some creative alternatives to "no" are "stop," "hot," "shut," "dirty," "hurt baby," or "down." Make up a universal "no" sound that immediately gets baby's attention. Our "stop" sound was a sudden loud "ah"; it halted Stephen in his tracks.

Gestures and Body Language

Besides baby's having more words at this stage, his body language, especially facial and arm gesturing, helps you know where you stand and what he needs. Baby may pull on your pants and raise his arms to get picked up. He gives you squirm cues in your arms to let you know he's ready to get down. If your baby intensely needs to get your attention, he may grab your nose or chin and turn your face toward his. This expressive body language matures long before the ability to say intelligible words. Perhaps a baby at this stage feels, "If you can't read my words, read my body."

Word and Voice Associations

By this stage, baby may be able to associate voices and names with people.

Who's on the telephone? Baby may now associate the voice with the person on the phone. One day when eleven-month-old Matthew heard my voice on the phone he turned and looked toward the door. My voice triggered the mental flash card of daddy coming through the door.

What's my name? Besides responding consistently to his own name, baby may now associate the name with the person. When seated at our busy family table, Matthew, by ten months of age, would catch the drift of the conversation. When I asked, "Where's Bob?" he would look at brother Bob.

Fun and Games with New Words and Gestures

Here are some favorite word games that will help you get a feel for how much body and verbal language your baby understands.

Waving bye-bye. In the previous stage baby probably could imitate your gestures for waving bye-bye. In this stage he might even initiate it. Baby learns to associate the sound-gesture "bye-bye" with departing actions, such as going out the door. You have repeated the bye-bye game so often that your baby imitates your

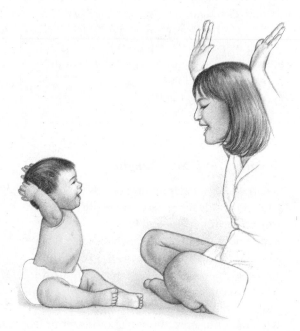

"So big!"

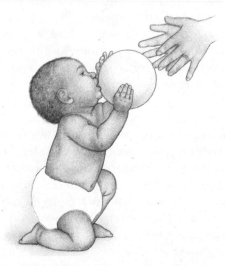

Babies at this stage love ball games and can usually follow simple requests like "Give the ball to mommy."

KEEP THE GAME GOING

When playing word games such as waving bye-bye and pat-a-cake, periodically give only half the message, such as the gesture without the sound or the sound without the gesture, and let baby complete the action. For example, say "pat-a-cake" without touching baby's hands, and let your sound trigger his memory pattern to clap his hands. Then be sure to reinforce baby's memory by clapping back. Keep these games going as long as you can, but remember that most babies at this stage have an attention span of less than one minute. When you feel that baby is really tuned in to what you are saying, keep his interest. For example, if you point to a bird in the sky and say "bird," and you notice baby also looks at the sky and utters what sounds like "bird," acknowledge how correctly baby perceived this sound, saying with a smile, "Yes, that's a bird!" This acknowledgment is the beginning of a mental skill that develops better in the next stage — baby's ability to make himself understood and to feel that his words are understood. While you are playing language games with your baby, notice that sometimes baby pauses as if to think whose turn it is. Language is now becoming more of a cognitive skill with baby thinking about what you are saying and about his reply.

waving. Now try saying "bye-bye" without waving or waving without saying "bye-bye." Once baby has learned the sound-gesture association he may wave when hearing the sound or say something that sounds like "bye-bye" when he sees you wave. Gestures and sounds trigger the mental associations that help baby put the two together.

Imitating gestures. By now baby is a master imitator. Favorites are gesture games incorporating hands and arms, facial expressions, and simple words — for example, so-big, and don't forget the oldie but goodie, pat-a-cake.

Peekaboo. A baby at this stage really gets into a game of peekaboo. Place a card in front of your face or a handkerchief over your head, meanwhile maintaining voice contact as you disappear, saying "Where's mommy?" As you remove the card from your face or baby pulls the handkerchief off your head and you reappear, notice the delight and laughter on baby's face. Reverse peekaboo is also fun. Drape a diaper over baby's head and say, "Where's baby?" As baby removes the covering and reappears, burst out with a "There he is!" Peekabo games stimulate baby's developing memory. Baby stores the image of the disappearing parent momentarily in his memory, and when you reappear he takes great delight in confirming that the image he sees is an accurate representation of the image he stored.

More ball games. Babies love the game of pitch-the-ball-and-go-fetch-it. One-step requests — "Get the ball for daddy!" — are inconsistently followed at this stage. A few months later baby may consistently follow one-step and even two-step commands: "Get the ball and throw it to daddy."

►**BALL TIPS:** *Babies like small, lightweight plastic balls. A Ping-Pong ball is a favorite because it makes an interesting noise when bouncing on the floor, it moves quickly, and babies can grab hold of it and control it easily. Babies also like large foam balls or soft, lightweight rubber balls that they can hold with two hands and throw or roll to you. Some babies at this stage may begin throwing a lightweight ball over their heads.*

CARING FOR YOUR BABY'S FEET

Caring for your baby's feet is just one more part of loving and caring for your entire baby. To help you get your baby off on the right foot, here are answers to the most common questions parents ask about their baby's feet and footwear.

When should I buy shoes for my baby?

Between nine and twelve months of age, when babies begin to pull themselves up and stand on their own, parents should begin thinking seriously about their baby's footwear needs.

Why does my baby need shoes?

Shoes help protect your baby's tender feet from the rough surfaces, splinters, and sharp objects that often lie in wait for the young adventurer. When your baby is learning to walk, she looks ahead, not down, and these uncautious little feet are likely to tread on anything.

Will shoes help my baby walk?

The flat, even bottoms of a shoe provide stability for a young tenderfoot. Usually I advise parents to let their baby take the first few steps barefoot and, once baby is walking well, make their first trip to the shoe store. A few beginning walkers, however, walk better and stumble less when wearing a well-fitting flexible shoe.

How can I tell if baby has outgrown her shoes?

Check your baby's feet periodically. Curled toes, blisters, indentations, or red burnlike marks on the soles of your baby's feet (friction rubs) are signs of an ill-fitting shoe. Most toddlers outgrow shoes before they outwear them. The average toddler outgrows her shoes around every three months. Here are signs that your baby has outgrown the shoes:

Toe room. While your child is standing, you can feel his pinkie, or little toe, pressing against the inside of the shoe. You should be able to press a distance of around a half inch (1½ centimeters) between baby's farthest-forward toe and the front of the shoe.

Throat room. The leather across the throat looks very tight and there is no give when you pinch it. A well-fitting shoe should allow you to pinch a small fold of material at the throat of the shoe.

The counter. The back of the shoe hangs over the heel either on the inner or outer side of the shoe.

WHAT TO LOOK FOR IN A BABY SHOE

The sole. As a general guide, the earlier the stage of walking, the thinner and more flexible the sole should be. Before buying a shoe, bend it in your hand to test its flexibility. Then watch your baby walk. The shoe should bend at the ball of the foot as your baby takes each step. Whether to get rubber soles or leather soles is a matter of which is most flexible. The rubber soles on some sneakers are thicker and stiffer than leather soles. Also, rubber soles tend to be more rounded, whereas the flatter leather soles tend to provide more stability. *Avoid stiff shoes for young feet.* If you have difficulty bending the shoe in your hand, leave it in the shoe store. Your baby will have even more difficulty bending the stiff shoe with his feet. Stiff soles may catch on the walking surface, causing a nasty fall.

The counter (back of the shoe). To ensure proper fit, the counter should be firm. Try this test. Squeeze the counter between your thumb and forefinger. If it feels too soft, it will weaken with wear, causing the shoe to slip off.

The heel. Beginning with your baby's first shoe, a slight heel is advisable to help prevent dangerous backward falls.

The top and sides. The throat of the shoe (the area across the top of the shoe just below the laces) and the sides should crease easily when your baby takes a step. If they don't, it means your baby's footwear is not flexible enough, and the foot can't bend naturally while baby walks.

Construction. Stick with natural materials — leather or canvas — that breathe, letting air get to baby's perspiring feet. Avoid synthetic materials, such as vinyl, which don't breathe.

Selecting a good shoe fitter is one of the most important steps in buying your baby's shoes. A qualified shoe fitter measures both feet while baby is standing, looking for flexibility at the ball of the foot while baby walks, and checks for toe room and heel slippage. And don't forget to consult the walker. Let baby test-stride the new shoes around the store.

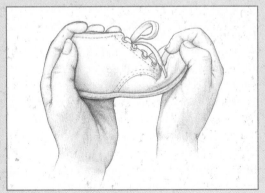

Squeezing the counter for firmness.

Testing flexibility.

22

The Second Year: From Babyhood to Toddlerhood

Enter the official toddler. The three master skills of this age, walking, talking, and thinking, are baby's ticket to advance from babyhood to toddlerhood.

Wave bye-bye to the sitting-still stage. Now you have a baby on the move. During the second year baby progresses from walking to running to climbing as he scurries around the house, flitting from one experience to the next. He seems to have wheels on his feet and is driven to get his hands on everything in grabbing distance, learning something from everything he touches. Knobs are to be turned, buttons pushed, and drawers pulled out. This is the age to explore and experiment. The maintenance stage of babyhood eases up as the supervision stage comes on strong.

Language fuels the fire of a curious house rover. Now baby has the capability to express what he wants, and the added power to direct his widening world. Increasing mental abilities add more excitement to the toddler adventure. Rather than impulsively rushing into a solution by trial and error, baby is able to figure out things in his head first.

But toddlerhood has its ups and downs. Separation anxiety adds some balance to baby's intense drive to explore and experiment. One minute baby will shadow you for security; the next minute he darts away from you in hot pursuit of some intriguing object. The ambivalence of dependence and independence and the desire to explore bring on emotional bursts of delight, laughter, fears, anger, and temper tantrums when overloaded. Baby not only experiences feelings but now has the ability to express them. Even though baby wants to "do it myself," reality tells him he can't.

While mental and motor growth surge, physical growth slows during the second year. During the first year the average baby may add 14 pounds and 10 inches (6.4 kilograms and 25 centimeters) to his growth; during the second year baby may add only 5 pounds and 5 inches (2.3 kilograms and 13 centimeters). This growth deceleration brings about a corresponding decrease in appetite, justifying the toddler label of "picky eater." Not only does baby take in fewer calories, but he runs off much of the first year's baby fat, becoming a leaner-looking baby.

TWELVE TO FIFTEEN MONTHS: BIG STEPS

Get ready. The walking show is about to begin. But while most babies can walk fifty feet (fifteen meters) by fifteen months, some are just beginning to take their first steps. Some babies walk everywhere, and some walk halfway across the room and then revert to crawling, especially if in hot pursuit of a desired toy or the family pet. Either is "normal" for this age.

Walking Stronger and Longer

First walks are aptly described as "drunken sailor" gait. Baby weaves and bobbles, teeters and staggers, waddles, falls, and crawls and then gets back up again to repeat the performance. Watch how baby orchestrates his arms, legs, and trunk muscles to balance and counterbalance and attempts to walk a straight line. As baby ambles across the room, notice that he bends his trunk slightly forward, thrusts arms out in front, and waddles with his legs wide apart. After a month or two of practicing these first steps, baby progresses from a wide-based, stiff-legged plop-plop gait to a more rhythmic knee-bending and heel-toe step with feet closer together, advancing to a determined marching type of gait.

Get-up-and-go maneuvers. Two master maneuvers at this stage help baby click into gear for a better walking start. Previously when baby wanted to go from crawling to walking he needed first to get to a standing position by scaling up a piece of furniture or the wall. Now baby can go directly from crawl to stand, bypassing the scaling stage. Watch your baby progress through the crawl-squat-stand-walk maneuver. Baby is sitting with his toys and suddenly decides to make rounds throughout the house. First he assumes the bear-crawl position (on hands

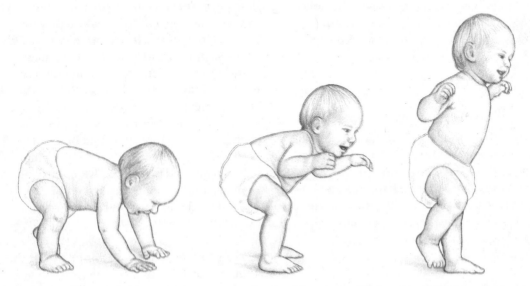

Now baby is able to go from a sitting to a standing position using the crawl-to-squat-to-walk maneuver.

and feet). Next, using his feet as the fulcrum of balance, baby lunges the weight of his bottom backward and moves his torso to assume the squatting position, resembling a quarterback about to say "hike." Then he straightens up his trunk to a standing position and off he goes. At first the steps in this maneuver are jerky and staccato, but gradually they become fluid. This is the master motor maneuver that gets baby from sitting to walking throughout most of the second year and the one that he uses to regain his stance after falling.

Entertainment steps. As baby masters walking forward, backward, and in circles, she begins to use walking games to entertain her admiring audience. With a sly look on her face she begins her antics. The helicopter game of wheeling around in circles with arms outstretched, ending in a dizzy fall, is a favorite. Another favorite game is looking through her legs. In the bear-crawl position, baby discovers she can peer through her outstretched legs and look at the world upside down. She holds that pose briefly, as though to say, "Hmmm, this view is different," and then raises herself to the standing position to toddle on.

Walk and Play

As with all developmental skills, mastery leads to enjoyment. A baby enjoys walking around holding on to a toy such as a foam ball. Walking under a table that just clears his head is another favorite challenge. As balance improves, baby enjoys stooping over to pick up a toy with one hand while stretching out the other for balance.

Babies still like assisted walking at this stage. Here is a fun game of walking together:

Stand facing each other, holding a foam ball in your hands, and get baby to hold on to it also. Begin walking backward, causing baby to walk toward you. Walk faster and faster, and notice baby chuckle as he tries to keep up the pace.

Toys for walkers. Push-pull toys are near the top of the list of favorite toddler toys. Watch baby mow the grass, toddling behind his toy lawn mower, or shop, pushing a cart. Ride-on toys are fun at this age, too. Baby can now sit astride a riding toy and maintain his balance for a few feet of locomotion on wheels. Because his balance is still precarious on these little bikes, parents should avoid letting baby ride on hard surfaces such as concrete. In addition, you should make sure the toy has a wide base of support and a low seat.

Play shelves. Easy-temperament babies, even at this stage, may be content to stand and play with toys on shelves. Impulsive babies, on the other hand, may stand and fling every toy in grabbing distance and may not be ready for ordered toys and play for many more months. If you place toys on shelves approximately twelve to eighteen inches (thirty to forty-five centimeters) off the floor, baby can toddle over to his own shelf and learn about taking off and putting on. He can select his toy and even use the shelving to help him stand and brace himself while he examines the toy. This gives him a complete and new perspective on playing. Expect baby to sometimes sweep his hand like a windshield wiper across the shelf, knocking off the toys.

Parents' little helper. To your surprise the kitchen may be baby's favorite playroom, a place where baby can use his new skills to "help" mom and dad. A play activity that comes about as a result of baby's standing skills is helping unload the dishwasher. Baby pulls himself to a stand when the dishwasher door is open, and he gets especially excited if he can reach the silverware basket. Because silverware attracts babies, sharp knives and other dangerous utensils must be kept out of reach, and of course you must supervise his "on-the-job training."

Walking together. Babies still like a social walk between parents, holding on with both hands, or alongside one parent holding on with one hand. Babies especially enjoy walking up and down the steps with the assistance of a parent, since most babies have not mastered solo stair climbing at this stage.

Joint ventures. Take exploratory walks around the house holding your toddler by one or both hands. As you navigate from room to room, show the young investigator how to safely use various pieces of furniture (only those that are safe for toddler climbing) and other interesting items on his level.

Hand Skills for Play and Self-help

Besides baby's being able to get around by walking, his rapidly developing awareness of his body parts and how to use them leads to the development of self-help skills.

Uses Tools

A favorite self-help activity is the use of tools, especially common household "tools," which baby has grown accustomed to seeing you use and now wishes to imitate: toothbrushes, hairbrushes, telephones, spoons and forks, plates, and cups. At the dinner table baby usually isn't as interested in eating the food as he is in using the tools.

Cooperates in Dressing and Grooming

Another self-help activity is trying to dress and undress. In the earlier stages, putting on and taking off clothes was often a wrestling match. While babies still squirm at one year, dressing them is usually a bit easier. Your toddler may put her foot out for her shoe, push her arm through her sleeve, pull her shirt over her head. She may even learn to blow her own nose or comb her own hair.

CLOSING OUT PLAY

Toddlers become so engrossed in their play that they protest when asked to stop playing and depart. Instead of just picking up your baby when it's time to eat, to get ready for bed, or to leave someone's home, here's a departure tip we have used successfully with each of our children: A few minutes before it's time to go, tell him it's time to go (or eat or sleep) and begin to help baby sign off by waving bye-bye to each toy. "Bye-bye truck, bye-bye blocks. . . ." These departure gestures help baby properly close out this play activity as if finishing a chapter in a book. This also helps parents realize that toddlers are little persons with strong wills who need creative discipline.

Cooperation is the result not only of increasing hand skills, but also of the increasing desire to imitate grown-ups and to "do it myself." You can help your baby increase her attention span during dressing and grooming by talking about the steps involved in what you are doing: "Now let's put your shoes on . . . give daddy your foot." Another way to ease dressing hassles is to make the clothes interesting and easy to put on: zippers, baggy sleeves and loose necklines, bright colors and eye-catching patterns. It helps, too, to make a game out of getting dressed. Play peekaboo, and ask "Where's baby?" when placing the shirt over your tot's head, followed by "There she is!" when her head pops through. Exercising baby's legs, "bicycling," as you put on baby's trousers helps baby's lower half cooperate. "This little piggy . . ." and a shared giggle ease the hassle of putting on shoes. Baby may lift her foot to put her pant leg on or raise her arms before you take off her shirt if you give short clear directions like "foot in" or "arms up."

Toys and Activities for New Hand Skills

Container play. Watch your baby opening and closing and reopening the cabinet doors and then hauling out all of the plastic containers and lids and sitting there on the floor with them spread around, trying to fit them together, and his skills coach cheering, "Put it in, take it out." Notice how he talks and sings to them and gives them orders and waves them around. Graduated cylinders, such as measuring-cup sets, help baby to develop the concept of relationships of sizes, how little containers fit into big. Baby becomes more aware of the relationships among playthings such as lids and containers and particularly

BABY'S OWN CABINET

To save wear and tear from your toddler's banging on your latched kitchen-cabinet doors, give him his own cabinet to toddle to and open as he wishes. Fill the shelf with container-type toys (graduated plastic cylinders, pots and pans, and a few of his favorites) and rotate the stock of toys frequently to hold your toddler's interest. Giving your explorer his own doors to open and a place to go may keep him from exploring less-safe areas.

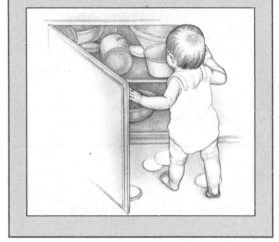

enjoys playing with lids. There is more interest in dumping out contents than putting the contents back in. Your toddler will join you, however, in putting the contents back in the container if you initiate this play activity and show him how the game is played.

Shapes and matching. Form boards are favorites. At around one year of age, the baby looks selectively at the round block and round hole, but misses usually outnumber hits. He may bang around the hole and seem to recognize the association between the block and the right-sized space, but he has neither the fine motor coordination nor the attentive patience to fit one into the other. Begin with a round-hole board because it's much easier for a toddler to put round shapes into round holes. As baby's matching skills and attention span increase, progress to the square pegs, which require baby to orient the peg's corners to the square hole.

Labeling: During container play and form board matching, if you demonstrate the correct matching, most babies by fifteen months can adaptively match the blocks and holes. You can help your baby enjoy and match containers and blocks by giving encouraging instructions such as "That's right, put the block in" while pointing to the correct space. Your baby will increasingly demonstrate the ability to follow your directions during play activities. This giving of directions ("Put the

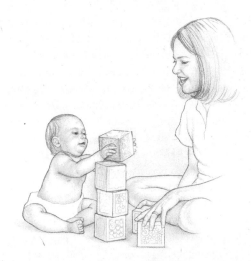

As baby gets bigger, blocks get bigger. Try four-inch rubber blocks that baby can either hold and stack with both hands or grab single-handed. Stacking three to four blocks and toppling the tower is a favorite sit-and-play activity.

block in") accompanied by the appropriate pointing gestures is called *labeling,* a language feature that increases baby's interest in play and encourages repetition of the specific activity. Emphasize play activities that encourage decision making. Set up the activity for baby and let him follow through.

Toy of the month. My vote for the household hand toy of the month is a shaving cream cap. Imagine all the fun things baby can do with this simple cap: bang it, transfer it, watch it drop, pick it up with thumb and forefinger or with one whole hand around the circumference or side; and in the bathtub, pour water from it, watch it submerge, reappear, and float.

Now if you want to do some mental games with the cap, drop it over the side of the bathtub and let baby watch it land on the

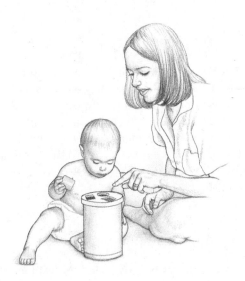

Your child will increasingly be able to follow directions during play.

floor. Then pick up the cap and hide it under your hand so that the cap is out of sight. Watch baby first look at the floor where he last saw the cap. Then show him the cap in your open hand. Close the hand over the cap and watch him reach for the hand with the cap. Then put your hands behind your back and change the cap to the other hand. Baby will reach for the hand that he previously saw the cap under, indicating a fairly accurate short-term memory at this age.

"Don't Touch"

The mind says to the hands, "Touch everything you can get your hands on, fill me with new touches. That's how I learn." And the legs, friends of the mind, are willing to take the hands where they want to go. But someone from above is always shouting "no!" Such is the world of the curious toddler. Here are alternatives for the baby who's into everything.

Touch-mes and touch-me-nots. Accompany the young explorer on his next trip around the house, showing him what things he can touch. Encourage safe touches: "Oh, look at pretty flowers, touch nicely," and model a soft touch. Provide baby's own special drawers and special cabinets (leave one in every room if possible) to keep busy hands into the right stuff.

The trading game. Just as baby's hands are opening to grab the lamp cord, your mouth is opening for a reflex "no!" but as a veteran at keeping one step ahead of baby you quickly channel her interest into a more exciting toy, "Mary, look what's in the box. . . ." Mary turns to the surprise box, and the lamp is safe.

Elevate your world. Rather than playing guard and blaring constant noes, raise your

---

SAFETY TIP

Possession meaning ownership begins as baby tenaciously holds on to a prized toy. If baby grabs a dangerous item, such as a knife, resist the impulse to snatch it out of his hand. Baby might protest, and one or both of you get cut. Instead, grab and gently squeeze baby's *wrist* with one hand to keep him from tightening his grip. (Try this maneuver by grabbing your own wrist and notice how wrist compression inhibits the fingers from closing.) Now say, "Give it to mommy," and substitute an equally enticing but safe toy while removing the dangerous one. Babies cannot yet understand why you are removing the dangerous object from their hand. Substituting toys is also handy for solving play squabbles and the inevitable "my toy" scene of possessive toddlerhood.

---

breakable world a few feet for a few years. Put up the dog dish and hide the wastebasket. Hearing "No, don't touch" too often creates a negative atmosphere in the house. The toddler may feel that everything is off-limits. This dampens baby's instincts to explore, therefore to learn. Direct your baby toward the hands-on approach with the right touches. (See "The Twelve-Inch Rule," page 556.)

Language Development

The second year is aptly called the walkie-talkie stage. Both verbal and body language take giant steps. You will notice two parts to your baby's language development: expressive language — intelligible words, what baby says — and receptive language, what baby understands. In all stages of development receptive speech is months ahead of expressive. In the early part of the second year baby says little but understands all.

First Words

Many babies don't voice a lot of new words at this stage, perhaps because they devote most of their developmental energy to walking. Once steps are mastered, words also take off. The average baby may speak only four to six intelligible words by fifteen months. Favorite first words are

- *b* words: ball, ba-ba (bottle), bird, bye-bye
- *c* words: cat, car
- *d* words: dog, dada
- *g* words: go

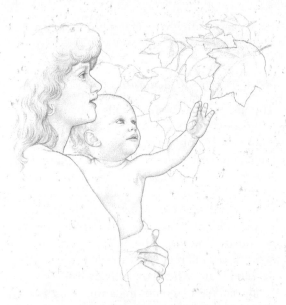

Giving names to things as you go about your daily activities will help baby's language skills.

Baby may not yet say the whole word, but may utter only the initial sound to give you a hint of what he's saying, as if he expects you to fill in the blanks: "ba" for "ball," "buh" for "bird," "ca" for "car." But the accompanying pointing gestures leave no doubt what word he means. Beginning toddler speech usually has all the right tones and inflections, only the mature words are missing.

First "noes." Baby can express "no" or a related negative expression, "na-na-na," and, in case you missed the cue, reinforce his wish by shaking his head or pushing your hand away when you try to feed or give him medicine.

Using labels. Continue putting a label on each person and thing that fills your toddler's everyday world. You point to the truck, give it a name, and your nearby little parrot

echoes a sound that, at least to your trained ear, resembles what you said, "Tuck." Take nature walks. Stroll with your toddler in the park or woods, stopping frequently to name things. Take cues from your baby. When he points to an insect, give it a name, "bug." When baby echoes "buh," agree, "Yes, that's a bug." When baby points to the moon and utters "moo," respond, "Yes, that's a moon." Reinforcing that you correctly understand him motivates baby to be a better parrot. That's how babies learn to talk.

The young parrot. The great imitator loves noise games, such as blowing bubbles or making raspberry sounds. He loves to mimic animal sounds, like the "woof-woof" of the family dog, or character sounds on TV. Use baby's desire to imitate to your advantage. At this age Matthew hated getting his nose wiped. So we let him participate in the procedure, by saying, "Blow your nose as I blow mine." Then we helped him mop up with a gentle wipe.

Be Alert to Your Toddler's Cues

Though you may be physically exhausted from coexploring with young Christopher Columbus, a combination of good language and good parenting skills makes living with a toddler easier because your baby can finally tell you what he wants. For example, baby tugs at your sleeve or brings you his coat to go outside or brings you a CD to play. Listening to your toddler is the most important activity for skill building and self-esteem development. When you actively listen you establish lifelong communication skills between yourself and your child. Give him the same respect you would give any adult who talks to you. He may be little, but he has big things to say. And remember, the main reason a toddler learns to whine is that when you don't listen the first (or second or third) time, his voice reflects his frustration, and the whine pitch "works." You are also modeling to him that you don't expect him to listen the first time. He'll do as you do, not as you say.

"Asks" for help. Besides saying intelligible words, baby uses gestures and body language to seek assistance. When frustrated because she can't get the lid off a container or a toy is stuck, baby shouts "help me" noises or toddles over and yanks at your sleeve for assistance. These sounds and body language say to you, "Come help me pry this toy loose," as she hands you the toy, expecting adult help.

"Feed me." Besides cues for help during play, baby gives feeding cues. Baby may pull up your blouse to breastfeed or ask for "ba-ba" (bottle) and point to it. And even

your own meals are not without some intervention from the toddler sitting next to you. As you take a spoonful of food, your toddler may grab your hand to redirect the food his way. The ability to use sounds and body language to get help and meet needs is a valuable social milestone.

Showing moods. Along with using sounds and actions to signal needs, baby can now use specific facial language to reflect moods: downcast eyes, lips overlapping a fussy pucker, furrowed forehead, and jutting jaw. All these baby-face contortions convey an "I'm upset" feeling.

Word Associations

Baby begins to connect what he hears with what he sees, realizing that everything in his widening world has a label.

Associates words and pictures. Words make looking at books and TV more fun. Watch for the day baby will toddle over to the TV, point to the dog, and holler, "Gog, gog!"

Words make minding easier. Picture this scene. It's time for a snack, but your toddler is busily into a pile of toys. Rather than pry away a protesting baby, suggest, "Let's go get a cracker." The word "cracker" triggers a pattern of association in her mind: "Cracker in a box in the kitchen," as baby trots off to the kitchen toward the cracker box.

A word for the wise. Words make thinking easier. Now that every thing and person in baby's intimate world has a label on it, he can store lots of mental pictures and recall them when hearing the label. We have used this cognitive ability to make traveling in the car seat smoother. Matthew has always adored his older brother Peter. One day as fifteen-month-old Matthew was fussing in his car seat we pacified him by saying, "We're going to see Peter." The word "Peter" triggered the mental association of a favorite person, and he stopped fussing to think about Peter. Baby's growing vocabulary and growing mind work together to make the toddler a very interesting little person to talk with and be with.

Following Directions

In addition to saying and imitating more words at this stage, baby more consistently understands one-step requests such as "Go get ball," and retrieves the ball from the pile of toys. In a later stage she may be able to understand and remember two-step and more complicated requests: "Get the ball in the kitchen and bring it to daddy."

Sign Language

Besides understanding more words, the toddler begins to associate gestures with the meaning of words. During this stage, Matthew would grab and bear hug our indestructible family cat. We would rescue the cat and show Matthew a kinder approach, "Be *gentle* to the cat," as we took his hand and showed him how to handle the cat. He understood our gentle gesture by the tone of our voice and actions of our hands. And this helped him understand when we needed to clean his face or wipe his nose, because we would tell him, "Mama be gentle" (and then be sure we were).

Show-and-tell

A precious scene well worth recording is toddlers greeting each other. Watch what happens when you put an affectionate kissing toddler with a more reserved one. Mr. Affectionate embraces Miss Reserved in a beautiful gesture of tenderness. Meanwhile you monitor these advances to be sure your baby doesn't love too hard. As Miss Reserved draws back, Mr. Affectionate tightens his grip and comes on too strong. One baby cries and the other is confused, and a struggle follows. As a watchful parent you intervene with an encouraging "Love the baby" as you teach both babies a softer touch. To teach a baby proper social graces, take baby's hand and demonstrate with both words and gestures the touch you want your baby to learn.

A House Person

Toddlers now become more aware of household sounds and their sources. The doorbell rings, and she toddles in that direction. The buzzer on the stove sounds, and she changes course toward that sound; the telephone rings, and she runs to say hello. It's fascinating to watch how this little person is so aware of her big and noisy world.

FIFTEEN TO EIGHTEEN MONTHS: BIG WORDS

In this stage of development babies do all the things they did in the previous one, but they do them better.

Moving Faster

Baby continues to experiment with his newly found walking skills. He pivots and circles, walks backward, and walks up steps (still holding on to a railing or person). As is true with most developmental skills, baby's desires exceed his skills; his mind travels faster than his feet. Both falls and frustrations remind the growing wanderer that he's still a baby.

First running. Like the first steps, baby's first runs are likely to be stiff legged, short, and end in frequent falls. When baby first shows the desire to progress from walking to running, take him to a wide, long, well-padded area and turn him loose. Once baby learns to bend his knees more and lift his feet higher, he walks and runs faster and trips less.

Stop and stoop. Baby may be walking briskly across the room and notice a tempting toy on the floor. He stoops, picks it up, and is on his way. Adding the skill of stooping and picking up makes walking around the house gathering treasures fun for the young adventurer.

➤ *SAFETY TIP: Every skill has its ups and downs. Now that baby can stoop and pick up, shadow baby when out walking around cluttered terrains. The curious scavenger may pick up objects such as cigarette butts.*

Mountain climbing. No chair, tabletop, or sofa is beyond the reach of the young climber. Respect the urge to climb by providing a safe climbing environment.

- Tuck seats under the table to deter a table-top explorer.

- Keep climbable furniture away from dangerous objects. A chair close to a stove invites disaster. A toddler can push a step stool or child's chair over to the stove.

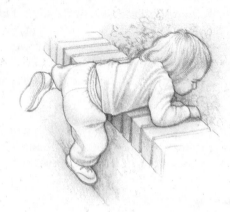

Baby's urge to climb won't be denied, so be sure to provide a safe area.

- Be especially vigilant for the toddler who climbs and stands on the seat of a chair and leans to peer over the back while he holds on. A trip to the emergency room is soon to follow.

- Create a safe climbing area. To satisfy the beginning climber we keep a fold-out futon and piles of foam squares and cushions in our family room. A climbing yard is also fun for the young scrambler, and piles of old tires make a safe obstacle course. Another winner is a short ladder and slide, which satisfy two favorite toddler desires: the urge to climb and the urge to slide.

Pull up a chair. By this stage most babies can feed themselves. Get baby a toddler-sized chair and watch how he navigates into it. He may first climb onto it but soon realizes this is neither comfortable nor safe, and the chair topples over. Then he learns to hold it with both hands behind as he backs his bottom into the chair. We gave one of our babies a tiny, lightweight canvas director's chair, which he carried behind him for a few yards after he

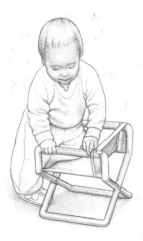

Scaled-down chairs and tables are a real toddler pleaser.

learned to negotiate sitting in it. Perhaps once he had mastered getting seated in the chair, he didn't want to let go and start over.

Remember that it's safer and more fun to bring the adult world down to baby's size. A toddler-size table and chair to contain the busy baby plus attention-holding toys such as interlocking blocks may keep the house rover sitting still awhile.

First rides. Toddlers seldom sit still, but they do sit and ride. Choose a riding toy with four wheels and a wide base that baby can easily handle. Before purchasing it, take baby to the toy store for a test drive. If he is learning to drive, let his first rides be on a soft carpet to cushion the falls.

First pitch. As with blocks, as baby gets bigger, balls get bigger. Watch your baby throw a ball by getting up on one knee with one foot planted on the ground and *pitch with the whole arm,* an improvement over the forearm fling of the previous stage.

Throw and kick. Attention baseball and soccer scouts! Now baby can do both sports. She can throw a ball from the hands-at-chest or overhead position with more force. Think about the learning value of a simple ball. As the young pitcher learns the most efficient windup, she needs to figure out when to release the ball, in which direction, with how much force, and what body parts to put into the throw.

GETTING PHYSICAL

Babies and parents love playing physical games. Favorites include the following:

Give me five. The best of hand-slapping games has many variations: one handed, two handed, high five, low five, and "too slow five," as baby misses your moving hands. This is a good game to spring on baby suddenly to introduce him to interaction or to redirect undesirable behavior.

Riding high. Baby loves riding on dad's shoulders, but be sure to duck as you go through doorways and under chandeliers, and avoid carrying baby under ceiling fans.

Ticktock. Hold baby by both feet and swing back and forth like a pendulum.

Other favorites. Ring-around-the-rosy, climb-on-pop, climb-over-pop, ride-horsey-on-daddy, hide-and-seek, and mimicking adult antics are other games toddlers enjoy.

Kicking balls around the yard is a favorite game. First kicks are likely to be more misses than kicks. Initially baby may approach the ball timidly and barely connect. Other times, the kick may end in a fall and a surprised look on baby's face, as if the holder moved the ball from the placekicker.

Bring out the big tools. Babies love activities and playthings that allow them to imitate an adult life-style in miniature. Toddlers have the skills to push, pull, pound, and pour. As a toddler, Matthew spent hours pushing along his toy lawn mower in imitation of daddy cutting the grass. Pull toys and push toys, such as baby buggies, are fun. Pound toys with toy hammers and pegs are good for the beginning carpenter. With a small sprinkling can, baby waters the plants.

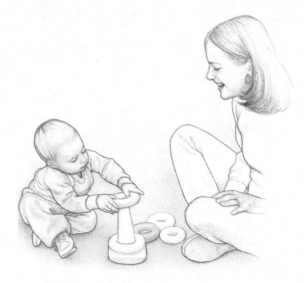

Increasing hand skills set the stage for more challenging toys, which also challenge the toddler's growing mental ability.

Activities and Challenges for Hand Skills

As baby's hand skills increase, toys become more challenging. Besides stacking more and larger blocks higher — usually four is tops for the young master builder — babies like interlocking blocks and those that stick and stack.

Sorting shapes. Graduated cylinders and rings are play-tested favorites that capitalize on baby's emerging cognitive skill of figuring out a sequence in her head before attempting it with her hands. Watch the decision-making and attention-holding expression on your baby's face as she puts graduated rings on a pole. Initially she may impulsively fling any ring onto the pole without regard for size. As her mental and hand skills mature together, she puts the largest ring on the bottom.

Hand-held toys. The combination of a keener mind and more skillful hands helps the toddler figure out and correctly use hand-held items. Previously, hand things were for banging. Now, for example, she can use a safe fork and spoon to feed herself.

Besides wanting his toys, baby wants to use adult hand "toys." A razor is very enticing, particularly when baby sees all the gooey fun dad has with it. Drawers are a red flag to your baby bull, especially those you put your "toys" in. To keep baby out of your drawers, give him his own and rotate its toy stock to hold his interest.

First art. Crayon marks on your walls are telltale signs of a scribbling toddler on the loose. For his first art lesson give baby an easily held, nontoxic crayon and a large white piece of paper. Either hold or tape the paper down.

Trying to hold the paper with one hand while creating his first masterpiece with the other is frustrating to the budding artist. First art is random lines, called scribbles. Baby holds the crayon fistlike, makes back and forth lines and an occasional wiper blade–like semicircle, and, to sign his art, stabs the tip of the crayon into the paper.

Let baby enjoy simply messing around with crayon and paper before sharing your artistic skills with him. Once baby controls his waving arms and begins to think before scrawling (watch the decisive look on his face), it's time for another art lesson. Encourage baby to imitate your sketches. First draw a simple vertical line and show baby, hand on hand, how to match your line. Then draw a horizontal line and encourage baby to copy. Next, draw a V shape, a semicircle, and eventually graduate to a full circle, which baby may not match until after the second birthday when true drawing begins.

Language Development

Toddler language development can be summed up in baby's favorite word — *more*.

More words. Baby's speech explodes from an average ten words at fifteen months to as many as fifty by twenty-four months, though many sounds are still unintelligible except to parents. A fun exercise to chart your baby's speech development is a word-a-day chart. Write down the new word your baby says today.

More intelligible. Baby's starter words progress from half to whole words as baby adds the right ending. "Ba" becomes "ball."

More syllables. Baby's speech lengthens from pronouncing short one-syllable words — "uh" and "cat" — to putting short words together: "all done," "bye-bye," "night-night," "no-no." Baby may now attempt multisyllable words, and what comes out of his mouth may top the laugh meter. Our favorite was "Ben-ben-ben" — toddler lingo for "Benjamin."

Understands more. Toddlers begin to seem more tuned in to the conversations around them. We call this secondhand language. One day Martha casually mentioned to Erin, Matthew's older sibling, that she should go upstairs and get the laundry because it was laundry day. I noticed fifteen-month-old Matthew marching very purposefully over to the laundry basket. He picked out several articles of clothing from the basket and marched back to Martha. He had caught the gist of the conversation although he was not directly part of it.

First Sentences

A baby's early phrases and sentences resemble a budget telegram or news headlines — only nouns or only nouns and action verbs, such as "Bye-bye car" or "Go bye-bye." Baby associates "bye-bye" with leaving the house (which he learns from your gestures when you depart) and "car" with the moving object that transports him from one world to the other. Baby may even begin to open a two-word sentence with "I," such as "I go." This language gives him the conversational skills to express an "I" desire, and it affords him a tool by which he can use his adult companions as resources to help him get his desire. One day I was playing a little kissing game with Matthew, kissing him on the leg and on the toes. When I stopped, he looked at me and said, "More . . . kiss . . . toes." Baby spurts out skeletons of the entire sentence and leaves the listener to fill in the missing words.

Responds to Words Without Gestures

Not only do toddlers speak in cue words, they also think this way. When I would say "go," eighteen-month-old Matthew would get his sweater and run to the door. To a toddler, language is a combination of gestures and verbal sounds. In the previous stage of development most babies would not follow a request unless accompanied by *both* a sound and a gesture (that is, pointing and saying, "Give it to daddy"). By eighteen months babies can understand most verbal cues without the accompanying gestures.

Social Talk

Baby becomes better at putting word labels on favorite everyday activities, especially during feeding, and continues giving both verbal and body language feeding cues. The toddler may pull up your blouse to breast-feed, asking for "nur" (nurse) or "num-num" (breast). He may ask for "ba-ba" (bottle) and point to it. Babies often get into social greetings, such as saying "hi-yo" (hello) when picking up the ringing telephone. He may even surprise you with an occasional "ta-too," for "thank you." Many of the words that you said hundreds of times in the previous stage now come back to you during social exchanges that take place during daily activities such as dressing. One day as I was undressing Matthew for bed he tugged at his shirt and said, "Up"; then he tugged at his pants and said, "Off." He had filed away the association of these words with these actions and could recall them.

New Concepts

Words make teaching safety and caring for baby easier. Many babies by this age learn the meaning of "hot." When you say, "Food is hot," baby may avoid touching it and look respectfully at the food while whispering what sounds like "hot," imitating the way you emphasize the danger by speaking in a long, drawn-out, whispering sort of inflection. When you say, "Let's change diaper," baby may acknowledge that he understands by looking down at his diaper, tugging at it, and either walking toward you or running away.

In addition, a toddler at this age can often point to and name his siblings. Older brothers and sisters naturally reinforce speech for the toddler by constantly encouraging baby to "say it again."

The concept of "other" is a major cognitive and verbal achievement. Beginning with body parts, baby may be able to point to an ear when you say, "Where's ear?" and then point to the opposite ear when adding "Where's other ear?"

First Songs

Singing adds a delightful musical touch to baby's speech explosion. Baby may begin humming while engrossed in her happy little world of sound and play. Capture these merry sounds on tape while you can. These are the sounds you wish that baby would never outgrow.

Gesticulating

Combining words and actions is a language skill that mushrooms midway through the second year: "up" accompanied by the arm-raising "Pick me up" gesture; "shhhhh" accompanied by an index finger by the mouth to gesture hush; and the inevitable "no-no-no!" accompanied by a firm and often comical shake of the head, or if firmly grounded in a negative response, baby scrunches up her eyebrows and puckers her lips in a scolding facial gesture and waves her finger at you while saying "No-no-no!" Perhaps she is mimicking her own scoldings. Babies also love gesture games like so-big. Even when baby can't come up with all the words for what she needs, her gestures are so much more understandable at this stage. For instance, while sitting at the table Matthew was presented with a dish that contained a little bit of leftover cranberry sauce. He gestured with his hands and vocalized some sounds that conveyed to us "I need a spoon." Although he didn't say any of those words, his meaning was very clear. If you are doubtful about what baby enjoys doing, watch and listen to her body language. One time I was patting Matthew on his tush, and when I stopped, he reached behind and patted himself a few times, giving me the message that he wanted me to continue the patting.

Parents' Speech Changes

As baby begins talking more like an adult, you may notice yourself talking less like a baby. You may resume speaking in a normal tone of conversation rather than in baby talk, as baby understands what you are saying to him without exaggerated inflections and a high-pitched tone of motherese.

ENRICHING YOUR TODDLER'S LANGUAGE

Most parents have a natural intuition about their toddler's language development and need no instruction manual. The "method" a mother (or father) uses flows naturally as part of intuitive parenting. These tips are only to reinforce and add variety to what you are, in all likelihood, already doing.

Look at and talk about picture books together. This is one of the primary ways in which children develop their word-object association. As your child advances, you can select increasingly stimulating books and prompt his recall of names by pointing to an illustration and saying, "What's this?" Show him the whole page of assorted objects and ask, "Where is the ball?" Associate the figures in the book with the same figures in real life. As you point to a tree in a book, also point to the real tree in the yard. Your child will develop a mental image as to what characteristics constitute the label "tree."

Expand a word or gesture into an idea. For example, if your child asks, "What's that?" and then points to a bird, you answer, "That's a bird," and add, "and birds fly in the sky." You have not only answered his question, but you have also given him a word-associated idea. When you notice your baby's interest in a sound, such as an airplane in the sky, pick baby up and point to the airplane and give it a name, "Airplane in the sky." Put as many labels on as many objects and persons as you can. This helps make baby's mental filing system of object labeling easier. Babies seldom speak in full sentences with all the words until the latter half of the second year, but rather continue to use cue words within each sentence. Picking up on cue words is particularly important for the child with lazy speech habits who gets what he wants by *pointing* all the time.

Play word games and sing action songs. These make learning language fun. Babies love to play games about their own body parts and learn quickly what their toes are after they have played this-little-piggy several times. Rhythm games that employ counting and finger play, such as one-two-buckle-my-shoe, and actions songs such as "Pop Goes the Weasel" are particularly helpful for encouraging gestures and cue words. Eventually baby will be able to complete the song when you sing the opening word as a cue.

Talk about what you do. In the earlier months you probably talked baby through every step of the diaper change. Now it's easy to mechanically go through maintenance exercises such as diapering and bathing without much dialogue. But continue the chatter: "Now we lift up your arm . . . now we wash your hands . . ." and so on.

Speak in questions. Toddlers seem to enjoy the inflections and intonations of your voice when you ask a question. A query implies that you welcome a response of some kind, and the toddler usually obliges.

Don't use too much disconnected chatter. Your child will tune you out. Instead, speak slowly in simple sentences and pause frequently to give your child time to reflect on the message.

Give your child choices. For example, "Matthew, do you want an apple or an orange?" This encourages him to reply and stimulates decision making.

Make eye contact and address your child by name. As a pediatrician, I find that looking intently into a suspicious toddler's eyes during a physical examination has a calming effect. If you can maintain eye contact with a child, you can maintain his attention. You want your child to be comfortable looking into another person's eyes when he addresses them. The ability to be comfortable with eye-to-eye contact is a language-enrichment exercise that benefits your child throughout his life. Also, addressing your child by his name when opening the dialogue teaches your baby a valuable social lesson — the importance of one's own name. And this teaches him to use names when speaking to others.

Go easy on correcting a toddler's speech. Remember, the main goal of toddler language is to communicate an idea, not a word. Much of a toddler's speech may be unintelligible under the age of two. This is normal. It is important for some babies to babble awhile and experiment with sounds without outside attempts to refine them. These toddlers are simply storing their language information for a sudden rush of intelligible words and phrases at around two years of age. If you sense your child is having trouble with certain words, make a special effort to repeat these sounds frequently yourself and capitalize on your child's desire to imitate. Correct by repetition, not by embarrassment. Remember, speech is primarily a skill to be *enjoyed* rather than a task to be learned. The more your child enjoys communicating, the better she will learn to speak.

DOES YOUR CHILD WALK FUNNY?

Toddlers' walking styles are as variable as their personalities. Most begin walking with feet turned out, a position that improves balance. Next, as you are beginning to worry about turned-out feet, baby exchanges one worry for another and turns the feet inward and becomes pigeon-toed. You can put off your mother's suggestion to take baby to an orthopedic specialist. Most toddler's legs and feet straighten by themselves by three years.

Toeing in. In the first two years nearly all babies toe in. This is due to two conditions:

*   The normal bowing of the legs left over from the fetal position in the womb.

*   Normal flatfeet. Babies seldom develop much of an arch until the age of three years. To compensate, babies turn their feet inward while walking, in effect to make an arch and better distribute their weight.

The normal developmental timetable for feet and legs is as follows:

*   bowed legs from birth to three years
*   toeing out, ballerina style, when beginning to walk
*   toeing in from eighteen months to two to three years
*   walking with feet straight after three years
*   knock-kneed from three years to teens

If your toddler runs without tripping, don't worry about turned-in feet. This should self-correct. If, however, your child is tripping over his feet more and more, orthopedic treatment may be necessary, usually beginning between eighteen months and two years. (Rarely needed treatment usually consists of a brace placed between special shoes to keep the feet turned out; the brace is worn while sleeping.)

Besides curving in of the lower legs, called *internal tibial torsion,* or ITT (twisting of

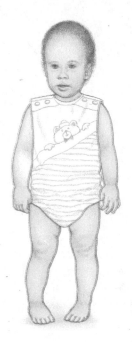

Nearly all babies are pigeon-toed in the first two years.

the major lower leg bone), another reason for toeing in is *internal femoral torsion* (twisting inward of the upper leg bones). Here's how to tell the difference: Watch your child standing. If the kneecaps are facing straight forward, the toeing in is most likely due to ITT. If the kneecaps turn toward each other (kissing kneecaps), that's internal femoral torsion.

Encouraging correct sleeping and sitting positions can lessen both deformities.

*   The saying "As the twig is bent, so grows the tree" certainly applies to baby's legs. Discourage your child from sleeping in the fetal position (see Figure A, page 550). If baby persists in sleeping in this postion, try sewing the pajama legs together.

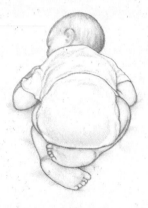

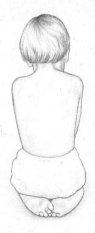

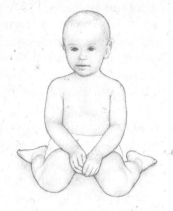

Figure A. The fetal sleeping position.

Figure B. The tucked-under sitting position.

Figure C. The W sitting position.

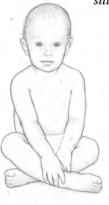

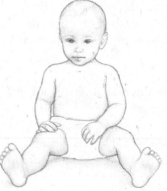

Figure D. Sitting cross-legged.

Figure E. Sitting with feet straight out.

- Try to keep your toddler from tucking his feet and legs beneath him while sitting; this aggravates internal tibial torsion (see Figure B).

- To lessen internal femoral torsion, discourage your child from sitting in the W position (Figure C), but encourage sitting cross-legged (Figure D) or sitting with his feet straight out (Figure E).

Flatfeet. These pancake-bottom feet probably won't last long; usually by three years the arch appears. Persistent flatfeet beyond age three may or may not need support. Here's how to tell if flatfeet are a problem. From behind, observe your child standing barefoot on a hard surface. Draw a line or place a ruler along the Achilles tendon to the floor. If the line is straight, flatfeet seldom bother a child, and they require no treatment. If the line bends inward (called pronation), your child may be helped by *orthotics* — plastic inserts that are placed in regular shoes. These devices support the arch and heel and align the ankle-bones and leg bones. Although controversy exists, some podiatrists feel that treating a child with severe pronation with orthotics from approximately three years through seven years may minimize leg pains and the risk of later bone and joint deformities.

Toe walking. Most toddlers go through a brief period of toe walking, heaven knows why! This is usually a habit or a bit of monkeying around. If it persists, your doctor should examine your child's calf muscles and Achilles tendons for tightness.

Limping and walking funny. It's important to notice unusual walking habits in your child and report them to the doctor. *Limping must always be taken seriously in a child and warrants a thorough medical exam.* If your baby walks funny (for example, waddles like a duck or drags one foot), report your observation to baby's doctor.

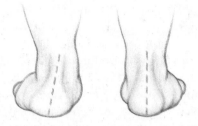

To determine if flatfeet are a problem, observe the line of the Achilles tendon while your child is standing on a hard surface. An inward-curving line (left) may indicate a need for orthotics; a straight line (right) usually indicates that no treatment is necessary.

Refusing to walk. If your previously normal walker suddenly refuses to walk, as happens occasionally, report this to baby's doctor. Take notes based on the following:

- Can you recall anything that may have triggered the refusal to walk, such as an injury or scare after a recent fall? Record the details of the day's activities before the walking strike.

- Do a parent exam: Undress baby. Feel and look all over the legs and feet for bruising, redness, swelling, and areas of tenderness as you carefully squeeze all the leg bones and anklebones. Compare one leg with the other; move the hip, knee, and ankle joints. Does the child wince in pain while you do? Examine and tap around the soles for splinters and pieces of glass.

- Is baby sick? Has she been running unexplained fevers?

- Have there been any recent emotionally traumatic events?

Take your baby (and your notes) to the doctor for a thorough exam.

Growing pains. These common toddler pains, which are experienced when the child is otherwise well, are hard to describe and difficult to localize. They usually occur in the evening and in both legs and are never accompanied by a limp. They are soothed by massaging the sore legs, and the child grows out of them. I believe many of these pains are muscle strains left over from daylong jumping and twisting. Also, I have observed children whose pains subsided after an arch and heel lift was put into their shoes, taking some of the strain off leg muscles during standing and walking, especially in a child with pronated flatfeet.

EIGHTEEN TO TWENTY-FOUR MONTHS: BIG THOUGHTS

Baby is now more aware of who he is, where he is, what he can do, and, frustratingly, what he cannot do — yet. The main reason for this surge of awareness is the rapid development of the ability to think and reason — cognitive development. This section will put to rest the adage "You can't reason with a toddler."

Around eighteen months baby's motor, verbal, and mental skills take off. Baby runs faster, speaks more clearly, and thinks better. The master developmental skill at this age, and the one that makes the motor, language, and social skills work better, is baby's mental development. Now he can figure out concepts in his head before he does or says something. These skills make the toddler a more fun person to live with.

Motor Skills: Running, Climbing, Jumping

Moving from walking to running is a motor highlight of this stage. It's as though someone installed a faster engine and put better wheels on this little machine, and baby is determined to use this new power full throttle.

Clear the Runway

Prepare for this scene: You and your baby are taking a walk. You open the door, step outside, and, like a jet plane, baby darts from you and takes off. You sprint after your baby.

What started out as a casual stroll becomes a race. Baby enjoys the chase but does not enjoy the frequent falls as the refugee, looking back at his pursuer, loses his balance and falls. The beginning jogger loves wide aisles and long halls (supermarket, theater, church). These are his runways, and he is determined to use them. Perhaps this is why toddlers — and often their parents — slim down during this stage.

Besides having faster wheels, another reason that babies dart off from the security of their parents is that the safety net of separation anxiety often wears off by eighteen months. If you are exhausted from chasing the beginning runner as soon as he lets go of your hand, try this. While he is still within hearing distance, yell "Bye-bye, [name]" and walk in the opposite direction. This often causes baby to stop and reassess whether or not he wants to stray that far from the home base. If his home base is moving in the other

---

EASY ON THE ELBOWS

You're in a supermarket, and your child darts from you, or it's time to go and your child throws a tantrum. You grab your runaway by the wrist. He yanks one way, you pull the other, and the elbow, which was not made for this tug-of-war, pops out of the socket. Result: Your child won't use his arm as it hangs limply at his side. This is a *pulled elbow*, which your doctor or emergency room physician can easily pop back into place, without any lasting harm. During swinging play or if you must grab your child by the lower arm, holding *both* arms is unlikely to strain the elbow.

direction, he may turn about and run back to you.

Not only does the beginning runner scurry faster, she runs more safely than in the previous stage, when baby still needed her head up and forward to keep her balance. Now she can look down at her flying feet and dodge the things in her way.

Climbing

Upstairs and downstairs. Toward the second birthday baby may go up the stairs without holding on but still will do one step at a time with both feet instead of alternating feet on each step. By twenty-four months most babies can also go downstairs while holding on.

Crib worries. The master climber may try, and succeed in, climbing out of the crib. When he can do this with the mattress in its lowest position, this is a sign that he is no longer safe left alone in his crib. He is now ready to graduate to a toddler bed.

Jumping for Joy

Baby gets cocky with his motor skills and starts jumping around. He may stand on one foot for a second or two while holding on and even progress to freestanding on one foot momentarily. Jumping and having fun with new steps naturally lead to moving in rhythm. Turn on the dance music, and the show begins. Baby turns circles, lifts and stomps feet, and delights in watching his own steps. Babies love to mimic adult antics and enjoy playing the up-and-down game as you bend at the knees, saying "Down," and then rise "up." Toddlers also love repetition. They like to repeat over and over tasks that they have mastered — jumping off a wall, coming

to a safe landing, and "do again," to the exasperation of the waiting parent who is already late.

Playing on the Move

First gymnastics. Baby now has an overall awareness of what acrobatics can do for his body. Somersaults are a favorite. *Gymnastics for two* is a fun way to teach baby various moves while also toning yourself.

First wheels. Vehicle fascination peaks around two years of age. Between two and two and a half, your child progresses from scooting about on a four-wheeled riding toy to a tricycle. For ideal size, your child should be able to just barely touch the pavement with the tips of his shoes when seated on the tricycle. He usually propels himself forward with his tiptoes before learning to pedal, and

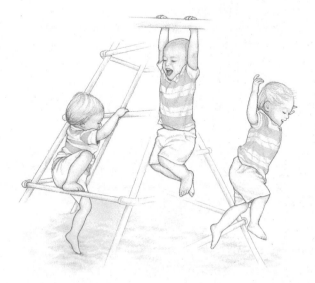

Baby's developing motor skills may leave him literally jumping for joy.

touching the ground gives him more control of the vehicle.

Ball playing. Playing with a ball remains a favorite activity, and you can tell a lot about your toddler's cognitive development by playing ball with him. For example, one day two-year-old Matthew and I were playing with the soccer ball in the driveway. He ran after the rolling ball, but when he stopped to kick it he found the ball had rolled past him. He then figured out that if he ran slightly ahead of the ball and turned around, he could stop and control the ball in order to kick it. This is the stage in which your baby may astonish you with his ability to think and plan ahead during play activities.

The master mover. Want to rearrange your furniture? Call Toddler Moving Company. Babies love to move furniture around, especially chairs on smooth floors. Be prepared for distress calls when the frustrated mover gets stuck. When baby gets bored with moving larger-than-baby-size furniture, he picks on fur-

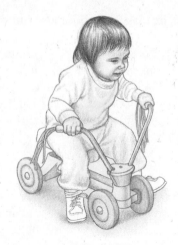

Before she reaches tricycle age, your toddler will enjoy scooting about on a four-wheeler.

niture his own size. Wastebaskets are a favorite target as baby grabs and flings their contents.

➤ *SAFETY TIP: Baby's rearranging can make a room unsafe — for example, putting chairs next to windows or stools next to balconies. Since you don't want to nail down your furniture or your toddler, keep liftable objects above his reach and keep a watchful eye on the mover.*

Parents' little helper. This may be the last stage when your child is such a willing helper, but you get what you don't pay for — a little mess. Encourage your aide to assist in "housework," making cookies, watering plants with a small sprinkling can. To get some useful help give your child a "special pail" and let him roam around the house and yard collecting clutter. There is a bit of a pack-rat tendency in toddlers anyway.

Redirecting play. We live in a busy home. Eight children who often have playmates

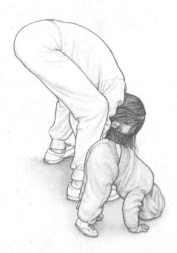

Gymnastics for two is fun for mom and baby.

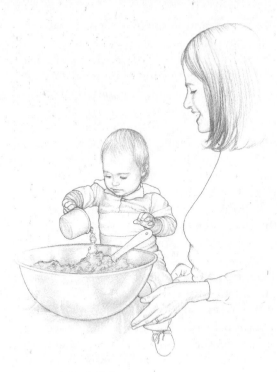

Mommy's little helper.

one or two valued toys, are much better than a pile of toys in a toy box, which encourages flinging frenzies. Child-size furniture and his own table and chair allow your child to be comfortable sitting for a longer period of time, thus encouraging task completion and concentration. Low-level wooden pegs, where he can hang his own clothing, encourage a sense of responsibility for belongings.

Busy Hands

Blocks. The favorite activity of stacking blocks continues into the two-year-old stage, but blocks are still getting bigger as baby gets bigger. The master builder loves stacking big foam or corrugated cardboard blocks taller than his height and then falling over them.

Knobs and buttons beware. This stage is literally a turning point for curious toddlers. They love to turn knobs and push buttons. If

who all have noisy toys. It's easy to turn down the volume of teenage noise, but noisy and dangerous toddlers sometimes need to be redirected. If your child likes to pound, get him rubber hammers. If she likes to bang, a toy xylophone may save furniture dings. If he's a thrower, Ping-Pong and foam balls get high marks.

Order in the house. Even though your toddler is always on the go, the two-year-old begins to show an appreciation for order. Respect this by providing appropriate storage and space. An orderly playroom with eye-level shelves helps to unclutter his world. Work and play surfaces should be from eighteen to twenty inches high. Low shelves with one-foot-square compartments, each containing

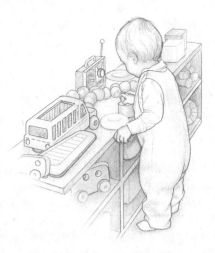

Even at two years of age, your child has an appreciation for order; convenient areas for play and storage will help cultivate this.

THE TWELVE-INCH RULE

Toddlers are fascinated by what's on top of tables, counters, and desks. They frequently reach an exploring hand over table edges in search of things to grab. Be table-edge watchful. Get into the habit of pushing dangerous items back at least twelve inches (thirty centimeters) from the edge, out of the reach of curious hands.

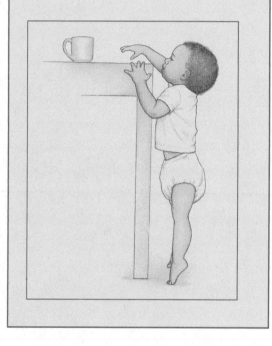

your TV suddenly blasts, you know you have a curious toddler at large. Babies are especially attracted to turning knobs and pushing buttons on radios, stereos, and televisions, which produce a change in sound. The cause and effect of turning knobs and making sounds fascinate baby, and he may continue to stand in front of your electronic toys pushing and turning all the moving parts to see what happens.

Supervise his exploration so he can learn without damaging your equipment. Talk about it. "On" and "off" can be his job. He'll be thrilled with the power this gives him. If he abuses his power you may choose to remove knobs or move the equipment to higher ground for a while. Better yet, get baby his own knobs and buttons to turn and push. Used radios and flashlights (from garage sales) are proven winners. Make-things-happen toys, such as push-down and pop-up toys, are interest-holding favorites.

Turning pages. Babies love turning pages in a book but prior to this stage usually grab two or three pages at a time. Around eighteen months baby may begin to turn one page at a time, especially if you show him how and have books with thick, tearproof cardboard pages.

More toddler art. By the time your toddler is two, you may have a collection of kid art plastered all over your kitchen walls and refrigerator. As baby scribbles a maze of lines or maybe even an occasional circle, she takes great pride in her work and expects applause and to have her creations hung in a place of honor.

Lid play. Babies love playing with lids and may begin screwing them on and off at this stage. We have found a shoe box and lid to be a perfect match for a toddler's hands.

Puzzles. For the older toddler who loves the challenge of matching and has the patience to try all the fits, puzzles are a hit. If your baby has a low frustration tolerance, sit next to him as he tackles an inset puzzle. Let him try himself, but if frustration signs are escalating, bring show-and-tell to the rescue.

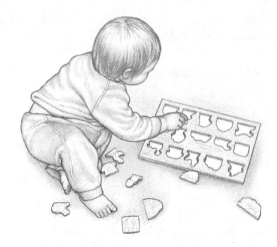

Puzzles can be fun for youngsters who enjoy a mental challenge.

Language Development

This is the new-word-a-day stage. Your toddler not only adds new words but adds new ways of using familiar words.

Babies develop speech at different rates. Some show a steady word-a-day increase in their vocabulary, some jabber in bursts of new words, and others don't say much until near the end of the second year, as if storing up a lot of words for the opening two-year speech. How many words a baby says is not as important as how he communicates. Some babies, even at two years, are in the "says little — understands all — communicates well" stage of speech development. They still primarily use body language to express a want.

As in all stages of language development, in this stage you're building more than a vocabulary, you're building a relationship. You are not just teaching words, you are teaching trust.

Put a Label on It

The toddler increasingly learns that everything and every person in the world has a name. As you walk around the house or drive in the car, give everything a label. Naming everything you drive past also helps settle the restless toddler. Words build memory, and it is easier to store a labeled than an unlabeled object in the child's growing memory file.

Spot-check to see if your child remembers the name of household objects by frequently asking "What's that?" as you point to items such as the piano. If he responds "Pee-no," add a reinforcing "Yes!" to praise baby for getting the right word and also add "That's a pi-a-no" as you model the correct pronunciation, but not in a corrective tone.

The question-and-answer game. Be prepared for a barrage of the classic toddler learning phrase, "What's that?" Once baby learns that everything has a name, she naturally wants to learn what all the names are. As you play the name-that-thing game, if you see your baby looking intently at an object, quickly put a label on it — "That's a box." Return to the box a few minutes later and check baby's memory, asking, "What's that?" as you point to the box. If baby points to an object but doesn't know its name, baby is signaling for you to fill in the missing word. Use favorite questions that guarantee a humorous response, like "What does dog say?"

Provide a running commentary. Babies learn that *actions* have words, too. Talk about daily rituals such as bathing and changing and eating. "Now we lift our arms, now we put them down." Toddlers easily master action

KEEPING A SPEECH DIARY

You can chart your baby's speech progress by recording words and phrases your baby says at each stage of development. In addition to recording the words, record the length and complexity of the sentences and especially the long words that he humorously messes up. Even more exciting is to keep a thought diary: what you guess baby is thinking by what he says and does. Reading and playing back this record when baby is older helps you relive one of the most exciting stages of baby's development.

words: "up," "down," "off," "go." And they love action phrases such as "Hug the mommy."

Read my lips. The two-year-old is a near-perfect parrot and soon becomes an accomplished lip-reader. During this stage when Stephen and I would be at head-to-head level, I noticed that he watched my lips during most of the conversation until he had a handle on the words I was saying.

The pointer. What about the baby who has good body language communication but says only a few clear words? He grunts "uh-uh" as he points to the cookie jar, and you understand he wants a cookie. Question the pointer: "Tell mommy what you want. Do you want a cookie?" As he shakes his head with an affirmative yes, acknowledge his body language: "Yes, I understand you want a cookie." Don't put pressure on the pointer to

speak, but let him hear the right words to complement his gestures.

Right Associations

Language helps a toddler express that he understands how certain actions go together. Baby may grab her coat and hat and wave bye-bye. The doorbell rings, and baby says "Door." Your baby may bring you your purse and say, "Money." Toddlers store patterns of association in their minds, and words help them express these.

Babies now also associate pictures and books with familiar objects and persons in their environment. By two, some may even differentiate boys and girls and correctly point to each sex in a book or in person.

Misunderstandings. Expect humorous word confusions as baby mismatches thoughts and words. Matthew was into Band-Aids. One day we were talking about his sister's headband, and he called it a Band-Aid because of the common root word "band." Idiomatic and figurative language are particularly confusing. For example, I was telling Stephen, "I really blew it," and he started blowing at imaginary candles (we have lots of birthdays in our family).

Nuances. Babies not only learn that objects have names. They also learn that the things that objects do have names: Plates get "hot"; popsicles are "cold"; and even these properties have further divisions. Notice the intense look on your baby's face as she struggles to get the right word. Sometimes a baby is about to say a word, realizes it's not the word she wants, and then changes it. For example, when feeling water temperature, a toddler may say, "Hot . . . no . . . warm!" In the previous stage she could understand only hot and cold. Now, she's aware of nuances of temperature, such as warm.

The theme doesn't fit. One night Matthew heard us talking about going out and naturally surmised that he would be going along. As we tried to put on his pajamas, he protested, "No, no!" He had computed that if he was going out, why was he being dressed for bed? He accepted the explanation, once he understood it.

Baby Talk

Challenge words. Babies become bored with words like "dog" and "cat." They enjoy being challenged by tough words. "Helicopter" was Matthew's favorite at this age; "dinosaur," a close second. Oh, sure, baby will mess it up, but often the messed-up version is more fun to hear.

Communicates preferences. Gone are the pointing grunts, almost. By age two, baby can communicate nearly all of his daily wants with words: "Go outside," "Play ball," "Want cookie." When given choices — a valuable learning exercise — baby can communicate preferences. At eighteen months Matthew was asked if he wanted to take a walk outside with me or take a bath with mommy. He couldn't give me a verbal answer, but he understood he had a choice. When I picked him up to take him outside, he used the squirm cues of his body language to lunge toward Martha and convey his preference. By the time he was two, when given a choice, he responded in words such as "go outside" or "mommy."

Read my words. In this stage of speech development not only are you teaching baby to understand your language, you are learning to interpret his, and baby expects that. As baby learns how to talk, you learn how to listen. Many toddlers still do not articulate many of their words correctly at this stage, but they do refine their ability to use correct inflections when communicating a word. "My-nun" means "raisin," and you will know this by the inflection in his voice. Good parenting skills include being able to decode the toddler's jargon and give him the feedback that he is truly understood by his caretakers.

Naming Games

Name those parts. By eighteen months most babies can name all their body parts and enjoy traveling around their body playing "Where's nose?" and so on. Upon hearing the cue word "nose," baby may point to his nose. Now you can add, "Where's mommy's nose?" and see if baby points to your nose. "Eyes" and "foot" are also on the favorite parts list. "Belly button" may not yet merit a point. During diapering or bathing baby may grab his penis or her vulva — this is a good time to start labeling ("That's your penis [vulva]"). Body-part naming becomes an attention-holding game because you are engaging the normally egocentric toddler in talking about himself. It's a good game when you're stuck with a restless baby without any toys as props.

Name those persons. Many two-year-olds can say their own first name and sometimes their last name. Baby may even name siblings and familiar caregivers or match the picture of a person and say the right name. Hold baby up to a wall full of pictures of familiar family members and play name-that-face. Put this on your list of what to do when there's nothing to do.

Social Interactions

Use my name. A beautiful feature of advanced second-year speech is starting sentences with direct address; "Mommy, I want . . ." or "Daddy, go . . ." Baby uses your name and that of familiar caregivers more if you have modeled opening your comments with baby's name and given eye contact as an added touch.

Happy words. Note the happy-to-see-you words your baby has when you return after an absence. Matthew would jump up and down hollering "yay" when we came home.

Giving orders. By two years old, most babies have the verbal and gesture language to direct their social interactions. "Jimmy wants to come over and play. Is that OK?" you ask your toddler. You may get a smiling answer, "'K." Baby may push you away from his toys with a "Go away" or "Move" if you are in his way. Amazed by his power to push people around with words, he also whines less during socializing. Baby can now ask for things at the table — juice, milk, and so on — and can go to the pantry or refrigerator in search of more food as a clue that he is still hungry.

Don't conclude, "This young upstart is bossing me around." Giving orders like "Come here" or "Get water" has nothing to do with who's in charge. Babies talk like that. Babies also try on new words and phrases to test adult reactions. If you like the words, affirm them; if not, change them. Babies think like that.

Little Persons with Big Ears

The astute awareness of the two-year-old is beautifully illustrated in his grasp of ambient language, that is, conversations that go on around him. In the previous stage baby began to understand the gist of the conversation. Now he verbally chimes in. One day Martha asked me a question that required a yes or no answer. Matthew, who was sitting next to us, immediately looked me square in the eye and said, "No!" We were astonished that he was, first of all, tuned in to our conversation and, second, that he was so ready with an answer (the correct one as it turned out) to a question that had not even been addressed to him.

GENITAL AWARENESS

The normal exploration of body parts, noticeable as thumb-sucking and finger play in the first year, progresses to penis pulling and vagina probing during the second year. The normal curiosity progresses to the experience of genital sensitivity and the pleasure of self-stimulation. Like thumb-sucking, the ability to use body parts for pleasure is a normal fact of growing up.

Handle genital play like nosepicking: Discourage it in public (consider family areas public) and gently distract the child when the actions are obvious. Avoid delivering the "dirty" speech. Part of a growing child's healthy sexuality is to be comfortable with and to value all of his or her body. And don't forget the "private parts" talk between two and three years.

Another time Matthew was just finishing his lunch when his brother Peter asked if anyone had seen his soccer ball. Matthew quickly finished eating and then started looking for the ball. Peter repeated the question, "Where's the soccer ball?" Matthew shrugged his shoulders and raised his hands in a puzzled gesture, as if to say "I don't know," then he gestured to Peter to come with him to look in the family room. From this dialogue we learned three things about Matthew's development. He now paid attention to what was going on, he had body language to express his desire to join in the search, and, finally, his mind was capable of re-creating the missing ball scene. Again, we learn how babies think by how they act.

This increased awareness should make parents more careful about what they say around baby. Recently in my office I observed how a twenty-one-month-old child reacted to a conversation we were having about whether or not her parents should leave her for a week's vacation. While not yet having the verbal ability to say, "No, don't leave me; take me with you," she exhibited a worried look that communicated to us only too well that she understood there was a plot afoot that she didn't like.

To determine your own baby's level of conversation awareness, try encouraging him to finish the sentence you begin. We call it the fill-in-the-missing-word-game. For example, after shopping one day, we found we had left one of Matthew's toys in the store. As we got into the car, I said, "Matthew, I guess we'll have to go back to the store and look for the . . ." He piped up, "Duck!"

Finishing Touches

The period leading up to baby's second birthday is like finishing school for toddler language. Sentences remain telegraphic but get longer and more accurate. "More" progresses to "More peace" (as he hears you say "please" repeatedly) to "Want more" to "I want more." When going into a dark room, initially baby may point to the light switch and holler "On"; later he adds "light" and eventually lengthens the sentence to "Turn light on." It seems that baby conceptualizes the full sentence and then gradually fills in the whole thought with words.

Language makes baby care easier. Baby often takes the lead in conversation. "Look" is a common opener in baby talk. Baby may say "off" and mime to signal he wants you to remove his diaper. And, of course, the "I do it" stage begins.

One-step, two-step. A noticeable maturity in baby's language comprehension is progressing from following a one-step to a two-step request: "Go get the pretzel, and bring it to daddy." Baby now has the memory and the attention span to go specifically and get a pretzel (amid many other objects in the kitchen) and remember to bring it to daddy once he has found it.

Let me tell you how I feel. Besides words to express wants, babies at this stage have words to express feelings. Babies become aware of "owsies," or scrapes and bruises. And, of course, baby pleads for the magical Band-Aid to repair his body. Toddlers normally overreact to bodily injuries.

Babies still don't have many words to express disappointment when being left, but the "I miss mommy" looks are unmistakable. When and how long to leave your baby is a difficult decision, especially when trying out a new caregiver. Learn to read your baby's body language for signs of approval or disapproval.

Developing Memory

Baby's improving memory helps him at this stage begin to think out an action before he acts, making toddler behavior less impulsive. I marveled at our son Stephen's ability to think ahead at nineteen months. One day I watched him holding a cup of yogurt as he approached the stairs. I saw in his expression that he was thinking through the process, and, just as he rounded the corner to start climbing the stairs, he reached out and handed the cup to me as though he had, ahead of time, recognized the fact that he could not negotiate the stairs with it in his hands. He gave the cup to me, understanding that his dessert would be safe in my care until I delivered it to him at the top of the stairs.

The ability to think before acting is most clearly illustrated in a toddler's normal daily play. Our other children enjoyed playing ball with Stephen. One day as he and his older brother Peter were sitting a few feet away from each other throwing a ball back and forth, the cat perched between them, right in the trajectory of the ball. Stephen realized he would hit the cat if he threw the ball in that particular direction, so he moved over to be able to throw the ball to Peter without doing so.

Your baby's increasingly vivid memory also helps him make more correct associations of how things belong together: The ball goes with the baseball bat, the crayons with the paper. The ability to make right associations is best illustrated by the way a child correctly matches apparel at this stage — who belongs to what. Try this fun experiment: Place a pair of daddy's, mommy's, baby's, and older sibling's shoes on the floor in the same room and ask your toddler to get daddy's shoes. Notice how your baby matches which shoes belong to whom. Laundry day is another opportunity to test associating abilities. As you take the clothes out of the dryer, initially label them with the owner's name: "Daddy's shirt . . . [baby's name] shirt . . ." After you have initiated this naming game, notice how your toddler can correctly match the person with the apparel as you take each piece out of the dryer.

The toddler's ability to remember, associate, and think before he acts makes teaching safety easier at this stage. Feeling the heat emanate from the stove elicits the verbal reaction of "hot," so that a toddler can now understand "hot" and "hurt," concepts that lessen the impulsive urge to touch hot objects. Parents often feel more comfortable teaching safety to a child of this age because they feel that they are finally beginning to get through to him on what he can safely touch and play with and what he cannot.

Growing together with your baby is what infant — and parent — development is all about.

23

Bothersome but Normal Toddler Behaviors

You may have noticed that up till now we have seldom mentioned the word "discipline." Actually, the *entire book* is about discipline, for as we said in the first chapter, true discipline is the product of a trusting relationship between parent and child. One of the benefits of the attachment style of parenting is that it helps you to really *know* your child, to be attuned to what is behind his actions, and to work *with* him to help channel his behavior in desirable directions.

THE REAL MEANING OF DISCIPLINE

During baby's eighteen-month checkup mothers often ask, "Should I begin disciplining my baby now?" What these mothers don't realize is that everything they have been doing with their baby is discipline. We believe that discipline begins at birth and evolves with each interaction you have with your baby, from the first cry to the first "no," and that discipline has different meanings at different stages.

Discipline Begins at Birth

Discipline begins as a relationship, not a list of methods. The first stage of discipline — the attachment stage — begins at birth and develops as you and your baby grow together. The big three of attachment parenting (breastfeeding, wearing baby, and responding to baby's cues) are actually your first disciplinary actions. A baby who is on the receiving end of attachment parenting feels right, and a person who feels right is more likely to act right. An attachment-parented baby is more receptive to authority because he operates from a foundation of trust. This baby spends the early months of his life learning that the world is a responsive and trusting place to be.

Parents who practice this style of parenting develop an inner sense of their baby's preferences and capabilities at each stage of development. They refine their ability to get behind the eyes and into the mind of their baby and understand the reasons for their infant's behavior. Connected parents and infants grow naturally into a disciplined relationship. As the relationship matures, attachment parents are better able to convey what behavior they expect of their child and the child is better able to understand these expectations. The parents are able to give better discipline and the baby is better able to receive it. With each interaction, parents become more confident in their own methods, not someone else's borrowed out of desperation from a book or "expert" adviser. By being open and responsive to their baby, parents do not let themselves become locked into a set of methods, instead realizing that discipline must evolve and adjust to changing family circumstances and the child's developmental stages.

This first stage of discipline is one of nurturing in which parents and infant have an interdependence — a *mutual* shaping of each other's behavior that helps them to know and trust one another. On this foundation both the connected parent and the connected infant can more comfortably graduate to the next stage of discipline — setting limits.

HEADSTRONG MIND-SET

The toddler has a clear image in his own mind of what he wants to do, and he doesn't easily accept alternatives. In adult jargon we call this a mind-set. The two-year-old is particularly known for having a *strong* mind-set when associating persons, places, and events, meriting the description "stubborn" or "headstrong." These babies like set routines and are unwilling to accept any breach in the routine without protest.

A very important social principle that masterful negotiators have long appreciated is that if you want to win people over to your mind-set, you first meet them where they are, and then gradually carry them to where you want them to be. Parents can use this valuable

negotiating principle in overcoming a common and very frustrating hassle — taking toddlers to the supermarket. Develop a supermarket routine and then try to stick with it. Stephen liked certain fruit popsicles and had fixed in his little mind that as he was wheeled through the maze of supermarket aisles, he would eventually be rewarded with a popsicle at a certain aisle, which he had learned to remember and anticipate. A periodic reassuring "We're going to get that popsicle" often buys you time to get your week's shopping done en route to the tantrum-saving treat!

"Mine" and "me" are by-products of the mind-set stage. Two-year-olds stake out their territory and often refuse to share space with their sibling. In fact, "sharing" may not yet be a part of your toddler's social repertoire. Thus squabbles and temper tantrums should be expected around this age.

Setting Limits

In our family we believe in consistent boundaries, not only for the discipline of the children, but for the sanity of the parents. At this stage, discipline is the skill of conveying to your child what behavior you expect, the benefits of desirable behavior, what behavior you will not tolerate, and the consequences of misbehavior. It also involves having the wisdom to consistently carry this out. Discipline is not something you do to a baby, it is working with a baby; the deeper your nurturing during the attachment phase of discipline, the firmer you can afford to be in setting limits. Toddlers and children derive a sense of security from knowing their limits.

Appreciate normal toddler development. In Chapter 22 we discussed how toddlers normally behave. By understanding infant development in general, and your baby's in particular, you will not expect too much or too little of your baby. Being around more experienced mothers and their babies also helps. (By the time your child is four years old, you will have the equivalent of a college degree in *your* child's discipline.) Babies need boundaries that take into account their capabilities at each stage of development. A twelve-month-old will need and expect different boundaries than a two-year-old. Around nine months baby starts showing she has an opinion, and it doesn't always agree with yours. Remember, a strong will is a sign of health. Baby needs a strong will to achieve all of the milestones of the following months and years. If she had no will, how would she ever be able to take all of the tumbles and spills and get right back up to try again?

"I've told my two-year-old over and over again not to pull the cat's tail. He just doesn't listen to me!" Sound familiar? Many of your directives don't seem to sink in, not because your child is being defiant, but because toddlers under two don't yet have the cognitive ability to *internalize* your discipline directives. When you say, "No street" to your two-year-old, he may act like he's never heard it before. Yet when he's three, he's likely to give you the look, "Oh, yes, I remember." The ability to internalize discipline is why age three is much easier to discipline than two.

Develop the wisdom to say no. As your toddler progresses from a lap baby to a house explorer, your role broadens to include that of boundary setter. When babies have clear boundaries they can proceed with growth and development instead of wasting energy dealing with uncertainty. As parents we are to be in charge of our children, but not to

the extent that we control them like puppets. Rather than being threatened by the independence of the toddler stage, a wise parent will find ways to channel the child's behavior.

Convey who's in charge. Be consistent in your discipline, and remember that lasting discipline requires persistent effort. Your child is about to handle a forbidden object. Rather than shouting from your easy chair, go to him, take him by the hand, look him squarely in the eye, demand his attention, and show the young adventurer why this behavior is not permitted. Sound firm and offer an alternative. Try to remember the golden rule of discipline and treat your child the way you would like to be treated. Even a toddler in an obstinate mood will find it hard to resist warmth and fun.

Keep your requests simple. Conversational dialogue is great for socialization, but wordiness can get in the way of your toddler's processing exactly what behavior you expect of him.

Martha notes: While sitting with Stephen over my morning cup of coffee as he finished his cereal, I realized he was interested in my cup. I very chattingly explained over and over that he shouldn't touch, that it was mama's cup, not Stephen's. Finally, as he was on the verge of tears because I was restraining him, it occurred to me that I had failed to use the one word he understands best — "hot." When I finally communicated to him in glowing tones "h-o-o-t-t," he repeated the word with respect and stopped his single-minded efforts to scald himself.

Put balance into your discipline. Give your child enough slack so he can safely test

MAKING DANGER DISCIPLINE STICK

Early in our parenting career, I felt that spanking was justified to teach a child about life-threatening situations, such as a two-year-old's running out into the street. I believed it was necessary to make an impression on mind and body that the child must never do this; and I reasoned that psychology must take a backseat to safety. With each child, we became increasingly more disciplined ourselves. And now we realize that there are much better ways to correct a child than spanking. Here's an example.

Martha notes: When our two-year-old was in the front yard, I kept my eyes on him like a hawk. If he ventured too close to the street, I put on my best street tirade, "No!! Street!!" and I grabbed him from the gutter and carried on and on — vocalizing my fear of his being in the street. I was not yelling at him or angry; I was expressing genuine fear, giving voice to that inner alarm that goes off in every mother's heart when her child could be hurt. It was very important that he believe me, so I didn't hold back. And it worked! He acquired a deep respect for the street and always looked for permission, knowing I would take his hand and we would cross together. A few times I had to reinforce this healthy fear by issuing a loud warning sound. I save this sound for times when an immediate response is needed for safety. This sound is hard to describe in writing, but it is a very sharp, forceful "Ahhh!" I have never used it casually, and I don't use it often. Day-to-day, moment-by-moment situations need to be handled more normally.

the waters. Give him a chance to mess up. If you routinely keep the rope too tight, he'll never fully learn what he can do and he will never fail. It is from his parent-supported failures that he will learn. Rather than prohibiting a child from climbing, for example, make the environment a safe one in which to climb.

Create a child-considered environment. One of your roles as disciplinarian is to be on safety patrol, keeping one reach ahead of those lightning-fast little hands. You may find it easier to simply raise everything movable up a few feet for a few years, rather than constantly raising your voice to a monotonous "No!" And reserve noes for the big things. (See alternatives for saying no, page 527.)

These insights are only starter tips. We advise you to do your own "study." Consult with parents whose concepts of discipline you admire. Ask them to suggest books on discipline (yes, books can be helpful to *supplement* your knowledge, but don't let them replace your own experience). Becoming a wise disciplinarian will make life easier for yourself and is a valuable inheritance to leave your children.

TOY SQUABBLES

"My two-year-old seems so aggressive during play. He's always pushing other children around and grabbing their toys." Sound familiar? Mix lots of kids (or just two) together with lots of toys in a small room, and you have the recipe for a clash. When it comes to play, first be sure you understand the difference between aggression, meaning infringing on someone else's territory, and assertiveness — protecting your own turf. It's sometimes difficult to draw the line between the two.

The Law of the Jungle

One approach is to throw your child into the pack and let him struggle for survival. The one who shoves the hardest and grabs the most keeps the toys. This scene is an aggressor's heaven. But the more passive baby either withdraws from social play because he can't handle the aggression or rises to the occasion and fights back. In other words, the soft get hard, and the hard get harder. In older children's lingo, they become street smart. The aggressive child learns that aggression pays, and the gentler child learns that gentleness doesn't. Soften this scene.

Orchestrate Your Child's Play Setting

It's not wise to control your child's play, but you can monitor the setting. The "mine" stage of toy possessiveness is a normal passing phase of toddler play, and you can help lessen annoying play conflicts.

Match playmates. Pairing two aggressors is a guaranteed fight, but if that's the case, sit between them and show how much more fun it is to play nicely.

Act as referee. Sometimes you have to be the referee, handing each child a toy, setting a timer, and then announcing round two — a strategy called *trading*: "Now it's time to trade toys."

Model gentleness. Acting as a role model is especially important if one child is throwing potentially dangerous projectiles, like metal cars. Say, "A car is for rolling," as you show the child how to play with a car.

Sharing. If sharing is a major problem, ask parents of other children to bring a few of their own toys when they come to visit. Capitalize on the grass-is-always-greener attitude: Children like to play with another child's toys. As your child grabs his playmate's toy, his playmate grabs his toy. He soon learns to give a toy to get a toy. Possession means ownership at this stage, and sharing does not come naturally to children, unless, of course, they see that giving up one toy gets them another.

Discourage grabbing. It also helps to teach nongrabbing ways of give and take. (Model "Give it to mama" when he is very young rather than just taking something quickly or forcefully.) Many children don't object to the sharing aspect, but rather to the aggressive removal of a toy from their possession. It seems so final in their eyes, especially when they see the glint of victory in the eyes of the grabber.

If toy squabbles continue, separate the players.

TEMPER TANTRUMS

When was the last time you pitched a good fit? Adults have tantrums, too, but we excuse them as letting off steam. When our desire to do or have something or our anger at making a wrong decision or losing a valued item exceeds our ability to simply shrug it off, we release our emotions by stomping our feet, slamming doors, throwing things, pounding fists on a table, and shouting with rage. Then you feel better (usually) and go about your business. Sounds childish? But it's also adultish. Add this normal behavior of any emotional person to the ambivalent feelings of a growing toddler, and you have the makings of a temper tantrum.

Two basic feelings prompt most temper tantrums. A child has an intense curiosity and a desire to perform an act, but very often the desire is greater than the capability. This leads to intense frustration, which is released in a healthy tantrum. Second, newly found power and the desire for "bigness" propel him toward a certain act, when suddenly someone from above, especially someone he loves, descends upon him with a "no." Acceptance of an outside force contrary to his own will is very difficult. It is a conflict he cannot handle without a fight. He wants to be big, but reality tells him how small he is; he is angry but does not yet have the language to express his anger, so he does so in actions. Because he cannot yet handle emotions with reason, he chooses to cope with his inner emotions by a display of outward emotions, which we call a tantrum.

Handling Tantrums

Temper tantrums become a problem for both the parent and the child. How should you handle such episodes? First, realize that you can't "handle" them; you can only respect them. They reflect your child's emotions, which *he* has to learn to handle. You are not responsible for the cause or the treatment of these outrages. Your role is to support your child. Too much interference deprives him of his power and a release from inner tension, whereas not enough support leaves him to cope all by himself without the reserves to do so. This can be an exhausting and frightening experience for both the child and the parents. Here are some ways to turn down the heat.

Learn What Sets Off the Fire

Keep a tantrum diary. Know what sets your child off. Is he hungry, tired? Are there circumstances that he can't handle? What triggers undesirable behavior? For example, if your toddler cannot handle the supermarket scene, shop during off hours and leave baby with your spouse.

Watch for pre-tantrum signs. If you notice that a few minutes before the flare-up, your baby is usually bored, doesn't seem connected to anyone or anything, whines, broods, or asks for something he can't have, intervene when you hear these grumbles, before the little volcano erupts.

Keep Cool

Model calmness. As baby sees, baby does. If your baby sees you tantrum, expect him to imitate your behavior. Older children can handle a behavior outburst from parents and siblings because they can understand an explanation of the behavior, and you eventually end it with an apology and a therapeutic laugh. Toddlers may be confused when witnessing too many angry explosions and feel this is standard operating behavior within the family.

Who's having the tantrum? "He knows how to push my buttons," stated a mother

REDIRECTING IMPULSIVE BEHAVIOR

Babies learn by doing things. Their growing minds are driven to explore and try out new behaviors, both for their effect on caregivers and for the way they work for the children themselves. Beware the noncurious baby.

When a baby is in a mood or stage to try out a certain behavior, attempt to channel it into one that is tolerable to you and has learning value for baby. Distracting the volatile toddler when he is about to explode may thwart a blowup.

Does this scenario sound familiar? Baby is throwing a hard ball in the house and is about to do some damage. You shout, "No!" and snatch the ball from the toddler's tenacious hands. He erupts into a flailing, kicking, stomping, angry tirade and disintegrates into a curled-up heap on the floor beneath your feet.

Scratch this scene. Instead, as you retrieve the dangerous ball with one hand, offer a soft ball with the other and a tantrum-aborting, "Here's a fun ball." Or as baby begins his "no-no" pleadings for *his* ball, channel his throwing into a more suitable ballpark: "Let's go *outside* and play ball together." This is a win-win situation: You make your point, toddler gets to play ball.

First of all, know yourself. If your child's cries or tantrums make you angry or anxious ("push your buttons"), it is important for you to understand what went on in your past to cause this. Sometimes just knowing that there is a connection helps a parent deal with upset behavior in their children in a mature way. Often the issues run quite deep, especially when abuse of any kind was inflicted on a person as a child, and counseling becomes necessary. It is important to the emotional health of your child that you seek help in counseling or therapy so that you can understand yourself and your reactions to your toddler's disturbing behavior.

Don't take it personally. If baby's rage easily gets under your skin, remember you are responsible neither for baby's tantrum nor for stopping it. The "goodness" of the baby is not a reflection of your goodness as a parent. Tantrums are as common as frequent falls as a baby climbs the shaky ladder toward independence.

A private scene. Temper tantrums in public places are embarrassing, and it is often difficult to consider a child's feelings first. Your first thought is more likely to be, "What will people think of me as a parent?" If you feel trapped and embarrassed — in line at the supermarket, for example — rather than lashing out, calmly carry your child (kicking and screaming if necessary) to a private place such as a bathroom or your car where your child can perform his act and you can calmly perform yours without worrying about audience approval.

Stay cool in hot places. Toddlers throw fits at the worst times, and this "bad" behavior makes you look bad around your friends.

who asked us for counseling to better handle her toddler's rage. If you are a volatile person, it's easy for a toddler to set off your own explosion, ending up in a shouting match that neither person hears or wins. He is already out of control and needs you to stay in control.

Tantrums often occur when parents are in a hurry and preoccupied with non-baby-oriented tasks, such as preparing a dinner party, or when babies sense that parents are not tuned in to them. Undesirable behavior often takes place when we impose unrealistic expectations on a child. To expect a curious toddler to be the model of obedience in a supermarket, where he is surrounded by a smorgasbord of tempting delights, may be asking too much. Go when you both are rested and fed and make it a time for dialogue about your purchases, letting him help from the safety of his belted shopping-cart seat. Remember, he is a person. Schedule upsetting events, such as getting shots at a doctor's office, at your child's best behavioral time of the day. Expecting a child to be the model of good behavior at the end of the day when he is tired and hungry (and so are you) is asking too much.

Choose your battles wisely. To survive the tantrum stage, we divide toddler desires into "biggies" and "smallies." Staying in a car seat is a biggie. It is nonnegotiable, and all the tantrum theatrics in the world will not free the safely contained protester. But whether to wear a red or a blue shirt is a smallie. A clothing mismatch is not worth a fight. Offering choices may save face for both parent and child: "Do you want to wear the red or blue shirt?" (he wants the yellow) may settle the difference. In our home we do not have the time or energy to hassle about small things. If our child demands peanut butter on top of the jelly but refuses to eat the stuff when smeared the other way around, we are not afraid to accommodate a minor whim. If grandma wonders, this is not spoiling.

When to Retreat

If you sense that your child is consistently using tantrum behavior to get his own way, don't change from a reasonable "no" to a wimpy "yes." (Unless, of course, you realize it's a smallie after all.) This reinforces negative behavior. Between two and two and a half, when your child is old enough to understand the reasons behind your noes, regularly changing your mind reinforces negative tantrum behavior.

The Ostrich Approach

Should you ignore a tantrum? Most of the time the "ignore it" advice is unwise. Ignoring any behavior in your child deprives your child of a valuable support resource and deprives parents of an opportunity to improve their rapport with the tantrumer. Your simply being available during a tantrum gives your child a needed crutch. Temper tantrums bring out the best of our intuitive parenting. If your child is losing control and needs help to regain control, often a few soothing words or a little help ("I'll untie the knot, and you put on the shoe") may put him on the road to recovery. If he has chosen an impossible task, distract him or channel him into an easily achievable play direction. Keep your arms extended and your attitude accepting. Occasionally a very strong-willed child will lose control of himself during a tantrum. It often helps to simply hold him firmly but lovingly and explain, "You are angry, and you have lost control. I'm holding you because I love you." You may find that after a minute or more of struggling to free himself, he melts in your arms, as if to thank you for rescuing him from himself.

Just as adults want to share their misery with someone, toddlers seldom tantrum alone. I believe that most babies actually want and need help during a tantrum. The fact that babies have more tantrums in the presence of someone they love and trust should not be interpreted as manipulation; it is rather that they feel safe and trusting enough to lose it in the presence of their favorite support person. Often a toddler tantrums because she does not have the words yet to express her needs, thoughts, or feelings. She may resort to a tantrum in order to break through to you if you are being distant. In these cases, you can usually help by giving her the words, verbalizing for her what you think and feel she needs.

Tantrum-Prone Kids?

Some children are like volcanoes with pent-up emotions that need to erupt occasionally, spilling their feelings all over everyone, then settling down waiting for those around them to clean up the mess. High-need children are especially prone to tantrums when their desires are thwarted. Compliant children are easily directed into behaviors that take them away from their tantrums, whereas strong-willed children are not so easily distracted. Look at temper tantrums from behind the eyes of your growing child. He is trying to be assertive, independent, and curious without the ability to understand why he cannot safely hold the crystal vase. There is a conflict between what he wants and what he can safely have. He understands his wants, but does not understand his "can't haves." As you teach a child what behavioral limits you will accept and he learns what he can handle,

tantrums subside, but prepare to clash with the strong-willed child during this declaration-of-independence stage.

Most babies who lose control during a tantrum settle when you hold them and hug them tightly, snuggling chest to chest, teddy-bear style. The tantrum-prone child is likely to squirm and protest being restrained during a tantrum. If you feel this child needs to be held to regain control of himself, hold him on your lap facing *outward*. This hold is less restraining but still gives him the security he needs during a tantrum. This kind of holding literally can help you to see the situation from behind the eyes of your child: why a strong-willed child becomes frustrated when he can't pull two blocks apart or his toy gets stuck under the sofa. In this case sit with the child awhile and become a partner in his play frustrations. Give your child words for his feelings: "You are angry because . . ." Sharing emotions with a child is a prelude to one of the best ways to get through the shield of the older child who needs help but is not very transparent. Nothing opens up a child more than the feeling that someone truly wants to empathize with his position. If you think about it, adults may spend thousands of dollars with a therapist in order to be able to say, "I'm angry." You cannot reason with a toddler (or anyone) in the midst of a tantrum, so wait until he settles before beginning parental counseling. (Holding is therapy.)

Fortunately, toddlers have strong resilience for recovering from tantrums. They usually do not sulk for long periods, and a properly supported temper tantrum wears off quickly in the child, although it may leave parents exhausted. Temper tantrums are self-limiting. As soon as your child has developed language to express emotions, you will find that this disturbing behavior subsides.

Breath-Holding Spells

These are five-star tantrums that exhaust the child and frighten parents. They are common following an injury, such as head bumping or a fall. At the peak of rage a child may start to quiver his lower jaw and hold his breath, first turning red in the face from anger and then turning blue. At this point you are holding your own breath for what happens next. Just as you are about to panic, the child takes a deep breath (so do you), and all is well. While most babies resume normal breathing just as they are on the brink of passing out, some do become limp and faint. These most alarming of breath-holding episodes resemble convulsions. But immediately after fainting, the child resumes breathing and seems none the worse for wear. The spells rarely harm the child but leave parents a wreck. Try to intervene with soothing words and gestures and distracting activities before the tantrum escalates this far. These episodes usually stop between two and two and a half years of age, when the child is old enough to express her feelings in words.

BITING AND HITTING

Most of the playful nips and slaps, awful as they look and feel, are normal baby communications and not angry, aggressive behavior. Much of baby's behavior is oriented around hands and mouth, and it is only natural to use these as social tools. Baby likes experimenting with biting and hitting different surfaces, both for the feel it produces and the reaction

it gets. During tantrums toddlers often bite or hit parents or other trusted caregivers rather than a stranger. Don't take this personally. Babies do bite the hands that feed them.

Besides being social tools, biting and hitting are forms of undesirable aggressive behavior that may hurt all those on the receiving end of sharp teeth and clawlike scratching. Resist the temptation to reach for the muzzle and handcuffs. There are easier ways to tame the biter and hitter.

Teach alternatives. Give baby *words* and *gestures* to express feelings. Help him make a good social impression and not a lasting impression on your skin: "No bite . . . biting hurts mama!" Offer alternative social gestures: "Hug daddy . . . give me five."

Track the trigger. Keep a diary of what circumstances set off aggressive behavior, such as too many kids in a crowded space and end-of-the-day overload and tiredness. Get behind the eyes of your child to see what triggers the biting or hitting. Is she tired, bored, hungry, or in a setting where tempers flare?

Tame the play. If you detect a mean streak developing in your child, model gentle actions and play, such as hug the bear, pet the kitty, love the doll. A clue to a developing aggressive streak is seen in the child who consistently bangs toys and crashes cars together and bashes dolls. While this is normal play, it is important to balance aggressive play with gentle play. Also, talk about the difference between bear hugs (good for mom and dad) and bunny hugs (good for fellow toddlers).

Actively supervise. Keep an eye on biters and hitters in a play situation and let the other mothers know to be vigilant as well. If your child bites or hurts another child, immediately separate the children and isolate the biter for some time-out. Reinforce the isolation with appropriate admonitions, such as, "Biting hurts and it's wrong to hurt, and we're going to sit on the chair to think about why you should not bite." If he is verbal and understanding enough, encourage an "I'm sorry." Your child needs to connect biting with an immediate removal from the scene of the crime. This may be his first lesson that undesirable behavior leads to undesirable consequences.

Remove the spotlight. Biters (and hitters) often become the center of attraction: "Watch out, he bites!" If you conclude that baby is biting for attention, channel baby into more socially acceptable attention-getting habits. Praise his good behaviors and downgrade the importance of biting.

Model, model, model. A baby who lives with aggression becomes aggressive. One time I witnessed a toddler hitting his mother, whereupon she immediately lashed out, "Don't hit me," as she slapped his hand. It is obvious where the child got his hitting habits. Also, don't bite your child back. Putting one immature behavior on top of another only aggravates the problem. But it is important for a child to learn that biting hurts.

Show and tell. If he won't take your word for it, here is a technique that parents have used successfully to make the point: Press your child's forearm against his upper teeth as if he were biting himself, but not in a punitive, angry way. Reinforce his self-produced marks on his own arm with "See, biting

---

TIME-OUT

Most two-year-olds respond to this simple consequence of not listening to your correction. There is no need to be punitive or angry; in fact, that will interfere with the teaching value of time-out. A child needs to learn that performing a forbidden action results in a break in the action. Depending on the age and temperament of your child, a one-to-five-minute time-out sitting on a chair is all you need. If a child can't cooperate with the time-out, you can sit with him to supply the control. Some quiet time together may be what you both need anyway. You may wind up holding him in place; that's fine, and maybe you can even get him to verbalize feelings, or you can verbalize for him.

---

hurts!" Administer this self-biting lesson immediately after your child bites someone, so that he makes the connection that biting hurts.

Hurt relationships. Your little biter may cost you your best friend. The parents of a biter are disturbed and embarrassed; the parents of the bitee are naturally upset that their child has been hurt, and you all start fussing at one another. If your child bites or hits, prepare the other parents in the play group ahead of time, and ask their help in tempering your child's behavior. Chances are they have also gone through this aggressive stage with their children and would appreciate your candidness and may offer good advice.

This warning also conveys that you care that their children are not hurt.

A note for concerned parents of the bitee: Instead of laying a you-have-a-bad-child trip on the biter's parents (they feel sorry enough already), be understanding. Offer to help. This not only maintains a friendship but relieves the other parents of the "bad parent" feeling.

Once your child learns to talk better, he is likely to keep his teeth and his hands to himself, and this undesirable social behavior will subside.

BABY WON'T MIND

Ponder for a moment what the verb "to mind" means. When a baby won't mind, whose mind is he not minding? What really bothers you is that he won't join his mind-set with yours. When you ask him to turn one way, and he turns the other, he is minding, but it's his mind, not yours. Call this defiance? Not exactly. The child is not saying, "I won't!" — he is saying, "I don't want to." The stronger the will of the child, the stronger the protest. The compliant child more easily yields her mind to yours; the strong-minded child is less likely to switch minds readily. When her behavior says, "I don't want to," it's your job either to help her want to or to follow through with a physical assist (pick her up bodily) and calmly administer time-out.

It's three o'clock in the afternoon, you are visiting a friend, and your two-year-old is engrossed in play. Your mind reminds you it's time to rush for an appointment. You nicely but firmly ask your child to put away the toys and come along. She either puts on the deaf act, or by real or body language says, "No!"

You ask louder; she still doesn't budge. Then the shouting and grabbing scene begins as you tote the flailing toddler away. Toddlers do not easily switch channels at the instant whim of the parent. See "Closing Out Play," page 535, for a way that causes less wear and tear on parents and child.

SCREECHING AND WHINING

One day I was counseling a mother about normal toddler behavior. Her toddler started yelling. By reflex she immediately yelled, "Stop that yelling!" We both laughed after we realized how ridiculous this sounded. Yelling and screeching peak at this stage, not as deliberately annoying behavior, but because baby is trying out his voice for both the decibels he can reach and the effect his siren has on his audience. And babies seem to reserve their loudest shrieks for the quietest places.

Here's how we muted our screamers. Teach your child what language you will accept. "Give daddy your nice voice . . ." or model a softer voice to him by whispering. When Matthew first started screaming, we took him outside into the yard and jumped up and down and screamed together as a game. Next time he began screaming in the house we again took him into the yard and repeated the screaming act. After that, whenever he would start to scream, we quickly interjected in a soft voice, "Only scream on the grass." We'd planted in his mind — at a stage in which babies make mental matches of what activity goes where — that screaming and grass (outside) go together, and any other relationship doesn't fit. The noisy stage soon passed as Matthew forgot the screaming and the grass.

PULLING UP PUT-DOWNS

Kids are sometimes not nice to other kids, and adults are sometimes not nice to children. While parents need not always protect their child from life's little digs, some children are supersensitive to attacks on their self-esteem or are going through a sensitive stage — just at the time when they may or may not have much self-esteem. In our family if an older child lays a "That's dumb!" on a younger sib, we quickly intervene: "That's a put-down!" Pulling up put-downs is where intuitive parenting gets results.

Sometimes a seemingly harmless correction may be perceived as a put-down by a fragile child. One day in my office, Tommy was pulling on the scale tray (I had completed his checkup, and he was bored, not part of the doctor-parent conversation). I respectfully asked Tommy not to pull on the scale and even offered a face-saving "please." Tommy obeyed, but just as he was about to disintegrate from a perceived put-down, his mother offered a rescuing, "Because you're so strong!" Tommy perked up, and so did I at the esteem-preserving insight of a connected mother.

Even though I thought I handled the situation in a psychologically suitable manner, I had only book knowledge; the mother had kid knowledge.

Early screeches and yells have shock value, causing all those within earshot to stop and pay attention. Similarly, toddlers whine because it works; if that is the only way baby can break through to you, whining is likely to continue.

Children need to learn that pleasant sounds get pleasant responses. When your toddler addresses you in his usual and pleasant voice, give a prompt response so that he learns that this is the best voice for quick action. Sometimes babies need reminding about which voice gets the best response. As soon as your child starts to whine, quickly get her to change her communication channels by interjecting, "[name], you have such a nice voice. Use your nice voice." After rehearsing this social drill many times, a parent can quickly head off a beginning whine by saying, "Nice voice, please." Besides learning that whining doesn't work, your child becomes more language fluent, and whining will be a sound of the past.

THUMB-SUCKING

Some babies are born with a callused thumb. In the privacy of the womb they sucked it, and no one noticed. Babies have an insatiable need to suck, and a love affair with the ever-present thumb is normal. In addition to parental comforting, the ability to self-soothe is a normal part of growing up. As is the case with the use of pacifiers, thumb-sucking bothers adults more than it harms children, perhaps because of the unwarranted worry: "Is my child lacking love and security if he sucks his thumb?" Many a happy, well-adjusted baby spends a good deal of his early years with his thumb in his mouth.

Thumb-sucking in the first two years seldom causes orthodontic problems. Beyond the age of two or three, habitual thumb-sucking can cause upper teeth to protrude. In our experience, foul-tasting paints on the thumb, restraints, or mittens seldom work. And if your child is old enough to harm his teeth by thumb-sucking, he is most likely old enough to understand that thumb-sucking may harm his teeth. The all-night thumb-suckers are the ones to worry about. As an alternative to the thumb, give your child a large cuddle toy (for example, a large teddy bear that he can get his arm around and then cannot have access to his thumb). Check on him several times a night for a while and remove the sleeping sucker's thumb. To redirect the daytime thumb-sucker, keep both his hands busy, and as soon as the mouth and thumb are about to connect, channel your child into a play activity that requires the use of both thumbs. In our office if I wish to unplug the thumb from the mouth, I entice the child to "give me one five" and then "give me two fives!" Avoid nagging your child — constant verbal reminders may actually reinforce the sucking by focusing attention on the behavior.

For parents who wish to redirect the thumb and the future orthodontist payments, consider the following preventive medicine. The only study we were able to find about lowering the risk of later thumb-sucking was a comparison between fifty children who were habitual thumb-suckers and fifty children who were not. Is there a profile of the young thumb-sucker? The researchers showed that thumb-suckers tended to be bottlefed rather than breastfed. The thumb chums were more often fed on schedule than on demand. Ninety-six percent of the thumb-

> ## DISCIPLINE: GIVING YOUR CHILD THE TOOLS TO SUCCEED IN LIFE
> To learn more about giving your toddlers and school-age children self-discipline tools, see these related books in our Parenting Library: *The Discipline Book: Everything You Need to Know to Have a Better-Behaved Child, From Birth to Age Ten,* and *The Successful Child: What Parents Can Do to Help Kids Turn Out Well.*

suckers had been left to fall asleep alone. The non-thumb-suckers had a different profile. The later the child was weaned, the less likely he was to suck his thumb. And children who did not suck their thumbs had been nurtured to sleep, often at the mother's breast, and not left alone to fall asleep. These researchers postulated that sleep is a regressive activity during which the infant returns to the more primitive activities he enjoyed in the womb, such as sucking and hand-to-mouth actions. They believed that if an infant was allowed to breastfeed to sleep, the sucking drive would be satisfied, and the pattern of thumb-sucking to sleep would not get started. This fits in with one of our own observations — a need filled in early infancy disappears; a need that is not filled does not go away but reappears, sometimes as an undesirable habit. In our own practice, we have noticed that babies who are breastfed to sleep, offered unrestricted night feedings, and not weaned before their time are much less likely to become habitual thumb-suckers. What a natural and inexpensive braces-saving technique!

24

Toilet Training

We all long for the day when we have changed the last diaper, but with mixed feelings. It also means waving bye-bye to the beautiful stage of babyhood.

Toilet training is a *partnership,* with proper roles assigned to each person. You can lead a baby to the bathroom, but you can't make him go. And you have not failed Parenting 101 if your baby is the last one on the block to be dry. As with eating and sleeping, you can't and shouldn't force a baby to be dry or clean, but you can set the conditions that help baby train himself. The bottom line is helping your baby achieve a healthy toileting attitude.

To approach toilet training as an exciting interaction rather than a dreaded task, consider this event an initiation into your role as instructor. From baby's viewpoint, toileting is his initiation into "bigness" — a rite of passage from toddlerhood into preschoolerhood. (This explains why the desire to stay little makes some procrastinators resist.)

FACTS YOU SHOULD KNOW

Toilet training is a complex skill. Before you rush baby to the potty at the first squat, consider what's involved in learning toileting skills. First, baby has to be aware of the pressure sensations of bowel and bladder. Then he must make the connection between these sensations and what's happening inside his body. Next he learns to respond to these urges by hurrying to the potty, where he must know how to remove his clothes, how to situate himself comfortably on this new kind of seat, how to hold his urges until all systems are go. With all these steps, it's no wonder many babies are still in diapers well into the third year.

Bladder and bowel muscles. The muscles surrounding the opening of the bladder and bowel (I call them doughnut muscles when explaining the elimination process to six-year-old bed wetters) need to be controlled to open and close at the proper time. Bowel training usually precedes bladder training, mainly because the doughnut muscles surrounding the bowel are not as impatient as those around the bladder. When a baby senses the urge to defecate, he has more time to respond before soiling his diapers. A solid substance is easier to control than liquid. When the bladder is full, the urge to go is sudden, strong, and hard to control.

The usual sequence of gaining bowel and bladder control is (1) nighttime bowel control; (2) daytime bowel control; (3) daytime bladder control; (4) nighttime bladder control.

Changing elimination patterns. Babies naturally experience a sort of self-training beginning in the early months. The many-stools-a-day pattern of the first month gradually changes to one or two stools a day by one year and one a day by two years. The number of daily bowel movements decreases, but the volume increases (bowel and bladder patterns vary considerably). By six months to a year many babies no longer have a nighttime bowel movement. Even the interval between wet diapers naturally increases over the first two years.

Gender and ease of training. Girls are rumored to be trained earlier than boys. This observation reflects more the sex of the trainer than the trainee. Culturally, toilet training has been left to mothers; naturally, women feel more comfortable training girls, and baby girls are more likely to imitate their mommies. Picture mommy standing and trying to show baby Bert how to urinate. By imitation, babies learn that girls sit and boys

stand, but in the beginning boys can sit, avoiding sprays and dribbles on walls and floor. When your son figures out he can stand just like daddy, he will.

BETTER LATE THAN EARLY

The pressure is off parents to toilet train early. Gone are the days when toilet training was equated with good mothering. In those days, the earlier the baby was eating three squares a day, weaned, toilet trained, and independent, the "better" the mother was. And it's no wonder. Hand washing and line drying the laundry were enough reason to push anyone to potty train their baby as soon as possible.

Diapering is certainly not the hassle it used to be. Diaper pins are going the way of the clothespin, and even fumbling fathers can manage the new, easy-to-put-on-and-fasten diapers. Disposables have made travel easier, and many a modern mother wants to hug the diaper-service delivery person. Also, we now understand more about how a baby's elimination system works. We now know that the nerves and muscles governing defecation and urination do not mature in most babies until eighteen to twenty-four months. As an added fact supporting later training, babies who begin toilet training later achieve control faster than those hurried to the toilet earlier.

A STEP-BY-STEP APPROACH TO TOILET TRAINING

In explaining how this system works, we do not mean to imply that you lazily leave baby alone until he is old enough to order his

---

QUICK CHANGES

Change baby promptly so that he gets used to feeling clean and dry. And when he can comprehend, point out how nice it feels to be clean and dry. A baby who is accustomed to the clean, dry feel is less likely to enter the go-and-won't-tell stage.

own potty-chair. Some training is necessary on the parents' part, and some learning is needed by the baby. The following step-by-step approach will help you achieve this partnership of toilet training according to the developmental readiness of your individual baby. And temperament of mother and baby play a role in readiness, too. A down-to-business baby tends to learn quickly, may even "train himself," especially if he has a mother who thinks the same way, but who is wise enough not to pressure. A laid-back baby with a casual mother may still be in diapers at three and no one worries. With a laid-back baby and a down-to-business mother things get more interesting, and it is to this mother-baby pair that we dedicate the rest of the chapter.

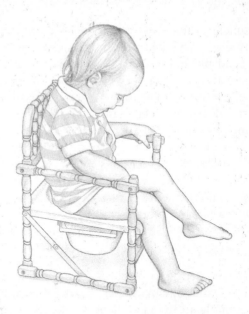

Toilet training is baby's initiation into "bigness."

Step One: Make Sure Baby Is Ready

As when determining readiness for solid foods, watch your baby, not the calendar, for the following "I'm ready to learn" signs of developmental readiness:

- imitates your toileting
- verbally communicates other sensations, such as hunger
- understands simple requests, such as "Go get ball"
- begins to push diapers off when wet or soiled, or comes to tell you he's dirty
- climbs onto the potty-chair or toilet
- stays dry longer, at least three hours
- investigates his or her body equipment

Watch Baby for About-to-Go Signals

Observe external signs that he feels the pressure inside: squatting, grabbing diapers, crossing legs; grunting and grimacing; and retreating to the corner or behind the couch like a mother cat about to deliver. These signs tell you that baby is developmentally mature enough to be aware of what's going on inside his body.

In all smoothly acquired developmental skills, mind and body work together in a

---

READING BABY'S BODY LANGUAGE

- *About to go:* retreats to quiet place, stops play, quiets, squats
- *Going:* grabs diaper, grunts, crosses legs
- *Gone:* peers at diaper bulge, senses different feel, resumes play or verbalizes production

timely fashion. Between eighteen months and two years, baby has language skills to understand and communicate, his desire is to imitate and please, he strives for independence, and he can run fast to the toilet. There are also developmental phases when toilet training is untimely. If your toddler is going through a generally negative mood in which he resists all interventions and his vocabulary is limited to the two-letter word "no," hold on to your techniques a few more weeks and catch him at a more receptive time.

Serendipity

Occasionally a baby will be so ready that he will learn quite by chance, or so it seems. For example, fresh out of diapers, mother says casually, "Oh well, just put on brother's pants for now." Three days later you realize he's done it! This does happen, and your mother-in-law would be so impressed. But don't hold your breath.

Step Two: Make Sure You're Ready

Are you ready? Choose a time to train when you are not preoccupied with other commitments: during an older child's high-need period, work stress, a week before childbirth (a new baby in the house tends to cause regressions anyway), and so on. Also, warm-weather training works best — you don't have snowsuits to contend with.

"Tools" that you will need include:

- sense of humor
- endless patience
- creative marketing

- potty-chair
- training pants

Here are some other training aids and techniques to consider:

Show-and-tell. Capitalize on a prime developmental interest at this stage — the desire to imitate. Let baby watch you go potty and explain what you are doing. Girls naturally do better in the bathroom classroom with mommies, boys with daddies, but same-sex training is not crucial.

Peer pressure. If baby has a friend in training, arrange for her to watch what her friend does. If baby is in day care, her teammates may show her a trick or two. In fact, some preschools won't accept children in diapers, so the pressure is already on to make the grade at such a tender age.

Potty props. Some parents use a doll that wets to model the steps to toilet training. Baby sees where the "urine" comes from, removes the doll's diapers, places the doll on the potty seat, changes diapers, removes and empties the potty-chair bowl into the toilet, and flushes the toilet. The combination of live models (parents and peers) and a doll model makes toilet training easier.

Book learning. Besides live models and doll models there are clever books that show pictures and show a child in training. By the time your child has been exposed to all these models of toilet-trained characters, he should get the message "If they can do it, so can I." Try the book *You Can Go to the Potty,* by William and Martha Sears and Christie Watts Kelly (Little, Brown, 2002).

Step Three: Teach Baby Where to Go and What to Call It

Once you've determined that baby is developmentally ready and you are ready to invest the time, class begins.

A Place to Go

Teacher's next decision is whether to get baby's own potty-chair or an adapter for the toilet. Pupil's decision is which one, if any, he prefers. Most babies prefer their own potty-chair. How comfortable and willing would you be to perform on a spa-sized toilet? Child-sized furniture makes the development of any skill easier. Potty-chairs securely contain babies, and with a potty-chair baby can plant her feet squarely on the floor, instead of dangling them in midair from the adult toilet. (Dangling feet tighten rectal muscles; planted feet relax these muscles.) Also, potty-chairs can be carried from room to room and even put in the car for travel.

Picking a Potty

Toddlers are most likely to use the potty they choose. There are as many varieties of potty-chairs as there are contours of babies' bottoms. Choose one wisely. Baby may prize it, much like his first riding toy. When purchasing baby's first potty, consider the following:

Baby's opinion. Take baby to the store with you for a test sit, as when picking out a toy or his own table and chair. See how comfortable your fully clothed baby is using it as a chair before using it as a potty.

Ease of cleaning. Be sure the catch bowl lifts out easily. A catch bowl removable from the top is easier to clean than one removable from the rear or side.

Safety. Beware of sharp edges or hinges on the seat that can pinch baby's fingers or bottom.

Stability. Be sure the chair doesn't tip easily when baby squirms. Since you will be using it on slippery surfaces (such as kitchen or bathroom tiles), it should have rubber tips on the bottom to keep it from sliding.

Design. Your toddler may enjoy trying one of these new designs:

- Musical pots. To entice the squirmy toddler to stay put, some first-class seats even play music while baby sits.

- Multiple-use potty-chairs. These clever designs contain three parts — a potty-chair for the rookie, an adapter seat that fits on an adult toilet for the graduate, and a step stool for the veteran ready to go it alone.

Toileting Talk

Teach your toddler words for the body parts and for the actions. Putting a label on what baby does makes any developmental skill easier.

First, a lesson in naming body parts. Give baby the proper names for proper parts (penis, testicles, vulva, vagina), but don't expect him or her to use them accurately until two and a half or three years of age. Say these words as comfortably as you would "arm" or "hand," so baby does not pick up vibrations that you are uneasy about these mysterious parts.

Now that the action is ready to begin, give baby easy words and phrases such as "go potty," and later get more specific — for example, "go pee-pee" or "poo-poo." Avoid words that imply shame: "stinky," or "Did you *dirty* your diapers?" Use terms that you are comfortable with and baby can say and understand. "Urination" and "defecation" are beyond toddlers.

Step Four: Teach Baby the Connection Between Feeling and Going

The next step is to help your baby make the connection between what he feels and what he has to do. In a nutshell, toilet training is teaching baby to make a series of connections between the urge to go and going to the potty, and between sitting on the potty and going in the potty. Let's go through this process.

Feeling and Going

The first training goal is to help baby make the connection between what he feels and what he needs to do. When baby shows about-to-go signs (for example, squatting, quietly retreating), interject a reminding "Go potty" as you usher the willing baby to the potty. Once you plant the connection *feel pressure—go potty* in baby's mind, in time he will go potty without your triggering his memory.

Many toddlers achieve nighttime dryness during the second year of life. Morning is a good time to suggest using the potty. The bladder is full. The child will learn what a full bladder feels like and associate a full bladder with using the potty. This easy morning routine will make the rest of the day of potty training easier.

> ## DRESS FOR THE OCCASION
>
> Dress baby for a quick change, making it easy for baby. If he has to struggle to remove complicated clothing en route from urge to potty, he is likely to let go before getting unhooked, unbuckled, unbuttoned, and so on, and you have a double mess, a soiled baby and soiled clothing. Elastic waistbands and quick-release Velcro fasteners are a must. In warm weather, very loose training pants are all baby needs around home. Use easily pulled-down pants or shorts when in public.

Feeling and Telling

Tell baby what to tell you. As soon as you notice the about-to-go signs, query, "Go poo-poo? *Tell* mommy!" (or "*Tell* daddy!") You are planting another mental connection: When he feels the urge, he says the words.

Once baby masters these two connections — urge to go with running to the potty and urge to go with asking for help by saying, "Go potty" — the rookie trainee is ready to advance. Notice the proper role-playing: You set the game plan, but it's up to baby whether or not he chooses to play. If after many rehearsals baby isn't getting the message, wait and try again.

Potty Times

The next connection to teach your trainee is that when you sit him on the potty, he goes. This is called a *conditioned reflex*. But it won't work unless baby is nearly ready to go.

The key is to catch him at the time or times when he is about to go, and sit him on the potty *before* he makes the deposit in his diapers. He will then associate sitting on a potty with having a bowel movement and, eventually, with urinating.

►**SPECIAL NOTE:** *The urine deflector should be removed while your little boy is getting seated so that he doesn't get hung up on it.*

Short of shadowing your baby all day long to catch him in the act, here's how to get some elimination-time clues. Make a potty time chart. For a week or two, record the time or times of the day when your baby has a bowel movement. If you detect a pattern, say after breakfast, put him on the potty each day at that time. Provide baby with an attention-holding book and let him exert his squatter's rights to sit until he goes. If you do not see a pattern, put baby on the potty every two hours, or as often and as long as your time and patience permit.

A physiologic aid for bowel training, called the gastrocolic reflex, may help predict when your baby will have a BM. A full stomach stimulates the colon to empty around twenty to thirty minutes after a meal. Try potty sitting after each meal until baby's patience runs out. Best odds for a predictable daily BM are after breakfast. Another value of this daily routine is that it teaches baby to listen to his bodily urges. It's a physiologic fact that bowel signals not promptly attended to will subside, and this can lead to constipation.

Understand that a child (like an adult) does not push out a bowel movement unless the colon is contracting. The colon has a natural rhythm that causes it to contract for several minutes a few times a day. It is this contract-ing that causes the urge to go to the bathroom. Therefore, it will not work to sit your child on the potty and tell him to push until he has a bowel movement unless the colon is naturally contracting at the time.

Even when you and baby and potty misconnect, and baby goes in his diapers, take baby into the potty-chair room and empty the contents into baby's toilet. At least this will teach him where his productions go. Typically, you are first catching your baby in the act in order to train him to eventually catch himself in the act.

Bare-Bottom Drills — An Undress Rehearsal

Covering up the evidence delays toilet training. Diapers keep baby from making the connection between the urge to release and what he needs to do about it, and they do for baby what baby needs to learn to do for himself.

Outdoor training. For warm-weather training, if you have a private yard, bare bottoms make training easier. Remove your toddler's diaper and let him run around the yard bare bottomed, covered mostly by a long T-shirt if you wish (T-shirts from an older child make good cover-ups). When the urge to go hits, he stops, maybe squats, because he suddenly realizes what's going on. Amazed by this revelation, baby may talk about what he's doing, "Go pee-pee" or "Go poo-poo," or look toward you for "What do I do now, coach?" guidance, or let go puppylike with his puddle or load.

Now it's your move. Watch how baby handles this uncovered elimination. He may look confused, proud, or even upset, especially if he soiled his legs. Praise his productions and clean up matter-of-factly. (If he protests bare-bottom drills, wait awhile and try again.)

Have the potty-chair available so you can put the BM in there, to show him where it goes. Then next time if you catch him squatting, show him how to sit on the potty instead. Don't resign as toileting coach if your baby plays with what he produces. Avoid showing disgust, as this only plants counterproductive connections that something is wrong with what comes out of him, so he'd better not let go anymore.

Indoor training. After trying outdoor drills for a week or so, you are ready to venture back indoors. Remember what you learned from the yard scene. Bare bottoms promote quick learning. The early days of indoor bare-bottom training should be spent, as much as possible, on a noncarpeted floor — easier to detect and easier to clean. You may need a few days of catching baby in the act and offering the reminder "Go potty" as baby enjoys his new diaper freedom.

Step Five: Graduate Baby from Diapers to Training Pants

After baby has been daytime dry for a couple of weeks, he's ready to graduate from diapers to "pull-ups." Pull-ups are there to catch accidents, not to be used as diapers. As long as baby is still going frequently in diapers, use diapers. Progress to pull-ups when the accidents are fewer, and then graduate to training pants when the accidents seldom occur.

Training Pants

Training pants look like superabsorbent padded underwear and are used in transition from diapers to pants. You can make your own or get extra absorbency by sewing a piece of cloth diaper into oversized underwear or into regular training pants. Be enthusiastic about this step up, but be careful what you call them. "Big boy" or "big girl" pants is a loaded term, especially if your toddler is not sure he or she wants to be big. This dilemma occurs with hurrying the older child into pants to make room on the changing table for a new baby. When the older child sees all the attention the diapered baby gets, he may not want to be a big boy. We prefer to call them *special pants.* Buy around six pairs, and be sure they are loose fitting for quick slip down by impatient hands.

When Accidents Happen

Expect soiled and wet pants when baby gets his signals crossed. This is normal when learning a new skill. Prepare for accidents during intense play when babies are so preoccupied that they miss their bladder or bowel signals. Babies become so engrossed in what is going on outside that they forget what's occurring inside. Trainees in these big-league pants may need an occasional bare-bottom reminder to keep their mind on their body.

Step Six: Teach Your Child to Wipe, Flush, Dress, and Wash Hands

As a final class, teach your baby how to wipe, flush, dress, and wash hands. Teach little girls to wipe from front to back (keeping germs that may cause a urinary infection away from the urethra). Don't be too quick to expect your child to wipe himself. A two-year-old seldom has the manual dexterity to adequately wipe, and some children may not be ready to do this until age four or five. This extra pressure after finally succeeding at being potty trained may cause the reluctant toddler to regress. Wait until potty training is consistently under way before teaching your child how to wipe. Moistened flushable wipes are more comfortable on the bottom than toilet paper.

Flushing is a matter of preference for the child. Some children fear the loud swoosh of the flush as their production disappears into a swirling hole. Others consider flushing part of the whole package and insist on doing the honors. Be prepared for an increase in your water bill from the frequent flusher who likes the sound-and-water show at the pull of the handle. Invest in a seat latch to be sure the right stuff gets flushed.

Praise Success, Overlook "Failure," Relax

There is no place for punishment in toilet training, just as you wouldn't scold the begin-

ning walker for tripping. Serious long-term emotional problems can result from angry scolding or punitive attitudes toward accidents or resistance. If you are struggling with your child over toileting and recognize negative feelings toward your child, get some help from trusted advisers or even a counselor. Your goal is for your child to emerge from toilet training with a healthy self-image. Then he or she can tackle the next phase of development, sexual identity, feeling good about himself or herself. Try to relax — what's one more year in diapers?

THE CHILD WHO WON'T GO

There are babies who refuse to announce their productions, hold on to what they have, and resist any attempt to toilet them. If you're still using a diaper service and the potty-chair remains unused, read on.

Late toilet training, like late walking, may be your child's normal developmental pattern and one shared by mom or dad when they were in training. The nerves and muscles involved in toileting may not yet be mature. Suspect this cause if your child has been on the late end of normal in other developmental milestones. Most children are well on their way to daytime bowel and bladder training by three years. If by that time you and your child have made no progress, consult your baby's doctor.

GAMES LITTLE BOYS PLAY

Remember, a sense of humor is tops on your list of tools for successful toilet training. Little boys like to

- "write" in the snow or dirt
- play crisscross pee with dad or an older brother
- sink floating pieces of toilet paper
- hit floating paper targets — these can be purchased as incentive gadgets

Beginning squirters do need a few lessons in target practice to improve their aim. Little boys are like that.

Not Willing to Move out of Diapers

If your child is over age three and you know he has achieved control, but he still refuses to go on the potty, try the "running out of diapers" approach. Show him the stack of diapers getting smaller every day: "Look, there are only ten diapers left." Count them down as you use them. When there is only one left, let him know that this is the last diaper and that you are not going to the store (if he asks). Time it so the last diaper is the first one of the day. When this last one is used up, you have the rest of the day to try the *bare-bottom drills* described above. Expect some protesting, and if it's extreme, you can "find" a small pile of diapers to use. Then try again in a few weeks.

Medical Reasons

A child won't perform any bodily function that hurts. Constipation is painful, often causing tiny tears in the rectum while the child is straining, which further makes the child hold on, and a painful cycle continues. Suspect this if your child squats, grunts, and painfully grimaces but produces nothing. (See causes and treatment of constipation, page 696.)

Bottom burns from food allergies are another culprit. Look for the telltale allergic ring and raw area around the anus. High-acid foods, such as citrus fruits, and lactic-acid-producing foods, such as dairy products, are the usual offenders. Diarrhea stools during the flu or after taking antibiotics may also temporarily hinder bowel control.

Are You Pushing Too Hard?

Class may have begun too early, during a negative stage, or teacher and pupil may be clashing. Consider backing off awhile and take inventory of the following emotional slumps that may slow training. Ask yourself what could be happening, or not happening, in your baby's life that makes him reluctant.

- Is baby going through a negative phase in which he is not receptive to anything new?

- Is there a disturbing situation in the family: a new baby, a major move, family stress, long working hours, a return to work, or an illness?

- Is your child angry? Anger shuts down proper functioning of all physiologic systems, especially toileting.

Take inventory of your parent-child attachment. Normally, children want to please, progress, and learn control of their bodies. I'm suspicious of the "Well, it's just a normal stubborn phase" defense. The problem may be deeper than the diaper.

This may be your child's way of maintaining control over one area of his life that you can't control. If you hold the reins tightly in other areas (choice of clothing, tidiness, choice of pastimes, and so on) don't be surprised if he becomes a holdout in this area. It may also be the only way he knows to stay little longer. This may be time to close the lid on the potty for a few weeks or months, tune in to your child, have some fun, build his self-esteem, and strengthen the bond. If your child is already emotionally upset and has shaky self-esteem, *be careful not to give the message that your child's value depends upon performance.* This number-one no-no in parenting is a sure strikeout, whether in toilet training or in Little League.

TOILET TRAINING QUICKLY: THE WEEKEND-TRAINING-CAMP METHOD

Most parents prefer gradually training their babies over several weeks or months and progressing at baby's own rate. But some would rather plunge right into an intensive course during a weekend off or during vacation time. A crash course in toilet training does work for certain parent-child pairs, but we don't advise this method for all babies. Some babies resist being pushed out of diapers too quickly, but others welcome help to master their body. The steps are the same as the more gradual method, just more concentrated.

Preliminaries

Select the right candidate. Only babies who are verbal, in a positive and receptive stage, and have a want-to-please attitude toward their trainers are suitable for this fast track.

Concentrate on the game. Approach this as a weekend of intensely relating with your baby, not as a contest, but as a game. You will be with your baby constantly during the waking hours, watching every clue of body language that hints of bowel or bladder signals. *Shelve all other commitments.* This is a special training session not open to the public.

Select the right season. Just as you don't schedule baseball games in midwinter, don't set P day when baby is in a negative stage. Choose good-mood weather, and you can always call the game if a bad mood prevails.

Schedule the game ahead of time. The day before, announce to baby that tomorrow is a *special day*: "We are going to play a special game," and repeat "special game" over and over during that day. (You will notice that we use the word "special" in most of our marketing tools. It works, perhaps because it has a special ring to it.)

Hold a pregame warm-up. Continue to emphasize that this is a special day and that you are going to do something special today: "We are going to play the game of no-more-diapers and use the toilet like mommy and daddy do." Throw in "like brother Jim" as an added incentive. Let baby catch your excitement. Babies get excited about what we get excited about.

Select the right uniform. Best is baby's birthday suit, weather permitting. Otherwise a long, loose shirt. No diapers, please. Show baby the training pants, his special pants. Show him how to put on the special pants, how to push them down and pull them up. Publicize this event. Take pictures, preferably Polaroid, and show them to your baby. Demonstrate the push-down and pull-up maneuver in front of a mirror. All the while keep a gamelike atmosphere. And if baby periodically loses interest or protests, take time out for a snack break.

Hand out the equipment. Bring out "special prizes." Like handing out party prizes, one by one unveil the tools of the trade: potty-chair (that you and baby picked out together at the store and kept in a box until P day), doll that wets and other props (see page 580), training pants, and reward stickers or other prizes.

TRAVELING WHILE IN TRAINING

Sometimes toilet training is easier while on vacation. You have more time and patience, baby is often a bare-bottomed beach bum, and you are not so concerned about messes. One of our children trained during a week-long beach vacation during which going without diapers was appropriate beach-wear. Or baby may relapse; if so, put any attempts to change his habits on hold until you return to your known environ-ment. If driving, take along P. Chair. It's handy for frequent pit stops for little blad-ders. We have precious pictures of our trainee sitting on his throne in the back of the family van doing his thing. A folding plastic adapter ring that fits adult toilet seats is useful for going in strange restrooms. Also, remember that a change in diet during family vacations is likely to bring about a change in bowel habits, either constipation or diarrhea, and a corresponding slump in training progress.

A message for young and old: Don't for-get to leave home with an empty bladder.

Practice Drills and Training Aids

The sitting drill. Practice sitting on the potty-chair "just like mommy and daddy." Put the potty-chair next to yours and sit together awhile and chat.

Instruction manuals. As you're sitting on your respective potty-chairs, read a picture book about potty training.

Get your signals straight. Give baby phrases such as "go potty," "go pee-pee," "go poo-poo."

Getting-on-potty-chair-and-what-to-do-there drill. Let him watch you (for real or just pretending) — an enthusiastic grunting sound can give him the idea.

A practice dummy. Go through a drill with a doll that wets, explaining each step of hav-ing the doll wet: removing pants, changing the doll, and emptying the potty-chair bowl into the toilet.

Play Begins

Meanwhile you have already scouted your star player and you know his moves. Squat-ting tells you it's BM time; clutching the front of the diaper (or where the diaper used to be) or looking down there is the about-to-wet signal. Watch for the player's signal. At the first squat interject a "Go potty" as you direct him toward the potty-chair, which is either on the kitchen floor or in the bathroom next to your toilet. Shadow baby all day issuing reminders of "Go potty" at each about-to-go signal. Keep his friend P. Chair in a central location. By repetition of the association between baby's about-to-go signs and your "Go potty" cues, baby makes the connection: "When I get the urge, I go to the potty."

Rewards

If baby consistently makes the right moves during the first day, chalk this up as beginner's luck. Also expect many false starts as baby learns that he can get mommy or daddy to come running at every squat. When you make the right call and take baby to the potty or, even better, he runs to the potty before he has to go and does his thing, reward each hit with a surprise. One mother who used this quick training successfully put reward stickers on the back of the potty-chair for each go.

Call the Game at Night

Don't expect nights free of diapering until several weeks after daytime training has been successful. And you're still in the right ballpark if your child needs nighttime diapers for many months or even years after day training is achieved.

If this instructive course isn't working, don't feel a failure as a teacher or demote the pupil. You may have a casual kid who needs a casual approach. The need for diapers does pass.

V

Keeping Your Baby Safe and Healthy

During the first two years you will earn your honorary medical degree. In this part of the book we will help you set up your own home health maintenance organization: designing a child-safe environment, showing you preventive measures to keep your child healthy, and pointing out ways to detect early signs of illness. Sick little people bring out the doctor or nurse in everyone. Our main goal in this section is to help you as parents form a medical partnership with your baby's doctor. For continued updates on new treatments and medicines visit www.AskDrSears.com.

25

Babyproofing Your Home

Suppose you had access to a medicine that would prevent one-third of childhood deaths? Well, parents have such a "medicine" — and it's free. It's called babyproofing the home. One in three childhood deaths is caused by an accident, and most of these are preventable.

The goal of this chapter is for you to learn how to babyproof your home, not your child. A toddler's curiosity will push him to explore his limits, get into cabinets, climb onto furniture, open containers, and try to get his little hands on anything and everything — including those things he isn't supposed to touch. This is normal toddler behavior. It enhances his development and should not be restricted too much. A toddler who is limited and restrained from exploring his environment can become more withdrawn and fearful of the world around him. This can also dampen his self-confidence. The toddler who, on the other hand, is allowed to safely roam around the house and explore and learn from his environment is likely to blossom into a curious, outgoing, self-assured child who feels safe in the world.

A general rule about babyproofing is that whatever is at the toddler's level should be fair game to him. Expecting the curious

toddler to keep his hands off the crystal vase that is sitting on a low coffee table is unrealistic. Of course, there will be many things that you can't raise out of baby's reach, such as lamp cords and electric outlets. This is where appropriate discipline comes into play. Teach baby there are "yes touches" and "no touches" throughout the home.

PROFILE OF AN ACCIDENT-PRONE CHILD

All babies are accident-prone, but some more than others. A baby's developmental pattern gives a clue to accident-proneness. An infant who progresses slowly but steadily through developmental milestones, such as crawling to standing to walking, is less likely to be accident-prone. This baby doesn't risk trying

> Safety items mentioned in this chapter can be purchased at infant furniture stores or from the resources listed on page 747.

an advanced step until he has securely mastered the step before. The impulsive baby, on the contrary, often speeds through developmental milestones more by trial and error than by calculated steps. The less cautious speeder rushes headlong toward a desired toy and is willing to accept a few stumbles in the relentless pursuit of his goal. This child is more likely to be known by name to your local emergency room staff.

"Mouthers" are also accident-prone. Some babies have such discerning tastes that anything plastic or metal meets a quick oral rejection. Other babies don't feel they really know an object unless they mouth it awhile. Watching how babies play gives you a clue as to who is a mouther and who isn't. The "researcher" picks up a small toy and studies it a bit before adding the oral test, whereas the mouther's first impulse is to go directly oral with the toy. This baby is more likely to have swallowing or choking accidents.

Finally, watch the "darter," who zips away from parents' watchful eyes and runs the stop sign of separation anxiety as if this stage doesn't exist. This baby is more accident-prone than the more dependent baby who frequently checks in at parental home base for "It's OK" signals before venturing into uncharted territory.

THE ACCIDENT-PRONE HOME

Not only are some babies more accident-prone, but certain life situations add another risk factor. Be especially vigilant about toddler accidents when you are

- running late for an appointment
- moving into a new home
- vacationing
- changing day-care centers
- changing caregivers
- experiencing the absence of a spouse
- going through marital stress or divorce
- bringing home a new baby
- caring for baby's ill sibling

►*SPECIAL SAFETY NOTE: Name the indispensable household utility that indirectly contributes to many childhood accidents around the home. Answer — the telephone. Many tragedies occur while a caregiver leaves baby unattended "just for a minute" to answer the phone. A cordless telephone is a wise investment, to keep yourself mobile so you can talk on the phone and keep up with your baby.*

HOME BABYPROOFING CHECKLISTS

Get down on your hands and knees and crawl from room to room looking at things from your baby's viewpoint and for things within a toddler's reach. If you have older children, let them join you on your safety tour, as it teaches them to be safety conscious for their younger siblings.

Keeping a Safe Medicine Cabinet

☐ Do you keep the cabinet latched?

☐ Do you keep safety caps on medicine packages, especially while using them around your baby?

☐ Do you keep medicines out of reach of your baby?

☐ Do you keep syrup of ipecac on hand?

☐ Do you dispose of out-of-date medicines?

☐ Are scissors, razor blades, pins, and so on out of reach?

Keeping a Safe Bathroom

☐ Do you have nonskid mats on the bottom of the tub and shower?

☐ Are tub faucets padded?

☐ Do bathroom rugs have slipproof backing?

☐ Are electrical appliances away from water?

☐ Are toiletries and cosmetics, especially nail polish and remover and aerosol sprays, out of baby's reach?

☐ Is your bathroom door kept closed? (To prevent a toddler from locking himself inside the bathroom, disengage the inside door lock, or place a hook lock high on the outside of the door to keep baby out or high on the inside for privacy.)

☐ Is the toilet seat down and latched? (Babies can drown head down in the toilet.)

☐ Do you have plastic cups and soap dishes — not glass?

☐ Do you drain water from the tub as soon as you are finished using it?

And, of course, never leave baby unattended in the bathtub. Besides being burned by turning on the tempting hot water knobs, an infant can drown in an inch of water.

MOST COMMON ACCIDENTS
ACCORDING TO DEVELOPMENTAL STAGE

Birth to Six Months (Rolling and Reaching)

- crib accidents
- falling off changing tables or out of infant seats
- burns: cups of coffee, tea, or hot water
- auto accidents, improper or no use of car seats

Six to Twelve Months (Crawling and Walking)

- toy accidents: sharp edges, strings, mouthable parts
- high-chair accidents
- falls against sharp table corners, stair edges
- cigarette burns
- grabbing accidents: burns from grabbing hot coffee, cuts from breakables
- walker and stroller accidents
- auto accidents

One to Two Years (Walking and Exploring)

- climbing accidents
- ingestion of poison
- exploring accidents: storage cupboards, medicine cabinets
- unguarded water hazards: pools, ponds, bathtubs, toilets, fountains
- cuts
- auto accidents, airbag injuries

Keeping a Safe Purse or Diaper Bag

Purses and diaper bags are a common source of infant poisonings and injuries. Curious infants and toddlers love to explore these tempting items. It is likely that at some point your unattended baby will find his way into your purse.

☐ Do you make sure there is no mace or pepper spray in your purse?

☐ If you have an air horn, do you leave it out of your purse? (It can damage baby's ears).

☐ Do you keep hairspray or other aerosols out of your purse?

☐ Do you keep your prenatal vitamins out of your purse?

☐ Do you make sure any medications you need to carry are in a babyproofed container?

☐ Do you keep a sharp comb, nail clippers, scissors, or any other sharp item out of your purse?

☐ Do you leave chokable items, like coins or buttons, out of your purse?

Keeping a Safe Kitchen

☐ Are glasses used by baby unbreakable?

☐ Do you routinely cook on back burners if your toddler is nearby, and keep pot handles turned toward the rear of the stove? Have you installed stove knob covers?

☐ Is there a fire extinguisher handy? (Choose a multipurpose extinguisher.)

☐ Are knives out of reach?

☐ If baby climbed onto the counter, would all potentially dangerous or poisonous items be out of reach?

☐ Are items that can break or cause choking on pantry shelves, out of baby's reach?

☐ Do you avoid using slippery rugs on a tile floor?

☐ Do you keep small appliances (blenders, toasters) unplugged?

☐ Do you have a special play cabinet and drawer set aside for your child?

☐ Do you have safety latches on cabinet and appliance doors? (These are easy to install.) Are cleansers, solvents, bleaches, and detergents behind a latched cabinet door, out of a toddler's reach?

☐ Do you make sure appliance cords and tablecloths are not left dangling over countertops?

☐ Do you keep chairs pushed in so your child can't climb onto the table?

Remember, "out of toddler's reach" may be higher than you think. Babies extend their reach by using chairs or boxes to climb up onto counters and tables.

Encouraging Safe Meals

☐ Do you keep toddlers from running around with food in their mouths? (Running with food risks choking.)

☐ Do you prepare foods safely? Whole hot dogs are unsafe because bitten-off chunks may lodge in a baby's windpipe. Slice lengthwise instead. Get into the habit of preparing sliced foods, which are less likely to cause choking than round or square chunks. Peel and slice apples and grapes, and mash or grind seeds and nuts. (See "Chokable Foods," page 229.)

Babyproofing the Nursery or Bedroom

☐ Is your baby's sleeping environment safe? (See the discussion of crib safety, page 603, and safe co-sleeping, page 341.)

☐ Do you use a safety strap on the changing table? (Never leave baby unattended lying on the changing table even with the safety strap.)

☐ Are baby-care items kept out of baby's grabbing distance when he's on the changing table?

Keeping a Fireproof and Burnproof House

☐ Are smoke alarms appropriately placed around your house? (Suggested places for installing include the ceiling in the entrance hall, the hallway outside bedrooms, the ceiling on each floor, the attic, the garage, and the basement. Do not place smoke detectors near air vents. To check operation, button test the detector quarterly. Replace batteries at least once a year on a preassigned day, such as a birthday or the day of fall time change, or when the detector emits its low-power warning.) You can install a child locator and smoke detector that attaches to the bedroom window; it emits a sound and

flashes red to alert firemen to a child's room.

☐ Do you have "tot finder" stickers — available from your local fire department — on children's bedroom doors? Place the stickers on the outside lower corner of the door (firemen search the house on their knees). Don't place them on a window, where they might advertise the location of the child's bedroom to undesirables.

☐ Do you remember not to leave cigarette lighters or matchboxes within a toddler's grabbing distance?

☐ Do you avoid smoking in bed or while lying on a couch and make sure not to leave lit cigarettes around?

☐ Is your baby's sleepwear flame-retardant?

☐ Do you make sure the fire is out or a screen is in place before leaving the fireplace unattended or going to bed?

☐ Is your electric portable space heater safe? Is it UL approved?

☐ If using an extension cord, does it have a high-enough power rating? Ask at the appliance store.

PUTTING OUT A FIRE

Teach children to do the following if their clothing catches on fire:

1. **Stop!** (Running fans the flame.)
2. **Drop!** (Fall to the ground immediately.)
3. **Roll!** (Roll or rock to smother the flames.)

☐ Do you know the location and operation of the main disconnect switch on your electrical switch box?

☐ Do you disconnect extension cords from the wall socket rather than leaving them plugged in? (Your baby could suffer an electrical burn by biting the cord or poking the extension-cord socket.)

☐ Is the temperature gauge on your water heater set below 120°F (49°C) to avoid scalding from tap water?

☐ Do you set down hot beverages out of a child's reach?

☐ Do you avoid heating baby bottles in a microwave? (This can cause hot spots.)

☐ Have you practiced your fire drill lately? (Teach children which exit routes to use; not to go back into a burning house after a toy; to stay low because smoke rises, crawling on hands and knees to a door or a window; not to open doors with hot doorknobs — there may be flames on the other side — but to escape through the window instead.)

Taking a Safety Walk Around the House

☐ Do you make sure your floor is clear of items that can cause choking or are dangerous, such as plastic bags, coins, plastic wrap, balloons, scissors, sewing tools, guns?

☐ Have you considered storing your coffee table for a few years to avoid stitches on your active baby's forehead?

☐ Do you keep plastic garment and grocery bags safely out of baby's reach?

☐ Do you check and reposition dangling strings, such as drapery cords, clotheslines, lamp cords? (Shorten drapery cords to adult-reach height; install shorteners on lamp cords.)

☐ Are your tablecloth corners folded under the tabletop so they don't dangle within baby's easy grabbing distance? (Placemats are safer.)

☐ Are you in the habit of pushing dangerous or breakable items toward the center of the table?

☐ Are area rugs removed from the path of a trippable toddler?

☐ Are the edges on your furniture (table corners, coffee-table corners, fireplace bricks) covered with rubber protectors? (Adhesive-backed weather stripping is useful for covering brick corners.)

☐ Are unused electrical outlets covered with dummy plugs?

☐ Do you routinely check electrical cords to make sure they aren't frayed?

☐ Are you aware of and have you removed toxic plants?

☐ Are firearms locked out of sight?

☐ Do you keep sliding glass doors closed? Or, when open, are the screens locked?

☐ Are glass doors marked with decals at toddler eye level to prevent run, bump, and break?

☐ Are windows properly locked and the screens behind them secure?

☐ Do you have metal screen guards in back of second-story or higher sliding glass windows? (Screen guards catch the screen and the child, in case your child pushes it open. If you have a screened-in porch, keep baby from leaning on the screens.)

☐ Are openings in balconies or porch railings safely enclosed with netting so baby can't squeeze through?

Now let's take a crawl or walk up the stairs:

☐ Are your stairs well lit, not slippery, and equipped with safe handrails? When your child learns to crawl, teach him to use the stairs safely. Sit below him as he explores and figures out how to crawl up and down. This way, when he manages to sneak around the guard gates, he will be less likely to fall.

☐ Are the stairs' edges protected with rubber stripping or carpet?

☐ Is clutter that can cause trips cleaned up?

☐ Is the carpet tacked down securely?

☐ Do you use a safety gate? (See discussion of safety gates, page 518.)

Now let's stroll out to the garage and down to the basement and laundry areas:

☐ Are power tools and sharp tools out of reach?

☐ Are paints, solvents, insecticides, detergents, bleach, and other chemicals out of reach?

☐ Are the washer and dryer doors kept closed?

☐ Is the switch or remote control for the automatic garage door opener out of baby's reach?

Keeping a Safe Yard

☐ Is your playground equipment sturdy and free of sharp corners and splinters?

☐ Are your swings and climbing equipment safe? (They should be installed at least six feet/two meters from obstructions such as fences or walls; the surface under them should be soft, to absorb the force of a fall. A swing set should be anchored firmly to the ground, and any exposed bolts or screws should be covered with plastic caps or taped over — try duct tape for a good all-around rough-edge cover. Swings with chair, sling, or saddle seats are the safest because they discourage children from standing up and help them to hold their bodies on the swing. Place swings at different heights for children of different ages. Keep the swing height as close to the ground as possible without catching baby's swinging feet. Remind the toddler and other children not to walk behind someone who's swinging. Avoid equipment with S-type hooks, sharp edges, or rings between five and ten inches/twelve and twenty-five centimeters in diameter, which can entrap the child's head.)

☐ Do you keep ropes or other items for climbing away from your children? These items are extremely dangerous and are responsible for a number of accidental child deaths each year when children use them to climb on a play set.

☐ Are garden hoses safely stored, not exposed in the hot sunshine? (The water in the hose may become hot enough to scald a curious child.)

☐ Do you avoid mowing the lawn with a power mower while baby is playing in the yard?

☐ Is your yard climbproof? Do you have safe climbing toys such as rubber tires?

Keeping a Safe Pool

☐ Is there an approved fence around your Jacuzzi or pool?

☐ Was your pool built by a professional according to city guidelines? New pools must now meet a large number of strict safety guidelines, including appropriate locks and alarms on all doors leading to the backyard and pool area.

☐ Do you use a firm, solid pool cover that will safely hold a child's weight? Soft, pliable covers are extremely dangerous, as a child or animal can get stuck and sink into the pool or be trapped under the cover.

☐ Are your children old enough and responsible enough for you to have a pool? If you are thinking of putting in a pool, consider waiting until your children are at least five years or older and you are not planning to have any more children. Older infants and toddlers account for most drownings.

☐ Is your Jacuzzi safe? Children can also drown in small Jacuzzis. Make sure there is a fence around it and an appropriate cover.

☐ Is your backyard secure from toddlers and young children entering unsupervised? Make sure any side yard gates, garage back doors, and sliding glass doors are appropriately locked. Many times a neighborhood child has drowned in someone else's pool.

☐ Always supervise your children as they play in the pool or Jacuzzi. Use this time as a good excuse to relax in a lounge chair while you keep your watchful eyes on the young swimmers, instead of trying to get things done inside while periodically glancing out the window.

☐ Do you have a motion sensor alarm in your pool to alert you if anyone falls in?

CHOOSING AND USING SAFE BABY EQUIPMENT

When selecting a toy or any piece of baby equipment, develop a safety mind-set. Think through how you (and baby) will use it before buying it.

Safe Toys

• Before buying or giving a baby a toy, check to make sure it has no small parts that could cause baby to choke — for example, doll shoes, buttons, beads, squeaker buttons in squeak toys, toys stuffed with small pellets. (Testing tubes for checking toy size are available at toy stores. If the part can fit through the tube, it can enter baby's airway. Blocks, balls, and other small toys should be no less than one and one-half inches/four centimeters in diameter.)

• Make sure toys have no sharp edges or splinters and inspect them frequently for loose parts. Perfectly safe new toys may become unsafe through wear and tear.

• Avoid toys with dangling strings longer than eight inches (twenty centimeters), or remove the strings.

HIGH-CHAIR SAFETY

- Position chair away from hazards such as stoves, windows, dangling drapery cords, and shelves.

- Be sure to use the safety belt that is attached to the chair. Do not depend on the tray to restrain the baby.

- Be sure the tray is properly latched on both sides, as babies tend to push against the tray when seated.

- Do not allow baby to stand in the chair.

- Be sure the chair has a wide base for stability, otherwise it may topple over when baby tries to climb into it. (Allow climbing only with supervision.)

- Periodically check for splinters, loose screws, and a wobbly base.

STROLLER SAFETY

- Choose a stroller with a wide base and rear wheels well behind the weight of the baby, so it will not tip when baby leans over to the side or rocks backward.

- If the stroller adjusts to a reclining position, be sure it will not tip backward when baby is lying down.

- Place shopping baskets directly over the front of the rear axle to prevent tipping.

- Test the brakes. Brakes on two wheels are safer than on one.

- Be sure that latching devices fasten securely. Latches can be accidentally tripped, causing a stroller to collapse. Strollers with two latching devices are safer than those with only one.

- When collapsing or opening a stroller, be careful of fingers — yours and baby's.

- Periodically do a loose nuts and bolts check and look for sharp edges and unsafe wheels.

PLAYPEN SAFETY

- If using a wooden playpen, make sure the bars are not so widely spaced that baby's head could get stuck. The same slat safety applies to playpens as to cribs (bars no more than two and three-eighths inches/six centimeters apart).

- If using a mesh playpen, check that the netting is small enough that it cannot catch the buttons on a child's clothing. Avoid mesh with large openings, which make easy toeholds for climbing.

- Never leave a child in a mesh playpen

with the side down. Baby can become trapped and can strangle in the pocket of mesh between the floor of the playpen and the lowered side.

- Avoid dangling strings from the sides of the playpen.

- Remove large toys or boxes or blocks that can be used as steps for climbing out.

- Cover exposed nuts and bolts.

- Secure latching mechanisms that may act like a scissors and pinch baby's fingers.

SAFETY INFORMATION

The Juvenile Products Manufacturers Association (JPMA) has safety-certification information on cribs, high chairs, walkers, strollers, and many other types of baby equipment. Send a self-addressed, stamped envelope to JPMA, 17000 Commerce Park-way, Suite C, Mt. Laurel, NJ 08054, tel. (856) 638-0420, fax (856) 439-0525, or visit their website, www.jpma.org. For additional information on toy safety and other infant products, visit the U.S. Consumer Product Safety Commission's website, www.cpsc.gov.

- Make sure unsafe toys are out of reach, such as balloons, beads, Legos, or pellet-like objects less than one and a half inches in diameter.

- Be sure to tell older children not to use loud toys such as cap guns around the baby; they may damage baby's hearing.

- Make sure toys fit baby's stage of development and temperament. If your baby is a thrower, get soft cloth or foam toys. Missile-type toys, such as darts and arrows, can cause eye injuries.

- Be careful of crib toys that are fastened between two side rails and hang over the crib, giving baby something to look at and reach for. These toys are recommended only from birth to five months and should be removed when baby is old enough to push up on hands and knees.

- Be careful of plastic toys that are thin, brittle, and likely to break easily, leaving sharp or jagged edges — airplane wings, for example. Before buying a toy, bend it a bit to see how breakable the plastic is.

- Be careful when balloons pop, especially at parties. Quickly gather up the pieces, and keep them away from babies who like to mouth objects and could possibly choke on the remnants of the popped balloon. Avoid letting babies play with uninflated balloons, as these can also cause choking. Always supervise play with an inflated balloon.

- Throw away plastic wrapping as quickly as possible when unpacking toys. Babies love to play with this type of wrapping, as well as with plastic garment bags, and may suffocate.

- Store toys properly. Avoid toy chests with attached lids that can fall on a child and cause injury and strangulation. Hinged lids should stay open by themselves, without propping. Instead of toy boxes, toy shelves are much safer and teach the developing child a sense of order.

- Don't let baby use a walker. Although these convenient "baby-sitters" may be tempting, a walker (a movable play chair with wheels that baby sits in and can use his legs to move around the house) is dangerous. Many pediatricians are lobbying the government to ban them. Not only are walkers responsible for many accidental deaths each year when babies fall down stairs or wander into areas that are not babyproofed, but they also interfere significantly with motor development of the legs and feet. Nonmobile exersaucers are a good alternative. See page 507 for more information.

Crib Safety

Crib accidents are high on the list of injuries to infants. Here are tips for selecting a safe crib.

- Look for a Consumer Product Safety Commission label stating that the crib conforms to commission standards.

- Make sure the crib is painted with lead-free paint. Those manufactured prior to 1974, when lead paint became illegal for cribs, may have been repainted several times with lead-containing paint.

- If baby is a chewer, cover the guardrails with nontoxic plastic chew guards.

- Check the drop sides. To prevent baby from releasing the drop sides, each one should be secured with two locking devices. Baby should not be able to release the drop sides from inside the crib.

- Check the space between the bars of the crib rail. The bars should be no more than two and three-eighths inches (six centimeters) apart, so that babies cannot get their heads caught between them. The bars of cribs made prior to 1979 may have wider spacing that does not conform to these standards.

- Rub your hands over all the wood surfaces, checking for cracks and splinters.

- Avoid cribs with ornate posts that have large crevices. Infants have strangled in

the concave space between the post and the crib. Shun cribs with decorative cutouts and knobs. A baby's clothes can get caught on these projections, causing strangulation. You can saw off the knobs and posts and sand the tops smooth.

- Check crib hardware for sharp points or edges, holes, or cracks where your baby's fingers could get pinched or stuck.

- Frequently check the mattress support system by rattling the metal hangers and by pushing the mattress on the top and then from the bottom. If the hanger support dislodges, it needs to be fixed or replaced. Be sure the four metal hangers supporting the mattress and support board are secured into their notches by safety clips.

- Resist hand-me-down or secondhand mattresses that may not fit your crib exactly. To check the fit of a crib mattress, push it into one corner. There should be no more than a one-and-one-half-inch (four-centimeter) gap between the mattress and the side or end of the crib. If you can fit more than two fingers between the mattress and the crib, the mattress is too small.

- Remember, the firmer the mattress, the safer.

- Make sure crib bumpers fit snugly around the entire perimeter of the crib and are secured by at least six ties or snaps. To prevent your baby from chewing on the straps and becoming entangled in them, trim off excess length. Remove bumpers and toys from the crib as soon as the child begins to pull himself or herself up on the crib rails, because they can be used as steps for climbing over the rail.

- Check crib toys, mobiles, pacifiers, and clothing worn in the crib to make sure they have no strings longer than eight inches (twenty centimeters).

- For the allergic infant or babies prone to a stuffy nose, avoid fuzzy animals and toys that can collect allergy-producing dust.

- Place the crib in a safe area in the room. It should not be against a window, near any dangling cords from blinds or draperies, or close to any furniture that the infant can use to climb out of the crib. When the baby gets older, give some thought to what could happen if your baby did climb out. The crib should be placed so that your baby will not fall against any sharp object or become entrapped or possibly strangled between the crib and an adjacent wall or piece of furniture.

- If your baby's crib is not in your bedroom or within hearing distance of every room in the house, buy a portable baby monitor — a valuable safety device.

Request pamphlets on crib safety by e-mailing the U.S. Consumer Product Safety Commission at publications@cpsc.gov or visit their website, www.cpsc.gov.

SAFE AND SANE CAR TRAVEL

How appropriate the bumper sticker is that reads, "If a mother's place is in the home, why am I always in the car?" Here are ways to make car travel safe and pleasant.

Rules for the Road

- Always wear a seat belt yourself and insist that all other passengers do so.

- Do not use an infant carrier or an infant seat in a car as a substitute for a car seat.

- Do not use an ordinary travel bed in a car as a substitute for a car seat.

- Do not strap two children or a parent and a child into one seat belt.

- Never let your baby ride in your arms while the car is moving. Avoid the temptation to not place baby in a car seat "because we're only traveling a few blocks."

- Do not leave the rear door of a hatchback or station wagon open. This lets in exhaust fumes, and dangerous objects may come through the open door in a crash.

- Do not allow children to play with sharp objects such as pencils or metal toys while

LOOK BEHIND YOUR CAR

In your haste to make an appointment, you rush into your car, jam it into reverse, and speed out the driveway, not realizing what or *who* could be lurking behind the car. Children love to play around cars. As a precaution, get into the habit of walking behind your car before entering; better yet, do a full-circle walkaround. As an added precaution, you can install an extended rearview mirror that increases your field of vision behind the car.

the car is moving. These objects become projectiles if a car stops suddenly.

- Watch those little fingers. Finger injuries often occur when parents close the door without paying attention to where the child's hand is. Children commonly grab the vertical doorframe in between the front and rear doors as they climb out of the car, often at the same time as the driver is closing his or her own front door. Get in the habit of pausing before you close any car door and checking where everyone's little hands are.

- Do not put groceries or loose potential projectiles next to baby in the car or even loose in the car. Put them in the trunk.

- Pregnant mothers should also use seat belts. Until your child is born, you are his or her "car seat." You are protecting two lives. Keep the lap belt below your uterus, across the pelvic bone, to avoid injury to your baby from the seat belt.

Air Bag Safety

Before air bags became standard, children could sit in the front seat safely, although the rear seat was considered safer. Now, however, air bags are standard in almost all new cars. Children under age twelve should never sit in the front seat if there is an air bag because of the risk of facial burns and severe or fatal neck injuries. Infants in car seats should never sit in the front seat with an air bag, even if in a rear-facing car seat. Some cars come with the option to deactivate the air bag. Although that makes the front seat safe for children, remember that the backseat is safer.

Choosing and Using a Car Seat

- Make baby's first ride a safe ride by purchasing and properly installing a car seat before taking baby home from the hospital.

- Decide where in the car to put your baby. The center of the rear seat is the safest place for baby. It is unsafe to have a child of any age in the front seat if there is an air bag. Even if there is no air bag in the front, the middle backseat is still the safest place for baby. Practically speaking, parents traveling alone with a child frequently take their eyes off the road or turn around to check that their child in the backseat is all right. Attach a mirror to the visor to easily view baby in the backseat. You may be tempted to put a rear-facing infant in the front seat, so you can better keep an eye on him. This is not recommended. If you are uncomfortable having your rear-facing infant out of your sight in the backseat, you may elect to place him in the front seat, *if there is no air bag.* Keep in mind, however, that while you may feel safer doing this because you can keep a closer eye on baby, this position in the car places baby at a slightly higher risk of injury if an accident occurs.

For children using a booster seat the safest place is the backseat restrained by a shoulder strap, even if this means sitting by a door. Many parents think that sitting in the middle backseat with a lap belt only is safer than sitting by a door with a shoulder belt. This is not true. Lap-only seat belts can be dangerous. A child restrained by a lap belt in the middle backseat is more likely to be injured during an accident than a child restrained by a shoulder belt beside a door.

- Use a car seat only in a seat that faces forward.

- Read the instructional manual for anchoring and attaching the seat belt correctly. Be sure your car seat can be used with the particular seat belts in your car. Pull the seat belt tight, then test its security by pulling the car seat forward. If you can easily tip it over, tighten or reposition. Use the locking clip (provided with newer car seats) if your car's shoulder/lap belt latch plate slides freely; otherwise the seat will not be anchored securely. Automatic seat belts will not safely anchor a car seat. Regularly inspect seat belts and connections for wear and tear. Also be sure the car seat fits in your car. The seats of some cars have such an unusual contour or slope that some car seats will not safely fit.

- Position the car seat at the correct angle. If the position is too upright, baby's head may plop forward; too far back and the car-seat back may not contain baby in the event of a crash. Some car seats come with a correct-position indicator.

- Support baby's wobbly head, especially in the first few months. You can use rolled-up towels, diapers, or commercially made car-seat inserts. A folded baby sling makes an ideal horseshoe-shaped head support for a tiny infant in a car seat.

- To avoid burning little skin, cover plastic or metal parts if the car has been sitting in the hot sun. Car-seat covers protect your infant's skin against hot or cold surfaces as well as cushioning baby.

- For cold weather, if you do not have a fitted car-seat cover, drape a blanket over the seat and cut holes in it for the harness strap and buckle to come through.

- Do not wear your baby in a cloth carrier in your car. Keep him in the car seat at all times. If baby is crying and hysterical, it is safer to pull off the road, stop, and comfort your baby rather than remove baby from the car seat.

- Be sure the seat belt straps are flat and not twisted.

- Position harness straps correctly. You should be able to only fit two fingers or fewer between the straps and baby. The chest clip that connects the two shoulder straps should be at armpit level.

- Be sure to adjust the car seat shoulder straps to a higher position as your baby grows taller, according to the manufacturer's guidelines.

- Five-point harness restraints (with straps over each shoulder, around the lap on both sides, and between the legs) are safer than three-point harnesses (with straps only over each shoulder and between the legs).

- Never use a lap-only seat belt. These significantly increase the chance of injury. Whatever stage your child is at, whether she is in a car seat or a booster seat or using a seat belt only, always use shoulder restraints.

- If your car seat is involved in a significant crash, buy a new one, even if the seat appears to be undamaged.

- Try before you buy. Be sure the car seat you have chosen can be properly installed in your car.

- The National Highway Traffic Safety Administration estimates that 80 percent of car seats are installed or used incorrectly. This means that four out of five people reading this may have their kids improperly restrained. Any local police

SETTLING TRAVELING TUMMIES

Motion sickness results from the brain's receiving confusing messages from the senses. For example, when your baby is buried in the backseat, his eyes see only the stationary seat back, but the motion sensors of the inner ear tell the brain the body is moving. The equilibrium center in the inner ear is more sensitive in some babies than others. Try these stomach settlers.

- Plan your route to use straight freeways: avoid going through busy towns. Frequent stops and starts and winding roads upset tiny tummies.

- Travel at nap time. Sleep settles queasy insides. The best time to depart is just before a nap, so you can hope to arrive at your destination with a comfortable and well-rested baby.

- Tank up baby, but not a full tank. Give baby a light meal before departure (nonfatty and nondairy foods — cereal, pasta, fruit), and take along stomach-friendly snacks: cookies, crackers, a cool drink in a carton with a straw.

- Tank up the car beforehand. Babies are sensitive to exhaust and fumes at gas stations.

- Provide a seat with a view — babies get carsick if they can't see out a window — but don't compromise safety for a view.

- Play games that keep baby focused on objects far away. Billboards, buildings, and mountains are much more tummy friendly during travel than close-up coloring books.

- Fresh air is a tummy rumble's best friend. Open a window on each side of the car for cross ventilation. Leave your air pollutants (cigarette smoke, perfumes) at home.

- Medications for motion sickness are not recommended under a year of age, but they may be used safely thereafter. Check first with your doctor in case there are medical reasons for your child not to take these. Dramamine is a safe and effective over-the-counter medication to quell the nausea, vomiting, and dizziness associated with motion sickness. The dosage for an infant from one to two years is a half-teaspoon, given one-half to one hour before travel; for the child two to three years the dosage is one teaspoon (five milliliters). It should not be given more frequently than once every six hours. Seasickness patches (Scopolamine) should not be used on infants.

station will provide a free car seat inspection. Visit one today.

- Let older children model "buckling up" for the toddler. Be sure they understand the nonnegotiable rule that the car does not start until all the buckles are snapped.

- If you're planning to use the car seat for plane travel, be sure your seat is certified for use in aircraft.

- If you are borrowing or buying a used car seat, check the label to be sure that it conforms to government safety standards.

- Choose a car seat appropriate for your child's age, weight, and height (see below).

Infants from Birth to Twenty Pounds (9 kilos)

Safety seats for this age and weight are rear facing and recline at an angle of forty-five degrees. With this design, most of the forward force of a collision is transferred to the seat belt holding the seat. The rear-facing, semiupright position allows the remaining force to be distributed throughout the baby's back to bones and muscles. Be sure to secure baby snugly in the seat with the safety harness. There are two types of starter car seats: infant seats and convertible seats.

Infant seats. These are tublike seats for infants weighing less than twenty pounds (nine kilograms); some have the added advantage of doubling as a carrier to transport a sleeping baby outside the car, and can be used as an infant seat inside the house. Infant car seats are designed only to be used in the rear-facing position.

One word of caution when using car seats with a detachable base: Infants can easily fall out of these when being carried if the handle is not locked in place. Several manufacturers have had to recall this type of car seat because of failures of the handle's locking mechanism. If you use this type of car seat/carrier, be sure to register your purchase with the manufacturer so you can be notified in the event of a recall.

Convertible car seats. Heavier, taller, and more expensive than the infant seat, convertible seats can be used from birth up to forty pounds (eighteen kilograms); so you do not have to buy a second car seat. But these are cumbersome. The weight and design of convertible seats make their use as an out-of-car transport seat impractical. And some of the convertible car seats seem too big for a baby under three months. Most manufacturers recommend you keep baby facing the rear until he reaches twenty pounds and one year of age. If the seat is turned forward too early in baby's development, his heavy, wobbly head could lurch forward. Rear facing is the safest position.

There are several different options for convertible car seats:

- five-point harness — safer, but more buckles to buckle up
- T-shield — more convenient (one buckle only) but only three points
- overhead shield — again, more convenient, and some come with a five-point harness.

One drawback of T-shields and overhead shields is that if baby is playing with a toy during a collision, the toy can injure baby's face as the force of the impact moves his head forward and down. Using these types of seats may mean sacrificing safety for convenience.

Be sure you are familiar with the height specifications for your car seat. If the top of your infant's *head extends higher than the back of the car seat,* it may be time to buy a larger one. Tall babies may outgrow their infant seat before they are one year or twenty pounds. Read your manual carefully, as this information will be different for every car seat.

Infants from Twenty to Forty Pounds (9 to 18 kilos) and One to Four Years

When baby reaches *both* one year of age *and* twenty pounds (nine kilos), it is time to change to a forward-facing position. If you have a large, convertible car seat that baby still fits in, continue to use this. If at this point you need a new seat, instead of buying a convertible type of seat that accommodates an infant as well, buy one that is for older infants only that will last you all the way to age four and beyond. Again, pay attention to the type of restraint system described above and decide which system is best for you. Keep in mind, five-point restraints are considered safer than the more convenient three-point restraints. Toddlers should remain in a car seat until they are *both* four years old *and* forty pounds (eighteen kilos).

Children from Forty to Eighty Pounds (18 to 36 kilos) and Four to Eight Years

It is recommended that children remain in a booster seat from four to eight years of age or until they reach eighty pounds. These booster seats come in two forms — a "bottom only" seat and a complete booster seat with a back. The car's shoulder and lap belt is used to restrain the child. Car seat laws vary from state to state. Some states currently have the eight years, eighty-pound requirement and some do not. Lawmakers are trying to make these guidelines nationwide. Automobile safety studies show clearly that children are safer in a shoulder-belted booster seat until they are either eight years old or weigh eighty pounds. I suggest parents follow this guideline.

There is also a new height guideline for booster seats: If a child reaches four feet nine inches before they are eight years old or eighty pounds, they should no longer use a booster seat.

New LATCH System for Car Seats

"LATCH" stands for Lower Anchors and Tethers for Children. New tether straps connect from the top and sides of the car seat to metal hooks anchored to the car behind and next to the car seat. Most cars built after 2001 are equipped with a top anchor, and most 2003 models have two sets of lower anchors in the back seat. Car seats made after 2001 come with tether straps that connect to both the top and lower anchor hooks, and some older car seats have a top tether strap. The new LATCH system secures the car seat instead of using seat belts. Follow the manufacturer's instructions carefully to make sure you are using this new system correctly.

SUMMARY OF CAR SEAT GUIDELINES

Rear-facing infant seats
- birth to age one *and* at least twenty pounds (9 kilos).

Forward-facing car seats
- Age one to age four *and* twenty to forty pounds (9 to 18 kilos)

Booster seats
- Age four to age eight *and* forty to eighty pounds *and* under four feet nine inches

Seat belts
- Over four feet nine inches tall, regardless of age and weight. A child taller than this is too tall for a seat belt to fit properly in a booster seat.

SAFETY GUIDELINES

These are the current safety guidelines at the time this book was published. For more information or updates on child-restraint safety guidelines, including car seat recalls, visit the NHTSA (National Highway Transportation Safety Administration) website, www.nhtsa.dotgov or call (888) 327-4236. For a list of child passenger safety seat inspection locations near you, go to www.seatcheck.org or call (866) 732-8243.

When Baby Protests the Car Seat

Develop a mind-set that car travel and a safety seat go together. This is nonnegotiable and without exception. If baby protests using the car seat, try the following tips.

- Some toddlers start to throw a fit as soon as they even approach the car. Give your toddler a snack to hold before you get to the car. He may concentrate on this, and before he even knows it, you'll have him buckled in and ready to go.

- For the toddler who screams hysterically no matter what you do, try to stay calm. Reassure him in a quiet voice as you gently secure him in the car seat. Give him the message that there really is no choice. Never let him think that fussing will make you change your mind about the car ride. He should come around soon.

- Make sure your toddler understands he should never undo the buckles of his car seat.

- If possible, time your car travel for when baby travels easiest. Some babies settle best early in the morning. Others do better traveling during nap time.

- Bring along a bag of soft toys such as a stuffed animal or toys that attach to the car seat. Cloth books are a winner.

- To solve the crying-baby-in-the-car-seat dilemma, travel with two adults in the car as often as possible. One adult sits in the back next to baby, the other adult drives.

- Avoid the urge to take baby out of the car seat and comfort him by feeding "just for a moment" while the car is moving.

- Have an older sibling sit next to baby in the backseat and entertain the car-seated baby during the trip.

- Sing songs to your baby and point out interesting sights that you pass by. We made up jingles that celebrated the safety issue ("buckle up for safety"). The unhappy child knew we understood her feelings, at least. And we'd usually get her to laugh.

- Play favorite tapes and have a few surprise tapes set aside for use in a pinch.

- Toddlers often get upset by not being able to see out the window. If this is the case, choose a car seat that props baby up high enough to learn from the outside moving world.

- Don't discount the value of a parent's voice chatting with the little traveler in the little seat. If you ignore the passenger, he has time to get bored and disgruntled.

Keeping Travel Pleasant

- Feed and toilet your toddler before the trip. A baby with dry pants and a full tummy is a more pleasant passenger.

- Treat travel like infant feeding: short, frequent trips rather than lengthy ones. When driving long distances, make frequent pit stops.

- Take along musical tapes, old favorites and new surprises. Start the tape right after buckling baby in and starting the car.

- Nonchokable nibbles, for example, rice cakes, may settle the hungry traveler. Do not allow the little rider to suck on anything with a stick, like a lollipop or popsicle. A swerve or an accident could jam the stick into baby's throat.

CYCLING WITH INFANTS

If you are a cycling family, you can safely take along the little cycler, but observe these rules of the road:

- Always put a helmet on the young passenger, even in a trailer or jogging cart.

- Do *not* carry infants under six months on a bicycle. They are unable to sit up and their heads may be too wobbly, especially with a helmet.

- Usually between nine months and a year infants are able to sit in a special child-carrier seat that is mounted over the rear wheel of an adult bicycle. Be sure to use the built-in safety harness and footrests that keep the child's feet away from the spokes.

- Ride only on bike paths or safe streets, not in busy traffic.

Teach children that helmets and wheels belong safely together. Whenever cycling with an infant in a carrier seat, pulling baby in a cart behind your bike, or even with your child's first sidewalk ventures on his tricycle, always use an approved safety helmet. If you teach your child the value of using a safety helmet at an early age, the head-protecting mind-set will grow up with him, making it a natural part of his life on wheels later on.

PLANTPROOFING YOUR HOME

You walk into your plant-adorned living room and see your toddler sucking on a leaf. Is it poisonous? Suddenly, you realize you don't know. Fearing the worst, you rush the baby to your local emergency room. The admitting nurse asks you why you came. You answer, "He ate a leaf." "What kind of leaf?" the nurse inquires. Embarrassed, you realize that in your haste you left the plant at home. You backtrack and now rush the plant to the emergency room. "What is it?" the nurse further inquires. Red-faced, you admit, "I don't know." The plant without a name is hurriedly circled around the emergency room staff, each person offering an "I thinks it's a . . . ," but no one is sure.

RECOMMENDED SHOPPING LIST FOR CHILD SAFETY PRODUCTS

- ☐ Car seat
- ☐ Safety latches for drawers and cabinets
- ☐ Cordless phone
- ☐ Safety plugs for electrical outlets
- ☐ Edge cushions for table corners, fireplace hearths
- ☐ Small-object testing tube
- ☐ Nonskid rugs

- ☐ Doorknob covers
- ☐ Cushioned covers for tub spout
- ☐ Stove knob covers
- ☐ Stairway gates
- ☐ Lid lock for toilet seats
- ☐ Guardrail that fits under adult mattress
- ☐ Intercom or baby monitor

- ☐ Netting for railings and balconies
- ☐ Tot-finder decals
- ☐ Screen guards
- ☐ Rubber stripping for stairs
- ☐ Flame-retardant sleepwear
- ☐ Fire extinguisher
- ☐ Smoke detectors

RESOURCES FOR BABYPROOFING YOUR HOME

The Perfectly Safe Catalog
5701 Mayfair Road
North Canton, OH 44720
(800) 898-3696; www.perfectlysafe.com

The Injury Prevention Program (TIPP).
Materials for accident-proofing your child's

environment. Available from the American Academy of Pediatrics. (800) 433-9016

The Family Guide to Car Seats. A helpful brochure listing all of the approved car seats. Available from the American Academy of Pediatrics at the above phone number.

RESOURCES FOR INFORMATION ABOUT CHILDHOOD POISONINGS

Baby-Safe Houseplants and Cut Flowers, by John I. and Delores M. Alber (Genus Books, 1991).

Handbook of Common Poisoning in Children. 2d ed. (American Academy of Pediatrics, 1983).

AMA Handbook of Poisonous and Injurious Plants, by Kenneth F. Lampe

and Mary Ann McCann (American Medical Association, 1985).

Regional poison control centers. Contact your local hospital or emergency medical system for the telephone number. Or call the nationwide poison control phone number, (800) 222-1222, to be connected to a center near you.

Know Your Plants

Understand what is meant by the term "poisonous plant." Many plants are poisonous, but some are more poisonous than others. Many plants are labeled "poisonous" when the only problems they cause are a sore mouth, an upset stomach, and vomiting with no lasting harm. Others may be fatal. Fortunately, the leaves of many toxic plants have such a bitter taste that babies seldom ingest a mouthful. When purchasing a plant, be sure the name tag is attached and leave it attached. Ask a knowledgeable person whether or not the plant is poisonous and, if so, how poisonous. If the plant has no name and no information on toxicity, don't buy it. If given or giving a plant, leave the identification tag attached. If you're the recipient, ask where the plant was purchased. Check out your leafy friend before admission to the family. If the plant has no tag, take a sample cutting to a nursery for identification.

➤ *SAFETY TIP: Some plants are so toxic that they should not be allowed in the house or yard — oleander, for example. Others may be only mildly harmful and may be safely kept out of reach. Be aware, however, that "out of reach" implies that children can't climb up to the top shelf, which they can, and that leaves don't fall to the toddler at floor level, which they do.*

Teach Your Child Not to Eat House and Garden Plants

While you can make your own home plant safe, homes you visit may not be so child centered. For example, grandmother may now adorn her house with all the plants she loves but couldn't have when you were a child because they aren't safe. By two years of age children can comprehend the meaning of such precautions as "hot," "hurt," "owie," "make sick." But don't rely on baby to remember your mouth-off-plants policy. Supervision is still the only prevention.

If Your Baby Eats a Plant

Even if your baby eats only a leaf, follow these steps.

Check baby. Check baby's hands and mouth for plant pieces — clues to whether or not baby ate a piece of plant. Oftentimes the bitter taste of the leaves prompts baby to immediately spit out the leaf without ingesting any. Check the hands, eyes, and lips for redness or blistering. Check the tongue and inside the mouth for cuts, redness, blistering, or swelling.

Check the plant. If uncertain which plant in the house baby sampled, ask your child to show you his "favorite" and, after you get his confidence, "which one you ate." Don't act scared or tentative, or baby will clam up. If still uncertain, examine the most reachable plants; look for broken leaves, spilled dirt, or any signs of child tampering.

Call poison control. If the plant is suspicious or poisonous, call your poison control center. When calling, give the full botanical name of the plant from the tag, or as much as you know. Take the plant or a sample cutting with you to the phone to offer a description. If the plant is definitely poisonous, the poison control center may advise you to give your baby ipecac syrup and juice or water immediately (see page 734 for instructions).

Take your child and the plant to the emergency room. When still uncertain but suspicious, take your *child and plant* to the emergency room. If you aren't sure what the plant is, it is best, if possible, to have someone take a plant cutting to a nearby nursery for identification while you go to the hospital. Have your associate phone the emergency room with the plant information while you're en route, if you are not already there. Except for causing a sore throat, nausea, vomiting, and a sore stomach, plants rarely are seriously toxic within minutes. The safest place, however, to be when in doubt is at your hospital emergency room.

Poisonous plants resource: See www. AskDr.Sears.com for a list of worry and no-worry plants.

ENVIRONMENTAL POLLUTANTS: GETTING THE LEAD OUT

Lead poisoning from eating lead-based paint chips resulted in a government ban on lead-based paint in 1978. Painted homes built after 1980 are required by law to use lead-free paint. So the problem should be over. Not so. While the signs of lead poisoning have long been recognized, recent research has shown that even small levels of lead in a child's blood may cause subtle developmental delays and behavioral problems or even brain damage. Lead is now dubbed "the silent hazard."

What Lead Does

This toxic material enters the bloodstream, and the body, mistaking it for calcium, welcomes it into vital cells such as those in bone marrow, the kidneys, and the brain, where it interferes with the enzymes necessary for these organs to function normally. Lead poisoning shows these features:

- colicky abdominal pain
- constipation, diminished appetite
- hyperirritability
- paleness from anemia
- growth delay
- developmental delay
- poor attention span
- convulsions

How Lead Gets In

Children do not get lead poisoning from chewing on pencils. Pencil paint is non-leaded, and the "lead" is harmless graphite. The lead that poisons children comes from old paint, gasoline emissions, contaminated soil, contaminated water, and lead pottery. Candy imported from third world countries may contain lead.

Getting the Lead Out

Look for the following high-risk sources of lead in your child's environment, and follow our suggestions to reduce the risk. Note, too, that children with nutritional deficiencies of iron, calcium, and zinc are more susceptible to lead poisoning, another example of how good nutrition is preventive medicine.

Old paint chips. Even though houses and apartments painted after 1980 should, by law,

COMMON NONHARMFUL OR MILDLY HARMFUL HOUSEHOLD SUBSTANCES

Accidental ingestion of the following does not usually require treatment. *Caution: This list is meant only as a guide. Consult your physician or poison control center for more information.*

antacids
antibiotics (if only a few tablets or teaspoons)
baby shampoo and lotion
bath oil
bath soap
blusher
bubble bath
calamine lotion
candles
caps (for toy pistols)
chalk
cigarettes[1]
cologne
cosmetics[2]
crayons[3]
dehumidifier packet
deodorant

deodorizers
detergent[4]
Elmer's glue
eye makeup
fabric softener
fishbowl additives
glue and paste
hand lotion and cream
incense
ink (markers and pens)
kitty litter
laxatives
lipstick
Lysol disinfectant (not toilet bowl cleaner)
makeup
matches

mercury from a broken thermometer
modeling clay
mouthwash[5]
oral contraceptives
pencil lead
petroleum jelly (Vaseline)
Play-Doh
putty and Silly Putty
shampoo
shaving cream
suntan preparations
sweetening agents
thyroid tablets
vitamins with or without fluoride[6]
zinc oxide

[1]*Although one cigarette theoretically contains enough nicotine to be toxic, ingested tobacco is not easily absorbed from the intestines. The child frequently vomits and gets rid of much of the tobacco.*

[2]*Most cosmetics are generally not harmful. However, permanent wave neutralizer and fingernail polish are extremely harmful. Even inhaling fumes from nail polish as it is being applied may be harmful to a child.*

[3]*Crayons labeled "AP," "CP," or "CS 130–46" are nontoxic.*

[4]*Most household laundry detergents, cleansers, and dish detergents are not toxic. However, bleaches, ammonias, toilet bowl cleaners, and automatic dishwasher granules and liquids are highly toxic.*

[5]*Mouthwash contains a large amount of alcohol and therefore can harm a child if ingested in large quantities.*

[6]*Iron and fluoride in vitamins may be toxic if ingested in large amounts.*

have lead-free paint, older homes and renovated homes may have new paint over old. Paint chips containing some of the old paint are inviting to the child who likes to mouth tiny pieces of anything. Even more toxic is the *lead dust* created from friction on paint chippings in areas of wear like windowsills, door frames, and baseboards. A lead-based paint chip the size of a postage stamp may contain ten thousand times the safe level of lead if eaten by a child. Exploring little hands wipe along the window ledge and suck the toxic lead dust off their fingertips. And ingesting only a few specks of this dust or a chip a day all during infancy can cause lead poisoning. To remove old paint dust from windowsills and other areas of wear, wipe with a high-phosphate detergent.

Renovation projects. If you are having an old home renovated, be sure the contractor knows how to thoroughly remove all the old paint residue. Also, keep your child out of the house during paint-stripping time. Following renovation, rent a HEPAvac (high-efficiency particulate-air-filtered vacuum) to remove leaded paint dust from the renovated area. Pay particular attention to old porches, which are notorious for providing millions of tiny flakes and paint dust for sticky little fingers.

Contaminated water. If you drink water from a well or live in an older home where pipes may have been soldered with lead, have your tap water tested by an EPA-certified laboratory or your local water department if it provides such a service. For information on how to get your water tested for lead, call the EPA safe drinking water hotline, (800) 426–4791, or visit www.epa.gov/safewater.

If your tap water is high in lead, in addition to replacing the plumbing, if that is a possibility, use cold water for cooking (hot water removes more of the lead from the pipes), use bottled water for drinking and cooking, and obtain a water filter that is proven to remove lead.

Water drawn from the tap first thing in the morning has the greatest lead concentration. This is important to know since many parents prepare a daily supply of formula in the morning. If your pipes are suspicious or your water has been proven to contain lead, run the cold water for at least two minutes to flush out the pipes before using the tap water to prepare formula.

Polluted air. If you live downwind from highways or major intersections, test your child's lead level at least a couple of times a year if moving is not an option.

Contaminated soil. Discourage your child from mouthing soil, especially if you live in renovated areas where old buildings have been torn down.

Other sources and precautions. Newsprint used to contain lead, but newer inks are lead-free and considered nontoxic, so parents don't have to worry about baby's mouthing newspapers and magazines. Avoid storing food or liquid in lead crystal or imported ceramics. And don't forget old toys and furniture that may be family heirlooms. As a final point, pregnant women and breastfeeding women should be especially vigilant to avoid exposure to lead. Pregnancy is not the time to strip the old paint from baby's future nursery, as the lead could pass from mother's bloodstream into the fetus. Before buying a home or renting an apartment, have the paint and water checked for lead content.

Testing Your Child for Lead

If your child has any of the above exposure risks, mention them to your doctor, who may order a blood lead test. In high-risk areas baby should be routinely tested at twelve and twenty-four months. Because of the recent finding that even low levels of lead can cause subtle developmental delay, the blood level at which a child may be at risk for damage is being lowered, from twenty-five micrograms per deciliter to ten micrograms.

The Treatment of Lead Poisoning

Treatment of lead poisoning (injecting medicines into the child's bloodstream to remove the lead) is expensive, painful, and cannot remove all of the lead. Some effects are irreversible. Prevention is the answer. Though environmentalists give much attention to preserving the wildlife in our forests, perhaps the most endangered species is the children in our cities.

26

Keeping Your Baby Healthy

Two facts of parenting life are that babies get sick and parents worry. How frequently and severely a baby gets ill depends primarily upon the baby's susceptibility to illness, not on your parenting. But there are basic things you can do to lessen your baby's chances of getting sick and to speed recovery when your baby does become ill. Here's how to begin your medical partnership with your doctor.

HEALTH MAINTENANCE BEGINS AT HOME

Learning to read your *well* baby helps you more intuitively recognize and help your sick baby. The attachment style of parenting really helps you shine in detecting and treating a sick child. A sensitive response to your baby's cries, and the hours of holding and nursing, all increase your ability to read your baby. You develop a feel for your baby when she is well so that you are instinctively alerted at the first sign of illness: "She's acting different," or "Her cries are different, I know she hurts somewhere." It's not as important to know *what's* wrong as it is to know *something's* wrong.

Becoming Dr. Mom and Dr. Dad

One of the most intuitive parents in my practice was a totally blind mother, Nancy. Because she could not see her baby, she went completely by sound and feel. Her baby got various skin rashes that caused her to frequent my office. Early in our rash-diagnosing challenge, Nancy brought baby Eric in for a rash I couldn't see. But mother said, "I feel it." Sure enough, the next day I could see it. Another intuitive mother told me that she could detect when her baby's throat was hurting because "I can feel she sucks differently." And another attachment mother once told me how she could tell her baby was beginning an ear infection because her baby did not want to put her head down and breast-feed on that side. This deep sensitivity to their babies earn these mothers an honorary degree of *Dr. Mom.*

Attached mothers and trusting babies help the doctor, too. Over the years of examining well and sick babies I have noticed that babies who are the product of responsive parenting radiate an attitude of trust, especially when they are ill. They are so used to getting their needs met that when they are ill, they trust that the doctor will make them well. They protest less during examinations, resulting in less wear and tear on the doctor and the baby. It seems that these babies operate from some inner trust that tells them that the doctor who puts a stick in their mouth, pokes their tummy, and shines the light in their ear is really on their side. And baby's cooperative trust helps the doctor make a more accurate diagnosis. For example, a screaming baby can cause a reddened eardrum and a confusing ear exam.

A close parent-infant attachment makes it easier for parents to care for the sick child. Many illnesses in infancy fall into the category of "I don't know what's wrong with your baby, so let's wait a day or two and see what changes occur." Take for example the baby who has a fever of unknown origin — FUO. (Or, as my former professor of pediatrics used to chide, "failure to uncover the obvious.") In this case I tell the parents that I suspect that this is just a harmless virus and their baby will get better in a few days, but "call me if the symptoms change." That last admonition is loaded. I am, in effect, releasing the sick baby to Dr. Mom and Dr. Dad and trusting that they will report back if their baby's condition worsens. But what are the credentials of these home doctors? They are sensitive to their baby, they can read their baby's cues, and they have such an intuitive feel for their baby that they almost hurt where their baby hurts. This sick baby is in good hands.

Good Food Promotes Good Health

Putting the right food into your baby can help keep the wrong germs out. The relation between good food and good health has received much press for adults, but it's even more important for babies. Most noteworthy of these nutritional advances is the return to breastfeeding, especially breastfeeding well into the toddler years, when babies contract the most illnesses. Breast milk is good medicine primarily in two ways: It lessens allergies, and it reduces infections. For example, when a breastfed baby gets a diarrhea illness, or intestinal infection, inflamed intestines may not tolerate formula but welcome breast milk. Breastfed babies suffer fewer diarrhea illnesses, especially the more severe illnesses requiring hospitalization, than their formula-fed friends. Breastfeeding has kept many babies out of hospitals. When a formula-fed baby has a severe diarrhea illness, it is usually necessary to stop or dilute the formula for a few days. This plus the fact that some babies refuse to take a bottle when sick requires that some babies be hospitalized for dehydration from the diarrhea. Seldom so the breastfed baby who usually continues to feed avidly when sick. It is *rarely* necessary or advisable to stop breastfeeding during a diarrhea episode.

Not only does breast milk help keep babies healthy, it keeps them comfortable. The comforting effects of baby's favorite pacifier are welcome when he is sick or hurting. And the mothering hormones stimulated by sucking help Dr. Mom give added tender loving care.

Separate Babies and Germs

Within reason and practicality, don't let germs and babies play together. While no baby can grow up in a germ-free bubble, you can avoid unnecessary exposure to germ-carrying kids. Infectious diarrhea and colds

SMOKING AND BABIES DON'T MIX

What happens to babies when they are exposed to cigarette smoke? Here are some shocking figures that should help you kick the habit forever. Babies and children who are exposed to cigarette smoke have a much higher incidence of pneumonia, asthma, ear infections, bronchitis, sinus infections, eye irritation, and croup. If that is not enough to help convince you to take your last puff, try this tragic statistic: Babies of smoking mothers and fathers have a seven times greater chance of dying from sudden infant death syndrome. If you still feel you can afford to smoke, try this statistic: Children of smoking parents have two to three times more visits to the doctor, usually from respiratory infections or allergy-related illnesses. Also, if you want to raise a healthy heart, children who are exposed to passive smoke in the home have lower blood levels of HDL, the good cholesterol that helps protect against coronary artery disease. Consider as well some long-term effects. Children of smoking parents are more likely to become smokers themselves. And a recent study found that growing up in a home in which two parents smoked could double the child's risk of lung cancer later in life.

are the two most commonly shared illnesses. If your baby's playmates have these contagious illnesses, your home should be off limits to them until they are no longer contagious. Require your baby's place of day care to enforce strict rules about potentially contagious children playing with healthy children. Ditto other places where bunches of babies play together, such as church nurseries.

Clear the Air

Contaminated air (pollutants and cigarette smoke) irritates baby's sensitive breathing passages, which rebel by secreting mucus. Germs love to bathe in the secretions in the nose, sinuses, and airways. Also, avoid household pollutants (perfumes, hair sprays, exhaust fumes, dust from remodeling) if your baby is sensitive to nasal irritants.

WELL-BABY CHECKUPS

Besides attachment parenting, good nutrition, healthy playmates, and clean air, another way to improve your baby's health is to follow your doctor's schedule for well-baby exams. Here's the schedule we use in our office, similar to the one advised by the American Academy of Pediatrics:

- monthly for the first six months for first-born babies; every other month for the first six months for subsequent babies
- at nine, twelve, fifteen, eighteen, and twenty-four months
- yearly thereafter

Well-baby exams are good for baby and for parents. During these exams expect to discuss:

- growth and development at each stage
- good nutrition
- preventive medicine and accident prevention

And to have:

- immunizations
- a thorough exam to detect normal or abnormal development
- height, weight, head measurements
- periodic lab tests: hemoglobin for anemia and urinalysis
- hearing and vision evaluations (when necessary)
- questions answered about parenting
- help with specific medical problems

During these checkups, besides helping you and your baby, your doctor grows in his or her knowledge of your well child — a useful reference point for when your child is sick. The current system of well-baby care is the best medical bargain around. Consider what your family gets for around six hundred dollars the first year (at this writing the average well-baby cost for a year, excluding laboratory tests and shots): access to your doctor twenty-four hours a day year-round, telephone consultation when needed, a hands-on feel for your baby's growth and development, and early detection of illnesses or abnormalities that, if undetected, may have lifelong consequences. Well-baby checkups are a wise investment in family health.

Getting the Most out of Your Doctor's Appointment

To get the maximum benefit from your time with the doctor, both parents should plan to attend. Many doctors offer extended hours to accommodate employed parents.

Before you go, make a list of the questions and problems you wish to discuss. It's a good

---

TELEPHONE COMMUNICATION TIPS

- Respect your doctor's time with his or her own family by limiting after-hours calls to especially worrisome situations in which you fear your baby will get worse before your doctor's office reopens.

- Have your pharmacy's phone number ready.

- Be prepared to communicate accurately your child's illness: when and how it began; if it has gotten better, worse, or is the same; what treatments you have tried and the response; how worried you are; and, above all, *how sick your child seems*. Your doctor must offer a medical opinion based only on your description.

- If you feel your doctor is not appreciating the seriousness of your concerns, repeat your concerns. I find the most direct approach is best: "Doctor, my child seems very sick, I'm very worried, and I would like him examined."

- Be sure you understand your doctor's phone advice and write it down.

- Don't hesitate to *call back* if your child gets seriously worse.

idea to memorize the list, as you may accidentally leave it at home. If you have an especially worrisome or complicated concern, such as a behavioral problem, request an "extended visit" when making an appointment. Respect the fact that your doctor allots the usual amount of time for each scheduled checkup in order to be on time for the other patients.

There is in every intuitive mother an inner warning light that flashes, "I know something is wrong with my baby and I'm going to keep after the doctor until the cause is found." With vague signs and symptoms (for example, colicky behavior, unexplained fevers, tiredness, poor weight gain) your doctor may not be able to pinpoint the exact cause of the problem, especially on the first office visit. Be sure to convey your degree of concern to the doctor, who is trying to decide how extensively to investigate your child's illness. You are a valuable part of the medical team. The intensity of your worry is often just what is needed to help the doctor make a judgment to further investigate your child.

Making Checkups Easier on Everybody

Trying to examine a screaming child is wearing on baby, parents, and doctor and makes a precise exam next to impossible. Here's how to help. Remember, you mirror the state of the world to your baby. If you are apprehensive, baby is likely to share your anxiety. Avoid worry-producing statements such as "The doctor won't hurt you" or "The shot will only hurt a little." The child may only perceive the word "hurt" and the very thought relates hurting with the doctor — an association that mushrooms into an all-out scene even before you sign in. Make a good first impression. Greet the doctor cheerfully. Carry on a "We're glad to be here" conversation before the exam begins. According to child's logic, if doctor is OK to you, he or she is OK to the child. If your child clings to you like Velcro at the first sight of the doctor, immediately put on your happy face. Rather than reinforcing the cling by holding your child even tighter (this tells the child there really is something to be afraid of but mommy will rescue her), loosen your grip so the child will loosen hers. Finally, request (if this is not already your doctor's custom) that your baby remain on your lap, at least during the initial part of the exam. I have found that this yields a more thorough exam and creates less wear and tear on everybody.

IMMUNIZATIONS: WHY, WHAT, AND WHEN

Next on our keep-healthy list is one of the most important public health benefits — immunizations, or "baby shots." First, I wish to clear up the confusion that the media have "injected" into vulnerable parents who wish to do the best for their baby and yet receive conflicting advice about immunizations. Parents face the dilemma of wanting to vaccinate their babies for fear of baby getting the disease, but are afraid baby may have a bad reaction to the shot. Here is a general overview of vaccines and the illnesses they prevent, as well as a discussion of side effects and other concerns about vaccinations.

How do vaccines work? A vaccine is made from parts of the disease's germ itself or a changed germ, and it stimulates the body to produce antibodies to the germ without causing the disease. If the real germ enters the

RECOMMENDED CHILDHOOD IMMUNIZATIONS

The following is a list of the 2002 immunizations recommended by the American Academy of Pediatrics and a brief explanation of their corresponding illnesses.

DTaP	*Diphtheria*, a severe respiratory illness that is extremely rare in the United States, but not uncommon in third world countries.
	Tetanus, a disease that causes paralysis when a deep, dirty wound is allowed to fester.
	Pertussis, or whooping cough, a respiratory illness that causes severe coughing fits lasting several weeks. In young infants it can be life threatening. It is an uncommon illness, even in the United States. The little "a" in DTaP stands for *acellular,* a newer form of the vaccine, which is less reactive than the older DPT vaccine.
DT or dT	The DTaP vaccine, but without the pertussis. It is used as a booster for older children and adults.
Hepatitis (Hep B)	A virus that causes severe and potentially lifelong liver damage and occasionally liver cancer. Transmitted by sexual contact, prolonged intimate contact, and exposure to infected blood through needles, it is very rare in infants and children. An infected mom can pass it to her newborn at the time of delivery.
Hib	Hemophilus Influenza B, which causes meningitis and blood infections. These conditions are now rare due to the vaccination.
Polio (IPV)	A virus that can sometimes cause paralysis. No cases have occurred in the United States for twenty years, and most other developed countries are also polio free. Polio still occurs in Africa and parts of Asia. Note that the older oral form of this vaccine is no longer used in many developed countries because it can very rarely cause polio. The injected form does not cause polio.
MMR	*Measles,* a rarely fatal virus that causes a rash, fever, and severe cough. It is fairly rare in the United States and other developed countries.
	Mumps, a virus that causes fever, tonsillitis, swollen cheek glands, and a rash. In older children and adults it can cause sterility and, very rarely, can be fatal.
	Rubella, or German measles, a virus that causes fever and a rash. Virtually harmless to infants and children, it can, however, cause birth defects if a nonimmune pregnant woman is exposed to it.

(continued)

Chicken Pox (Varicella)	A virus that causes fever and blistery spots. It is fatal in only about one in seventy thousand cases. Since the vaccine's introduction in the early 1990s, reported cases have decreased about 75 percent.
Pneumococcus (Prevnar)	A bacterium that causes meningitis, pneumonia, and blood infections. It is not a rare disease and is responsible for hundreds to thousands of deaths in the United States each year. This is a new vaccine, and since its release in 2000 the number of reported pneumococcus cases is already declining.
Hepatitis A (Hep A)	A very different disease from Hepatitis B, Hep A is a virus that causes mild flu symptoms, mild inflammation of the liver, and yellow skin in infants and children, with virtually no long-term effects. It can be more severe in teenagers and adults. It is transmitted through contaminated food or water. The vaccine is not recommended for all kids. It is optional in high-risk areas.
TB skin test	This is not actually a vaccine. It is a test used to determine if someone was ever exposed to tuberculosis (a serious lung infection) and has the germ living quietly in their body.

body, baby then already has antibodies against the germ and doesn't get the illness, or he may get only a mild form of the disease. Sometimes the effects of the vaccine wear off, requiring a booster shot to restimulate the body to keep the antibodies coming.

Vaccine Reactions

Many infants will not have any observable side effects from vaccinations. Some, however, will experience an adverse reaction. In most cases reactions are mild.

Common Vaccine Reactions. Here are the most commonly seen side effects that may occur after any of the shots. There is gener-

ally no need to call your doctor for these mild reactions.

- Fever. It is not uncommon to have a fever of around 101°F (38.3°C) for a day or two after a vaccination. It is also not unusual to have a fever as high as 103°F (39.5°C). This is generally not a cause for concern.

- Redness and swelling at the injection site. Some infants will have slight redness or mild swelling where the injection was given. Some will have a larger area of redness and swelling the size of one or two silver dollars. This too is OK.

- Fussiness or sleepiness. Infants may show one of either extreme for one or two days. This is not a cause for concern as long as

IMMUNIZATION SCHEDULE FOR 2002

This is the 2002 immunization schedule recommended by the American Academy of Pediatrics. Since these schedules may change and new vaccines may be added, consult your doctor or our website, www.AskDrSears.com, for the most up-to-date information.

Immunizations usually coincide with well-baby checkups. The recommended schedule calls for up to four injections at one time. Some doctors may give only two shots at a time and have you come back between checkups for "shot only" visits to catch up. Combination vaccines (combined DTaP, IPV, and Hib, for example) are being developed to decrease the number of injections. If your child misses a shot in a series, there is no need to begin the series all over, even if several years have passed. Any of the vaccines may be given simultaneously without increasing the risk of side effects.

Age	Immunization
Birth	Hep B
1 month	Hep B
2 months	DTaP, Hib, IPV, Prevnar
4 months	DTaP, Hib, IPV, Prevnar
6 months	DTaP, Hib, Prevnar, Hep B
12 months	MMR, Varicella
15 months	Hib, Prevnar
18 months	DTaP, IPV
2 years	Hep A (optional)
3 years	Hep A (second dose)
5 years	MMR, DTaP, IPV
15 years	dT

This schedule is not set in stone. Your doctor may use a variation of this schedule. Most shots do not have to be given at the exact age or time interval above. The shots may be spread out over a longer period of time at the parent's and doctor's discretion. The Hep B shot, for example, may be delayed until two months, then repeated at four months and nine months. The schedule may be altered somewhat, especially with the new combo vaccines.

your infant is consolable and arousable periodically.

- Lump at injection site. It is common to feel a marble-size, firm lump for up to several months. This is a small calcified bruise within the muscle, and it is harmless.

More Serious Vaccine Reactions. Rarely, an infant experiences a more severe reaction to a vaccine. Here is how to recognize a

---

TAKING THE STING OUT OF SHOTS

To lessen shot fears, hold baby securely on your lap or against your chest; offer a momentary massage to relax baby's leg or arm (relaxed muscles hurt less during an injection). Don't act anxious yourself. Shot fears are contagious, especially from mother to baby. Applying an ice pack just before the shot can numb the site. After the injection is given, immediately *distract* baby with a toy or a cheerful gesture and words, such as "Bye-bye, doctor!"

---

reaction that should be reported to your doctor right away.

- High fever of 105°F (40.6°C).

- Extreme, inconsolable, high-pitched continuous crying for three or more hours.

- Lethargy. This means that your infant is difficult to arouse and is less responsive to stimulation than usual.

- Convulsions. These are extremely rare but warrant immediate medical attention.

Any of these four reactions can indicate that the vaccine has caused a condition called encephalitis, or inflammation of the brain. This is not an infection (like meningitis), is not treatable, and usually resolves without any long-term effects. If such a reaction occurs, your doctor will discuss with you whether the suspected vaccine should be repeated in the future.

Vaccine-specific Reactions

There are a few reactions that occur only after a specific vaccine.

- MMR. One to two weeks following vaccination, approximately 5 percent of infants experience a rash, fever, or swollen glands that may last a few days. Less commonly, joint pain and stiffness may occur for a few days. The child is not contagious during these harmless reactions, and they resolve within several days.

- Varicella (chicken pox). Some children experience flu-like symptoms for several days after vaccination. This can occur right away or may take several weeks to appear. Only rarely, a child may get a mild case of minimally contagious chicken pox following the shot.

Treating Vaccine Reactions

If your infant or child has a reaction, try the following to ease the discomfort:

- Give acetaminophen or ibuprofen for pain or fever (see pages 657–660 for dosage). One is not necessarily any better than the other. You can safely give these medications for a few days if needed. Some doctors recommend giving a dose before a shot to minimize the reactions. Others feel you should just wait and see if your infant reacts, then give the medicine if necessary. Since most infants do not have the severe reactions that used to be more common, it may be better to wait and see how your child does. If your child does tend to get a fever after a vaccination, then you can routinely pretreat for subsequent shots.

- Use other fever-reducing methods (see page 655).

- Apply an ice pack to the swollen, red injection site.

Vaccine Myths and Controversies

Some well-meaning parents take the time to do research over the Internet and read literature about the safety of vaccines. Unfortunately, there is a lot of misinformation circulated about the dangers of vaccines, such as that vaccines don't work, vaccines cause brain damage, a child can actually get the disease from the vaccine, vaccines cause autism — the list goes on. Here is a brief explanation of some of these myths and misconceptions:

A child can get paralytic polio from the polio vaccine.

This is one myth that actually used to be true. The old oral polio vaccine that is no longer routinely used in the United States caused paralysis in around nine American infants each year. For this reason, doctors switched to using only the injectable polio vaccine in the late 1990s, which does not cause this side effect. With the oral form, it was also possible, though rare, for another person to catch polio from a vaccinated infant's stools. The injectable polio does not have this risk either.

The pertussis part of the DTP vaccine can cause brain damage.

There is a great deal of misinformation in the general public regarding the safety of the pertussis component of this vaccine. All this bad press is due to the older "whole cell" pertussis vaccine that is no longer being used in the United States. This older vaccine caused more severe reactions in a higher percentage of kids than most other vaccines do. With the older vaccine there were reports of encephalitis (see above, under "More Serious Vaccine Reactions") occurring after this vaccine, as well as seizures and shock. Rarely, a small number of children were severely disabled after such events. It has never been proven that the vaccine was responsible for these reactions, but the medical community was suspicious enough that in the mid 1990s doctors in the United States stopped using this vaccine. Instead, the newer *acellular* form of the pertussis DTaP vaccine is now being used everywhere in the United States. Many components of the cell of the pertussis bacterium that were most reactive have been removed from the vaccine. Severe reactions to this safer vaccine are now extremely rare, and most infants experience no side effects at all. Some countries around the world stopped using the DPT or DTaP vaccine due to public fears and immediately saw a resurgence of whooping cough and an increase in deaths from the disease. This has prompted them to start using the vaccine again.

Vaccines cause autism.

This controversy mainly involves the MMR vaccine. A researcher in England found that many children with autism had the measles virus present in the lining of their intestines. He speculated that this may have come from the vaccine and that this was a contributing factor to the autism. In addition, there has been an increasing number of children with autism in recent decades, coinciding with the introduction of some vaccines. Medical investigators who have studied the research surrounding this issue have not been able to find evidence that the measles vaccine causes autism. It is known that many factors, including heredity, environmental contaminants, and nutrition, among others, contribute to autism. The American Academy of Pediatrics, the U.S. Advisory Committee on Immunization Practices, and the FDA continue to review all available research and conduct detailed studies, and to date they have found no evidence that the MMR vaccine causes autism.

Vaccines don't always work.

This is actually true. However, no one has ever claimed that vaccines are effective 100 percent of the time. Most vaccines provide between 80 percent and 95 percent protection. This means that if one hundred vaccinated people are exposed to a disease, between five and twenty of them will catch it. This is much better than all the people catching the illness. This high level of protection ensures that these diseases will not run rampant through our population. Also, if a vaccinated child does get the illness, it is likely to be much less severe than if the child had not been vaccinated.

Vaccines contain mercury.

This was true until 2001. The FDA realized that, while the miniscule amount of mercury in each vaccine was probably harmless, the cumulative amount of mercury in all the vaccines given over the first two years of life may be too much. This caused a big media scare (and probably rightly so) and prompted vaccine manufacturers to take the mercury out of almost all the vaccines. A few brands still have mercury in them, but the vast majority do not. Ask your doctor to give your child mercury-free vaccines.

Risks and Benefits of Vaccines

Every vaccine — for that matter every foreign substance (even a new food) that is put into the body — carries both risks and benefits. When evaluating any medicine or vaccine, we need to weigh the benefits against the risks.

Nearly all vaccines have a low risk-to-benefit ratio, meaning that the risk is small compared with the benefits. There are several vaccines that are no longer used because the benefits no longer outweigh the risks now that there are safer alternatives, such as the oral polio and the whole cell pertussis vaccines. Another example is the smallpox vaccine. This was discontinued in the 1970s because smallpox was virtually eradicated, and the vaccine itself was causing some very serious illnesses.

The present vaccine schedule carries very little risk. The benefits of preventing these diseases, all of which are potentially fatal, far outweigh the tiny risk of the vaccines. It is easy to forget about a disease when we don't live with it anymore. Nearly every grandparent who grew up in the prevaccine era can remember some child lying in an iron lung, suffering from polio. As an intern in pediatrics, I often encountered the seal-like sounds and barking coughs of very ill babies in the whooping cough ward. Vivid in my memory are the babies with brain damage from measles encephalitis before the measles vaccine. And let's not forget the babies with birth defects from their mothers' exposure to German measles during pregnancy. We don't have many of these villains with us anymore, thanks to vaccines.

Contraindications to Vaccination

While immunizations are safe for most infants and children, there are certain circumstances in which the risk of a vaccine is greater than the risk of catching the illness itself.

Here are situations in which your child should absolutely not receive a particular vaccine.

- If your child had encephalopathy following a previous vaccination. This is a more severe form of encephalitis (described above), in which the person is in a coma-like state, completely unresponsive, and may have continuous seizures. This can last for hours or even days. This has occurred only rarely in children around the time of a vaccination, and a causal relationship with the vaccine has not been found. Yet it's still wise to avoid the vaccine in the future.

- If your child had a severe allergic reaction (moderate to severe hives, wheezing, or difficulty breathing) following a vaccination.

- If your child is known to be allergic to one of the vaccine ingredients.

Here are some situations in which you and your doctor should discuss whether or not to give a particular vaccine. You must weigh the risk of the disease for your child's age against the risk of a repeated reaction and strongly consider not repeating the vaccine if any of the following occurred.

- Encephalitis following a previous vaccination.

- Convulsions following a previous vaccination. This used to be considered an absolute contraindication, but it is not anymore.

- Your child has a particular immune deficiency.

- Any other reaction that you or your doctor consider to be severe.

Here are some conditions that used to be contraindications, but are now considered safe for vaccination:

- Stable seizure disorder.

- Egg allergy. You can now give the MMR vaccine safely even if your child is allergic to eggs.

Vaccinating Under Special Circumstances

If Baby Has a Cold

If your baby is scheduled to receive a vaccine but has a mild cold without a fever and is not sick, he may safely get a vaccine. Deferring vaccines because of minor illnesses and catching up later is unnecessary and unwise. Some babies have colds so frequently during the first two years that they never catch up on their shots if they are postponed. If, on the other hand, your baby has a bad cough, green mucus from the nose, recent vomiting, moderate to severe diarrhea, and especially a fever, and is generally acting sick, wait until he recovers before he gets the shot.

Vaccinating After Exposure to Certain Illnesses

Some diseases that your child is not routinely immunized against may have a vaccine that will prevent the disease if your child is exposed.

Hepatitis A. As explained above, this is a generally benign illness in younger children.

Therefore, vaccination after exposure to this disease is not necessary. For teenagers and adults, however, this can be a more severe disease. There are two types of vaccinations: *Hep A immune globulins,* active antibodies to the disease that will act right away; and *Hep A vaccine,* a vaccine that stimulates your body to make its own antibodies. These are both helpful vaccinations if given within a few days of exposure.

Chicken pox. If you are exposed to this disease and have not had the vaccine or the illness before, getting the Varicella vaccine within three days of exposure may prevent the illness or make it less severe. Parents may choose, however, to just let the illness run its course naturally. There is also a Varicella immune globulin, like Hep A, but it is used only for people with immune deficiencies.

Rabies. This virus is transmitted through the bite of an infected animal. Animals that pose the highest risk include bats, raccoons, skunks, foxes, bears, opossums, weasels, wolves, and woodchucks. This infection is almost always fatal if not treated. There is both an immune globulin and a vaccine to prevent this illness if you are exposed to it.

Measles. Vaccinated individuals have excellent protection if exposed to someone who is sick with measles. No further precautions are necessary. However, any susceptible person (unvaccinated children or older adults who no longer have protection) exposed to measles can benefit from receiving either the routine vaccination if given within seventy-two hours of exposure or a measles immune globulin (as described above under Hep A) if given within six days of exposure.

Vaccines for Foreign Travel

Vaccines for foreign travel include those for cholera, typhoid, yellow fever, and hepatitis A, and medication to prevent malaria. Because requirements change frequently, contact the Centers for Disease Control Traveler's Hotline at (877) FYI-TRIP or visit their website, www.cdc.gov/travel, for up-to-date information.

TREATING LITTLE PEOPLE

Infants, like adults, need help when hurt. But unlike adults, they often can't tell you where it hurts or what they need. The bump on the arm may need only the kiss-and-make-better treatment, but an infant who acts sick needs more. Sick children naturally become clingy, turning to the person they trust. They also expect you to know and fix what's wrong. Be prepared for a child's behavior to deteriorate when she is sick. Don't take it personally if the child hits the arm that holds her. Sick little people need big patience.

Sick Signs to Know

While preverbal children cannot tell you where they hurt, babies' bodies are honest mirrors reflecting their illness. They act sick when they are sick. Here are some signs that will help you determine how sick your baby may be.

Fever. As a general but not foolproof guide, a baby who doesn't have a fever probably does not have a serious illness. On the other hand, just because baby *does* have a fever does not necessarily mean she has a serious bacterial infection. Fever is only a sign that your child is fighting an illness; it does not always reflect the severity or the cause of the illness. Some harmless, and untreatable, viruses can cause a fever as high as 105°F (40.6°C), whereas some bacterial infections may cause a fever of only 101°F (38°C). Fever is defined as a temperature over 101°F (38°C). See pages 647–662 for a complete discussion of fevers.

Peakedness. This is mother lingo for a sick-looking kid: droopy, puffy eyes; sad expression; pale skin; and a loss of that happy sparkle in the face that you love to see.

Listlessness. Most babies don't move around much when they are sick. They act sluggish, as if redirecting their energy into healing. They spend a lot of time in your arms or lying quietly on the couch. They remain quiet, periodically drifting off to sleep, then awakening for a brief period when they may seem a little better. This listless behavior is typical of many nonserious illnesses.

Lethargy. Parents need to understand the difference between true lethargy and listlessness, as described above. Many worried parents tell their doctor that their child is "lethargic," when in reality the behavior they are discussing is only listlessness. Listless symptoms are usually an indication that things are not too serious. True lethargy, on the other hand, is a sign that something may be seriously wrong with the child. A lethargic child doesn't make eye contact, doesn't really acknowledge that the parent is there, may open his eyes only briefly, and does not perk up and respond to verbal or physical stimulation. Instead, he lies limp and unmoving,

seemingly unaware of what is going on around him. When communicating to your doctor, try to use these two different terms accurately. This will help your doctor decide the best course of action.

Behavior changes. Babies usually act either listless or fussy during an illness, especially when there is a fever. This is expected and shouldn't necessarily be viewed as a sign that the child is seriously ill. If baby perks up and seems to feel somewhat better when the fever is down, a serious illness is less likely. If, however, baby is truly lethargic, as described above, notify your doctor. In addition, if baby is continuously irritable and inconsolable, as described below, you should notify your doctor.

Lower your standards for behavior during an illness. A baby who doesn't feel good doesn't act good. Get a reading on your baby's pain tolerance. Some babies loudly protest a tiny owie; others don't broadcast their hurts.

Irritability. This term refers to a baby who cries continuously for many hours and is virtually inconsolable, no matter what you do. While all babies have inconsolable periods associated with colic or teething, these episodes generally do not last for more than a few hours. Babies are also fussy on and off during any illness. Normal fussiness, however, can be periodically consoled. True irritability can be a sign that your baby has a serious illness. Your doctor should be notified right away.

Poor appetite. This is expected during almost any illness. Do not worry if your infant doesn't eat well for a few days. Babies generally do take in enough fluid to sustain themselves. An infant can go for several days without eating at all during an illness, as long as there is enough fluid intake.

Dehydration. Many parents get worried that their infant will become dehydrated during an illness. While babies may become mildly dry during any sickness, decreased fluid intake for several days during a normal cough, cold, and fever rarely is significant enough to worry about. True dehydration occurs only when an infant or child has persistent vomiting and/or severe, frequent diarrhea. For more on dehydration, see page 686.

Rash. Rashes are very common during a variety of illnesses. They usually indicate that the illness is a nontreatable virus, although occasionally they can signify a bacterial infection. They are rarely a reason to panic and page the doctor after hours or to rush to the emergency room. See page 426 for a discussion of rashes.

The body speeds up. When baby is sick, especially with a fever, he will breathe fast, and you may feel a fast, pounding heartbeat (too fast to count easily). These are baby's natural resources for healing and releasing excess heat. But normally these fast signs slow when the fever comes down. A fast heartbeat and fast breathing that continue even after the fever breaks suggest a more serious illness.

Intestinal protest. Diarrhea accompanies many viral infections. Vomiting accompanies many throat, chest, kidney, and ear infections. And baby may show a double-end response of vomiting and diarrhea with an intestinal infection. Except for wanting to breastfeed more often, most babies do not eat much

---

FEEDING A BABY BEFORE ANESTHESIA

Until recently it has been customary not to allow babies to be fed for eight hours prior to anesthesia, for fear they might aspirate stomach contents into the lungs. New studies, however, show that starving before anesthesia is not necessary and may even be detrimental. Pediatric anesthesiologists now recommend feeding baby juice, formula, or breast milk up to four hours prior to anesthesia. Because breast milk is cleared rapidly from the stomach, breastfeeding up to four hours (some anesthesiologists permit two hours) before anesthesia is both safe and comforting to baby.

---

when sick. While periodic vomiting is normal when ill, persistent vomiting (especially with increasing lethargy) is a worrisome sign and merits reporting to your doctor.

TLC — Helping Your Baby Feel Better

The following are proven home remedies. Most are treated in more detail in the next chapter.

Rest. The wisdom of the body says rest when sick, as if to divert energy into healing. Social and economic pressures often prevent adults from listening to their body's counsel, but babies are freer and wiser; they rest when sick, without any prompting on your part. Achy heads, sore tummies, and congested chests don't like being jostled. Engage in quiet nesting interaction, a massage or back rub, a quiet story, songs, or a video for two with baby nestled in the arms or lap of his favorite nurse.

Outside help. Babies don't have to stay indoors when sick. Fresh air is good for the baby and keeps the housebound parent-nurse from going stir-crazy. Dry, stuffy air aggravates congested breathing passages, so ventilate the room well. Drafts don't cause colds. Fresh air and sunshine are good for the patient — and the nurse. Take baby out in a sling or stroller and enjoy the mental and physical lift that nature provides.

Drink, drink, drink! Babies need more fluids when sick. Fever, sweating, panting, vomiting, diarrhea, sneezing, coughing, tearing, and a diminished desire to eat or drink all lead to dehydration (excessive loss of body fluid). This condition itself makes an already sick baby sicker. Try these drinking tips:

- The *sips-and-chips* method: Small, frequent sips are best. Too much fluid taken too fast is likely to come right back up. Popsicles (homemade juice or nutritious fruit bars) and ice chips are proven winners.

- Clear soups: Medical research has validated grandmother's wisdom — chicken soup is good for colds (researchers feel that the steam to clear the nose and the fluid to prevent dehydration are the active ingredients in this magical potion). However, highly salted or bouillon-based soups can aggravate dehydration. Lightly salted canned soups are all right; homemade is best.

Feeding an illness. Babies may not eat when sick, but they need extra fluids to prevent dehydration and extra calories to fuel the increased energy demands. The answer is liquid food. Try these sick-child feeding tips:

- Offer small, more-frequent feedings — *half as much twice as often.*

- Smoothies can be made with fruit juice, a little sorbet, protein powder, yogurt, pureed fresh or frozen fruit, and a spoonful of honey for a child over one year. Encourage sipping slowly through a straw. This cold fruit drink is a welcome friend to a sore throat.

- Homemade vegetable and chicken soup and freshly cooked soft vegetables may easily slither past a sore throat.

Healthy sugars. The last thing you want is frequent blood-sugar swings in an already irritable and miserable child. Encourage fruit sugars and pasta as good sources of slow-release sugars. And it is OK to temporarily relax your no-sugar standards if all that a sick child will eat or drink are the sweet popsicles, gelatin desserts, or ice cream that you normally forbid.

GIVING MEDICINES

Every profession has its drawbacks, and in the otherwise joyful aspects of baby care, giving medicine ranks near the bottom of parents' job satisfaction list. Of course, medicine won't work unless it's administered correctly, and it won't work if given to the floor or your blouse.

Know Your Medicine

The following items are what every home pharmacist should ask or know about baby's medications:

- Ask your doctor to explain prescription medicines or any recommended over-the-counter medicines. What is the nature of the medicine? Is it an antibiotic, decongestant, cough syrup? Understand why you are giving it to your baby.

- Find out the medicine's adverse effects, if any. Ask your doctor what signs to look for. For example, a hivelike rash means baby is allergic to the medicine. Vomiting and diarrhea or a tummy ache doesn't imply an allergy but may require a different preparation or dosage, or even a different medicine. Report any reactions to your doctor.

- For future reference, record any adverse reactions, keeping a record of what medicines your baby can't tolerate or won't accept. Mention these to the prescribing doctor who may not have easy access to your baby's chart.

- If your baby has a chronic condition and is taking medicines regularly, remind the doctor what medicines baby is currently taking. Ask if it is safe to take these medicines together. Most commonly prescribed medicines for babies may be taken together. Over-the-counter medicine may be given along with antibiotics.

- Understand how the medicine should be stored. Most over-the-counter medicines can be stored on the shelf, yet many antibiotics must be refrigerated. Ask the pharmacist. Also, know which medicines keep for what period of time, and be sure to check the expiration date on the label. Discard expired medicines.

Giving Medicines Correctly

Observe the following tips when giving your baby medicines:

- Be sure you understand the dosage schedule: how much, how often, how long to give, and before, with, or after meals. Most medicines are best given just before a meal. Giving medicines with or after a meal risks losing both the medicine and the meal.

- Most prescription medicines are given three or four times a day, but rarely should you awaken a sleeping baby at night to give medicine. Theoretically medicines work best when spaced around the clock. Practically, unless advised otherwise by your doctor, they can be spaced during waking hours.

- If the instructions on the bottle differ from what you recall your doctor or pharmacist said, call to confirm.

- Measure carefully. Be as precise as possible when measuring the medicine. Most medicines for children are prescribed by the teaspoon. It is best to use a measuring spoon or a calibrated medicine dropper rather than a household teaspoon when measuring medicine for children. One teaspoon equals five cubic centimeters (cc) or five milliliters (ml). There are a variety of medicine spoons, cups, and calibrated dropperlike devices available for giving liquid medicine to children. Your pharmacist can help you select one.

- Keep a medicine reminder chart on your calendar or kitchen counter or a

STOCKING YOUR HOME FIRST AID KIT

- ☐ Acetaminophen pain reliever, liquid and suppositories
- ☐ Adhesive tape
- ☐ Alcohol swabs
- ☐ Antibiotic ointment
- ☐ Antiseptic solution (Hibiclens, Betadine)
- ☐ Band-Aids
- ☐ Cotton balls
- ☐ Cotton-tip applicators (Q Tips)
- ☐ Flashlight
- ☐ Gauze: four-inch (ten-centimeter) individual squares, nonstick pads, and a roll of gauze
- ☐ Hydrogen peroxide
- ☐ Instant ice packs
- ☐ Ipecac syrup
- ☐ Measuring cups and measuring spoons or calibrated dropper
- ☐ Nasal aspirator
- ☐ Nose drops (saline) or saline nasal spray
- ☐ Scissors (blunt ends)
- ☐ Steri-strips (butterfly adhesive bandages)
- ☐ Thermometer (glass or digital)
- ☐ Tongue depressors
- ☐ Tweezers

timer to go off every four to six hours. Forgetting doses is the most common error and a reason for baby's not responding to the medicine. If you are a forgetful parent (and we all are) ask your doctor if the same or a similar medication could be given *once* or *twice* a day instead of three or four times a day. Some medicines come in more concentrated form so you can give a smaller volume.

- Most medicines, especially those labeled "suspension," need vigorous shaking before using.

- Give the whole course of treatment. Avoid the temptation to stop the medicine because your baby feels better. Antibiotics, for example, often relieve symptoms within a day or two, but it takes the full course of treatment to eradicate the bacteria and keep the illness from recurring.

- Understand what you can safely mix with medicine. While nearly all children's medicines mix safely with a spoonful of jam or a sweet treat, some do not. For example, the efficacy of penicillin medications may be lessened if taken with a highly acidic juice, such as orange juice. Check with your friendly neighborhood pharmacist about which drinks can safely be used as a chaser. Resist the temptation to add medicine to a bottle of juice or formula, since baby may not consume the entire bottle. Most medicines mix safely with an ounce or so of formula or breast milk, but the taste won't be entirely masked and you'll just have that much more of the stuff to coax down.

Easing Medicine Down

As Mary Poppins sings, "A spoonful of sugar helps the medicine go down." Add a large measure of creative marketing as the finishing touch. Try these tricks.

Match the medicine to the mouth. The same medication may come in a variety of flavors and forms. Stick to your baby's preferences. Generic brands may have a harsher taste.

Numb the tongue. Letting your child suck on a popsicle for a few minutes can numb the taste buds.

Try magic paste. Most babies prefer liquid, but if your baby is a spitter or a sprayer, ask your doctor if the medication comes in a chewable tablet form. Crush the tablet between two spoons and add a drop or two of water to make a thick paste. Apply a little bit (a fingertipful) of the paste at a time to the inside of your baby's cheek, and it will be swallowed without a struggle. The flavor of chewable tablets is usually more pleasant. This is even true of acetaminophen.

Make a cheek pocket. This is our family secret for giving medicine to veteran spitters (be sure you have the medicine within reach and ready to go before you start this procedure): Cradle baby's head in the crook of your arm. With the same hand, encircle baby's cheek and use your middle or index finger to pull out the corner of his mouth, making a pocket in his cheek. With the other hand drop the medicine into this cheek pocket a little at a time. This hold keeps baby's mouth open and his head still. Best of all, the traction on baby's cheek with your finger keeps him from spitting the medicine back out. Maintain the

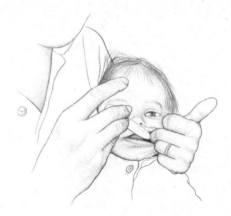

The "cheek pocket" technique helps prevent baby's spitting out medicine.

traction until all the medicine has gone down. Necessity is the mother of invention, or in this case the father. I discovered this technique when Martha, the queen medicine giver in our family, left me alone at medicine time with eighteen-month-old Stephen.

Use the art of camouflage. You can bury a crushed pill in a sandwich — jam it into the jam, place the paste under the peanut butter — or chase it with a small amount of milk, formula, or juice. Make the medicine as palatable as possible without fibbing that the medication is "candy." I even stuck a chewable pill into an ice cream sandwich for my kids.

Try spoons, droppers, and other medicine helpers. A shallow plastic medicine teaspoon (calibrated and available at pharmacies) is easier to use than a teaspoon. To wipe the remaining medicine from the spoon, use the upper lip sweep, sweeping the bowl against the inside of your baby's lip as you pull the spoon from your baby's mouth. A calibrated medicine dropper inserted into the side of baby's mouth, between cheek and gum, is a proven medicine-giving aid. Squirt in a few drops at a time in between swallows. Some babies accept medicines best from a tiny plastic cup, which can also be used to catch and recycle the dribbles.

Aim wisely. Try to avoid sensitive areas in the mouth. The taste buds are concentrated toward the front and center of baby's tongue. The roof of the mouth and the back of the tongue are gag-sensitive areas. Best is the side pocket between gum and cheek, to the rear of the mouth.

Sit on your child. At first glance, this may sound a little harsh. But if your goal is to get the medicine down, this will work. Lay your child down on her back and sit on the floor with the child's head between your legs, and the child's arms restrained under your thighs. If your child kicks, you can use your legs to keep her legs still. The child's head will be secure, and you will have both hands free to administer the medication. For the child who refuses to swallow and tries to spit the medicine back out, you can gently plug her nose. This will prompt her to swallow.

Dr. Bob notes: Be sure to speak to your child in a calm, soothing voice so she knows you aren't angry or punishing her by using this method. Again, if this sounds too harsh to you, then don't do it. But sometimes there is no other alternative — the medicine has to go in.

What If Baby Spits Up the Medicine?

Most medications are absorbed by the intestines within a half hour to forty-five minutes. If your baby has retained the medicine that long, it is usually unnecessary to make up the dose. If baby spits up the medicine immediately, repeat the dosage — unless precise dosing is necessary, as is the case with some heart and asthma medicines. If the child spits up an antibiotic within ten minutes after administration, repeat the dose.

Sometimes you are in a bind when a baby is too sick to retain oral medicine and spits up every dose. This is common with oral fever medications, such as acetaminophen. In this case use the fever-lowering medicine in *suppository* form. Also, your doctor may prescribe an antivomiting suppository to be given twenty to thirty minutes before an oral dosage, which may help the oral medicine stay down.

If your baby becomes so sick that he can't keep an antibiotic down (too lethargic to take, too much vomiting to retain), this is a sign that the medical condition may have worsened and a call to your doctor is warranted. Oftentimes an injection of an antibiotic may get the child well enough to take the medicine orally. Some antibiotics, available only by injection, work terrifically fast, but they are very expensive.

REDUCING THE RISK OF SUDDEN INFANT DEATH SYNDROME

Until recently the traditional wisdom about sudden infant death syndrome (SIDS) was: "No one knows why it occurs, and there's nothing parents can do to prevent it." New research challenges this dismal view. For parents who worry about this tragedy, here is the current thinking about SIDS and, more important, what you can do to lower the risk.

Before proceeding further, we want to offer a caution: The following discussion is meant to inform, not to offend; to inspire, not to scare. By understanding the details of this grim mystery, parents will worry less. By knowing they can participate in their own risk-lowering program, parents need not feel so helpless. We don't want to imply that if you don't take the precautions we recommend, your baby might die — or that if you do, he won't. Besides, SIDS is rare (see box "SIDS Facts"). But our suggestions may lower the risk of SIDS for your baby. They are based on the most up-to-date research about SIDS, as well as on our own experiments. All of these risk-lowering tips have been well researched. Until more research helps us better understand and prevent this tragedy, we give you our best shot.

Background of the Risk-Lowering Program

Our SIDS risk-lowering hypothesis is this: *By taking certain health precautions and by practicing the attachment style of parenting, parents can lower the risk of SIDS.* Specifically, here are the practical recommendations to support this hypothesis:

1. Get good prenatal care.
2. Don't smoke around your baby.
3. Put baby to sleep on his back or side.
4. Breastfeed your baby.
5. Avoid overheating baby during sleep.
6. Avail yourself of health care for baby.
7. Keep baby's sleeping environment safe.
8. Practice attachment parenting.
9. Sleep with your baby.

Some of these measures may seem like commonsense precautions. They are. Others may seem new to you, so we will discuss each in detail. But to help you understand how we arrived at these recommendations, we will first review how our understanding of SIDS evolved.

My own involvement in the subject began in the early years of my pediatric practice. During checkups I would usually ask new parents if they had any worries. "SIDS," they would confide. "Why does it happen?"

"I don't know," was my feeble answer.

"Is there anything we can do to prevent it?" they persisted.

"Not that I know of," I evaded.

Every time I finished this unhelpful dialogue I felt that I had let parents down. For there to be no way to lower the risk seemed defeatist. I was especially shaken when trying to console parents who had lost a baby to SIDS. I grieved for their loss, and I grieved for my inability to explain why it occurred and what they might do to lower the risk of such a tragedy happening again. As a parent I wanted a list of things I could do to keep SIDS from claiming our babies. As a physician I wanted a list that was well researched. And I set out to compile that list.

Over the next twenty years I studied the most reputable investigations of SIDS. Contrary to popular belief, SIDS is not a complete mystery. There is a lot known about what SIDS is, and what it is not. But only recently has the valuable insight made it out of the research laboratory and into the homes of parents. I also discovered that there was a general reluctance of all baby books to tackle this delicate issue from a preventive viewpoint. But, in my experience, and I assume in the experience of those who read this book, *informed* parents worry less, not more.

In these studies of SIDS, two facts stood out: It occurs *during sleep,* and it occurs

SIDS FACTS

Sudden infant death syndrome (also known as crib death) is defined as the sudden death of an infant under one year of age that remains unexplained after the performance of a complete postmortem investigation, including an autopsy, an examination of the scene of death, and a review of the case history. In the United States, SIDS occurs in less than one in one thousand babies, usually between two and six months of age, and has a peak incidence between two and four months. Ninety-five percent of SIDS deaths occur by six months. This tragedy occurs most commonly between midnight and 6:00 A.M. It is more common in the months of December and January. Around three thousand babies die in the United States from SIDS each year, and it is the leading cause of death between one month and one year.

While most babies dying of SIDS have shown no previous warning signs or risk factors, some infants have a slightly higher risk of SIDS than others. These include:

- premature infants
- infants who have had stop-breathing episodes (apnea) in the early weeks of life
- infants who have had an ALTE (apparent life-threatening event), such as a stop-breathing episode in which the baby was pale, blue, and limp (the older term for this was near-miss SIDS)
- babies whose mothers had little or no prenatal care
- infants in a poor socioeconomic environment

It is noteworthy that even babies in these high-risk groups have less than a 1 percent chance of SIDS. SIDS is not caused by immunizations or choking; and it is not contagious.

The cause of SIDS is presently unknown. There are many theories, but none proven. The prevailing concept is that SIDS is a sleep disorder. Studies suggest that a baby at risk of SIDS is born with some physiological differences. On the outside, these babies look healthy and act just like any other baby, but on the inside these at-risk babies have an immature breathing-regulating system. Deep within everyone's brain lies a master control center designed to receive stimuli and regulate breathing. For example, your furnace has a master control center that is set to click on and off whenever the temperature goes below or above a preset level. Similarly, the breathing center in the brain is preset to maintain a healthy level of oxygen in the blood. When the oxygen level in the blood falls too low, or the carbon dioxide goes too high (as happens when a person stops breathing or holds his breath), the breathing center automatically clicks on to stimulate breathing. This protective mechanism is supposed to function even when one is in a deep sleep. But in some infants, for some unknown reason, breathing does not automatically restart. In short, some SIDS babies have a disorder of arousal from sleep.

most frequently *between two and four months* of age. SIDS may have various causes, but wouldn't it seem reasonable to think that for most infants SIDS could be a basic sleep disorder? And why was the age two to four months so vulnerable? I set out to answer these questions. I found two groups of investigators — basic science researchers, who were studying the possible physiological characteristics of SIDS babies, and statistics collectors, who looked for patterns and risk factors of SIDS. While both of these approaches were necessary to unravel this puzzle, I felt yet another approach was needed. I wanted to know how certain sleeping arrangements might affect an infant at risk of SIDS, especially during the high-risk situation (sleep) and during the high-risk period (the first six months). I wanted to fill in this research gap.

Since SIDS seems to be a disorder of sleep, I wondered if a parent, most often the mother, could affect the arousability of her infant by changing their sleeping arrangement. I developed a hypothesis: *Sleeping with a baby may reduce the risk of SIDS.* Here is the first case we studied to test this hypothesis. A baby at high risk of SIDS was being monitored in her crib at home. When she was around three months of age, stop-breathing alarms began going off with increasing frequency. But when mother took baby into her bed and slept next to her, the episodes of alarm sounding ceased. When the baby was moved back into separate sleeping quarters, the alarms resumed.

In 1986 I was invited to present this case, and the whole hypothesis, at the International Congress of Pediatrics in Honolulu. The title of my presentation was "The Protective Effects of Sharing Sleep: Can It Prevent SIDS?" I wanted my presentation to stimulate research to prove or disprove my theory. Over the next few years, research organizations began showing more interest and support in studying a relationship between parenting styles and SIDS. The National Institutes of Health began funding studies on mother-infant sleeping pairs. Beginning in 1988, there was a surge in SIDS-prevention research. In early 1992, two blessings further helped us study our hypothesis: Improved computer technology for home sleep studies became available, and a new baby entered the Sears bedroom laboratory. We will discuss our exciting findings and others later.

From this background the following SIDS risk-lowering program evolved.

Nine Ways to Lower Your Baby's Risk of SIDS

Based on the current SIDS research — including our own theories — here are some ways you can reduce a baby's risk of SIDS.

1. Get Good Prenatal Care

Strive for a healthy pregnancy and obtain good prenatal care. SIDS has been shown to be higher in babies whose mothers smoked or took addicting drugs during pregnancy and those who lacked good prenatal care. The reasons for these risk factors are unknown, but they probably stem from chronic oxygen deprivation and the increased risk of prematurity in these babies.

2. Don't Smoke Around Your Baby

Studies show that smoking is the highest risk factor and the one that all researchers agree increases the chance of SIDS. The risk is proportional to baby's exposure to smoke and the number of cigarettes smoked each day. New Zealand studies show that infants of smoking mothers and fathers have a seven times greater risk of dying of SIDS. The mechanism of this preventable association is not completely understood. It's probably a combination of many factors. Babies exposed to smoke are more likely to have congested breathing passages. Researchers have recently found that children of smoking parents have certain chemicals in their blood that indicate they have been chronically oxygen deprived. (See page 620 for more effects of passive smoke on babies.)

3. Put Baby to Sleep on His Back

Conventional wisdom used to say that it is safer to put babies to sleep in the prone (tummy-down) position. The rationale behind this time-honored advice is that if an infant spits up or vomits, the material will run out of the mouth by gravity, whereas if baby is supine (on the back) it may lodge in his throat and be breathed into his lungs. But new studies question this old advice. According to SIDS researchers, it is extremely unlikely that a baby will choke on spit-up when sleeping on his back. In the past decade, worldwide Back to Sleep campaigns have reduced the incidence of SIDS by 40 to 50 percent.

Why sleeping on the back or side may lower the risk of SIDS is unknown. The most plausible theory is that back-sleeping babies arouse more easily from sleep. Another theory is that babies are less likely to become overheated. Lying on the side or back leaves the internal organs more exposed so they can radiate heat more readily than when on the tummy. Another possibility is that when

---

BABIES WHO SHOULD SLEEP PRONE

Be sure to check with your doctor to see if your baby has any medical conditions that warrant putting baby to sleep on his tummy. Babies who *should* sleep prone are:

- Premature babies still in the hospital; sleeping on the tummy increases breathing efficiency in prematures.

- Babies who suffer from gastro-esophageal reflux; these babies are best placed tummy down with head elevated thirty degrees (see page 394).

- Babies with small jawbones or other structural abnormalities of the airway.

---

sleeping facedown, a baby may press his head into the soft surface, which then forms a pocket around his face, allowing carbon dioxide to accumulate and baby to rebreathe his own exhaled air. I wish to reassure parents that in no way should they conclude that if they put their baby to sleep on his tummy he is going to die. Studies only show a *statistical* increase in SIDS risk.

Should babies sleep on back or side? One reason some authorities prefer the back position is the concern that babies put to sleep on their side may roll over on their tummy. But in our experience, babies usually roll from side to back, not side to tummy, possibly because their outstretched arms act as a barrier from rolling onto the tummy. We have found that in the early months our babies sleep best on their side. Also, when placing baby to sleep on his side, pull his underneath arm forward to make it less likely that baby will roll onto his tummy.

BACK IS BEST FOR BABY'S SLEEP
Now you lay me down to sleep
On my back for safest keep.
It's tummy time when I'm awake,
but back is best for sleeping breaks.

Keep quilts, toys, and pillows out of my bed.
Never put covers over or beneath my head.
Cigarettes are bad for me.
Please keep my environment smoke-free.

These may be many rules to know,
but minding them will help me grow!
Remember this rhyme when caring for kids,
and help reduce the risk of SIDS.

From SIDS Alliance, www.sidsalliance.org

4. Breastfeed Your Baby

New research confirms what I have long suspected: The incidence of SIDS is lower in breastfed babies. In a New Zealand study, SIDS was three times higher in nonbreastfed babies. Older studies from New Zealand have also shown that SIDS occurred less in breastfed babies. Even large-scale studies from the U.S. National Institute of Child Health and Human Development (NICHD) found SIDS babies were breastfed significantly less often, and, if breastfed, were weaned earlier.

Why breastfeeding may lower the risk of SIDS is unknown, but I suspect it is a combination of the following factors. The infection-fighting factors in breast milk result in fewer upper respiratory infections that can compromise breathing, and the nonallergenicity of breast milk could keep breathing passages less congested. Also, it could be that the

breastfed baby might have sleep cycles that enable him to be more easily aroused in response to a life-threatening event.

Could it be the nature of breast milk itself? Gastroesophageal reflux (GERD, see page 388) can increase the risk of SIDS. Milk regurgitated into upper airways can trigger a stop-breathing reflex. Reflux occurs less often in breastfed babies. Could the swallowing and breathing mechanisms of breastfeeding babies be better coordinated? We do know that breastfed babies suck and swallow differently than those who are bottlefed. Breastfed babies also usually feed more frequently than their formula-fed friends. Therefore, they could get more practice at coordinating their swallowing and breathing mechanisms. Finally, breastfeeding babies, especially if they sleep next to the mother at night, show different sleep patterns, more frequent sucking, and usually sleep on their side, facing mother. Could these also be safer sleep patterns? The effect of breastfeeding on mother's sleep and the effect of breast milk itself on an infant's physiology are poorly understood; further study of these fields, I believe, will eventually shed light on the puzzle of SIDS.

5. Avoid Overheating Baby During Sleep

Babies who become overheated from over-bundling have a higher risk of SIDS. Be particularly careful of overheating if baby sleeps next to you. The parent's body acts as a heat source. If baby is dressed to sleep alone and then during the night you put her in bed with you, change her dress appropriately. Studies have shown higher incidence of SIDS in countries that heavily bundle babies as opposed to those in which babies are loosely and lightly bundled and the room is appropriately heated. Signs of overbundling are sweating, damp hair, heat rash, rapid breathing, restlessness, and sometimes fever. Both overheating and overcooling have detrimental effects on breathing.

6. Avail Yourself of Health Care for Baby

While SIDS spares no one group of babies, the incidence is higher among the socio-economically underprivileged. If you are overwhelmed with domestic and financial stresses and your ability to mother your baby is compromised, seek help from your doctor and the social welfare agencies in your community. Studies have shown that increasing parenting skills can decrease SIDS. An interesting study in Sheffield, England, validated that mothers can be their baby's best emergency medical system. Researchers divided a large number of high-risk babies into two groups. After birth one group received biweekly home visits by a public health nurse. Their mothers were educated in mothering skills, nutrition, hygiene, and recognizing when their infants were sick. The mothers in the second group received no special attention. The SIDS rate was three times greater in this second group.

7. Keep Baby's Sleeping Environment Safe

Remember that nearly all babies who die of SIDS die in their sleep. If putting baby to sleep on an adult mattress, place him on his *back*. Always use a firm mattress. Use the same precautions when traveling or in any strange sleeping environment. (See also "Safe Co-sleeping," page 341, and "Crib Safety," page 603.)

8. Practice Attachment Parenting

Have we been paying a price for replacing a style of parenting that has endured for thousands of years? I believe, and research supports, that three key elements of attachment parenting — breastfeeding on cue, sharing sleep, and wearing baby — promote organization of the baby and sensitivity in the parents. In the early months, baby's central nervous system and breathing-regulating mechanisms are immature and somewhat disorganized, as are their sleep-wake patterns. Attachment parenting promotes an overall regulation of baby's physiological systems and this carries over into regulating his breathing mechanism.

Attachment parents develop a radarlike awareness of their baby. One day I was writing at my desk when my emergency beeper sounded, beckoning me to the hospital emergency room to evaluate a five-month-old baby who had stopped breathing. The parents and baby were visiting friends. Bedtime came and mother put baby down in their friends' upstairs bedroom. The party was noisy when, unexpectedly, mother's sensitivity alarm sounded. She felt, "My baby is very sensitive to noise. Why isn't he waking up? I'd better check." She found him pale and not breathing. She summoned her husband to revive the baby with mouth-to-mouth resuscitation. The child is alive and well.

9. Sleep with Your Baby

Here is where the controversy begins. Does sleep sharing decrease or increase the risk of SIDS, or does it make no difference? We believe sleeping with your baby can *reduce* the chance of SIDS. But some researchers have the opposite opinion. Overlying (rolling over onto your baby, which we have discussed on page 341) is nearly always associated with abnormal sleeping circumstances, such as the parent's being under the influence of drugs or alcohol, or too many children in one bed, or not taking the precautions mentioned in item 7 above. The New Zealand cot-death study that sparked many of these precautions also considers sleep sharing a risk factor, and these findings are creeping into the press, alarming parents into believing that if they allow their baby into their bed they put him at risk for SIDS. Could a normal nighttime parenting style that has endured for centuries be all of a sudden unsafe? The real lesson to be drawn, we believe, is not to discourage parents from sleeping with their baby but to show them how to do so safely.

Convincing research suggests that infants at risk of SIDS have a diminished arousal response during sleep. It follows that anything that increases the infant's arousability from sleep or the mother's awareness of her infant during sleep may decrease the risk of SIDS. That's exactly what sleeping with your baby can do.

How Sleep Sharing Can Lower the Risk of SIDS

In the early months of life, much of a baby's night is spent in active sleep — the state in which babies are most easily aroused. This state may "protect" the infant against stop-breathing episodes. From one to six months, the time of primary concern for SIDS, the percentage of active sleep decreases and quiet, or deep, sleep increases. This is called sleep maturity, when babies reach that long-awaited nocturnal milestone — sleeping through the night. That's the good news. The concern arises, however, that as baby learns to sleep more deeply, perhaps the risk of SIDS increases, since sleeping deeper does not always mean sleeping safer. Offsetting this worry is the fact that at the same time baby is sleeping deeper, his compensatory cardiopulmonary regulating system is maturing, so that by six months the breathing centers are more likely to restart should breathing stop. But between one and six months, when sleep is deepening and the compensatory mechanisms are not yet mature, there is a *vulnerable period* when babies are most at risk for SIDS. Sleep sharing fills in this gap.

Mother as a Pacemaker

Picture what happens when mother and baby sleep side by side. Put baby next to a warm body and that person acts as a "breathing pacemaker" during these vulnerable early months of life when baby's self-start mechanism is immature. The sleep-sharing pair develop what we call sleep harmony. Mother sleeps like a baby until baby is mature enough to sleep like an adult. Both members of the sleep-sharing pair develop synchronous sleep stages, perhaps not perfectly in step but close enough to be mutually aware of the other's presence and mutually affecting the other's physiology, but without disturbing each other's sleep. Because of this mutual sensitivity, the presence of the mother raises baby's threshold of arousability, a protective benefit should a stop-breathing episode occur.

Even when SIDS has occurred in sleep-sharing pairs (and it has), the mother has the comfort of knowing that she was there. This sleeping arrangement does not imply that mother is expected to be a guardian angel during every sleeping hour for the first six months, or that she is an inadequate parent if she chooses not to do so. This takes the joy out of nighttime parenting and replaces it with fear. We're simply talking about forgetting cultural norms and doing what comes naturally for you. And don't fear that you must never let your baby sleep alone and that you must go to bed early with baby every night. Also, the time of day in which SIDS is most likely to occur is after midnight. Remember, SIDS is a relatively rare occurrence and this section is written in answer to the question, "Is there anything I can do to lower my baby's risk of SIDS?"

The Evidence for Our Sleep-Sharing Hypothesis

Testimonies from nighttime parents. Over my years in pediatric practice, I have been impressed by stories from numerous parents about their sensitivity while sharing sleep. Many times mothers would relate, "I wake up just before my baby does; I nurse him and we both drift back to sleep." To many parents there is no doubt that a mutual awareness occurs while sleeping with their baby. In fact, it was these insights that prompted me to develop this SIDS-prevention hypothesis. Purists will argue that this is only anecdotal evidence, but I have grown to value the wisdom of an intuitive parent as much as the methods of the most meticulous scientist.

Our experience. We logged more than sixteen years of sleeping with babies. As I have watched our own sleeping beauties, I was impressed by how sleeping babies automatically gravitate toward mother. They usually sleep face-to-face with their mother and spend much of their time on their side. Is there more physiology going on here than meets the eye? Perhaps the face-to-face position allows mother's breath to stimulate baby. I noticed that when I lightly breathed on our babies' cheeks, they would take a deep breath. Could there be sensors in a baby's nose that detect another's breath and stimulate baby to breathe? Then there's the reach-out-and-touch-someone observation. While sleeping close by, our babies would extend an arm, touch Martha, take a deep breath, and resettle. In essence, there seems to be a mutual awareness without a mutual disturbance.

Our experiments. When we were writing the first edition of this book, we were sleeping with our four-month-old daughter, Lauren. On seven occasions we continuously measured Lauren's pulse, blood oxygen, breathing movements, air flow, and sleep patterns in two settings: sleeping next to Martha one night and sleeping in another room the second night. The instrumentation was painless and Lauren literally slept right through. Our studies vividly demonstrated a mutual sensitivity. When Lauren slept next to Martha, her breathing physiology improved. The oxygen level in her blood was higher in the sleep-sharing arrangement. Our studies and others are too preliminary to draw conclusions about SIDS prevention, but at this point we are confident to conclude: *The presence of the mother sleeping next to her baby does influence her baby's physiology.*

Current research. Dr. James McKenna, director of the Mother-Baby Behavioral Sleep Laboratory at the University of Notre Dame, has studied sleep-sharing pairs for more than ten years and has come to the following conclusions:

- Sleep-sharing pairs show more synchronous arousals than when sleeping separately. When one member of the pair stirs, coughs, or changes sleeping stages, the other member also changes, often without waking.

- Each member of the pair tends to often, but not always, be in the *same stage* of sleep for longer periods if they sleep together.

- Sleep-sharing babies spend less time in each cycle of deep sleep. Lest mothers worry they will get less deep sleep, preliminary studies show that sleep-sharing mothers do not get less total deep sleep.

- Sleep-sharing infants arouse more often and spend more time breastfeeding than solitary sleepers. Yet, the sleep-sharing mothers do not report awakening more frequently.

- Sleep-sharing infants tend to sleep more often on their backs or sides and less often on their tummies, a factor itself that could lower the SIDS risk.

- A lot of mutual touch and interaction occurs between the sleep-sharers. What one sleeper does affects the nighttime behavior of the other.

Studies of infant sleep-wake patterns. Experiments have shown that babies who sleep next to mother, especially if breastfeeding, awaken more frequently than infants who do not. In one study researchers compared sleep-wake patterns in infants of different nighttime parenting styles. Group one breastfed on cue during the day and night and slept with their babies. Group two breastfed their babies but tended to wean earlier and sleep separately. The third group neither breastfed nor slept with their babies. Babies who breastfed and shared sleep with the mother awakened more frequently and slept shorter stretches at a time; those who breastfed but did not sleep with the mother slept longer; and the babies who neither breastfed nor slept with the mother slept the longest. Could babies who sleep alone be training themselves, before their time, to sleep too long and too deeply?

SIDS rates in sleep-sharing cultures. The incidence of SIDS is lowest in populations that traditionally share sleep, but the SIDS rates may increase in these populations when their cultural environment changes. For example, SIDS rates are low in Asian immigrants to the United States, but a recent California study showed that the longer these immigrant groups lived in the United States, the higher their rate of SIDS, as perhaps these populations adopted more detached parenting styles.

From the preceding evidence, draw your own conclusion: If there were fewer cribs, would there be fewer crib deaths?

Certainly I do not wish to lead parents to believe that any of these precautions and parenting styles will absolutely prevent their baby from succumbing to SIDS. The best we can hope for is to do whatever possible to lower the risk. And, if a baby does die of SIDS, it may be of some comfort to parents to feel in their hearts that they did everything they could to prevent this tragedy. (For more information about SIDS, see "Resources," page 747.)

27

The Most Common Medical Problems: Self-help Home Care

We have chosen from our gallery of infant illnesses the most frequent medical problems that babies are likely to have during the first two years. Besides helping you get a working knowledge of what bothers your baby the most, we will give you tools to make home treatment easier on your child, your doctor, and yourself.

PARENTING THE BABY WITH FEVER

During your baby's first two years you may spend more time treating and worrying about fever than any other concern. Babies get hot, and parents get worried. Here's how to treat both.

Fever Facts

What is a fever? Babies' normal body temperatures vary from 97° to 100°F (36° to 37.8°C). The average *oral* temperature in babies is 98.6°F (37°C). The axillary (armpit) temperature may be one-half to one degree lower than oral, and the rectal temperature may be one-half to one degree higher than oral, but there is nothing magical about these figures. Every baby has his or her own normal body temperature. Daily temperatures can regularly fluctuate one to one and a half degrees above and below the normal. A well baby can have a temperature of 97°F upon awakening in the early morning and a temperature of 100°F in late afternoon or after a tantrum or strenuous exercise. Here is how we rate fevers *(all temperatures in this section are rectal unless otherwise stated):*

- low-grade fever — temperature between 100.4°F and 100.9°F (37.2°C to 38.3°C)
- moderate fever — temperature between 101°F and 102.9°F (38.4°F to 39.4°C)
- high fever — temperature higher than 103°F (39.5°C)

It is best to know your baby's normal temperature. When baby is well, take and record his temperature upon his awakening. Do this again in late afternoon when he is quiet. These are your baby's average temperatures. Any temperature greater than these indicates a fever.

Why Fever?

Fever is a *symptom* of an underlying illness, not an illness itself. Fever is the normal and healthy response of the body to an infection. But we all have a fever phobia. Fever worry accounts for 50 percent of phone calls to doctors and 20 percent of emergency room visits. And many parents mistakenly believe that fever will harm their baby.

Fever usually means there is a fight going on within your baby's body. When germs and germ-fighting white blood cells clash, these cells produce substances called *pyrogens,* which cause the following effects in the body: First, they stimulate the body's defenses to fight germs. Then they travel to the hypothalamus, a tiny organ in the brain that acts as the body's thermostat to maintain a reasonably constant body temperature. These pyrogens stimulate the hypothalamus to raise its set point, allowing the body to operate at a higher temperature. The body responds by using its available resources to get rid of the excess heat produced: The blood vessels dilate, increasing heat loss through the skin and resulting in flushed cheeks. The heart beats faster to pump more blood to the skin. Baby breathes faster to release warm air, similar to the way a dog pants to cool off during warm summer months, and the baby sweats to cool by evaporation, although sweating is more common in the older child. So if fever helps fight infection, why fight fever?

Fever is both friend and foe. The pyrogens released during fever slow the multiplication of viruses and bacteria, increase production of antibodies to these germs, and increase the number of white blood cells to fight the infection. But fever also bothers babies, making them upset and irritable on top of the discomfort from their illness. Also, rapidly rising temperatures may cause convulsions or fever fits. (More about these problems later.)

➤ **SPECIAL NOTE:** *Because of discoveries showing that fever-producing substances in the body help fight infection, parents became reluctant to lower their baby's fever for fear of lessening the body's natural defenses. Newer research, however, has shown that fever-lowering medicines work directly on the body's thermostat to lower temperature but do not interfere with the body's infection-fighting defenses, which carry on their biological work even when fever-lowering medicines are given.*

EAR THERMOMETERS

Anyone who has tried to take the underarm (or worse, rectal) temperature of a squirming, screaming toddler will tell you it is next to impossible. When ear thermometers came along, they were thought to be the answer to every parent's prayers. Unfortunately, they have not lived up to expectations. Ear thermometers are notorious for giving erroneous readings, measuring a temperature of 95°F when you know your baby has a slight fever, or scaring you with a reading of 105°F when in reality the fever is only 102°F. We utilize this convenient tool in our office because it is a quick and easy way to tell if someone has a fever; but if we want to know accurately just how high the fever is, we use a regular glass underarm thermometer.

Taking Temperatures

Temperature-taking technology is changing as fast as quick-and-easy diapering, so perhaps the glass thermometer will someday take its place in the baby-antiques museum next to diaper pins. Digital-display thermometers are quick, easy, accurate, and inexpensive. Forehead tapes (also called temperature strips) are easy but less accurate. The newest ear thermometers are the fastest and easiest way to take a temperature, but they sacrifice accuracy for convenience. The glass thermometer that grandmother used may still be the most reliable. Here's how to select a thermometer and use it.

Choosing a Thermometer

The two types of glass thermometers are rectal and oral. The only difference is the business end. Rectal thermometers have a short, stubby end for safe and easy insertion; an oral thermometer has a long, thin end for greater surface area to be in contact with the tongue and is marked "oral." Either type may be used to take underarm temperatures, but only the rectal type is safe to be inserted into the rectum. Since a rectal thermometer may be used for both underarm and rectal temperature taking, there is no need to buy an oral thermometer for babies. The oral thermometer is impractical in the squirming toddler, and seldom do children under the age of four cooperate with having a thermometer in their mouth. Rectal or underarm temperature taking is the safest; rectal the most accurate. Test read a thermometer before purchasing it, as some are easier to read than others. Glass thermometers without mercury are now available.

▶*TEMPERATURE-TAKING TIP: For normal, everyday temperature taking, start with the underarm method, instead of the more traumatic rectal method. An underarm temperature will give you an accurate enough reading of your infant's status. The only time a rectal temperature is most useful is during the first two months of life, when you really need to know exactly how high the fever is. Even during this early age, however, start with an underarm reading. If it is normal, then you can stop there. If it registers a fever, then you should confirm this with a rectal temperature before calling your doctor.*

The Rectal Method

Some toddlers are very upset by the rectal method because of the discomfort. Respect

---

THE KISS-AND-GUESS METHOD

Fever can play tricks on skin. Usually when body temperature goes up, blood vessels in the skin dilate and the skin gets flushed and feels hot to the touch or kiss. But sometimes skin may feel only slightly warm despite hot insides. Hot spots that register fever to touch are baby's forehead and upper abdomen. Studies have shown that parents are right 75 percent of the time when they conclude their child has a fever by feeling the forehead. (A better percentage than with forehead tapes.) Get used to baby's "normal" feel. Besides the "hotness" of baby's skin, watch for other signs of fever: flushed cheeks, fast heartbeat, breathing faster with hot breath, and sweating.

this reluctance and never force a child to submit to the rectal method.

Getting baby settled. Trying to insert a thermometer into a wiggly baby's bottom may raise both your temperatures. Also, a screaming baby is likely to be a hotter baby. Giving baby a breast, a pacifier, or a reassuring song before and during T time often works.

Getting the thermometer settled. Hold the thermometer at the top and, using a wrist-snapping action, shake down the liquid column below 96°F (35.6°C). A mess-saving tip: Slippery thermometers fly out of anxious hands. Shake it over a bed or rug. And stock a spare thermometer in your medicine cabinet just in case of an accident. Generously coat the bulb end with a lubricant.

Positioning baby. Drape baby bottom up with her tummy on your lap and her legs

dangling gently to relax the buttocks. Or lay baby on the floor or changing table in the diaper-changing position, grasping both ankles and flexing the legs toward the abdomen. The target will appear right in front of you. The tummy-over-lap position allows easier restraint, while the back-lying position allows face-to-face interaction and better insertion.

Taking the temperature. Spread the buttocks apart with one hand while gently inserting the thermometer bulb about one inch (2½ centimeters) into the rectum with the other hand. Hold the thermometer between your index and middle fingers, cigarettelike, with the palm of your hand and your fingers grasping your baby's buttocks. This hold keeps the thermometer in place and keeps your baby from squirming. Never leave a baby alone with the thermometer in place.

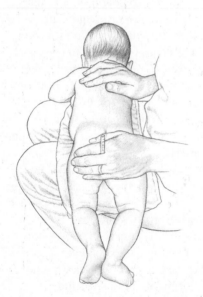
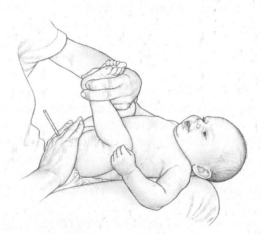

Taking rectal temperatures: two approaches.

Timing. Try to keep the glass thermometer in place for three minutes. If your baby is protesting, a *one-minute reading* will be within a degree of the true rectal temperature. Some digital thermometers give an accurate reading in less than thirty seconds.

The Underarm Method

While not as accurate as a rectal reading, taking your baby's temperature in the armpit is easier and gives you a ballpark reading of the true temperature — which, in most cases, is all that is necessary. Underarm temperatures can be as much as two degrees lower than a true rectal temperature. Follow these steps.

Positioning baby. Sit your child on your lap, on the corner of the couch, or on a bed and hold her firmly with one arm around her shoulder. If baby is upset, you can easily place the thermometer after putting her to the breast in the cradle hold or when she is asleep.

Preparing the thermometer. Shake down the thermometer as described for the rectal method above.

Taking the temperature. Wipe her armpit dry. Lift her arm and gently place the bulb of the thermometer into the fold of the armpit.

Hold your child's arm flat against the chest, closing the armpit.

Timing. Allow at least three minutes to get an accurate underarm temperature.

When to Worry and When Not To

Here are some guidelines to help you decide when a fever may be cause for concern.

How high the fever goes. A higher fever does not always mean a sicker child. In fact, some minor viral illnesses produce the highest fevers (104–105°F/40–40.6°C). And each baby reacts individually to fever-producing illnesses. Some infants spike high fevers with slight infections, other babies get only slightly warm even with a serious illness. Unless it reaches 107°F (41.7°C), high fever does not harm babies. It does not fry brains. Your degree of worry should be related less to the degrees of fever and more to how sick your child acts.

How the fever begins. ("She seemed so well an hour ago, and now she is burning up.") Sudden-onset fevers tend to be viral illnesses, especially if baby does not appear very ill. A gradually rising fever, plus a steadily worsening baby, is of more concern.

CHARTING THE FEVER

Make a temperature chart listing the following information: time, temperature (rectal or axillary), treatment, and response to treatment. For example:

Time	Temperature	Treatment	Response
4 P.M.	102° (rectal)	1 dropperful acetaminophen	Temperature went down to 100° and baby was less irritable

How the fever behaves. If a mother tells me, "No matter what I do I can't get the fever down, and he seems just as sick before and after medication," this is more worrisome than the observation, "this fever goes up and down by itself, with or without treatment." But don't rely on the response of the fever to temperature-lowering medications as the only worry sign. Studies have shown that response to fever-lowering medications is an inconsistent predictor of the seriousness of the illness.

How the baby behaves. *How your baby acts is more important than how high his temperature is.* "He has a temperature of a hundred and four but is still happily playing" is not such a worrisome situation, but a baby who just wants to lie around though his temperature is only 102° is a worry. How your baby's illness behaves along with the fever is also a guide. "He seems just as sick even when the fever comes down a bit" is a worry sign. "He seems sick when the fever is high but well when it comes down" means you can worry less, but this sign is still no guarantee that your baby does not have a serious illness.

How your intuition reacts. The degree of your worry is more important to your doctor than the degree of fever. Be sure to convey to your doctor your inner sense that a serious illness may be brewing in your baby. Your alarm may be just what the doctor needs to help him or her make a decision about how quickly and extensively to respond to your child's fever.

➤*SPECIAL NOTE: The younger the baby, the more the worry. Fever in a three-month-old is much more worrisome than in a three-year-old. Tiny babies have tiny defenses against germs. Any fever in a baby under three months should be reported to your doctor. (See "Sick Signs to Know," page 630.)*

When to Call Your Doctor About Fever

Your observational assessment of the health of your baby is more important to your doctor than the degree of fever. Unless baby is obviously very ill, there is seldom a reason to call your doctor after hours at the first feel of a hot forehead. If baby's fever comes down with treatment (even if not all the way to normal) and his behavior perks up a bit, then you can probably wait until your doctor's office next opens (except as noted below). Before calling your doctor, try the fever-reducing methods listed on the next few pages, and make a fever chart as suggested on the previous page, because the doctor will want to know what you have already done and how your child responded to your treatment. After taking, recording, and treating your baby's fever, call your doctor in the following circumstances:

• Any rectal temperature of 100.4°F or higher in an infant less than three months of age that persists more than eight hours should be reported to your doctor. At this age if baby seems sick (lethargic, vomiting persistently, drowsy, not eating, pale), you should contact your doctor immediately, regardless of the hour of the day or night. If, however, baby does not seem that ill and the fever comes down easily by simply increasing fluids and unbundling baby, it is safe to wait a few hours, monitor the course of the temperature and the illness, and then report it to your doctor. Remem-

WORRYING ABOUT FEVER

When to Worry Less

- Baby not acting worse.
- Active, playing, responds normally to interaction.
- No difference in skin color other than flushed cheeks at height of fever.
- Smiling, alert, interested in surroundings, eyes wide open.
- Baby "back to normal self" when fever breaks.
- Cries vigorously but can be consoled.

When to Worry More

- Baby acting sicker by the hour or day.
- Increasingly lethargic, drowsy, less responsive.
- Pale or ashen skin color.
- Dull, anxious facial expressions.
- Baby seems no better when fever subsides.
- Cries inconsolably or moans and cry becoming weaker.

ber to take fever in a baby under three months seriously.

- If your baby is becoming increasingly drowsy, pale, and lethargic and does not respond to fever-lowering methods, call your doctor.

- If your baby has obvious signs of a bacterial infection such as ear pain, severe cough, sore throat, or painful urination associated with the fever, call your doctor.

- Before paging your doctor, confirm the fever with a glass thermometer. Don't page the doctor with only an ear thermometer reading, as it is not accurate enough.

➤**REMEMBER:** *Determine whether or not to call your doctor according to the severity of your baby's illness, not the degree of temperature.*

Reporting Your Baby's Fever to Your Doctor

When communicating with your doctor by phone or in his or her office, have the following fever information ready:

- How the fever began: Did it shoot up very fast in a previously well baby, or did it begin very gradually and increase slightly each day as your baby became sicker?

- What the fever's pattern has been: Show or tell your doctor about your fever chart.

FALSE-ALARM FEVERS

Before calling your doctor, take the extra clothing or blankets off baby. Overwrapping babies is a common cause of false-alarm fever.

- How the illness has progressed: Does your baby seem to be getting more sick, less sick, or is she staying the same?

- What the other symptoms are: Does your baby have any other symptoms: painful crying, diarrhea, sore throat, vomiting, snotty nose, cough?

- How worried you are.

The Doctor's Approach

The combination of a feverish baby, a worried parent, and a concerned physician occurs many times a day in the life of a busy doctor. Get behind your doctor's stethoscope and see fever from his or her viewpoint. Fever is only the symptom that brought you to the doctor's office. It is the cause of the fever that counts.

First, your doctor tries to make a general decision: worry or no worry. Is this a minor illness, such as a virus (for example, roseola, see page 714), that will go away within a few days with only fever-lowering treatments and a tincture of time? Or is this a bacterial infection that will need antibiotics? And another decision: If it's a bacterial infection, is it serious or not?

Next, while laying hands on your hot baby, your doctor listens to your history and looks at your fever chart — which you brought along, didn't you? Then the doctor checks your baby for any clues to the cause of the fever. Sometimes the diagnosis is obvious by your history or the physical findings. At other times, it's a toughie, needing more time and tests for the diagnosis. If your doctor doesn't suspect more than a virus, he or she may go over fever control with you and send you and your baby home with the following admonition: "Be sure to report in if your baby gets worse." Sometimes the diagnosis is not apparent on the first exam, but baby will reveal more clues each day as the illness progresses, such as telltale spots in the throat or an illness-specific rash. In general, a viral illness is not treated with antibiotics, but in some cases there may be a reason to use an antibiotic to prevent a secondary bacterial infection from developing.

Your doctor will come to one of three conclusions:

- Your doctor will identify a specific bacterial infection (such as in the ear, throat, lungs, sinuses, intestines, or skin) and treat it appropriately.

- Your doctor won't find any specific cause for the fever, and after determining that the symptoms do not appear to be serious will conclude that the illness is probably an untreatable virus (such as a cold, flu, or other viral syndrome) and recommend a period of observation.

- Your doctor won't find any specific cause for the fever but will determine that the child seems unusually ill and be concerned that there may be an internal bacterial infection (such as a bladder or kidney infection, a blood infection, meningitis, a bone infection, or a pneumonia that is undetectable with a stethoscope). Such signs that may lead the doctor to this conclusion include rapid pulse, labored breathing, extreme irritability, severe lethargy, and a variety of other signs.

If your doctor suspects a serious bacterial infection, but it is not evident on examination where the infection is, he or she may order some laboratory tests, such as a culture (material to grow the germ from the throat, blood, or urine), blood tests, a chest X ray, or a urinalysis. How the white blood cells behave, determined by doing a *blood count,* often gives a clue to the type and seriousness of the infection.

Dr. Jim advises: Remember, treat the child, not the fever. You do not necessarily have to treat the fever if your child is acting fine or seems only minimally bothered by the fever. If your child has a fever of 102°F but is sitting quietly, resting, and not complaining, then you don't have to give any medication.

A Step-by-Step Approach to Lowering Your Baby's Fever

Reducing temperature in your baby is similar to cooling a house. Suppose your home is too hot. First, you reset the thermostat to a lower temperature so that the furnace doesn't click on so quickly (or you turn down the furnace). This is how fever-lowering medicines such as ibuprofen and acetaminophen work. They lower temperature production by resetting the body's thermostat. Next, you open the windows to let out the excess heat. This is also how you cool your baby's body, by removing clothing and putting baby in a lukewarm bath. And you keep attending to these heat-reducing and heat-releasing procedures until your home, or your child, is comfortable.

Suppose, however, you open the windows without turning down the furnace or the thermostat. The furnace would keep producing heat to match the degree set on the thermostat, and the house would stay hot. Or suppose you turn down the furnace but don't open the windows — the house would cool, but not as quickly. The hot house and the hot baby need *both* mechanisms: to decrease heat production and increase heat release.

Step One: Give Fever-Lowering Medicine

Acetaminophen and ibuprofen are fever-lowering medications of choice for infants and children. Aspirin is rarely used in children due to its possible link to Reye's syndrome (see page 712), its irritating effect on the intestines, and its narrow dosage range between efficacy and toxicity — pharmacy talk meaning the dose that does any good is very close to the dose that does harm.

Acetaminophen and ibuprofen can begin to lower the temperature within one-half hour and exert the maximum effect of bringing a high temperature down an average of 3°F (1.7°C) by around two to four hours after administration. But seldom does acetaminophen or ibuprofen bring a high temperature down to normal. Here are other things you should know about these medicines:

- Fever-reducing medicines for babies are available in liquid (drops and syrup), chewable tablets, and suppository forms. Drops are usually easier for infants under a year, syrups for children one to three years, and chewable tablets for children over three years. Suppositories are useful for vomiting babies who are unable to keep down oral medicine, but their fever-lowering effects are more variable than with the other forms.

- Pay careful attention to which form you are using. For example, acetaminophen and ibuprofen *drops* and *syrup* have different concentrations. If you were to use the dropper (which is designed specifically for administering only drops) to give the syrup, you would be giving your baby too little; if you were to use a teaspoon to administer drops, you would be giving your baby too much.

656   KEEPING YOUR BABY SAFE AND HEALTHY

> ## "VIRAL SYNDROME"
>
> You take your child to the doctor to evaluate a fever. After examining your child, the doctor says your child probably just has a virus. It is not treatable with antibiotics and should get better within a few days. The doctor leaves, and you are left not really knowing exactly what is wrong with your child.
>
> "Viral syndrome" is a diagnosis we give when we can't find a visible bacterial cause for a fever and the child does not appear very ill. There are dozens of viruses out there. Some of these we can identify because they fit a specific pattern and rash (such as chicken pox, roseola, and measles). Other viruses cause fever with or without a rash and do not fit a distinguishing pattern. We can determine that a child has a virus, but we can't always diagnose which virus it is. Not to worry, these viruses resolve within several days without any complications.

- Acetaminophen or ibuprofen overdosage is unlikely in children, since it takes ten to fifteen times the recommended onetime dose to make baby sick. Studies have shown that many parents *underestimate* the correct dose of fever-lowering medicines for their baby.

- It is safe to give baby an initial onetime *double dose* of acetaminophen if baby is in severe pain or is uncomfortable from a high fever.

- It is not safe to give a double dose of ibuprofen.

- If you have given your infant one fever-reducing medicine (say, acetaminophen) and it doesn't work within an hour or two, you may safely give the other medicine (ibuprofen) without waiting for the first medicine to clear the baby's system.

Which is better, acetaminophen or ibuprofen? Most parents have heard that ibuprofen works better than acetaminophen. While this may be true for some children, it is not true for others. Try each medication and see which one works better for your child. Here is a comparison of the two:

Acetaminophen

- has been around longer, and therefore has a longer safety record
- is approved for use in newborns
- is milder on the stomach, and therefore may be easier for little tummies to keep down
- lasts only three to four hours
- is processed by the liver

Ibuprofen

- may work faster
- may work better for higher fevers
- lasts longer, up to six to eight hours
- was only recently approved for as young as three months of age, so safety record in young infants not as time tested
- is more irritating to stomach, so it's better if taken with food
- is processed by the kidneys
- has added benefit as an anti-inflammatory — it can help with swelling, inflammation, cramping, and some aches that acetaminophen can't help

ACETAMINOPHEN DOSAGE

When treating fever or pain, we like to use a strong but safe dose so your child will feel better sooner. We have designed this chart with narrow weight ranges so you can give the best dose. The usual dose is 7 milligrams per pound, or 15 milligrams per kilogram, of body weight. For example, a 23-pound infant would get 160 milligrams (7 × 23). An 11-kilogram infant would get 160 milligrams (15 × 11). Pay careful attention to which form you are using: Drops and liquid come in different concentrations. *Doses can be given every four to six hours. The maximum number of doses per day is five.*

Weight	Dosage in milligrams	Infant drops	Children's liquid	Children's soft chews 80 mg each	Junior strength caps or chews 160 mg each
9–10 lb 4–5 kg	60 mg	¾ dropper (0.6 ml)	⅓ tsp (1.8 ml)	N/A	N/A
11–16 lb 5–7.5 kg	80 mg	1 dropper (0.8 ml)	½ tsp (2.5 ml)	N/A	N/A
17–21 lb 7.5–10 kg	120 mg	1½ droppers (1.2 ml)	¾ tsp (3.75 ml)	N/A	N/A
22–26 lb 10–12 kg	160 mg	2 droppers (1.6 ml)	1 tsp (5 ml)	2 tablets	1 tablet
27–32 lb 12–15 kg	200 mg	2½ droppers (2 ml)	1¼ tsp (6.25 ml)	2½ tablets	1 tablet
33–37 lb 15–17 kg	240 mg	3 droppers (2.4 ml)	1½ tsp (7.5 ml)	3 tablets	1½ tablets
38–42 lb 17–20 kg	280 mg	3½ droppers (2.8 ml)	1¾ tsp (8.75 ml)	3½ tablets	1½ tablets
43–53 lb 20–25 kg	320 mg	4 droppers (3.2 ml)	2 tsp (10 ml)	4 tablets	2 tablets
54–64 lb 25–30 kg	400 mg	Use liquid or tablets	2½ tsp (12.5 ml)	5 tablets	2½ tablets

Weight	Dosage in milligrams	Infant drops	Children's liquid	Children's soft chews 80 mg each	Junior strength caps or chews 160 mg each
65–75 lb 30–35 kg	480 mg		3 tsp (15 ml)	6 tablets	3 tablets
76–86 lb 35–40 kg	560 mg		3½ tsp (17.5 ml)	7 tablets	3½ tablets
87–95 lb 40–45 kg	640 mg		4 tsp (20 ml)	8 tablets	4 tablets
>95 lbs >45 kg	Give adult dose				

Acetaminophen Suppositories Dosage

You will notice that these doses tend to be a little higher than oral doses. Higher suppository doses are safe for two reasons:

1. Suppositories are absorbed less consistently than oral doses.
2. Suppositories are meant for short-term use (only when your child cannot tolerate oral doses), and giving a little higher dose for one day is not harmful.

Doses can be given every four to six hours.

Weight	120 mg suppository	325 mg suppository
12–17 lb 6–7.5 kg	1 suppository	
18–23 lb 7.5–10 kg	1½ suppositories	
24–37 lb 11–17 kg	2 suppositories	
38–60 lb 17–27 kg		1 suppository
61–90 lb 27–40 kg		1½ suppositories
>90 lb >40 kg		2 suppositories

IBUPROFEN DOSAGE

Different dropper sizes: Some **infants'** ibuprofen brands come with a 1.25 ml dropper, and some brands come with a 1.875 ml syringe for dosing. The amount you are giving is the same; you are just giving it in a different-size dropper. The **children's** liquid is dosed in teaspoons. The usual dose of ibuprofen is 5 milligrams per pound (or 10 milligrams per kilogram) of body weight. For example, a 20-pound (9-kilogram) infant would get 100 milligrams. *Doses can be given every six hours. The maximum number of doses per day is four.*

Weight	Dosage in milligrams	Infant drops	Children's liquid	Children's chewable tablets 50 mg each	Junior strength caps or chews 100 mg each
9–10 lb >3 months 4–5 kg	25 mg	½ dropper (0.625 ml)	N/A	N/A	N/A
11–16 lb 5–7.5 kg	50 mg	1 dropper (1.25 ml)	½ tsp (2.5 ml)	N/A	N/A
17–21 lb 7.5–10 kg	75 mg	1½ droppers (1.25 ml + 0.625 ml)	¾ tsp (3.75 ml)	N/A	N/A
22–26 lb 10–12 kg	100 mg	2 droppers (2 × 1.25 ml)	1 tsp (5 ml)	2 tablets	1 tablet
27–32 lb 12–15 kg	125 mg	2½ droppers (2 × 1.25 ml + 0.625 ml)	1¼ tsp (6.25 ml)	2½ tablets	1 tablet
33–37 lb 15–17 kg	150 mg	3 droppers (3 × 1.25 ml)	1½ tsp (7.5 ml)	3 tablets	1½ tablets
38–42 lb 17–20 kg	175 mg	3½ droppers (3 × 1.25 ml + 0.625 ml)	1¾ tsp (8.75 ml)	3½ tablets	1½ tablets
43–53 lb 20–25 kg	200 mg	4 droppers (4 × 1.25 ml)	2 tsp (10 ml)	4 tablets	2 tablets

Weight	Dosage in milligrams	Infant drops	Children's liquid	Children's chewable tablets 50 mg each	Junior strength caps or chews 100 mg each
54–64 lb 25–30 kg	250 mg	Use liquid or tablets	2½ tsp (12.5 ml)	5 tablets	2½ tablets
65–75 lb 30–35 kg	300 mg		3 tsp (15 ml)	6 tablets	3 tablets
76–86 lb 35–40 kg	350 mg		3½ tsp (17.5 ml)	7 tablets	3½ tablets
87–95 lb 40–45 kg	400 mg		4 tsp (20 ml)	8 tablets	4 tablets
>95 lbs >45 kg	Give adult dose				

Step Two: Let the Heat Out

After giving your baby the proper dosage of medication and lowering heat production in the body, next you want to let the excess heat out. Here's how.

Dress for the temperature. Neither underclothe nor overclothe baby. Underdressing encourages shivering, while overdressing retains heat. In the summer it is best to let baby run around and sleep in diapers only, or at most in lightweight, loose-fitting cotton clothing. This allows excess heat to escape from your baby's body into the cooler air. One day I heard a mother and grandmother arguing in my waiting room about whether to bundle or undress a feverish baby. Grandmother was admonishing the new mother,

"Wrap him up with more clothes or he'll catch cold." The mother snapped back, "He already has a cold. The heat needs to get out."

This is one of the few instances where mother's wisdom prevailed over grandmother's. Overbundling keeps heat in, like putting a blanket over a hot house. I have seen babies with fevers come into my office bundled up like little Alaskans or baby burritos.

Keep cool. This applies to your environment, your baby, and yourself. Open a window in baby's room or use an air conditioner or fan. Cool air helps remove the heat that is radiating from your baby's hot body. A draft will not bother baby. Also, it is all right for a feverish child to go *outside*. The fresh air is good for her.

Give extra fluids. Fever makes the body thirsty. Sweating and rapid breathing cause the body to lose fluids that need replacing. Let your baby suck on nutritious popsicles and sip cool, clear liquids all day. Breastfeeding is a good source of fluids *and* comfort.

Feed the fever. When hot the body works faster to remove the extra heat and burns up fuel that needs replacing in the form of nutritious calories. Babies often do not want to eat when they are sick and feverish, but they must drink. Your baby may protest heavy, fatty foods. They are difficult to digest because intestinal activity seems to slow down during fever. Nibbling and sipping throughout the day is a healthy eating pattern for the feverish child. Calorie-filled smoothies combine the need for food and fluids — and they are cool.

A cool dip. If baby's temperature is 104°F (40°C) or higher, or if baby seems bothered

by the fever, put her in waist-high lukewarm water. Adjust the water temperature so that it is just warm enough to be comfortable for baby. Hot babies usually protest cold water, and it can make them shiver, increasing the body's temperature. Allowing water to remain on baby's hot body promotes cooling by evaporation. During the bath, rub baby's skin with a washcloth to stimulate circulation to the skin and increase heat loss. Prolong this sponging ritual as long as baby will tolerate it. It usually requires at least twenty minutes to bring the temperature down two degrees. After the bath, pat your baby's skin but leave a little bit of dampness to evaporate for an added cooling effect. If an hour or so after the bath your baby's temperature zooms back up, it's back into the tub for the bathing and sponging ritual.

Here are some other bath tips:

- Be sure to give your child fever-lowering medication *before* putting her in the bath. If she gets out of a cooling bath and starts to shiver, her temperature will go back up. Medications lessen this reaction.

- Putting a screaming baby into the tub only raises her temperature. Instead, try sitting in the tub with her, amusing baby with her favorite floating toys.

- Try standing with baby in a lukewarm shower — this may work even better than a bath.

- Do not use *alcohol baths* to lower fever. Alcohol may be absorbed through baby's skin or its vapors inhaled into the lungs, both possibly harming baby. Also, alcohol constricts the blood vessels in the skin, reducing heat loss and aggravating fever.

GETTING FEVER DOWN

- Give appropriate doses of medication every four waking hours.
- Push fluids.
- Keep the environment cool.
- Do not overclothe baby.
- Place the infant in a lukewarm bath if her temperature is 104°F (40°C) or higher.

Fever Fits (febrile seizures)

Fever itself is not dangerous and does not harm a baby unless it reaches 107°F (41.7°C), which is rare. The two main reasons for treating fever are to relieve the overall discomfort of feeling feverish and to avoid febrile convulsions. A baby's immature brain may react to sudden temperature fluctuation with a convulsion. It is not so much how high the temperature soars, but rather *how fast it rises* that causes convulsions. Younger infants are most susceptible to febrile convulsions; they are unusual in children over the age of five.

Some convulsions give warning *twitches* — a shaking arm, a twitching lip, or a vacant stare. As soon as you notice one of these signs, to the shower immediately you and baby go. A quick cooling may abort a temperature takeoff and prevent a total convulsion. Other times a full-blown convulsion occurs without any warning, and parents may not even realize baby has a fever. Baby shakes all over, his eyes roll back, his skin becomes pale, and he goes limp. While seeming like an eternity, most febrile convulsions last only ten to twenty seconds, not enough to harm baby, but they may leave parents shaking. Only convulsions that cause baby to turn blue for several minutes (very rare with febrile convulsions) are likely to harm a baby. Expect baby to fall asleep following a convulsion, but you to be wide-awake with worry.

The same fever spike that caused the first convulsion may return for a repeat performance within an hour or two. For this reason, administer fever-prevention remedies right after the convulsion. If baby is sleeping, give an appropriately dosed acetaminophen *suppository* and only lightly dress your sleeping baby. If baby is awake after the convulsion, encourage extra fluids (but no food if you suspect another convulsion coming, as baby may choke on the food during a convulsion); also give medications and a shower, an assisted tub bath, or an out-of-the-tub sponge bath if you sense another convulsion coming on. (See also "Convulsions," page 731.)

COLDS

Most babies get six to eight colds during the first two years. Get to know these germs well. Here is how to prevent, recognize, treat, and live with your infant's colds.

What Is a Cold?

What is this mysterious germ that causes babies to miss sleep, parents to miss work, and doctors to get phone calls? A cold, called an upper respiratory infection (URI) in medical terms, is caused by germs of either viral or bacterial type. These microbes infect the lining of the breathing passages: nose, sinuses, ears, throat, and bronchi in the lungs. Nesting in these moist membranes, the germs multiply. The lining reacts to this invasion by swelling and secreting mucus, accounting for the noisy breathing of colds. Mucus continues to pour out, giving the telltale runny nose. Mucus also pours inside, causing postnasal drip, a throat tickle, raspy sounds, and a cough. If germs advance farther into the caves of the breathing tunnels, similar swelling and mucus accumulates in the sinuses and ears. Finally, these germs make their deepest penetration into the bronchi of the lungs, where the swollen lining narrows the airways, causing noisy, wheezy breathing.

By this time the body is ready to fight back. Reflexes in the airways trigger coughing and sneezing, the body's guns, to blast the unwelcome mucus out. Usually after coughing, sneezing, and dripping for a few days, the body wins the fight, the cold leaves, and all in the house sleep well again. But sometimes these germs refuse to leave without more of a fight, and the body mobilizes higher-powered troops to wage a more explosive fight. White blood cells, the body's scavengers, advance to the scene of the invasion and attack the germs wallowing in the mucus. The by-product of this fight is a four-letter word that will irritate your baby and cause you to miss sleep and miss work. It is called, in medical language, mucopurulent discharge; in parent terms, snot.

Now, the problem with snot is that it is not easily pushed around like its earlier relative, the drip. It just stays there blocking the breathing roads. Then it thickens and takes on a coat of a different color — green. When the green flag goes up, it means other germs take advantage of this thick mess — a perfect culture medium for germs. Like fertilized weeds, the bacteria grow in the goo, and the green-yellow flag of infection is raised: green

snotty nose and yellow discharge from the eyes. As a sign that the body is mobilizing its big infection-fighting guns, fever arrives. At this point the battle is at a turning point. The body's defenses and home remedies alone may win, and the cold departs within the next few days, leaving behind only a residual sniffle and cough. Or the illness may escalate and the child act sicker. General Mom or Dad seeks reinforcements. The doctor prescribes an antibiotic that gets right to the heart of the matter and kills the germs. As this master fighter does its job, the snot thins into a drip, the swollen passages shrink, and baby breathes nicely again — and so do the parents. This is the story of a cold.

How Colds Are Caught

The saying "to catch a cold" is medically accurate, although it is more correct to say the cold catches you. Cold germs travel by droplet spread, meaning they ride on microscopic water balloons tossed into the air by a cough or sneeze, to be inhaled by other persons

---

SLOWING DOWN THE SPREAD OF RUNNY NOSES

- "Hose the nose" frequently. (See "Unstuffing Baby's Nose," page 665.)
- Teach your child to blow his own nose, using a tissue.
- Teach your child to cover her nose and mouth while coughing or sneezing using the "cold shoulder" technique: Show her how to turn her head toward her shoulder, while lifting her arm in front of her face, instead of covering nose and mouth

with her hands during a cough or sneeze. Coughing into the shoulder or upper arm is less likely to spread germs than coughing onto the hands.
- Wash your child's hands after nose wiping and coughing.
- Avoid nose-to-nose snuggling during a cold.
- Discourage your child from rubbing her nose and eyes during a cold.

within cold-catching distance. These droplets and their germ passengers also travel from hand to hand. So not only can we catch a cold, we can literally pick one up. Baby A rubs his own snotty nose with his hands, shakes his gooey hand with that of Baby B, who rubs his own nose, and the germ finds a new nose home to begin another invasion. This is why wise grandmother insisted that a snotty child wash his hands and cover his nose and mouth when coughing and sneezing. But grandmother was mistaken when she proclaimed that colds come from drafts, cold feet, uncovered heads, or not eating vegetables.

More About Colds

If your baby played with a sneezing friend yesterday and is coughing today, his friend didn't share this germ. Most cold germs take at least two to four days from exposure to symptoms, the *incubation period*. Search for where your child played a few days ago. After the six to eight colds of the first two years, a child's immunity builds up, and the doctor visits and missed workdays lessen. Expect more-frequent colds in the winter, from November through February. The cold weather is not to blame. A more likely explanation is that children are bunched closer together in the winter and stay indoors more, where the air is drier and stagnates (especially in centrally heated homes).

Besides runny noses, some colds cause a low-grade fever, generalized aches, watery eyes, diarrhea, and a generally unwell feeling. Most viruses make a gentle exit within a few days, leaving only a slight runny nose and a happily running child. Occasionally a cold lingers for two to three weeks with a nagging cough and runny nose, and then finally goes away. Sometimes, however, colds progress into more worrisome infections needing more vigorous treatment.

Treating Colds

Most of the discomfort from a cold is due to thick mucus obstructing narrow airways. Just as still water in a pond stagnates and becomes a breeding ground for all kinds of organisms, so do mucous secretions in children. Secretions trapped in the sinuses and middle ears provide an attractive nutrient for bacteria to multiply and eventually cause a bacterial infection. Treatment, therefore, is aimed at keeping secretions moving through clogged airways. Remember the golden rule of treating colds — keep the mucus *thin and moving*. Here's how.

Clearing the Nose

"Hose the nose." Since babies are usually unable to clear their own nose, you must do it for them. Follow the technique described in the box on the next page.

Teach baby to blow his nose. Most children under three have difficulty blowing their nose, but it's worth trying with your two-year-old. Teach him to blow out a candle, and then show him how to do it with his nose, and "that's the way you blow your nose." You can also try squeezing the child's lips closed while he blows, which will redirect the air to come out his nose. Then blow your nose and have baby hold the handkerchief in front of your nose while you blow. Next he does the same, and you blow noses together. "Blow, don't sniff" is the motto of the clean-nose club, but blow gently.

UNSTUFFING BABY'S NOSE

Babies can seldom blow their own nose. You have to clear the stuffy nasal passages for them. Here's how to "hose the nose."

Giving Nose Drops to Baby
Purchase saline nasal spray (a specially formulated saltwater mist solution available over-the-counter at a pharmacy). Hold baby upright. Squirt one spray into each nostril. Next, lay baby down for a minute with head lower than body. This allows the saltwater to loosen the thick secretions and stimulates baby to sneeze them to the front of the nose, where you are waiting to grab the thick stuff with your trusty nasal aspirator (veteran nose cleaners call this gadget their snot snatcher). Expect your baby to protest this intrusion into his nose; but little noses need to be unstuffed for breathing, especially during feeding.

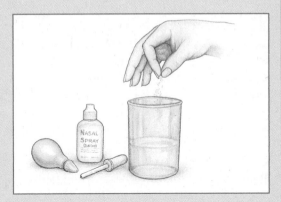

Home nasal care kit (left to right): bulb aspirator, commercial saline spray, medicine dropper, homemade saline solution (pinch of salt in a glass of water).

Or you can make your own saltwater nose drops. Put a pinch of salt (no more than one-quarter teaspoon) in an eight-ounce (240-milliliter) glass of warm tap water. With a plastic eyedropper, squirt a few drops into each nostril and proceed as above.

Be careful not to release the dropper bulb or spray bottle while it is still in baby's nose. This allows nasal secretions into the dropper or bottle, contaminating the fluid. Wash the area of the dropper or bottle that touched the nose. Because it's specially formulated, over-the-counter nasal spray is kinder to the lining of the nasal passages than home-made nose drops.

Using a Nasal Aspirator
To use the nasal aspirator, squeeze the rubber bulb, then insert the plastic or rubber tip into baby's nose firmly enough to form a seal, and slowly release, letting the suction draw out the mucous plugs. Do this two or three times in each nostril, or as often as your baby needs suctioning and will tolerate the procedure. After each use, suck soap and water into the aspirator and rinse well with plain water. Various shapes of nasal aspirators are available at your pharmacy.

> **Dr. Sears's home cold remedy:**
> **A "nose hose" + "steam clean" = easier breathing.**

Blowing or sniffing too hard may drive secretions into the sinuses or ears and prolong the cold. Teach your child to gently but effectively blow his nose. Babies seldom cough the secretions out. Instead, they swallow the goo and their stomach rebels. Vomiting following coughing is common in children.

Thinning the Secretions

Dry air and small breathing passages don't make good roommates. The breathing passages are lined with tiny filaments, called cilia, on which rides a layer of mucus. This protective system acts like miniature conveyor belts, removing lint and other particles from inspired air. Dry air, especially from central heating, acts like a sponge, soaking up moisture from all parts of the body — skin, hair, and especially the breathing passages. Dry air, in effect, stops these conveyor belts. The mucus accumulates in globs and acts as a culture medium for bacteria; this results in swollen, clogged airways and difficulty breathing.

"Steam clean" stuffy airways. Giving baby extra fluids during the day and running a vaporizer while he sleeps helps thin secretions, making them easier to sneeze or cough out. Or take baby into the bathroom, close the door, turn on the hot water in the shower, and enjoy a steam bath together. Steam opens clogged breathing passages and helps drain the secretions.

Maintaining the proper humidity in baby's sleeping environment will give the breathing passages the moisture they need. Allergists caution that a relative humidity over 50 percent may encourage the growth of molds and dust mites and trigger allergies, whereas respiratory therapists warn that humidity under 25 percent may clog the airways. Thus a room humidity of 30–50 percent is ideal. Check the humidity in the bedroom, using a hygrometer available at a hardware store. Having a higher humidity from a vaporizer in baby's bedroom for a few days during the worst part of a cold is OK. Be sure to air out the room during the day by opening the windows.

Although we prefer vaporizers for adding moisture to the air, humidifiers, if properly operated and *carefully* maintained, can also do a satisfactory job. Here are some tips for using vaporizers and humidifiers:

- Because vaporizers produce *hot* mist they pose a burn hazard. Carefully instruct toddlers and older children about this danger by showing them the hot steam and teaching them it is hot. Burns on the hand can be serious. Be sure to place the vaporizer out of baby's grabbing distance.

- Clean vaporizers and humidifiers according to the manufacturer's suggestions at least once a week; more often is preferable. One-half cup bleach to a gallon of water (125 milliliters bleach to 4 liters water) makes a good cleaning solution (better is whatever solution is advised by the manufacturer). Rinse well after cleaning.

- Change water daily and dry the vaporizer between uses.

- Use water (either distilled or tap) according to the manufacturer's suggestions.

- Place the vaporizer about two feet (sixty centimeters) from your infant and direct the jet across baby's nose to deliver concentrated humidity.

- Adding medicines: Eucalyptus-containing medications to open breathing passages

HUMIDIFIERS VERSUS VAPORIZERS

That blast of humid air you breathe may thin the secretions and ease breathing, but not all mist is clean or safe. Humidifier or vaporizer mist is produced three ways: shaking the water (ultrasonic), blowing it (impeller-type), and boiling it (a vaporizer). Here's what you should know about these appliances.

Humidifiers

Humidifiers produce a *cool* mist. The newest are the whisper-quiet, ultrasonic type, which use high-frequency sound to break up water into mist. This produces clean air (kills bacteria and mold) but may not produce safe air. New studies reveal that this ultrafine mist may also contain the pulverized impurities in mineral-laden tap water. These minute particles (for example, asbestos, lead, and other minerals) can be breathed into the airways and irritate the lower breathing passages. This potential danger can be minimized by buying an ultrasonic humidifier with a built-in particle filter or changeable demineralizing cartridges, or by using distilled water.

Impeller-type humidifiers are usually not as quiet as the ultrasonic, and these humidifiers are likely to harbor bacteria and mold and spew these germs into the air. Some of the newer impeller humidifiers contain filters.

Worst are the older rotating-drum and furnace-mounted humidifiers, which hold a pool of stagnant water. We discourage using this type.

Vaporizers

As their name implies, vaporizers produce a hot vapor and deliver a more concentrated amount of mist over a smaller area. Because the water is boiled inside, the steam produced kills bacteria and molds, and the minerals never leave the machine. For most respiratory illnesses, vaporizers are preferred over humidifiers for delivering moisture to breathing passages. A vaporizer also enables you to turn down central heat, thus minimizing its drying effects. A hot-mist vaporizer can keep a nursery-sized bedroom comfortably toasty while keeping little noses from drying out. There is one situation, however, where cool mist is better than hot steam, and this is during an illness called croup (see page 683 for more information).

---

are available to add to the vaporizer (not to the humidifier). Unless advised by your doctor, these are unnecessary for children.

- In a pinch you can rig your own "vaporizer" by closing the bathroom door and running a hot shower.

Understanding and Selecting Cold Medicines

How do you define "confusion"? Answer: Standing in a pharmacy surveying the "coughs and colds" shelf. There are many kinds of over-the-counter cold formulas, and their advertised ways of working can be grouped simply: They dry or thin secretions and squeeze or shrink mucus-producing vessels and glands lining the airway passages.

Medicated decongestant nose drops or sprays. These work by constricting the blood vessels in the lining of the nose and shrinking the swollen membranes, thus opening up the nose. In infants, even newborns, nose drops can be safely used, but they can also be abused. Infant nose-drop medications do give temporary relief by helping baby breathe. Infants are obligate nose breathers, meaning they do not easily breathe through their mouth when their nose is plugged, like adults do. They keep on struggling to breathe through an obstructed nose. Nose drops often open up a plugged nose within a few minutes, allowing the previously stuffy-nosed, restless infant to feed or fall asleep. But a word of caution: Use these drops no more than *three* times a day for *three* straight days, because they can cause a rebound effect when stopped — the constricted vessels dilate even more and produce even more congestion. For nose drops to work best (get down to the lining of the nose where they do their job), clear the nose first with the saline "hose the nose" method, then instill the drops. Unlike decongestant sprays, saline nasal sprays may be used as often as needed.

Decongestants. Taken orally, decongestants shrink the lining of the breathing passages by constricting the dilated blood vessels and lessening mucous secretion. But there may be a downside to overusing them. Remember our goal: to keep secretions thin and moving. Some research has shown that decongestants interfere with the action of cilia, the tiny hairs that line airway passages and push secretions along. This fact, together with the drying effect of decongestant-antihistamine combinations, may actually cause secretions to stagnate. Also, at a dosage high enough to decongest, these medications may rev up the system, causing a fast heart rate, hyperactivity, and sleeplessness. Oral decongestants are currently approved for use in infants as young as six months of age. We discourage their use in younger infants.

Antihistamines. As the name implies, antihistamines block the action of histamine, the substance that is produced when an allergen comes in contact with the allergy-susceptible lining of the breathing passages. Histamine releases secretions: runny nose, watery eyes, sneezing. Antihistamines may be effective if your child's symptoms are due to allergies, but may have little effect on a cold. Undesirable effects are drowsiness (unless it's nighttime), dizziness, and gastrointestinal upset. In babies and children antihistamines rarely excite the system instead of sedating the baby. Some preparations contain decongestant-antihistamine combinations, but unless your doctor tells you to use them, single-ingredient cold preparations are preferable for infants. Sometimes infants have both an allergy and a cold, and it is difficult to tell them apart or tell which came first (see page 426 for telling the difference between a cold and an allergy). In this case, a combination medicine may work well.

To help you decide which cold medicines may help your baby, try these suggestions:

- The first step is deciding whether or not to even use medicine. Treat the child, not the runny nose. If your child is breathing comfortably and the runny nose isn't bothering him, then it's okay to let it go. It's better to let the mucus come out.

- Limit the use of cold medicines to the following situations: if you are advised by your doctor to use them; if the congestion is truly bothering baby, that is, preventing sleeping or feeding; if baby tolerates these medicines without uncomfortable side effects (infant tolerances vary greatly); and if you objectively believe they work.

- Currently there is only one decongestant ingredient that is used in all over-the-counter medications. It is called pseudoephedrine. Therefore, it doesn't really matter what brand you use, as long as you use the right dose.

- There are several different antihistamines, and all are considered safe when used as directed. Drowsiness is common and may be unwanted during the daytime in older children.

- Combination decongestants and antihistamines are generally safe and effective, especially if you want the sedating effect to help your infant sleep day or night.

- These medications are available in combination with a cough medicine. These are appropriate when there are multiple symptoms that are bothersome.

- It is safe to use several different medications, as long as the purpose of the medicines does not overlap. For example, you can use a separate decongestant, a separate antihistamine, and a separate cough medicine. But you shouldn't use a combination cough plus decongestant medicine along with a separate decongestant medicine.

- Expectorants help loosen chest congestion. These can be useful in combination with decongestants and/or antihistamines if your child's cold is accompanied by a congested chest.

For most colds and most babies your nasal care kit is still the safest, least expensive, and most effective cold remedy — along with, of course, the tincture of time.

When to Call the Doctor

Most viral colds need only good nasal care, extra fluids, and time. A trip to the medicine shelf may be helpful, but a visit to your doctor's office is not always necessary. Yet oftentimes the cold lingers (the snot thickens), and you're faced with the decision of whether or not to take your baby to the doctor. Here's how to tell.

CONSULT DR. SEARS'S MEDICINE CABINET

For updates, dosages, and additional help in selecting appropriate cold remedies for infants and children, visit www.AskDrSears.com. Click on "Medicine Cabinet." Most cold and cough medications instruct consumers to consult their doctor for correct dosage for children under two years of age. Our online medicine cabinet will give you correct doses down to six months of age.

How much is the cold bothering baby? Is baby happy, playful, eating and sleeping well, with little or no fever? This cold is simply a noisy nuisance and needs only your home treatment.

What's coming out of baby's nose? If the secretions are clear and watery (runny nose), it's a no worry. If the discharge is becoming increasingly thick, yellow, or green (a snotty nose) and stays that way for several days, this is not necessarily a worry, especially if it is not accompanied by a fever and a cranky child. A nose tip: Don't be fooled by your child's snotty nose when she first wakes up in the morning. This is usual even with a simple cold, because the secretions have had a chance to thicken overnight. Hose the nose and see if the discharge clears. A green nose doesn't necessarily mean it's a bacterial infection. Many viral colds have a thick, green mucousy phase that may last seven days or more.

How is your child acting? If your child is generally happy, with little or no fever, and not seemingly ill, then you do not necessarily need to take him to the doctor, even if his nose is green.

Look into your baby's eyes. Eyes mirror health. If baby's eyes are still sparkly, don't worry. If they are glazed, be concerned. If yellow matter exudes from the corners of baby's eyes most of the day (not just in the morning), this usually merits a visit to the doctor.

►*SPECIAL NOTE: Discharging eyes plus a cold warrants a doctor's exam. This is a clue to a probable underlying sinus and/or ear infection. Discharging eyes plus reddened eyeballs and no snotty nose may be con-junctivitis and not a cold. These observations are why our office policy is not to treat discharging eyes over the phone if baby has a cold. (See also discussions of blocked tear ducts, page 105, and conjunctivitis, page 426.)*

What direction is the cold taking? Days one to three, the nose is running and the baby is running. But by day five the snot thickens and baby quiets; and other signs appear: fever, crankiness, and a peaked look. Off to the doctor go you and your baby. Colds without worry steadily get better over three to five days; colds for concern steadily get worse.

Other signs and symptoms. Common colds are mainly a nuisance because the nasal congestion obstructs breathing. Once the nose is cleared, baby should feel and act better. But a cranky child, snotty nose, fever, sleeplessness, sore throat, sore ears, severe cough, or puffy, discharging eyes are signs that more is brewing than a common cold.

What to Expect at Your Doctor's Office

When your doctor examines your baby for a cold, he or she tries first to make the decision if it is a viral cold that will go away without prescription medicine or a bacterial infection, which warrants an antibiotic. Next question is, If it is a bacterial infection, where is it hiding: nose, sinuses, throat, ears, or chest? If your doctor finds no signs of bacterial infection in any of these hiding places and baby doesn't seem that sick, he or she will advise you to continue home treatment, with the admonition: "Call me if baby gets worse." Remember this counsel. Colds often travel into sinuses, ears, or chest, and this requires a change in diagnosis and treatment.

How to Talk with Your Doctor About Baby's Cold

When communicating with your doctor by phone or in the office, have the following cold facts available:

- When did the cold begin?

- How has it progressed? Is it getting better, worse, or staying the same?

- How much is the cold bothering your child's sleep, play, and appetite?

- What is the nature of the nasal discharge? Is it clear and runny or thick, yellow, green, and snotty, and for how long has it been this way?

- Are there other signs and symptoms, such as fever, eye drainage, cough, earache, paleness, lethargy, sore throat, swollen glands, rash, persistent vomiting, or drowsiness?

Finally, be sure to communicate how sick you feel your child is and how worried you are. In pediatrics especially, doctors regard intuitive parents as partners in the diagnosis and treatment of their sick child. Your running commentary of the illness helps the doctor make the right diagnosis. Sometimes your child just happens to act well during the five-minute doctor visit but very sick before and after; in this case, your doctor may not have a true picture of how sick baby really is. Your history helps.

When Is a Cold Contagious?

A cold is most contagious in the very early stages, before you even realize your baby is sick. As a general guide the longer the cold persists, the less contagious it is. If your baby has a clear runny nose and no fever, is not acting sick, and is just noisy because of sniffling and coughing, it is seldom necessary to quarantine him. If, however, your baby is coughing profusely, has a snotty nose and yellow drainage from the eyes, is running a fever, and is generally ill, keep him away from other babies for a few days. If he is in a group where runny noses are the rule, wash his hands frequently and don't let him share mouthable toys.

COUGHS

Besides fevers, coughs rank at the top of the call-your-doctor list. Coughs present two problems: They are a nuisance, often keeping baby and everyone else awake, and the cough is a signal that something unwelcome is brewing in the lungs. Consider the following cough tips.

Rate the Cough

Most colds produce coughs as the baby's natural defense to dislodge the obstructive mucus from the breathing passages. Coughs

---

DR. SEARS'S ADVICE

- Happy child + clear nasal discharge = no worry.
- Increasingly unhappy child + increasingly snotty nose = time to visit the doctor.
- *Always* check with your doctor if your baby's cold is getting worse.

WORRYING ABOUT COUGHS

When Not to Worry

- Baby has no fever and appears well.
- Baby coughs during the day but sleeps well at night.
- The cough does not interfere with eating, playing, or sleeping.
- The cough is steadily improving.

When to Call the Doctor

- The cough begins suddenly, persists, and you feel the baby may have gotten something lodged in his throat.
- The cough wakes the baby at night.
- The cough is accompanied by severe allergies.
- Baby also has fever, chills, and is generally ill.
- Baby is coughing up thick, yellow-green mucus.
- The cough gets progressively worse.

---

divide into three categories: noisy coughs, nuisance coughs, and need-doctor coughs. If your baby has a cold and a hacking cough but eats well, plays well, and sleeps well, no concern or treatment is necessary. If baby is not acting sick during the day, but the cough keeps her awake during nap time and the night, this is a nuisance cough that may need treatment. If the cough is associated with fever, a fast heart rate, lethargy, vomiting, or coughing up green stuff, this is a need-doctor cough.

The Persistent Cough

For a week or two after the nose is clear, a cough may hang on, becoming a nuisance for the child and family. Most lingering coughs are caused by lingering viruses, especially with the story, "He doesn't act sick and the cough doesn't bother him, it just lingers." Allergies head the list of chronic cough causes, especially if accompanied by other allergic signs: runny nose, puffy eyes, wheezing. (See "Tracking and Treating Inhalant Allergies," page 698.) Don't forget a foreign body as a hidden cause of a persistent cough. The bronchus will not tolerate a resident peanut and, by coughing, will tell the world to get it out. Any cough that persists for more than two weeks merits a doctor's exam.

Coughs associated with the common cold are seldom contagious after the first few days of the illness, especially if baby is generally acting well.

Pneumonia

Many parents bring their kids into the office with cough and fever because they are worried about pneumonia. Pneumonia is actually fairly rare, and most deep, junky sounding coughs with fever are simple chest colds. Symptoms of pneumonia include rapid, labored breathing, chest pain, fever, vomiting, and a severe deep cough. Your doctor will be able to distinguish between a chest cold and pneumonia on examination.

Two Unique Coughing Situations

There are two illnesses that cause a very specific cough that you should be aware of.

Croup. This is a virus (not treatable with antibiotics) that causes a cough that sounds like a seal barking. It also causes raspy breathing and a hoarse voice. If this describes your child, see page 683.

Whooping cough. This is a bacterial illness that starts off like any normal cold and cough, then progresses into severe fits of uncontrollable and continuous coughing that last from thirty seconds to two minutes. What is unique about these fits is that the child can barely catch his breath during the attack, which causes his face to turn red, purple, and even blue if the fit is prolonged. When the child is finally able to take a breath, it sounds like a hollow, raspy "whooping" sound as the child gasps for air. If this describes your child, see page 716.

Calming Coughs

That hacking noise that keeps you on edge or gets baby ejected from day care does not always need to be stopped. This noisy nuisance can be a cold's best friend. Secretions accumulating in the lower airways trigger the cough reflex to dislodge the pesty mucus like some mighty wind clearing the roads. Without the cough, secretions would form mucous plugs that both obstruct air flow and serve as tiny culture packets for bacteria to grow. With these cough facts in mind, treat this special chest protector kindly. If the cough bothers baby, try the following.

Keep the secretions thin and moving. To make it easier for baby to cough up the mucus, try the home remedies that we advised in "Thinning the Secretions," page 666.

Clap on baby's back. Called chest physiotherapy, clapping at least ten times on each side of baby's back around four times a day may help dislodge mucus from the airways. Following an exam, if your doctor detects a certain place that the airways are obstructed, he or she may instruct you to clap most where the doctor's X marks the spot.

Clear the air. Allergens or irritants in the air, especially in baby's sleeping room, can cause a lingering cough and aggravate an existing cough caused by an infection. Definitely have a no-smoking rule when there is a baby in the house or car. (Also see "How to Allergyproof a Bedroom," page 700.)

Choose the right cough medicine. There are three kinds of cough remedies: suppressants, expectorants, and mixtures of both. These are different medicines for different coughs, and the wrong use may worsen the situation.

Daytime coughs usually do not bother a baby and often need only the remedies mentioned above. If the cough, however, interferes with baby's eating, napping, and playing, give an *expectorant-only* preparation. If the cough still interferes with baby's daytime functioning, try an *expectorant-suppressant* combination according to the dosage on the package or as prescribed by your doctor.

At night, if baby's sleep is not interrupted by the cough, use a vaporizer only, no medicine. If the cough prevents baby from going to sleep or staying asleep, try the same procedures as during the day: Give a combination expectorant-suppressant a half-hour before bedtime, and repeat in four to six hours if baby awakens coughing. It is best to allow baby to cough during the day but sleep well at night. Cough medicines, if used wisely and safely, may help baby and you sleep.

- *Suppressants* are cough stoppers that inhibit the cough reflex in the brain. The most commonly available over-the-counter preparation is *dextromethorphan,* identified by the suffix *-DM* added to the trade name. Since package labels do not give the DM dosage for children under two years of age, here is a safe dosage guide: 2 milligrams of DM per 10 pounds of body weight, or 2 milligrams per 5 kilograms. (For example, for a 20-pound toddler the dosage would be 4 milligrams of DM.) This dosage could be repeated in four to six hours during the night if the child persistently awakens. Side effects of nausea, dizziness, and drowsiness infrequently occur with DM-containing cough syrups. The most effective cough suppressant is the prescription narcotic codeine, which most doctors are wisely reluctant to prescribe for children because of the side effects of drowsiness or hyper-irritability. But if the over-the-counter DM isn't working and you have a choice between being up all night and getting a good night's sleep, then a codeine syrup may be just what the doctor ordered.

- *Expectorants* are cough looseners that liquefy the secretions, making them easier to cough up. Indirectly these may lessen the cough by thinning the secretions, but they do not directly stop the cough. They are safe, effective, and available over-the-counter as the active ingredient guaifenesin. It does not usually cause side effects.

- *Mixtures.* Some cough remedies, both over-the-counter and prescription, contain three ingredients: a decongestant and/or antihistamine, an expectorant, and a suppressant. Theoretically, a decongestant or an antihistamine should not be given to a coughing child, as it may thicken the secretions and make the phlegm more difficult to dislodge by the cough. In practice, however, if your child has nasal congestion, runny nose, and cough that are severe enough to keep her up all night, the benefit of a combination medicine probably outweighs this theoretical worry. The sedating effects of an antihistamine are usually welcome at night. The decongestant and the cough medicine will usually improve symptoms enough to get you all through the night. See www.AskDrSears.com's Medicine Cabinet for more on cough and cold medicines.

We often ask parents if their infant is able to successfully cough up the mucus out of their lungs. The answer is usually no, because they don't see anything coming up and out. Realize, however, that any infant or young child will naturally swallow any mucus that is coughed up. This is fine. It is better to get the mucus out of the lungs and swallow it than to leave it in the lungs, where it can become infected.

EAR INFECTIONS

A father whose infant is a frequent visitor to my office for ear infections recently opened his visit with, "My baby's ears are the most expensive part of his body to maintain." Correct, but when you consider the valuable speech and hearing that ears provide, they are well worth the price of good maintenance.

What Parents Need to Know About Infant Ears

Understanding how the ear structures work and how an infant's ears differ from an adult's ears will help you appreciate why babies are prone to ear infections and why it's important to treat them correctly. Let's travel with a germ from nose and mouth to ear to see how an ear infection develops. A germ enters the nose and throat and travels up the eustachian tube to the middle ear space. The eustachian tube connects the throat to the middle ear and serves to equalize pressure on both sides of the eardrum. Without this tube, your ears would be painful, popping, and feel plugged the way they temporarily do when you climb at high altitudes or fly. Besides being a pressure equalizer, this tube protects the middle ear, opening and closing appropriately and draining unwanted accumulations of fluid and germs.

The reason babies get more ear infections than older children depends on this tiny tube. Not only may it not open and close efficiently, a baby's eustachian tube is short, wide, and set more evenly with the throat — all characteristics that allow germs and secretions easy access to the ear from the throat. As baby grows, the eustachian tube lengthens, narrows, and is angled downward to the throat so secretions have to travel uphill to get to the ears.

During a cold or an allergy attack, fluid accumulates in all the breathing passages and in the middle ear. The same stuff that's in baby's nose is behind baby's eardrums. This is what has occurred when your doctor says, "Baby has fluid behind his eardrums." The medical term for this condition is *serous otitis media* (secretions in the middle ear). At this point in the cold, baby may not act sick. However, the feeling of pressure in the ear may awaken him and make him irritable. He may even be a bit off balance when walking because the fluid sloshing around in the middle ear affects the sense of balance. But usually at this stage babies act as if they only have a cold. The fluid may drain out by itself, baby's germ-fighting cells clearing up whatever germs may be in the fluid, and baby will get better. That's the good news.

Oftentimes, however, if the eustachian tube closes, this fluid in the middle ear becomes trapped. There is a general principle of the human body that fluid trapped anywhere usually gets infected. This trapped fluid serves as a nutrient for germs that grow in the fluid, making it thick like pus. This thick fluid puts pressure on the eardrum, producing pain, especially when baby is lying down. This is why ear infections make their

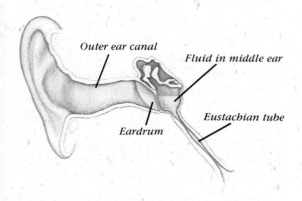

Outer ear canal

Fluid in middle ear

Eardrum

Eustachian tube

Structure of inner ear.

SIGNS SUGGESTING AN EAR INFECTION

- increasingly thick and snotty nasal secretions
- eye drainage
- crankiness and irritability
- frequent night waking or change in sleep pattern
- unwillingness to lie flat
- crying or screaming plus cold symptoms
- drainage from ear
- sudden worsening of a cold

untimely presentation at night when baby lies down and sometimes seem better by day. Pain, crankiness, and sleeplessness are the usual presenting symptoms, sometimes (but not always) associated with fever, a snotty nose, and vomiting. More subtle signs are seen in a breastfeeding baby who begins sucking differently and a baby who doesn't want to lie down. Ear pulling is not a reliable sign. Babies play with their ears, especially during teething.

Sometimes the pus under pressure bursts through the eardrum, and you notice purulent fluid draining from baby's ear canal — a snotty ear. This may occur during the night and be confused with nasal discharge. Baby usually feels better after the eardrum ruptures, since the pressure is released. Still take baby to the doctor for treatment the next morning. (In the pre-antibiotic era doctors used to lance eardrums to relieve the pressure and the excruciating pain.)

Meanwhile, at the Doctor's Office

The doctor looks into the baby's ear and notices a red bulging eardrum, which reflects why no one slept last night. Baby's doctor prescribes an antibiotic, the type and dosage depending on the severity of the infection and baby's past response to antibiotics. Then your doctor adds a very important reminder — "and we'll recheck your baby's ears in two or three weeks." Three important points to remember about ear infections: follow-up, follow-up, follow-up.

After a day or two on the antibiotic, baby should feel somewhat better. If there is no improvement within forty-eight hours, be sure to check with your doctor, even earlier if baby's condition worsens. Upon first sight of your baby's ear infection, the doctor tried to match the antibiotic to the infection, but only the baby's response will tell if this has been the right match. But don't expect immediate improvement; it may take twelve to twenty-

TUGGING AT EARS

Many parents bring their children into our office because they are pulling on their ears. There are no cold symptoms or fever, just ear pulling. Tugging on the ear *almost never* means an ear infection when there is no accompanying cold or fever. Teething is actually the most common cause of ear tugging. Baby is looking for some way to relieve the pain and pressure of teething. So if baby is pulling or digging at his ears, shows signs of teething, and there are no fever or cold symptoms, then there is probably no ear infection.

COMFORTING LITTLE AIRBORNE EARS

Here are some ways you can prevent or minimize ear discomfort when traveling with your baby by air. Breastfeed or bottlefeed, or give baby something to suck on or drink on takeoff and landing. If baby is sleeping on takeoff, no need to awaken. Takeoff does not seem to bother the ears as much as landing. When the plane is descending is the only time in the whole world you ever want to wake a sleeping baby. The eustachian tubes don't work well to equalize pressure when asleep. If baby has a cold or stuffy nose, use an oral decongestant or nose drops (recommended by your doctor) a half-hour before takeoff. To combat the dry cabin air, place a washcloth moistened with warm water in front of your baby's nose to humidify little breathing passages, or use saline nose drops.

four hours for the antibiotic to start to work. And the fever, if present, may last one or two days. Antibiotics do not lower fever. They treat germs, and when the germs leave, the fever breaks.

Suppose your baby feels better, even completely well, after three days into the antibiotic treatment. Tempted to stop the medicine now? Don't! The fluid and germs are most likely still hanging around and will flare up if you stop the treatment too soon.

Do all ear infections need antibiotics?
No. New research is showing that mild ear infections often resolve without antibiotics. There is a new trend to take a "wait and see" approach. If your child has a mild ear infection and isn't acting too sick, the doctor may choose to observe the baby over the next few days without prescribing an antibiotic. In this case, just treat the pain and any fever with medications and anesthetic eardrops. If, on the other hand, baby gets more fussy and the fever worsens or persists, an antibiotic may be warranted.

How Ear Infections Resolve

After an ear infection is treated, it will take one of four courses:

• The infection and the fluid will drain completely out of your child's ear within one to four weeks.

• The infection will resolve, but some non-infected fluid will remain in the middle-ear cavity for as long as three months.

• The infection will only partially resolve, and after several days without antibiotics it will regrow and turn into another infection. This can occur if the antibiotics are stopped too soon or if the infection is resistant to the antibiotics.

• The infection will be completely resistant to the antibiotic, your child's ear pain and fever will persist for two to three days on that treatment, and a stronger antibiotic may be needed.

It is important for your doctor to reevaluate the ears two to four weeks after an infection. This serves several purposes: to make sure the infection is clearing up; to make sure the middle-ear fluid is draining out (if the fluid stays around continuously for more than three months, your doctor needs to know); and to help determine if the next ear infection is a new one or a continuation of an old infection.

Why worry about ear fluid if it is not infected? One main worry about chronic middle-ear fluid is that it decreases hearing. While this isn't really a problem if it is temporary (a few weeks of hearing loss won't interfere significantly with speech development), going for several months with hearing loss can greatly affect language acquisition during the crucial learning years. Another more worrisome possibility is that the middle-ear fluid can thicken over a few months into a sticky gel, a condition called "glue ear." This "glue" interferes with the bones in the middle ear that transmit sound, and if left in the ear for too long can occasionally lead to a permanent decrease in hearing. Your doctor may use an instrument called a tympanogram (it looks just like an ear thermometer and is painless) to help measure the middle-ear pressure and evaluate how much middle-ear fluid is present.

This is why follow-up with the doctor is so important. If your doctor sees the middle-ear fluid persist for several months after an ear infection, he or she may refer you to an ear, nose, and throat (ENT) specialist, who may suggest inserting ear tubes to drain the fluid before it turns into glue ear. If, on the other hand, your doctor sees the fluid resolve completely, then glue ear is not a concern. And when your doctor sees your baby a few months later for his next ear infection, and normal ears have been documented in between the two infections, then you and your doctor don't need to worry that this condition may have been present over those few intervening months.

Preventing Ear Infections

Suppose this scene repeats itself with increasing frequency and severity over the next year, a common occurrence in pediatric practice. Here are ways to prevent or at least lessen the frequency and severity of ear infections.

Breastfeed as long as possible. Breastfed infants have fewer ear infections.

Control allergens. Allergens cause fluid, which serves as a culture medium for bacteria and infections, to build up in the middle ear. Be your baby's allergy detective to determine the most probable allergens your baby may be exposed to. The most common are inhalant allergies — cigarette smoke, dust, and animal dander. *Above all, don't smoke around babies.* Take particular precautions to rid your baby's sleeping environment of fuzzy and stuffed animals that collect dust (see page 700 for tips on defuzzing your baby's bedroom). Food allergies, particularly to dairy products, also contribute to ear infections.

Change baby's social situation. Is baby hanging around with snotty-nosed babies? Babies in day care do get more colds. Consider placing your baby in less crowded day care or consider a home day-care setup in which the provider has strict policies to either separate or send home sick children.

Feed baby upright. If your baby is bottle-fed, feed him upright, or at least at a forty-five-degree angle. This lessens the chance of milk or formula entering the eustachian tube from the throat and setting up inflammation within the tube and middle ear. Breastfeeding

HOW TO PREVENT EAR INFECTIONS

- Breastfeed.
- Control allergens.
- Minimize exposure to sick babies.
- Feed upright.
- Treat colds early.
- Keep nasal passages clear.
- Schedule frequent follow-up exams.
- Treat surgically with ear tubes.

lying down seldom predisposes baby to ear infections because the swallowing mechanism is different and breast milk is less irritating to the middle ear tissues. But if your breastfed infant is prone to recurrent ear infections, avoid feeding lying down.

Treat colds early. Note your child's usual cold-to-ear-infection sequence. If the typical pattern is a clear runny nose and a happy child, progressing to a snotty nose and a cranky child, then escalating into a full-blown ear infection a few days later, it would be wise to consult your doctor early, before the cold progresses to an ear infection.

Keep nasal passages clear. Steam treat (see page 666) and hose the nose (see page 665) to help drain snotty secretions.

Recurring Ear Infections

Suppose you have tried all the above preventive measures, your baby is still in and out of the doctor's office with recurrent ear infections, and she begins to show signs of deteriorating behavior, such as chronic irritability, which I call an ear personality. These behavior changes are common in babies with recurrent ear infections simply because they do not feel well or hear well and therefore do not act well. In fact one of the earliest changes parents notice after constant ear infections are brought under control is improvement in baby's behavior.

The entire prevention regimen, including maintenance antibiotics and surgical treatment, simply buys time until your child's immunity to germs increases and the eustachian tubes mature. Most children outgrow the tendency to recurring ear infections by age three to four years.

Long-Term Antibiotic Treatment

One tool in the prevention of recurrent ear infections is the use of a low-dosage, mild antibiotic once or twice a day for one to six months, especially during the winter months.

Parents are naturally uneasy about giving their child an antibiotic for so long a time, but consider the alternatives. A low dosage of a mild antibiotic is easier on baby's system than periodic progressively stronger antibiotics. The antibiotics that are used for prevention, similar to those that some children take daily for twenty years to prevent rheumatic fever, show no harmful effects. Without this prevention regimen the baby with recurrent ear infections may suffer temporary hearing loss at a time when good hearing is necessary for optimal speech development. Ear infections that occur too frequently and persist too long may even cause permanent hearing loss. Without this prevention regimen, surgical

PROGRESSION IN TREATMENT OF RECURRING EAR INFECTIONS

For proper management and prevention of ear infections, it is important to go through each step in a timely manner. When the first three steps are followed properly, the majority of babies with recurrent ear infections do not need step four, surgical treatment.

Step one: Treat each ear infection as it occurs. Continue treatment and careful follow-up with your doctor until the infection is completely resolved and baby's ears are normal. If the ear infections become more frequent, progress to:

Step two: Take preventive measures. As suggested earlier, try the prevention regimen of breastfeeding, controlling allergens, monitoring baby's exposure to sick children, feeding baby upright, treating colds early, and clearing baby's nasal passages. If the ear infections continue to occur, progress to:

Step three: Try a course of daily maintenance antibiotics. If you still frequent the doctor's office, move on to:

Step four: Treat surgically with the insertion of tubes.

treatment may be the next step for the child with recurrent ear infections.

Keeping the germs and the fluid out of the middle ear for an extended period of time also allows the middle ear structures, especially the eustachian tubes, to recover from the constant infections. Usually by this time a vicious circle has been set up whereby the eustachian tube has been so chronically damaged that it malfunctions, which predisposes to more ear infections. Oftentimes a preventive antibiotic treatment may keep the baby free of ear infection long enough for him to finally grow out of it. Except in allergic babies (and even this is questionable) decongestants and/or antihistamines have not been shown to be of any value in treating or preventing ear infections. And remember, antibiotics only kill germs. They do not drain fluid from the ears. Keeping your baby's nasal passages clear is good preventive medicine.

Surgical Intervention

Occasionally the prevention regimen does not work, and baby continues to get frequent ear infections. By this time the fluid in the middle ear has become thick, like glue, and requires surgical drainage. This operation is a *myringotomy,* during which, under light general anesthesia, an ear, nose, and throat specialist drains the gluelike fluid from the middle ear. At this time the doctor inserts a tiny plastic tube (about the size of the tip of a ballpoint pen) into the eardrum. These plastic tubes remain in place for around six months to a year, allowing accumulated fluid to drain out, thus lessening the frequency of middle ear infections and producing an immediate improvement in baby's hearing. This procedure requires about a half hour and is occasionally done in a doctor's office, but is most often done as outpatient surgery in the hospital. These tubes fall

DOES YOUR BABY HEAR?
HOW TO TELL

Here are some easy observations to make at various ages to check your baby's hearing. If the answer to many of the questions is no, have your baby's hearing checked by your doctor.

Age	Observation
	Does baby:
Birth– 3 months	☐ Startle or blink at sudden noises?
	☐ Stop crying when you talk?
	☐ Stop sucking when you talk?
	☐ Seem aware of your voice?
	☐ Awaken to sound, not only when the crib is jostled?
3–6 months	☐ Turn her head toward your voice?
	☐ Recognize and respond to your voice?
	☐ Smile when spoken to?
	☐ Coo when you talk?
	☐ Settle to music?
6–9 months	☐ Turn her head in search of a new sound?
	☐ Babble many sounds?
	☐ Vocalize different sounds for different needs?
9–12 months	☐ Turn when her name is called from behind?
	☐ Turn her head toward a speaker at the table?
	☐ Imitate your sounds?
	☐ Appear attentive during conversations?
12–18 months	☐ Respond to "no"; say "mama," "dada"?
	☐ Turn toward a familiar object or people when they are named?
	☐ Understand "Throw the ball"?
	☐ Run toward the door when you say "go"?
	☐ Wave when you say "bye-bye" without gesturing?
18–24 months	☐ Speak at least ten words?
	☐ Sometimes repeat your requests?
	☐ Point less and speak more words or sounds than in the previous stage?
	☐ Follow your requests without watching your face very closely while you are speaking? (Be suspicious of the child who rivets to your face during conversation; she may be lip-reading.)

out by themselves. The tiny hole left in the eardrums seals over by itself.

Self-help for Middle-of-the-Night Earaches

Doctors and parents have professions that require giving up the right to a full night's sleep. But it is seldom necessary to consult your doctor in the middle of the night if your baby awakens with an earache, unless he seems generally and seriously ill. The only treatment that your doctor could advise that you could not do yourself would be an antibiotic, and this will not immediately relieve the pain. Also, you may have difficulty finding a drugstore open in the wee hours of the morning.

Try these middle-of-the-night pain relievers until you can contact your doctor the next morning. You can even try these out during the day until prescribed antibiotics take effect.

- Give your baby acetaminophen or ibuprofen (see pages 657–660 for dosages). It is safe and appropriate to double the first dose of acetaminophen.

- Put some cooking oil, such as vegetable oil or olive oil, in a small glass and warm it by setting the glass in warm water. Squirt a few drops into the sore ear. Massage the outer edge of the ear canal to move the drops down toward the eardrum to relieve the pain.

- If your infant is prone to ear infections, keep the prescription pain-relieving drops Auralgan on hand.

- Encourage your baby to lie with the sore ear up, or sit your baby upright and try to help him go to sleep in that position. You may need to sit propped up in bed on a couple of pillows and allow your baby to fall asleep on your chest with the well ear toward your chest and the sore ear up.

- To promote drainage of secretions from the nasal passages (and possibly the eustachian tubes), give baby a steam bath (see page 666).

Treating Ear Infections with Antibiotics over the Phone

Doctors are reluctant to do this for several reasons. Even very painful ears are not necessarily infected. I have seen many children over the years with complaints of severe ear pain, and their ear exam is normal. Early mild ear infections don't necessarily need antibiotics. Better to make the trip to the doctor and possibly save your child a course of antibiotics. Visually confirming an ear infection will also help your doctor determine the status of the ear on follow-up appointments.

SINUS INFECTIONS

As germ-carrying air travels through the breathing passages, there are several out-of-the-way places where infections can occur. We just finished our trip through the middle ear. Next are the sinuses, small cavities in the facial bones along the sides of the nose, beneath the eyes, and above the eyebrows. Like the nose during a cold, the lining of the sinuses becomes inflamed as it secretes mucus. This mucus accumulates in the sinuses and drains into the nose and either drips forward, contributing to a runny nose, or flows back into the throat, causing a postnasal drip, throat tickle, and resultant cough when lying on the back. Instead of draining and clearing as with a cold, the fluid sometimes collects in sinuses, becoming stagnant and infected. Unlike earaches, runny noses, or sore throats, sinus infections have *subtle* signs and symptoms and are often overlooked because baby does not seem that sick. Realize that sinus infections rarely just appear out of the blue. It usually takes seven to ten days for the above process to create enough bacterial overgrowth to lead to a full-blown sinus infection. So if your child is experiencing some of the symptoms described below, don't run to the doctor on day one. Wait and see how things progress.

Symptoms

Because the sinuses are located inside the bones of the face and nose, your doctor can't actually visualize the infection like he or she can with an ear or throat infection. Your doctor will rely heavily on your description of symptoms, as well as an examination of the nose, ears, eyes, and face. Suspect a sinus infection when the following conditions are present:

- yellow or green nasal discharge for more than a week
- a lingering cold (more than a week or two), or a cold that keeps recurring as soon as antibiotics are finished
- dark circles under the eyes and puffy lower eyelids
- a pale and peaked face
- mucus drainage from the eyes
- a productive cough, usually worse at night
- odorous breath coming from the infected mucus in the back of the throat
- fatigue and low-grade fever
- headaches around the eyes, forehead, and cheeks

Treatment

Trends in antibiotic treatment for sinus infections have become more conservative recently. Research has shown that early and mild sinus infections may resolve with proper and vigorous nonantibiotic measures, such as "nose hosing" and "steam cleaning" (see pages 665 and 666).

Sinus infections when treated are treated like ear infections, but they are treated *longer*. It is not unusual for a child to need two to three weeks of antibiotics to completely clear up a sinus infection. In addition to antibiotics, it's important to clear baby's nose to help the secretions drain out of the sinuses. There are also safe and effective decongestant nasal sprays to open the nasal passages, allowing the sinuses to drain.

Sinus infections are more common in preschool and school-age children and adolescents, but even the small sinuses of infants get their fair share of cold germs.

CROUP

Croup (the medical term is laryngotracheitis) is a virus infection of the upper airway passages. What makes croup of such concern is the location of the infection. The vocal cords are already the narrowest part of the air passages, and any swelling from infection may narrow the airway enough to obstruct breathing.

Symptoms

Croup may begin without warning when baby suddenly sits up in bed with a barking cough, sounding like a seal. Or it may begin as a cold that gradually escalates into a croupy cough in addition to fever, hoarse voice, raspy breathing, and a sore throat. The main concern of parents is to recognize when croup is serious and when it is not.

Signs of Nonserious Croup

The behavior of your baby and how the croup progresses are the features to observe. If your baby is smiling, happy, playful, looking around, interested in the environment, and not obviously bothered by the croup, these are good signs. As a final reassurance, if your barking baby is able to lie down and sleep without repeated interruption, his breathing is not jeopardized. Don't worry if you hear mild raspy breathing as long as baby is sleeping comfortably. Mild croup rarely warrants an urgent call to your doctor, as it can easily be minimized with the measures below.

Signs of Serious Croup

Here's when to be concerned but not to panic. The baby whose airway is obstructed and who is unable to get enough air has a worried look on his face and is not interested in any play or interaction, as if concentrating all his energy on getting air. Baby won't lie down; he just sits up and barks, and he can't sleep. When you watch the little dent in baby's neck just above the breastbone, it caves in with each labored breath. This sign is called *indrawing*. When baby breathes in, you will hear a raspy drawn-out noise called *stridor*. These are potentially dangerous signs that need immediate medical attention.

Treating Croup

The first thing to do in treating croup is to relax your baby. Here's where parents' TLC really shines. Anxiety (baby's and parents') aggravates croup. If you can relax baby, his airway may also relax. Sit baby upright in your lap, play soft music, sing lullabies, read a story, or let baby watch soothing television. If breastfeeding, offer the great pacifier. (See discussion on relaxing the hospitalized child, page 187.)

Humidity helps clear baby's swollen breathing passages. Close the bathroom door, turn on the hot shower (or bathtub faucet), and sit with baby on the floor (if the room stays humid enough, as steam rises), or sit on the counter while you read a story. Open a window if possible. The cool air mixed with steam may work better than steam alone. You can also do this in the bedroom with a steam vaporizer. Let baby lie with his head on a pillow on your lap or propped up against you. You could instead place a vaporizer shooting steam directly over baby's nose, or make your own croup tent by placing a sheet over the crib and directing a cool-mist humidifier into the tent. In my experience croupy babies may resist the confines of a tent. Let baby fall asleep first in your arms and then position your sleeping baby upright in an infant seat inside the mist tent. Or you can even sleep for a while together in the steamy bathroom.

If baby has a fever, give an appropriate dosage of fever-lowering medicine (see pages 657–660). Let baby drink slow sips of juice, but it's not wise to feed solid food during a croup attack in case baby chokes or vomits and aspirates the food into his lungs. Serve soft foods, such as gelatin, until the worst is over. *Don't give over-the-counter medicines,* especially decongestants or antihistamines, without your doctor's advice. These may dry the narrowing air passages that the moisture is trying to open. One of the best treatments is taking baby out in the cool, moist night air (but don't tell grandmother). Take a slow car ride with the windows down. The misty night air is why babies with croup often improve en route to the hospital.

Even though antibiotics are not used to treat this viral illness, there is one prescription medication that can shrink the swelling in your baby's airways and vocal cords and greatly improve the breathing. This medicine is an oral steroid. Steroids sound scary to most parents, but all the bad things you hear about steroids occur from chronic use, not from a brief course of several days. When used in croup, the steroids work for about twenty-four hours and are typically given during the second and third nights (the worst part of the illness). But don't page your doctor in the middle of the night just to ask for a steroid prescription. It takes about eight hours for this medicine to work, so it will not help if given in the middle of the night.

When to Move Quickly

After trying the preceding treatment, assess in which direction your baby is going. If indrawing is lessening, color is returning to baby's pale cheeks, or baby initiates some interaction or wants to drift off to sleep (though still breathing noisily), continue with the steam and a watchful eye and ear. Watch for the following emergency signs, and if any of them occur, call the doctor and rush baby directly to the emergency room.

- The indrawing is becoming more labored, and baby's inhaling changes from a low-pitch stridor to a whistling sound.

- Baby becomes paler.

- Baby can't speak or cry from lack of breath.

- Baby is struggling more to get each breath.

- The indrawing is increasing, but the sound of breathing is decreasing.

En route to the emergency room, remember to leave the car windows open for humidity and ventilation, and try to settle baby with a calming song. Croup merits concern at all stages of severity. If at all in doubt which direction your baby's croup is taking, consult your doctor or take baby immediately to the local emergency room or children's hospital.

The Expected Course of Croup

The croupy, barky, raspy, feverish phase of croup generally lasts around five days. Croup usually improves during the day, only to flare up again each night. The second and third nights are typically worse than the first night. So it is important to check in with your doctor the morning after croup begins to see if an appointment is necessary. After these five days, most cases turn into a junky-sounding chest cough that lasts another week or so. Do not worry about this cough unless fever persists for more than five days or your child seems unusually ill.

DIARRHEA

If an infant has stools that are runnier than normal but no more frequent, then this is not really true diarrhea. Diarrhea, meaning liquid stools, refers more to the frequency of the bowel movements than to the consistency. During infancy the most common causes of diarrhea in order of frequency

SIGNS OF DEHYDRATION

Mild to Moderate Dehydration

- weight loss of 5 percent
- still playful, but quieter behavior
- dry mouth, fewer tears when crying
- urination less frequent than usual

Severe Dehydration

If your child has three or more of the following signs, or is acting unusually ill, you should seek medical attention.

- weight loss of 5–10 percent
- lethargic or hyperirritable behavior (see page 631)
- sunken eyes
- sunken soft spot in the head (in infant under one year)
- dry mouth, no tears when crying
- dry, pale, wrinkled skin
- infrequent urination (only two times a day or less)
- dark yellow urine

are gastrointestinal infections, colds, food intolerances, and antibiotic treatment. Throughout infancy, it is normal for the stools to periodically change in consistency or color, especially following a change of diet. Do not worry if your infant's stools become looser for a few days. This is just a normal variation in intestinal function. Teething is a common reason for a few days of runnier stools.

When the intestinal lining is infected, it heals very slowly. The lining contains millions of tiny projections through which liquidized food weaves and is absorbed. When infected, this brushlike lining is injured, along with the digestive enzymes it contains, allowing the food to pass through undigested. In fact, "diarrhea" comes from a Greek word meaning "to flow through."

The stools of diarrhea from gastroenteritis are frequent, watery, green, mucous, foul smelling, explosive, and occasionally blood tinged. Usually there is a raw red rash around the anus. In addition, baby often has other signs of a viral infection: a cold and a general unwell feeling and appearance.

Dehydration: When to Worry About Diarrhea

Most diarrhea illnesses are more of a nuisance than a medical problem and clear up easily with extra fluids and minor changes in the diet. The main concern with diarrhea is *dehydration.* Your baby's body contains just the right balance of salts (called electrolytes) and water. Healthy intestines and kidneys regulate this balance. A proper balance is necessary for organs to function. Diarrhea interrupts this balance, causing the body to lose water and electrolytes, or dehydrate. Add vomiting and you further increase the risk of dehydration.

Managing Your Baby's Diarrhea

Step one: Determine the cause. Have you changed baby's diet lately — for example, switched from formula to cow's milk, weaned from breast milk to formula, added new foods — or is baby overdosing on any one food, such as juice? (See page 690 for a discussion of juice diarrhea.) Loose, watery stools (usually without mucus or blood) in an otherwise well baby and a red ring around the anus (allergy ring) are signs of an intolerance to a recently introduced food. Go back to baby's previous diet and reduce or eliminate the suspected offender (see the discussion of food allergies, page 267). The stools should return to their previous characteristics within a week. Or does your baby have a cold and fever, and is he generally unwell in addition to having loose, mucous stools? If so, the diarrhea is probably due to an infection. Go on to the next step.

Step two: Determine the severity of the diarrhea and dehydration. Is baby playful and wet (eyes, mouth, diaper)? Perhaps except for more frequent messy diapers, you wouldn't know anything was amiss. In this case you don't have to change anything (except more diapers), and observe what direction the stools take.

To make sure the diarrhea is not causing dehydration, weigh baby daily, preferably undressed and in the morning before feeding, using the most accurate scale you can obtain. If you have access to an accurate infant scale, weigh your preferably undressed baby daily during a diarrhea illness. As a general guide: *no weight loss — no worry,* and no need to call your doctor yet. Both the degree and the rapidity of weight loss determine the severity

INFECTIOUS CAUSES OF DIARRHEA

Here are the most common causes of diarrhea. These conditions generally are not treated with antibiotics, except where noted.

Rotavirus. This is a very common cause of diarrhea, especially during late fall and winter. It is characterized by very foul smelling, watery, green or brown diarrhea that can persist for weeks. Fever and vomiting are common at the onset of the illness.

Other viruses, such as the flu, also commonly cause diarrhea.

Bacteria. These include E. coli, salmonella, and several others. Diarrhea may be accompanied by vomiting and fever. *Blood in the diarrhea* is a hallmark finding with bacterial intestinal infections. Even though these are bacterial infections, they are not always treated with antibiotics.

Parasites. These are usually contracted during foreign travel. The telltale sign of a parasite is very watery diarrhea that lasts beyond two weeks.

These conditions are all generally contagious as long as any diarrhea is present.

of dehydration. If your baby has not lost significant weight, she is not becoming dehydrated. However, if your child loses 5 percent of her baseline body weight (for example, a weight loss of one pound in a twenty-pound baby), she has experienced mild to moderate dehydration, and this merits a phone call to your doctor. A rapid weight loss is more of a concern than a gradual one. A twenty-pound infant who loses a pound of body weight over the period of a day is much more worrisome than one who loses the same amount of weight over a week's time. But infants usually appear very sick if they are losing weight rapidly; they do not act as sick if their weight loss has been gradual. *Ten percent* weight loss, especially if occurring within a few days, suggests serious dehydration, and you should call your doctor immediately, preferably even before this degree of weight loss occurs.

If you notice the stools are getting more frequent, greener, and more watery and explosive, and your baby begins to act sick, though still wet and playful, progress to the next step.

Step three: Eliminate irritating foods. If baby is also vomiting, *stop all solid foods, milk (except breast milk), and formula.* If baby is not vomiting and has only mild diarrhea, stop all dairy products, juices, and high-fat foods. If the diarrhea is severe (watery, explosive stools every two hours), stop all foods, milk, formula, and juice. *It is rarely necessary to stop breastfeeding.* Refrain from these foods and liquids for from twelve to twenty-four hours, depending on the severity of the diarrhea, while at the same time beginning *oral rehydration* (step four).

Step four: Prevent dehydration. If baby is not breastfeeding, substitute for baby's regular diet an *oral electrolyte solution* (for example, Pedialyte), available without prescription at your local pharmacy or supermarket. These solutions contain an ideal balance of water and electrolytes to replace what your baby is losing in the diarrhea. They also contain an amount of sugar that won't aggravate the diarrhea, especially those solutions made with *rice syrup.* If your child won't take an electrolyte solution, try white grape juice (the juice that is most friendly to inflamed intestines), diluted to half strength with water. Give small, frequent feedings, using the sips-and-chips method: sips of the solution and ice chips or popsicles made with the electrolyte solution. If your baby takes a bottle, instead of his normal formula offer half as much oral electrolyte solution twice as often. The minimum fluid requirement of the solution to offer your baby is *two ounces per pound* of body weight (130 milliliters per kilogram) per twenty-four hours. For example, if your baby weighs twenty pounds, offer forty ounces in twenty-four hours. When sick, many infants refuse to take this much, but try your best. If baby has vomiting and diarrhea (dubbed a "double-ender"), offer small sips even more frequently. Some infants may take only one to two teaspoons every five minutes in the first day or two of the illness.

If your baby is breastfeeding, let him feed as much as he wants. He'll get all the fluid he needs and will be comforted by the sucking. If he rejects the breast temporarily, offer him an oral electrolyte solution. Even if he vomits, allow him to feed — perhaps more slowly on a not-so-full breast. If the milk only stays down ten to twenty minutes, much of it will be absorbed, and it won't hurt baby to bring up breast milk. In fact, having something to bring up is probably more comfortable than dry heaves.

Step five: Resume regular feedings. According to the course of diarrhea and the sick level of your child, along with your doc-

KEEP A DIARRHEA RECORD

To keep track of your baby's illness, make a diarrhea chart. This record helps your doctor advise you on how soon to resume baby's regular diet and whether or not baby is becoming dehydrated. Charting helps you do your part in the medical partnership with your doctor.

Day	Weight	Number and Nature of Stools	Treatment	Course of Illness
1	20 lb.	8, green, watery	40 ounces Pedialyte	Vomiting stopped, slight fever, stools same.
2	19.5 lb.	6, no change	20 ounces Pedialyte, resumed full-strength formula (20 ounces and rice cereal and bits of banana)	Fever gone, baby more perky.

tor's advice, resume dilute formula (half formula and half oral electrolyte solution) or resume regular breastfeeding once the diarrhea slows down. Advance to full-strength formula around twenty-four hours later. Between twenty-four and forty-eight hours, resume baby's previous diet but continue small, frequent feedings for a few days. Avoid cow's milk as a beverage until the diarrhea subsides, but yogurt is all right. During the one-to-six-week recovery period from a severe intestinal infection, your doctor may advise using a non-lactose soy formula, since the healing intestines may not tolerate lactose. If baby's diarrhea relapses when resuming solids, back off a bit and return to the previous step. For a general guide, *as your baby's stools become more solid, so may the diet.*

Intestines heal slowly. It is very common for "nuisance diarrhea" to last for several weeks during the recovery phase of a viral intestinal infection. "The stools remain loose but baby remains well" may be the story for a month. If diarrhea persists, especially if accompanied by abdominal pain and poor weight gain, your doctor may wish to order several stool cultures, looking for a parasite, such as *Giardia.*

More Tips on Treating Infant Infectious Diarrhea

In light of new research, management of infant diarrhea has undergone three changes.

Routine use of oral electrolyte solution. Scratch previously recommended homemade solutions: gelatin, cola, ginger ale, juice, and sugar water. While all right if oral electrolyte solutions aren't available (it's wise to keep a

---

THE BRATY DIET

Here are five foods you can feed your infant that may help slow down the diarrhea: bananas, rice or rice cereal, applesauce, unbuttered toast or bread (if over age one), and yogurt.

---

bottle in your medicine cabinet), they are no longer recommended because their salt content is too low and the sugar content is too high and could possibly aggravate the diarrhea.

Earlier feedings. Starving diarrhea is not helpful. Earlier feedings provide needed nutrition and may accelerate healing. The American Academy of Pediatrics recommends the treatment described in step five: resuming full-strength formula by twenty-four hours and progressing to a regular diet by forty-eight hours. Even temporarily using the time-honored BRATY (bananas, rice cereal, applesauce, unbuttered toast, and yogurt) may be necessary only in severe cases.

Avoiding juice. Juice may not be the intestines' best friend. Many juices contain *sorbitol,* a sugar that is not absorbed in the intestines and that acts like a sponge, absorbing water from the intestinal lining into the stools, increasing their water content and thus aggravating the diarrhea. That's why prune juice is a laxative. Too much juice (especially pear, cherry, and apple) may cause diarrhea and is also a subtle cause of abdominal pain and bloating in toddlers who overdose on it. (These are general recommendations. It's best to check with your doctor,

since your child may need special dietary manipulations.)

What Not to Do for Diarrhea

Inflamed intestines need tender care. Here are some things that may aggravate the diarrhea.

- Don't stop breastfeeding. It is rarely necessary to stop breastfeeding, since human milk is not irritating, may even be therapeutic, and may be the only food and fluid a sick child will take or tolerate.

- Avoid boiling solutions, especially milk and sugar, since boiling may cause the water to evaporate, making the solution too strong and aggravating the dehydration.

- Do not withhold food for longer than forty-eight hours. Your child needs nutrition for healing, and a clear fluid diet alone may itself produce diarrhea, called starvation stools.

WHEN TO CALL YOUR DOCTOR

Call your doctor if

- dehydration is worsening
- baby has lost more than 5 percent of her body weight
- your child is becoming increasingly lethargic
- the fever remains high
- the vomiting continues
- baby is having increasingly severe abdominal pains

Medications for Diarrhea

Diarrhea is best treated with fluid replacement, using a commercial oral electrolyte solution and the BRATY diet, as previously described. Seldom are drugs necessary to treat diarrhea in infancy. In fact, narcotic medications, which are often used to control diarrhea in adults, are not safe for children. While these medications stop the diarrhea by slowing down the action of the intestines, this may actually worsen the condition, since it allows the germs and infected fluid to stagnate in the gut and increases the chance of these germs entering the child's bloodstream, where they can cause serious illness. Also these medications, while externally stopping the diarrhea, still allow the fluid to be lost into the intestines (internal diarrhea), producing a silent dehydration that may not be appreciated because the diarrhea appears to be lessening.

Baby may get diarrhea as a result of antibiotics; giving acidophilus powder and plain yogurt daily during antibiotic treatment and for a week after lessens diarrhea. This works by restoring the normal bacteria in the gut that are killed by antibiotics. Acidophilus or *Lactobacillus bifidus* is available at nutrition stores.

To prevent a rash, apply a barrier cream with every diaper change.

PROBIOTICS

Probiotics (meaning "for life") are bacteria that promote intestinal health. Also known as "good bacteria," these organisms coat the intestinal lining and fight off disease-causing bacteria by keeping them from penetrating the intestinal lining. This century-old idea of feeding the gut good bacteria to fight bad bacteria has recently received scientific validation. Probiotics (the most familiar is lactobacillus acidophilus, one of the main bacterial cultures in yogurt) come in a variety of pills, liquids, and powders, and are found at pharmacies and nutrition stores. Consult your baby's doctor for the dose and form best suited for your baby's intestines. Probiotics have been found useful in the following medical situations:

- following antibiotic therapy
- rotavirus-associated diarrhea
- lactose intolerance
- intestinal bacterial and viral infections
- chronic, allergic eczema in infants
- diarrhea from any cause
- bladder infections

VOMITING

"If it's not one end, it's the other," complained a mother about her baby's sensitive intestines. It's a fact of infant life that some of what goes into a baby will come back up. Here are the most common causes of vomiting in babies and what to do about it.

Vomiting in the First Month

Most vomiting in the first few months is simply the nuisance of *spitting up* (see page 104). Next on the regurgitation list is formula allergy or allergens in breast milk (see page 152). These are temporary nuisances that baby will outgrow. But there are some medical conditions that need special attention.

Pyloric Stenosis

The most serious cause of vomiting in infancy is intestinal obstruction, either partial or complete. A blockage in the intestines prevents the milk from getting through, and back up the esophagus it comes. The most common of these is pyloric stenosis.

Pyloric stenosis is the narrowing of the lower end of the stomach, called the pylorus. While the condition is seldom apparent in the first week or two after birth, the muscle that circles the pylorus gradually grows thicker until it squeezes the end of the stomach like a band. When the pylorus is only partially obstructed, the milk trickles through, and baby appears only to spit up. But toward the end of the first month, as the opening becomes narrower, the milk backs up in the stomach, and the stubborn stomach tries with great force to push the milk through the narrowed opening. Some leaks through, but most comes forcefully out as *projectile vomiting.* Baby may spray the milk a distance of two feet (sixty centimeters) across your lap. Whereas the normal spitter dribbles on the burp cloth on your shoulder, the projectile vomiter spews the contents a few feet away. Picture an overfilled water balloon with a knot tied loosely at both ends. You squeeze the balloon (the stomach contracts), and you keep squeezing until a knot loosens and squish, the water shoots out. This resembles what occurs in a baby with pyloric stenosis.

How to recognize pyloric stenosis. Signs that your baby may have pyloric stenosis are the following:

- persistent projectile vomiting
- weight loss or failure to gain weight
- signs of dehydration: wrinkly skin, dry mouth, dry eyes, and decreasing number of wet diapers
- stomach swollen like a big, tense balloon after feeding and deflated after vomiting
- increasing hunger and eager feeding, followed by vomiting and repeated vigorous feeding

Some normal babies may experience projectile vomiting once or twice a day if overfed, underburped, or jostled too much. But persistent projectile vomiting accompanied by weight loss and dehydration needs immediate medical attention.

Helping your doctor diagnose pyloric stenosis. If you suspect your baby may have this condition, make a doctor's appointment, but do not feed your baby for an hour or two before your appointment. (Unless baby is obviously dehydrated, this is not a medical emergency, and you can usually wait to see your doctor during regular office hours. This condition has been brewing for a week or two.) By the description of the frequency and nature of the vomiting, and your description of your concern as an intuitive abdomen watcher, your doctor will suspect this condition. To confirm pyloric stenosis your doctor may want to watch you feed your baby while looking for the ballooning of the tense stomach and feeling the pyloric muscle in spasm (it feels like an olive). Occasionally, if diagnosis is suspected but the abdominal signs are not definite, your doctor may order X rays of the stomach (an upper GI series) or an ultrasound of the pylorus to confirm the diagnosis.

COMMUNICATING WITH YOUR DOCTOR ABOUT VOMITING

When phoning your doctor, have answers ready for the following questions:

- How did the vomiting start: suddenly or gradually?

- What is the character of the vomitus? Is it clear, dark green, curdled, or sour? Is it spit-up or projectile?

- How often is your child vomiting?

- What amount of vomitus is produced each time?

- Are other household members sick with similar signs?

- Does baby's abdomen hurt? Where, and how much? Is it tense, balloon-like, soft, caved in?

- Does baby have any signs of dehydration? (See page 686.)

- How sick does your baby seem overall?

- Is baby's condition the same, getting better, or worse?

- What treatment have you tried?

- What other symptoms are present (diarrhea, fever, cough)?

Treatment. Following the confirmation of the diagnosis it is usual for baby to need a day or two of rehydration with intravenous fluids in the hospital before surgery. The operation to relieve the pyloric obstruction takes about a half hour and is done through a small incision in the upper abdomen. Improvement is immediate, and recovery time short.

Gastroesophageal Reflux

This condition is one of the most frequent causes of vomiting in the early months of life. See page 388 for a detailed discussion.

Vomiting in the Older Infant

Vomiting in older babies is usually caused by an intestinal infection, such as an intestinal flu called gastroenteritis (see page 686). Sometimes vomiting accompanies common serious illnesses such as ear infections, urinary tract infections, pneumonia, meningitis, encephalitis, and appendicitis. It can also result from swallowing the infected secretions of a sore throat. Vomiting due to intestinal infection is usually accompanied by cold symptoms, diarrhea, fever, and abdominal pain.

Treatment of Vomiting

Management is the same as for diarrhea (see page 687) and is mainly to prevent dehydration caused by the loss of fluid and body salts in the vomitus. The most effective way to ease the discomfort and prevent dehydration is to give your baby popsicles made with oral electrolyte solutions. This acts as a slow drip into baby's stomach. Offer small, frequent doses of fluid. Sometimes it is necessary to give baby *a teaspoon of liquid every five minutes;* any more than that may be rejected. If breastfeeding, offer one breast at a feeding and feed more frequently but for a shorter time.

Keep in mind it is normal for a child to vomit several times an hour for the first few

BLOOD IN VOMITUS

Don't be alarmed if you see an occasional blood-tinged vomitus. This commonly happens with retching types of vomiting because of tiny tears in the blood vessels lining the esophagus as the forceful fluid shoots by. This usually is not serious and subsides quickly if you give your baby cold liquids, especially ice chips and popsicles. Call your doctor if the amount of blood in the vomitus is increasing.

begins between four and twenty-four hours after the offending meal. Baby retches (dry heaves) and experiences chills, but there is usually no fever. You may also feel that baby has pain in his upper abdomen, but when you press on it, it is soft, not tender, and baby usually does not protest when you press on the lower abdomen. Give your child ice chips and popsicles made with oral electrolyte solutions and withhold all other food (breastfeeding is fine), and the symptoms of food poisoning will usually subside within six to eight hours, although it may persist for up to twenty-four hours. If baby is becoming dehydrated, call your doctor. (See "Signs of Dehydration," page 686.)

hours of any stomach or intestinal infection. Expect any fluids you put into your child to just come right back up again. One helpful tip during this initial severe phase is *total stomach rest.* Don't even try to get down any fluids until this phase is over. Some kids, on the other hand, prefer to have a little bit of liquid to throw up rather than to dry-heave for hours. Review the signs of dehydration (see page 686), and be especially watchful for dehydration if the vomiting lasts more than a day and is accompanied by diarrhea or if your child is becoming generally more ill. Prescription antivomiting medications are available if the vomiting does not subside with home remedies.

It is common for many vomiting illnesses to have a brief recurrence one or two days after the initial vomiting subsides. This may be a sign that too much food is being given too soon. Take a step back in your routine until this second round of vomiting stops.

Food Poisoning

More common in older children and adults than in babies, food poisoning generally

Intestinal Obstruction

When is vomiting a medical emergency? Rarely, intestines may become twisted or the small intestine may telescope into the large intestine (called an intussusception), and the intestines become obstructed. This is a medical emergency demanding immediate medical and surgical attention. Here are the general signs of intestinal obstruction:

- sudden onset of severe colicky abdominal pain
- persistent dark green–stained vomiting, sometimes projectile
- obvious discomfort and sometimes agonizing pain, but may be intermittent rather than constant
- absence of bowel movements
- pale and sweaty skin
- signs worsening rather than improving

When to call your doctor after hours for vomiting. It is rarely necessary to page your doctor after hours during the first few hours of vomiting.

Here are situations that do warrant a call to your doctor after hours:

- The vomiting is occurring several times an hour and you want to try a prescription anti-vomiting suppository (not generally used in infants under two years).

- Your child is severely dehydrated (see page 687).

- Your child has symptoms of intestinal obstruction (see above), meningitis, pneumonia, bladder infection, appendicitis (see page 706, "Childhood Illnesses at a Glance," for more on these), or you feel your child is seriously ill.

At the doctor's office. Your doctor may not be able to tell you exactly what the cause of the vomiting is. His or her main task is to make sure it is not one of the above worrisome causes, determine the degree of dehydration (and whether or not a trip to the ER for IV fluids is needed), and prescribe anti-vomiting suppositories if needed.

CONSTIPATION

Constipation refers to the compactness of the stools and the difficulty passing them, not the frequency of bowel movements. The consistency and number of stools varies according to age and from baby to baby. In general, newborns have several stools a day that are soft and the consistency of seedy mustard, especially if breastfed. Formula-fed infants usually have fewer and firmer stools. Some breast- or formula-fed infants may have a bowel movement only once every few days. As long as it passes fairly easily and without too much discomfort, this is *not*

considered constipation. Once solid food enters the diet, the stools become more formed and less frequent, and some babies may have a bowel movement without difficulty only once every three days, but daily is preferable.

Normally, as digested food travels down the intestines, water and nutrients are absorbed, and the waste material becomes stools. For a soft stool to form, enough water must remain in the waste material, and the lower intestinal and rectal muscles must contract and relax to move the stool along and out. Malfunction of either of these mechanisms, too little water or poor muscle movement, can cause constipation. Being plugged up with hard stool for three days can be very uncomfortable. In fact, we did not appreciate this until we strained along with one of our babies, who was constipated for the first two years of his life. As Martha would help him produce a bowel movement, she would proclaim, "I feel like a midwife."

Constipation often becomes a self-perpetuating problem. Hard stools cause pain on passage; consequently, baby holds on. The longer the stool remains, the harder it becomes — which makes it even more painful to pass. And the longer the large stool stretches the intestines, the weaker their muscle tone becomes. To complicate matters, passage of a hard stool through a narrow rectum often tears the rectal wall (called a rectal fissure), accounting for the streaks of blood. This painful tear prompts baby even more not to want to have a bowel movement.

To tell if your baby is constipated, look for the following signs:

- in a newborn, firm stools less than once a day with straining and difficulty passing them

- dry, hard, large stools and pain on passing them
- hard, pebblelike stools passed by a baby who strains during a bowel movement, drawing her legs up on her abdomen, grunting, and getting red faced
- streaks of blood along the outside of the stool
- abdominal discomfort along with hard, infrequent stools

Finding the Cause

New foods or milks can set off constipation. Has your baby begun new foods, switched from breast milk to formula, or formula to cow's milk? If you suspect a food or milk change as the culprit, return to the looser-stool diet. For bottlefed infants, consider experimenting with various formulas to find the one that is kindest to the stools. Also, give your formula-fed baby an extra bottle of water a day.

The cause could also be emotional. Is your toddler going through a negative phase or emotional upset that may cause reluctance to have a bowel movement? When a person is upset, his or her intestinal functions may be upset, showing either diarrhea or constipation.

Treating Constipation

Lessen constipating foods. White rice, white bread, rice cereal, bananas, apples, cooked carrots, milk, and cheese are potential constipators, though food effects vary widely among babies. (See "Constipation When Starting Solids," page 224).

Add fiber foods to baby's diet. Fiber softens the stools by drawing water into them, making them bulkier and easier to pass. Fiber foods for older babies are bran and barley cereals, graham crackers, whole-grain breads and crackers, and high-fiber vegetables such as peas, broccoli, and beans. Laxative fruits are apricots, prunes, pears, plums, and peaches.

Give baby more water. Here is the most often forgotten, least expensive, and most readily available stool softener. Extra water must accompany extra fiber. Otherwise, fiber can make stools harder rather than softer.

Try glycerin suppositories. As they are going through a phase of learning how to have a bowel movement, many babies in their early months grunt and draw up their legs to push out a stool. But the straining baby may appreciate a little outside help with a well-timed, well-placed glycerin suppository. Available without prescription at your pharmacy, these look like tiny rocket ships. If your baby is straining, insert one as far into the rectum as you can and hold baby's buttocks together for a few minutes to dissolve the glycerin. These are especially helpful to lubricate the rectum if baby has a rectal tear. Don't use for more than a few days without your doctor's advice. For newborns through six months, cut a pediatric suppository in half lengthwise.

Use a laxative. When using a laxative, try the most natural first. Begin with diluted prune juice (half and half with water), a tablespoon or two (15 to 30 milliliters) for the four-month-old and as much as eight ounces (240 milliliters) for the toddler. Try strained prunes or make a prune puree (stew your own or buy commercial), either straight or disguised (mixed with a favorite food), or spread it on a high-fiber cracker. Apricots and the four P's — prunes, pears, plums, and peaches — usually exert a laxative effect. If these seem insufficient, here are other ideas to try:

- Flaxseed meal and psyllium husks (basically, very fine flakes of psyllium bran) are natural-fiber stool softeners available at nutrition stores. These bland laxatives are sprinkled on cereal or combined with a fruit-and-yogurt mixture. Try two teaspoons a day for a six-month-old; for toddlers, try one or two tablespoons a day.

- Nonprescription laxatives such as Maltsupex (a malt-barley extract) may soften your infant's stool. In the baby from one to two years, give one tablespoon a day mixed with eight ounces water or juice. As the stools soften, cut back on the dose.

- One of the most successful laxatives we have prescribed in our pediatric practice is flaxseed oil. Whereas flaxseed meal contains both the oil and the fiber and is therefore also a useful laxative, young infants may prefer the smooth texture of the oil over the grainy texture of the meal. Besides being a natural laxative, this oil is a rich source of omega-3 fats and provides extra calories for those picky-eater toddlers. Start with one teaspoon per day for the six-month-old, or a tablespoon a day for a one- to two-year-old. Most infants and toddlers won't take flax oil straight, so mix it in pureed fruit, a fruit-and-yogurt smoothie, or in barley cereal. Unlike the commonly used laxative mineral oil, which provides no nutritional value and may take vitamins with it as it slides through the intestines, flax oil is a nutrient that facilitates the absorption of many vitamins. For this reason, we recommend flax oil over mineral oil as an effective and nutritious laxative for infants and children.

- Laxative suppositories (glycerin suppositories containing a laxative ingredient) may be used periodically if the constipation is severe and resistant to the preceding simpler measures. Another way to treat constipation from below is with liquid glycerin (Baby Lax) gently inserted by dropper into baby's rectum.

Try an enema. Baby Fleet enema may be tried if your toddler is miserably constipated and nothing else is working. It is available without prescription, and directions are on the package insert.

Be sure to continue to try dietary manipulations and natural food laxatives so your baby does not become dependent upon suppositories or other laxatives. Fortunately, as the wisdom of baby's body sorts out which foods are intestinal friendly and learns to respond more quickly to bowel signals, this uncomfortable problem will pass.

Chronic Constipation in the Older Toddler

The above principles and treatments apply to older toddlers as well as to infants. However, there are some differences in the physiology of the older toddler's colon that parents must understand when dealing with chronic constipation.

The normal colon. Normally the colon slowly fills up with stool. When it gets stretched to a certain point, the colon sends nerve signals to itself (and to the brain) that cause it to naturally contract to push the stool out. This is the sensation we get when we feel we need to have a bowel movement. This normally occurs one to three times each day.

The constipated colon. A chronically stretched colon, as occurs when stool is not routinely pushed out, will stop sending nerve signals to itself or to the brain. The child will therefore not get the urge to pass the stool. This is a chronic cycle that gets increasingly worse.

Treating chronic constipation. When using the above principles to soften the stool and increase bowel movements, continue the treatments for at least *two months.* Your goal is to help the colon shrink back down to its normal size, so that it will start sending signals again when it gets stretched. It takes two or three months for this resetting of the colon's stretch point to occur.

Dr. Jim notes: Don't force your child to sit for hours on the toilet. Your child can go only when the colon is naturally contracting. The best time to encourage a bowel movement is when you see your child trying to hold it in. This means he is getting a signal but fighting it. And remember, rectal muscles relax when the feet are planted squarely on the floor, whereas dangling feet tighten rectal muscles and make it harder to go.

TRACKING AND TREATING INHALANT ALLERGIES

Many of the substances in the air around baby are unwelcome in the breathing passages, and the body reacts by uncomfortable signs we call allergies. The fight that occurs when an allergen enters the body through the air is similar to the struggle described in detail under food allergies, page 267. Sneezes, wheezes, drips, and itches are frequent nuisances in the life of an allergic child. The good news is that parents can help.

Is Your Child Allergic? How to Tell

All of the common signs of allergies are listed on page 270. Inhalant allergies often have a seasonal variation, and the following signs and symptoms are the most frequent ones your child is likely to show:

- clear runny nose and watery eyes
- bouts of sneezing in quick succession
- constant sniffing
- nosebleeds
- a crease on the top of nose from frequent wiping (called the allergic salute)
- dark circles under the eyes (allergic shiners)
- frequent colds and/or ear infections
- night cough and a stuffy nose in the morning
- noisy breathing at night
- coughing during exercise
- lingering cough, often rattling or wheezy

Is it an allergy or a cold? In both cases little noses run and little chests cough. But if you have to decide whether your child is able to attend day care, see "Colds Versus Allergies," page 426. If you can't determine whether it's allergies or a cold from the immediate symptoms, then you will just have to give it time. If symptoms persist for more than several weeks, then allergies are more likely. It is not imperative that you distinguish between the two conditions in the short term, since treat-

<table>
<tr><td>

A TIP FOR ALLERGY DETECTIVES

If you suspect that your child is allergic to something in the environment but you are uncertain, take a vacation. If your child's usual allergic signs and symptoms subside or change, you can bet he is allergic to something around the house.

</td></tr>
</table>

ment to relieve the symptoms is the same. (See "Treating Colds," page 664.)

Tracking Down Your Baby's Allergies

Decide first how much of a problem your baby's allergies are. Are they simply a noisy nuisance that time and a ton of tissues will wipe away? If so, don't delve into the time-consuming world of allergy prevention. Or are the allergies interfering with your baby's normal growth, development, and behavior? As your baby's allergy detective, try to find out the most probable allergens that trigger the allergic signs. Here are the four most common categories of inhalant allergies and what to do about them.

Pollens. Suspect these if your baby's allergies are seasonal, occurring when the pollen count is high, during windy days, and when your allergic friends are also dripping and sneezing. If outside pollens are the suspect, try the following:

- Keep baby indoors on the windy days of pollen season. You can access local pollen count information on the Internet.

- Avoid places where pollens and other allergens are prevalent — for example, weedy and flowery fields.

- Keep the windows closed, at least in baby's sleeping room.

- To remove the pollen, bathe baby and wash her hair before bedtime; launder the pollen out of clothing.

- Consider air-conditioning and an air-filtering system for a bedroom or the whole house if the allergies are severe.

- When driving, keep windows closed.

- Don't hang bedding or clothes outside; they become pollen catchers.

Animal dander. Next, suspect the family cat, dog, bird, or the neighbor's pet. Does your baby sneeze, drip, or wheeze when playing with a pet? If a pet is suspected, at least banish him from the room where baby sleeps. Contrary to what you may think, it is not the animal hair that is allergenic, it is the dander (skin shedding) that triggers allergies. Oftentimes baby can play with his allergenic pet outdoors without suffering allergies but begins to sneeze as soon as the pair snuggle together indoors. Again, how much you need to separate baby and pet depends upon how much the allergies bother baby. If you have a strong family history of allergies or baby has other allergies, it would be wise, before acquiring a pet, to let baby and prospective pet hang around each other (indoors) for a test sniff. All dogs and cats are potentially allergenic, but some breeds seem more so than others. If you are a very allergic family, think goldfish.

Molds. The spores of plants that thrive in dark, cool, damp places are called mold or

HOW TO ALLERGYPROOF A BEDROOM

The Bedding

- Encase mattress, box springs, and pillow with dustproof zippered covers. Seal the zippers with tape.

- Avoid down or feather pillows and comforters. Also avoid kapok or foam-rubber pillows (foam may grow mold if damp). Purchase nonallergenic pillows and coverings made with polyester materials.

- Defuzz baby's immediate sleeping environment: Remove fuzzy stuffed animals and furry toys from baby's crib or bed and from the bedroom if baby is highly allergic. Tuck them away in a garbage bag in the garage. If your child is attached to a fuzzy favorite, choose one that can be frequently washed. Replace wool blankets and sleepwear with synthetics or cotton and wash frequently. Air and vacuum the mattress and wash pillowcases, mattress pads, and blankets in hot water at least every one or two weeks.

- Avoid stuffing items under the bed for storage.

- Move the crib or bed far away from the window (if open) and away from air vents.

Bedroom Furnishings

- Replace fabric and upholstered chairs with plastic, wood, or canvas.

- Use throw rugs on a wooden or linoleum floor and wash the rugs frequently. Avoid plush carpet if possible.

- Avoid ornate furniture with dust-collecting crevices.

- Avoid books or bookshelves, which are sure dust catchers.

- Don't use the bedroom as a storeroom.

- Avoid piling clothes about the room. Keep all dust-collecting clothes and other items in closets and keep the closet door closed.

- Roll-up window shades are preferable to the more dust-collecting blinds.

- Use easily washed cotton curtains — no draperies, please.

- Check how allergenic the furniture material is. A subtle allergen is the form board made with formaldehyde that may be used in the construction of beds or other furniture. Check with the manufacturer.

mildew. Molds are found in cellars, closets, attics, piles of clothing in corners, old mattresses, pillows and blankets, baskets, damp carpet, garbage cans, shower curtains, shower stalls, bathroom tiles (especially damp corners), and houseplants. A frequently overlooked source of molds spewing out into the bedroom is a humidifier (see discussion of humidifiers and vaporizers, page 667). Outdoor sites of molds are piles of damp, dead

Ventilation and Air Purifying

- Keep the door to the bedroom closed and the pet out.
- Keep the windows closed during pollen season.
- Put filters or cheesecloth over forced-air inlets; best is to close and seal them.
- Avoid electric fans; they collect and circulate dust.

- Consider an air filter; the best choice is one that shows the term HEPA (high efficiency particulate accumulator), which means it can remove dust mite sheddings, pollens, molds, spores, animal dander, and many of the irritants from smoke and fumes. The cost of air cleaners may be covered by your insurance if you have a doctor's prescription.

Cleaning Tips

- Do not vacuum when your baby is in the room, because vacuum cleaners spread dust. Air the room after vacuuming. Use a tank-type vacuum cleaner with a water filter to prevent some dust and mites from reentering the room. Best is a HEPA dustless vacuum cleaner, which both picks up and retains the invisible dust allergens.
- Wet dusting is better than dry.

- Damp-mop the floor with a mold-killing disinfectant, such as a bleach solution.
- Banish smokers from your home.
- Beware of other allergens and irritants in the air: cooking odors, deodorizers, air fresheners, fireplace smoke, houseplants, perfumes, baby powders, cosmetics, mothballs, and insect sprays.

Seldom do parents have to go to such great lengths to make their baby's environment allergy-free. But for highly allergic babies most of the above allergyproofing tips are required. Consult your doctor or pediatric allergist for other suggestions in tracking down and dealing with your baby's allergies.

grass, leaves, or stacked firewood. To demold your baby's sleeping or playing environment:

- Air out and clean all of the mold sites mentioned above. Use a mold-killing disinfec-

tant such as bleach (keep out of a toddler's reach) to clean mold areas.

- Close windows that are near mold-producing or pollen-shedding shrubs.

Also, clear damp piles of debris in the yard, and prune the shrubbery.

- Remove carpet and wallpaper that are damp from recent water leaks.

- If you run a humidifier during months of central heating, there's likely to be mold on the draperies or wallpaper. In this case, clean the drapery frequently and remove the wallpaper.

The extent of your mold mowing depends on the severity of baby's allergies. Most persons and a little bit of mold coexist well together. An environmental testing company can test your house to see if mold is a problem. In some cases, the mold is too extensive to clean up, and you may need to move. Usually, however, the company can assist you in cleaning up the mold enough to decrease your family's exposure to a healthy level.

Dust. The allergens on dust are caused by tiny insects called dust mites. These critters are like microscopic crumbs and live among the dust in carpets, bedding, and upholstered furniture. They thrive in warm, humid environments and feed on the flakes of skin humans continuously shed. The mites excrete tiny pellets that float through the air into a person's allergy-prone respiratory tract. It's this excrement that triggers allergies, not the dust or the mite itself. But lessening dust does help control the allergenic substances. Acarosan powder can be applied to carpets to kill dust mites and to neutralize their allergenic sheddings and make them easier to remove by vacuuming. Ask your allergist about this product.

A dust-free home is as impossible to achieve as a constantly clear nose. But there are ways to minimize dust and defuzz your baby's environment. Again, remember the severity of your defuzzing is proportional to the severity of baby's allergies. Don't overdo dust prevention for a mildly allergic child. Begin in the bedroom if your baby has a lot of nighttime breathing noises and awakens in the morning with a stuffy nose. (See pages 700–701 for how to allergyproof a bedroom.)

Allergies at School

If your child's symptoms are worse at school, here are several causes to consider:

- Cockroaches in lockers or other areas. Their feces can trigger allergies.

- Pets in the classroom. Sometimes the class gerbil, rabbit, or other rodent may be the culprit. Ask the teacher to have someone take the pet home for two weeks and see if your child's symptoms improve.

- Dust mites and mold. Talk to the school principal about how to detect and correct any possible sources.

- Plants and grasses. There may be specific grass or pollens present only at school. Unfortunately, it is difficult to prevent exposure to these.

Seeing an Allergy Specialist

If your child's symptoms do not improve after you have done your own investigating and prevention, an allergist can perform skin testing to see which specific things your child is allergic to. This will help you focus your preventive measures on specific allergens, instead of trying to prevent everything. Blood testing for allergies is also available, but it is not as accurate as skin testing.

Medications for Allergies

Decongestants, antihistamines, and combinations of these two are used more in older children and adults but are also available for babies. Follow the same precautions suggested previously for cold remedies (page 667). Better is to use the nonmedication tips for nasal hygiene and move secretions along (see page 664). Depending upon the severity of your baby's allergies, your doctor or allergist can suggest a safe and effective medical regimen.

ECZEMA

Eczema, or atopic dermatitis, is the most common rash of infancy and childhood. It is caused by a combination of a genetically hyperactive immune system that makes the skin react to foods and the environment, a genetic tendency toward dry skin, and specific allergens. The rash shows up as:

- Dry skin. You may feel tiny white bumps as you run your fingers across the rough skin.

- Dry patches. Scaly, dry, white, or bumpy red patches appear anywhere on the body.

- Flare-ups. From time to time, especially during winter, some areas of the skin become more irritated and flare up into raised, red, slightly oozing patches. These generally occur near skin creases, most commonly the inside of the elbows and behind the knees, but also on the neck, wrists, hands, and feet.

Treating Eczema

If the eczema appears in only a few mild patches and is not bothering your child, you can just leave it alone. If, on the other hand, it is more significant, then follow the recommendations below. Treatment is aimed at both lubricating the dry skin and removing allergic and irritating triggers.

Moisturize and Avoid Skin Irritants

Apply a hypoallergenic, unscented moisturizing lotion or cream to your child's skin two or more times each day. There are dozens of brand names, and no one is best for every child. Experiment with different lotions until you find one that works and is tolerated by your child. Try these tips for avoiding dry skin:

- Avoid hot baths. Bathe your child in luke-warm water.

- Do not let your child sit in soapy water or bubble baths.

- Gently pat the skin dry with a towel. Do not rub.

- Do not use soap, even liquid baby soap. This can dry the skin. Instead, use a hypoallergenic, unscented moisturizing bar like Dove.

- Maintain a humidity around 40 percent in your home. Use a humidity gauge if needed for accuracy. Run a humidifier, air conditioner, or both during dry weather. During the winter months, when using central heating, run a humidifier as needed.

- Avoid wool and synthetic materials. They can be more abrasive and irritating to the skin. Cotton clothing is best.

- Use cotton sheets and soft, cotton blankets.

- Wash new clothes before your child wears them. This will get out any chemicals from the manufacturing process.

- Use a mild, dye-free and perfume-free detergent such as Dreft, Ivory Snow, or All Clear. Liquid detergents rinse out better. Double rinse the wash to get out all the detergent. Avoid using dryer sheets.

- Bathe your child after she plays in the grass or engages in activities that make her sweaty.

- Apply a suntan lotion that doesn't irritate your child's skin. PABA-free is better.

- Dress your child in loose-fitting clothes with long sleeves and pants.

Feed and Water the Skin

In our pediatric office we have seen amazing results by feeding infants with eczema or dry skin a diet rich in omega-3 fats, or by increasing the omega 3's in the diet of a breastfeeding mother. (See www.dhadoc.com for information on the importance of omega-3 fats in infant nutrition.) Also, hydrate your infant by encouraging him to drink several extra glasses or bottles of water a day.

Investigate and Avoid Allergic Triggers

If you can pinpoint and avoid any allergens that may cause or worsen the eczema, then you should see a dramatic improvement in your child's eczema.

Food allergies. The six most common foods that trigger allergies are dairy products (milk, yogurt, cheese, butter), eggs, soy, peanuts, fish, and wheat. Eliminate all six foods for two to three weeks. If you see a dramatic improvement, re-introduce each food one at a time to determine which one is causing the allergy. Breastfeeding moms should also try this with their own diet if their infant has eczema. If using formula, try a different one. (See page 201 for types of formula.)

Environmental allergies. Dust, mold, pets, and seasonal outdoor allergies such as pollens are more likely to cause nasal allergies and asthma rather than eczema. They can, however, contribute to eczema.

Relieve the Itching

Follow these steps to minimize the itching:

- Hydrocortisone cream. During a flare-up, you can apply extra-strength over-the-counter hydrocortisone cream to problem areas twice a day for several days. Your doctor can also prescribe a stronger cream if needed. (Don't use prescription-strength cortisone cream on the sensitive skin of baby's face without the approval of your doctor.)

- Oral antihistamines. Available over the counter (for example, Benadryl) and by prescription, this medication can dramatically relieve the itching, especially at night.

- Keep your baby's fingernails cut short and clean them regularly.

Most children outgrow their eczema during childhood. Some, however, will continue to live with this condition into adulthood.

QUESTIONS PARENTS HAVE ABOUT AIDS

Compared with many other infectious diseases, AIDS is relatively uncommon among infants. But it's high on parents' worry lists. Despite the hype about AIDS in the media, 99.95 percent of the U.S. population are HIV-negative. It's estimated that HIV-positive mothers represent only around 0.01 percent of women giving birth in the United States. AIDS stands for "acquired immunodeficiency syndrome" and is caused by the human immunodeficiency virus, or HIV. This virus incapacitates the immune system, making the body vulnerable to overwhelming infections such as pneumonia and infections of the blood. In infants, AIDS may also cause abnormalities in brain development, failure to thrive, tumors, and is eventually fatal. Here are the most common questions parents have about AIDS.

How can my baby contract AIDS?

AIDS can only be transmitted in these ways:

- sexual intercourse
- blood transfusions
- infected hypodermic needle
- infected mother to her baby during pregnancy or possibly through breast milk

AIDS cannot be contracted from

- saliva
- tears
- coughing
- sneezing
- sweat
- utensils
- dishes
- toilet seats
- pets
- flies
- mosquitoes
- excrement
- swimming pools
- clothing

Can my baby get AIDS from playing with an AIDS-infected baby?

No. The AIDS virus does not spread through the air. As a testimony to how difficult it is to transfer the AIDS virus among children, studies have shown that children who live with AIDS-infected siblings have not been infected with AIDS, even though they share toys, toothbrushes, drinking glasses, and so on.

Could my baby contract AIDS at a day-care center?

Babies have caught just about every other infectious disease in a day-care center, but not AIDS. AIDS cannot be contracted by a hug or a kiss, and AIDS experts feel that transmitting AIDS through a child's bite would be extremely unlikely. Even if an AIDS-infected baby gets cut, the infected blood would have to be injected into the blood of another child, perhaps through an open wound. Though theoretically possible, this coincidence would be highly unlikely.

Can babies get AIDS from pets or toys?

No. The AIDS virus can only survive in a human body. Even toys that might be contaminated with infected blood can be disinfected with simple household bleach.

Can an AIDS-infected pregnant mother transmit AIDS to her preborn baby?

Yes, studies estimate she has approximately a 30–50 percent chance of such transmission, yet this transmission is often preventable with medication.

Could my baby get AIDS from a blood transfusion?

At present the risk is negligible. With current blood-screening techniques, the Red Cross estimates the chances range from one in forty thousand to one in one million. Since this risk will still bother you, if baby needs a blood transfusion blood can be donated by you or a family member or a friend with compatible blood type.

Can AIDS be transmitted from an infected mother to her baby through breast milk?

New insights have shown that HIV-positive mothers should not always be discouraged from breastfeeding their babies for fear of transmitting this infection through their milk. Though the science of HIV-transmission is clouded by emotion and politics, it seems that the risk of maternal-infant transmission through breastfeeding is much lower than previously suspected. The risk of transmit-

ting AIDS through breast milk is definitely lower than the risk of transmitting it through the blood during birth. In light of recent research, we advise an HIV-positive mother to consult an HIV specialist before concluding that she absolutely cannot breastfeed her baby.

CHILDHOOD ILLNESSES AT A GLANCE

Illness	Cause	Signs and Symptoms
Appendicitis	Inflammation	Abdominal pain; may begin as general pain in middle, then confines itself to lower-right part of abdomen; becomes increasingly severe; fever and lack of appetite usual; vomiting possible; extreme pain when lower-right abdomen is pushed on
Asthma (wheezing)	Food or environmental allergies; lung infections	Whistling, crackling sound during exhalation; may occur during inhalation if more severe; may worsen with exercise or during coughs and colds; may just be a tight, frequent cough without audible wheezing; may have other allergic signs; *asthma attack* is wheezing with fast, labored breathing and indrawn skin over the neck, ribs, and upper abdomen
Bladder infection	Bacteria	Three classic urinary signs: frequency — urination one or more times per hour; urgency — feeling of needing to urinate is extremely urgent; may have "accidents"; burning during urination. Accompanying fever, back or side pain, and vomiting may indicate more severe kidney infection
Boils	Bacteria, usually staphylococcus; may arise from an infected pimple	Raised, red, tender, warm swellings on skin; common on buttocks
Bronchiolitis (spasm and inflammation of small airways; usually in infants under 1 year)	Virus called RSV	Like "baby asthma," rapid, shallow, noisy, labored breathing; musical cough; paleness, fatigue, anxiety; cold symptoms

Would it be safe for me to be a foster parent for an AIDS-infected baby?

Yes. As in school or day care, the chance of an AIDS-infected baby transmitting the virus to family members, friends, or foster parents is, according to the American Academy of Pediatrics Task Force on Pediatric AIDS, "virtually nonexistent."

Researchers are prudently working to formulate both a safe and effective drug to cure AIDS and a vaccine to prevent it. For now, the best way to prevent AIDS in babies is to prevent it in adults.

Home Treatment	Medical Treatment	Of Special Note
...one; observation	Evaluation by doctor or ER: blood work, urine test, X ray, or ultrasound may or may not confirm diagnosis; surgery if confirmed or highly suspected	Consider other causes, such as severe gas pain, bladder infection, or severe constipation
...est, relaxation; upright sleep if ...ossible; steam treatments in bath-...oom; clap on chest to encourage ...oughing; for chronic asthma try ...ood-allergy and environmental-...llergy avoidance; for breastfed infants ...void dairy and other allergens in ...om's diet; change formula to soy or ...ther formula; non-prescription ...xpectorants	*For asthma attack:* prescription albuterol inhaler (to relax and expand lung airways) every 3–4 hours; steroid liquid or pills if severe. *For chronic asthma:* allergy avoidance and testing; daily preventive steroid or antihistamine inhaler; allergy medications	A few episodes of wheezing does not mean asthma; "asthma" means chronic or recurrent wheezing episodes
...lenty of fluids; 1 cup cranberry juice ...or a cranberry mixed juice) once ...r twice per day	Urinalysis and urine culture (if needed) to diagnose infection; antibiotics if infection suspected or confirmed; continue cranberry juice and fluids	Urinalysis may reveal infection; if not, urine culture may take up to 48 hours to confirm infection
...pply hot compresses 10 times daily ...or a few minutes to bring boil to head; ...ontinue a few days after boil pops ...nd drains; keep covered until ...rainage stops.	May incise and drain; prescription antibiotic ointment after draining; oral antibiotics may be needed	Avoid squeezing or picking to avoid scarring and spreading
...omfort and calm baby; induce sleep ...ith baby propped up 45 degrees; use ...arm mist; nonprescription expector-...nt to loosen chest congestion; increase ...uids, give small frequent feedings; ...ry chest clapping	Prescription albuterol (to relax and expand lung airways) can be liquid by mouth, inhaler with mask, or nebulizer (turns medicine into a mist that is inhaled); if severe, hospitalization with oxygen therapy	If baby is a "happy wheezer," no treatment may be needed; minor recurrences common with subsequent colds

CHILDHOOD ILLNESSES AT A GLANCE *(continued)*

Illness	Cause	Signs and Symptoms
Bronchitis (spasm and inflammation of the large airways; any age)	Usually virus or allergies; sometimes bacteria	Cold symptoms, low fever (101°-102°F/ 38.3°-38.9°C), deep, junky chest cough, worse at night, paleness, tiredness; child may also wheeze, as with asthma
Cellulitis (infection of the skin)	Bacterial infection, usually staphylococcus or streptococcus	Swollen, red, tender, warm area of skin usually on extremities or buttocks; often begins as puncture wound, scratch, or boil; local lymph glands swollen and tender; fever if more severe
Chicken pox	Virus (incubation 7-21 days)	Flulike symptoms, fever 101°F/38.3°C; rash on trunk begins like bites, rapidly forms blisters and spreads over trunk, face, mouth, then extremities; then scabs; rash in different stages at same time; itchy; new spots pop up daily for several days and go through these changes; difficult to diagnose on day 1 of rash; assume contagious while waiting 2 to 3 days to observe if spots change as above
Conjunctivitis (pinkeye)	Virus, bacteria, allergies, or environmental irritants	*Viral:* red eyes, occasional discharge. *Bacterial:* red eyes, persistent discharge, swollen eyelids. *Allergic:* red, itchy, tearing eyes, maybe white discharge. *Irritant:* red, burning, maybe white discharge
Diphtheria	Bacteria (incubation 2-5 days)	Severe, obstructive tonsillitis; white membrane covers tonsils; fever; difficulty breathing and swallowing
Epiglottitis (life-threatening swelling of the larynx [voice box], obstructing passage of air into windpipe)	Bacterial infection, usually *H. influenzae* (HIB)	Fever 103°F/39.4°C; baby looks panicky and acts sick, behaves as if choking (leans forwards, protrudes tongue, opens mouth, drools); prolonged seal-like noise during exhaling; indraws while inhaling; rapidly worsens
Fifth disease	Virus	Bright red rash begins on cheeks; "slapped cheek" look; lacelike red rash on trunk and extremities may fluctuate for 1-3 weeks; possible slight fever; sore joints; possible cold symptoms

...ome Treatment	Medical Treatment	Of Special Note
...est, relaxation; upright sleep if ...ossible; frequent steam treatments ...bathroom; steam vaporizer while ...eeping; clap on chest and encourage ...oughing; nonprescription expectorants ...uring day; multisymptom cough ...edicine at night	Prescription-strength cough medicine at night if needed; antibiotics for bacterial infection	Most bronchitis in infants and children is viral, so no antibiotics needed; if chest pains during coughing are prolonged or fever lasts several days may be bacterial
...pply hot compresses for a few minutes ...very 2 hours; elevate infected area; ...cetaminophen for fever and pain	Antibiotics; oral if mild, by injection twice daily if moderate, intravenous in hospital if severe; may need blood tests to evaluate severity	Mark borders of infection with pen; notify doctor if continuing to spread
...ut fingernails and wear long clothes to ...void scratching; for itching, use Aveeno ...atmeal baths, calamine lotion (do not ...pply to open sores on face — may scar); ...ive oral Benadryl for intense itching; ...ntibiotic ointment for infected sores	Prescription antihistamine for severe itching; antiviral medication may shorten course and severity if started within 72 hours (only for older children); antibiotics for widespread infected sores	Transmitted by prolonged close proximity; contagious until all sores are scabbed; sun exposure may increase scarring
...ash out eyes with saline eyedrops ...everal times each day; warm washcloth ...ompresses; for allergy, nonprescription ...ntihistamine eyedrops	*Viral:* saline eyedrops. *Bacterial:* prescription antibiotic drops or ointment. *Allergic:* prescription antihistamine eyedrops. *Irritant:* flush repeatedly with saline solution	Bacterial and viral both mildly contagious until redness and discharge gone; in newborns and infants, daily discharge without redness may be caused by plugged tear ducts (see page 105)
...ive fluids, popsicles, bland diet; ...se mist	Prevention with DTaP vaccine; antibiotics; hospitalization	Rare, especially in immunized countries
...*Medical emergency:* rush to hospital, ...all doctor; calm child and open ...indows in car en route; don't feed; ...t baby up to breathe	Hospitalization, ICU observation; antibiotics; oxygen, mist, intravenous, inhalation therapy; sometimes lifesaving tube put through mouth into airway; HIB vaccine lowers risk	Differs from croup (page 683): with epiglottitis, child sicker, higher fever, drooling, difficulty swallowing; child looks panicky and hungry for air; usually, but not always, occurs in child over 2 years; now rare because of HIB vaccine
...reat fever and any other symptoms ...s needed	None necessary	Keep away from pregnant women, as can cause miscarriages, especially in first trimester if exposed woman not immune; most contagious at onset of rash or fever until child no longer feeling ill; residual rash probably not contagious

CHILDHOOD ILLNESSES AT A GLANCE *(continued)*

Illness	Cause	Signs and Symptoms
Flu (influenza)	Virus (incubation period 1–3 days)	Fever (may be high), body aches, vomiting, diarrhea, sore throat, headache, cough, runny nose, red eyes; infant looks unwell, but illness not toxic; can begin quickly; worst symptoms slowly resolve over several days, cough and cold symptoms may linger
German measles (rubella, 3-day measles)	Rubella virus (incubation period 14–21 days)	Low-grade fever 100°–101°F/37.8°–38.3°C, baby *mildly* sick; flulike, slight cold; pinkish-red-spotted rash begins on face, spreads rapidly to trunk, and disappears by third day; swollen glands behind ears, nape of neck
Hand, foot, and mouth virus (herpangina virus)	Coxsakie virus (incubation 3–6 days)	Tiny blisterlike sores in mouth, on palms of hands, soles of feet; sore throat, painful swallowing; excessive drooling; inflamed gums; diarrhea; high fever up to 5 days; can be extremely painful; may have spots in only one place; lasts around 7 days; many cases involve larger grayish-white ulcers inside mouth
Hepatitis A (inflammation of the liver — very different from Hepatitis B and C, which are sexually transmitted diseases)	Virus (incubation 2–6 weeks, usually 4 weeks)	Depends on age. *Infancy–6 years:* mild flu symptoms (stomachache, vomiting, diarrhea); yellow skin; lasts a few days; no long-term problems. *6–12 years:* same as infant, but symptoms may be more severe and last longer, no long-term problems. *12 years–adult:* same symptoms but can last for a week or more; degree of liver inflammation and damage can be more severe; long-term liver damage rare but possible
Herpes simplex (stomatitis, cold sores, fever blisters)	Herpes virus (incubation 7 days); different strain from genital herpes	Painful, swollen, reddened, sometimes bleeding gums; tiny blisters on tongue, gums, lips, and around mouth; blisters break, leaving sores that heal in a week; low-grade fever; irritable; little appetite
Impetigo (infection of the skin)	Bacteria, streptococcus or staphylococcus	Pimple-size or coin-size spots, oozing, blisterlike, honey-colored crusts; usually below nose, around mouth, in diaper area

Home Treatment	Medical Treatment	Of Special Note
Give sips of liquids, ice chips, popsicles, oral electrolyte solutions, small frequent feedings, acetaminophen; treat most bothersome symptoms with multi-symptom cold and flu medication if needed	Flu vaccine strongly recommended for children with chronic illnesses: heart, lung; the vaccine is also useful in preventing the flu even in healthy infants over six months of age; antibiotic given if secondary infection; may lead to complications such as bronchitis, pneumonia, or ear infection; antiviral flu medicines not used in children; prescription suppositories to stop vomiting if needed	Doctor's exam helpful to rule out secondary infection; clue that it is the flu is presence of several of the above signs together
Treat like flu; baby not that sick	Prevention with MMR vaccine; exam to confirm diagnosis; may resemble other viruses; serial blood tests can confirm, yet this is rarely necessary	Keep away from pregnant women, as can cause birth defects (85 percent of women already immune); contagious from a few days before to 7 days after rash appears
Two main goals: to give pain and fever relief and to prevent dehydration; give acetaminophen as needed; push fluids, popsicles, Jell-O, ice cream, soft, bland foods; avoid acidic foods like citrus and tomato sauce; Benadryl liquid for calming effect	No antibiotics; prescription anesthetic mouth rinse for children old enough to rinse and spit	Child can act very ill, but condition is not serious or harmful; extremely contagious until fever and pain resolve; mild dehydration common but almost never needs medical intervention; child may go several days without eating
Same as for flu	Same as for flu; prevention with Hepatitis A vaccine; Hep A immune globulin also available for adults and older children (see page 629)	Transmitted from an infected person by contaminated food or direct contact (e.g., restaurant employee); water-borne outbreaks rare
Same as for hand, foot, and mouth disease; try yogurt and lactobacillus culture; do not use cortisone creams (eczema creams)	Same as for hand, foot, and mouth disease; prescription antiviral cream may shorten course of external sores (not inside mouth)	Virus lives inside nerve endings; tends to recur periodically throughout life; contagious when active
Cut fingernails, keep baby from scratching; keep covered to prevent spread; discourage picking raw skin, e.g., under nose; nonprescription antibiotic ointment	Prescription antibiotic ointment; oral antibiotic if severe	Not highly contagious if covered and while being treated by doctor, but don't let child touch other children with infected area

CHILDHOOD ILLNESSES AT A GLANCE *(continued)*

Illness	Cause	Signs and Symptoms
Lyme disease (named from town Old Lyme, Connecticut, where first diagnosed)	Spirochete germ from an infected tick bite (incubation 3–32 days)	Rash begins as single, red, raised ring with pale center around bite; circular spots spread to trunk and extremities; flulike symptoms; swollen glands near bite; sometimes conjunctivitis, sore throat; joint swelling or pain may appear weeks later
Measles (rubeola)	Virus (incubation 8–12 days)	Begins like a cold, then fever 104°F/40°C, cough; bloodshot eyes, sensitive to light; around fourth day rash (deep red, confluent) begins on face, spreads all over body; disappears first on face but lasts 5 days; child acts sickest when rash first appears
Meningitis (spinal meningitis, inflammation of lining of brain)	Bacteria or virus (incubation period depends on infectious agent, usually 10–14 days)	*Bacterial:* four classic symptoms — high fever, severe headache, vomiting, stiff rigid painful back of neck (worse when bending head down); other signs include lethargy, eyes sensitive to light, stiffening of back when legs pulled up to change diaper; bulging soft spot in head; child acts extremely ill. *Viral:* similar signs, but child does not appear as sick
Mumps (inflammation of salivary glands in neck)	Virus (incubation 7–10 days)	Begins like flu, usually also upset stomach; 2–3 days later tender swollen glands beneath earlobes; may begin on one side, then the other; "Chipmunk cheeks," may be painful to open jaw; lasts 7–10 days; possibly low fever; usually child doesn't act very sick
Pinworms	Intestinal worms, a parasite (incubation varies, can be months)	Night waking, restlessness; intense itching around anus or in vagina; worms look like threads, 1/3 inch (1 cm) long; travel out of rectum to deposit eggs around anus or vagina at night
Pneumonia (inflammation of lung tissue)	Bacteria or virus (incubation usually 7–14 days depending on germ)	Starts off as regular cough and cold, then worsens. *Bacterial:* 102°–104°F/38.9°–40°C, chills, rapid breathing, fast heart rate, productive cough, abdominal pain, chest pain, vomiting; baby progressively sicker. *Viral:* low fever, no chills; lingering cough; baby not that sick; may last 3–4 weeks
Reye's syndrome (inflammation of brain, liver)	Unknown, possibly toxins released by viral illness	Increasing lethargy, may progress to coma; persistent vomiting; fever; follows viral illnesses; seizures; *a serious disease*

ome Treatment	Medical Treatment	Of Special Note
emove tick carefully (see page 740); pply antiseptic to bite; contact doctor; ave tick in case later needed r analysis	Confirmation of diagnosis difficult, possibly blood tests to confirm; antibiotics necessary if confirmed	Suspected more often than confirmed; relatively uncommon disease
uarantine until rash gone; push fluids; se fever control	Prevention with MMR vaccine; treat complications: pneumonia, encephalitis, ear infection; confirmation of diagnosis by telltale white spots on inner cheeks	Often suspected but may be other virus; rash of measles *deep* red, covers most of face and trunk and child very sick; high fever
one; clue to diagnosis is painful, stiff ack of neck combined with several ther symptoms; if several symptoms re present but neck and back are fine, ss likely; call doctor immediately if ultiple symptoms present or child ery ill	Prevention with HIB and Prevnar vaccines; spinal tap to determine diagnosis. *Bacterial:* intravenous antibiotics for at least 7 days; monitoring for complications. *Viral:* treat like flu, no antibiotics	The earlier the diagnosis and treatment, the better the outcome; also depends on type of germ
ive bland diet, smoothies; apply cool ompresses to neck; give cetaminophen; call doctor if baby ecomes drowsy, persistently vomits, r has stiff neck	Prevention with MMR vaccine; treatment of rare complications: encephalitis, dehydration	Not to be confused with other swollen neck glands: mump glands very large, tender, and just beneath earlobe but above jawbone; other glandular infections occur *below* jawbone; contagious until swelling gone
se flashlight to see worms in anus at ight or place sticky tape around anus capture eggs, take to laboratory for entification; cut fingernails to iscourage scratching	Prescription medicine for each family member; take once but be sure to take another dose 2 weeks after first dose	More of nuisance than medical problem; only transmitted from person to person, not from pets or toys; child scratches, gets eggs beneath fingernails, shares with friend or puts into own mouth, eggs grow into worms in intestines, and cycle continues
ots of fluids; treat fever; steam eatments — have child breathe in eam deeply for 10 minutes; pound or ap on front, sides, and back of chest to icourage coughing; give expectorant guaifenesin) to loosen chest congestion; ve cough suppressant at night only needed	Oral antibiotics; chest X ray sometimes needed to confirm diagnosis; hospitalization only if moderate to severe labored breathing and oxygen needed	Provided it is treated early, no longer considered a serious disease; easily treatable with antibiotics and chest-pounding therapy; doctor can hear specific pneumonia sounds with stethoscope
otify doctor if baby shows rapidly *eteriorating state of consciousness*	Hospitalization; supportive treatment; treatment of brain swelling, liver involvement, seizure control	Aspirin implicated (but not proven) as cause when taken for chicken pox or influenza

CHILDHOOD ILLNESSES AT A GLANCE *(continued)*

Illness	Cause	Signs and Symptoms
Roseola	Virus (incubation 5–10 days)	Sudden onset of high fever 103°–105°F/39.4°–40.6°C in previously well baby, may cause febrile convulsions; fever decreases easily with treatment; baby does not act very ill, especially when fever goes down; fever breaks on third day; baby seems almost well, then faint pink rash appears on neck, trunk, and extremities, lasting 1 to 3 days
RSV (respiratory syncytial virus — inflammation of the lungs). See Bronchiolitis	Virus (incubation 5–8 days)	Like bronchiolitis: raspy cough, rapid breathing, wheezing, indrawing; one of the most common causes of "wheezing" or "bronchitis" during first 6 months
Scabies (skin infection)	Mite, microscopic size	Intense itching and scratching of flea-bite-size bumps; sometimes mites burrow under skin, leaving linear, bumpy rash; persists for weeks without treatment
Scarlet fever (scarlatina; basically, same illness as strep throat) — see "Sore throat," below	Not an infection itself; immune reaction to strep throat infection	Sunburnlike rash over face, trunk, and extremities, feels like sandpaper; mustachelike pallor around mouth; rash disappears in 5 days, leaving peeling areas; fever 101°–104°F/38.3°–40°C; tonsillitis, like strep throat; vomiting common; occurs during a strep throat infection
Sore throat (strep throat, viral sore throat)	Virus, bacteria (streptococcus) (incubation 2–5 days)	*Strep throat:* uncommon under age 3; red throat and tonsils; moderate to severe sore throat; painful swallowing; red spots on palate; may or may not have pus on tonsils; "strawberrylike" tongue; possible swollen tonsils and neck glands; fever; may have headache and stomachaches. *Viral sore throat:* more common cause of sore throat in infants and toddlers; may have similar signs as strep, but less severe; often accompanied by other general cold and flu symptoms
Tetanus (lockjaw)	Bacteria (incubation 3–21 days); caused by toxin from bacteria in deep, contaminated wound	Generalized muscle spasms, especially jaw muscles; convulsions
Tonsillitis (sore throat)	Often bacterial, sometimes viral	Similar to strep throat (see "Sore throat"), but tonsils are more swollen and usually have pus; more difficulty swallowing; usually acting sicker than with strep throat

Home Treatment	Medical Treatment	Of Special Note
Treat fever, push fluids; don't worry despite high fever if baby seems better when fever decreases	Control fever; diagnosis not confirmed until rash appears	Very common cause of fever in 6–18-month-olds; suspect in baby who has high fever that goes up and down but who doesn't act very sick; if antibiotic is given and rash later appears, it may be mistaken for allergic rash to the antibiotic
Same as for bronchiolitis; notify doctor if baby having difficulty breathing, becoming exhausted, or pale or blue around mouth	Possibly hospitalization; antivirus medication by special inhalation therapy in severe cases	Be concerned about any lingering cough and increasingly labored breathing in infant under 6 months; common cause of chronic progressive cough in newborn in first few months
Give cool baths; try Aveeno baths; cut fingernails; launder clothing and bedsheets; liquid Benadryl for itching	Prescription cream or lotion (use only as directed; overuse may be toxic); anti-itch medicines	Suspect if intense, itchy rash lasts for weeks; highly contagious from person to person, not from toys
Same as for sore throat; Aveeno oatmeal baths and Benadryl liquid for itching	Same as strep throat	No more serious than regular strep throat; no special precautions necessary
Push fluids, popsicles, soft, bland foods; treat pain with acetaminophen or ibuprofen, throat lozenges, anesthetic throat sprays if severe; gargle with warm salt water	*Strep throat:* quick strep test (results within 5 minutes) or throat culture (1–2 days) needed to confirm diagnosis; antibiotics if test positive. *Viral sore throat:* no antibiotics needed	*Strep throat:* contagious for 24–48 hours after treatment begun. *Viral sore throat:* contagious until fever is gone for 24 hours and pain is minimal. Clues to distinguish between the two: strep usually in ages 4 and up, sore throat is main symptom, and child generally acting sicker than with viral; viral more common in infants or preschool kids; sore throat along with various other cold and flu symptoms
Prevent by cleaning wounds with antiseptic and immunizing	Prevention with DPT vaccine; hospitalization; antibiotics	Uncommon
Same as for sore throat	Oral antibiotics usually given; oral steroids for extreme swelling	Contagious for 24–48 hours after treatment begun

CHILDHOOD ILLNESSES AT A GLANCE *(continued)*

Illness	Cause	Signs and Symptoms
Whooping cough (pertussis)	Bacteria (incubation usually 7–10 days; can be 20 days)	Begins like regular cold but lingers; cough worsens around 2 weeks later; severe coughing fits begin in which child has 30-second to 1-minute coughing fits producing thick mucus, excessive drool, red face, and often vomiting at end of fit, followed by long catch-up inhalation ("whooping" sound); child may turn pale or blue around mouth during coughing; usually no fever, and child seems unusually well between episodes, with no in-between coughing; episodes may occur a few times an hour or once every few hours

VISIT DR. SEARS ONLINE

For more detailed information on common and not-so-common childhood illnesses, visit www.AskDrSears.com.

ome Treatment

ush fluids; try cool mist, chest
apping, expectorant cough syrups;
all doctor if cough persists, child
ecomes exhausted, has difficulty
reathing, or is turning blue during
pisodes

Medical Treatment

Prevention with DTaP vaccine; diagnosis
based mostly on parent's description of
cough or doctor observing an episode;
antibiotics important to prevent epidemic
spread, household contacts usually treated
as well; expectorants may help;
hospitalization if child is turning blue
with coughing fits

Of Special Note

Most serious under 6 months;
older toddlers and children
usually do not suffer complications; contagious until treated for
5 days; coughing episodes may
persist for weeks after treatment

28

Lifesaving Procedures and First Aid for Common Emergencies

Susan, a prematurely gray-haired mother of an accident-prone toddler, once asked, "Where can I find a live-in doctor? Will I ever survive these toddler years?" When accidents happen, and they can, even in the safest homes and to the smartest babies, you, mom and dad, are baby's first emergency medical system. Here is a crash course on how to save your baby's life.

THE THREE *P*'S

If an emergency happens, and it most likely will, preparing your home, your skills, and your mind keeps you a childsaving step ahead.

Prevent. Accidentproof your environment, as much as possible, by following the home babyproofing guide in Chapter 25.

Prepare. Take an infant-CPR and first aid course and a refresher course every two years. These are offered by your local Red Cross or hospital. If not, get a group of parents together and hire a certified instructor from your local emergency medical system.

Just as a childbirth class prepares you for your baby's birth, a CPR (cardiopulmonary resuscitation) class prepares you for your baby's life. Junior-high- and high-school-age children should also take a CPR class, especially if they frequently baby-sit for younger children. At least watch a CPR video together as a family. Discuss and practice what you learn from the class and the video. Require that your regular baby-sitter take a CPR course, and if your baby is in day care, be certain the day-care providers are trained in CPR.

Practice. Periodically rehearse in your mind and by acting out what you would do if . . . Rehearse what you learned in the CPR class. Practice on dolls or cushions, not babies. Prethink a plan of action and store this strategy in your mind like a flash card to be clicked into, almost by reflex, in an act-fast situation.

In this chapter we will outline the techniques you need to know to be a skillful and fast lifesaver in a number of emergency situations.

▶ *SPECIAL NOTE: The following instructions do not substitute for taking a first aid or CPR course.*

CHOKING

Choking means that baby is trying to dislodge material from a partially obstructed airway or is frantically trying to get air in, past the obstruction. It is one of the most common causes of death in children.

What Not to Do

If baby can cough, cry, or speak and is obviously breathing, the airway is not obstructed. It takes moving air to make sounds. Baby's own gag-and-cough reflex will usually dislodge the piece. In this case, doing any of the intervention procedures is unnecessary and potentially dangerous. Instead, remain on standby offering baby the emotional support of a calm, reassuring "It's OK" so that baby doesn't panic. Remember, you are a when-to-worry mirror to baby. *If you panic, baby panics.* Unless you can easily see the obstructing object, do not use a blind finger sweep to grope for it; doing this may push the object farther back in the throat.

When to Intervene

If baby shows the following signs, his airway is obstructed:

- gasping for breath or turning blue
- fainting (and you suspect choking)
- displaying an "I'm choking" expression: wide eyes, open mouth, drooling, a panicky look
- for an older child, showing the universal choking sign by clasping his throat

If Your Baby Is Choking: Two Techniques

If your child shows any of the signs just listed, there are two approaches you can take: *the Heimlich maneuver* (also called

---

SWALLOWED OBJECTS

From hand to mouth is standard operating procedure for a baby but a worry for parents. Babies sometimes swallow small objects such as coins, which nearly always pass through the intestines and are eliminated in one to three days without causing any harm. If your baby is not coughing, not drooling excessively, not experiencing any abdominal pain, and seems perfectly well, it is seldom necessary to share your discovery with your doctor.

But there are times when you need to worry. Sometimes objects such as rock candy or a large coin may lodge in baby's esophagus, the tube running from the mouth to the stomach. An object stuck in the esophagus is much less serious than one stuck in the windpipe, but it may still compromise baby's ability to swallow and sometimes even the ability to breathe. Here are the call-doctor-right-away signs: *excessive drooling, pain where the object is stuck* (usually only an older child can locate the site of the pain), and *inability to swallow.*

abdominal thrusts) for infants over one year, and the *back blow–chest thrust technique* for infants under one year. The Heimlich maneuver is not recommended for infants under a year because it can possibly cause a contusion to vital abdominal organs. In the past there has been spirited controversy over whether the back blow–chest thrust method or the Heimlich maneuver is better for the infant between one and two years, but now there is general agreement on the superiority of abdominal thrusts (Heimlich) for older children and adults. Parents usually feel more comfortable and therefore make fewer mistakes with the back blows; but as of 2000 a safety committee of the American Academy of Pediatrics recommended the infant version of the Heimlich maneuver in infants over a year old. It may be necessary to use both the back blow–chest thrust and abdominal-thrust methods.

▶*SPECIAL NOTE: No matter which method you use, pull out all the stops. Don't give up. The foreign body may dissolve or become smaller, or the airway may relax, making dislodgment easier. If your baby chokes in a public place, shout for help, especially if you don't know CPR. There may be a guardian angel off-duty fireman or paramedic (or someone else who knows CPR) who will assist while called-for help is on the way. Act fast, but make every action count.*

THE BACK BLOW–CHEST THRUST TECHNIQUE (FOR INFANTS UNDER ONE YEAR)

Step one: Five back blows. Straddle baby facedown along your forearm in a slightly head-down position. Support baby's chin in your cupped hand. Apply five quick, forceful back blows between baby's shoulder blades with the heel of your hand. Meanwhile shout for help: "My baby is choking — dial 911!" If you are alone, do steps one to four, then run with baby to the phone (see step five).

Step two: Chest thrusts. If baby has not dislodged the object (evidence is coughing or crying, or you see the piece shoot out) and is still not breathing, flip him over on your thigh. Deal five quick, forceful chest thrusts to baby's breastbone. To find the right place, imagine a line between the two nipples. The right area to depress is one finger's width

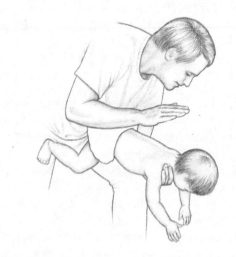

Back blows.

below where this line intersects the breastbone. Use two or three fingers to quickly
depress the breastbone to a depth of one-half
to one inch (1½ to 2½ centimeters), allowing
the breastbone to return to its normal position between thrusts without moving your
fingers.

Step three: Tongue-jaw lift. If baby is still
not breathing, check for a visible obstruction.
Depress baby's tongue with your thumb,
and holding the tongue and jaw between
thumb and forefinger, lift the jaw up and
open to inspect the back of baby's throat.
This draws the tongue away from the back
of the throat and may relieve the obstruction. If you see the obstruction, sweep it
out with a finger encircling the object, but
avoid blind groping that could push the
object farther back.

Step four: Mouth-to-mouth breathing.
If baby is still not breathing, give two
breaths by the mouth-to-mouth or mouth-
to-mouth-and-nose technique (see pages
723–724). If baby's chest rises with each
breath, you know the airway is clear. Continue ventilation until baby is breathing on
his own.

Step five: Repeat the sequence. Repeat
steps one to four while calling or waiting for
trained emergency help. With practice, this
entire sequence can be performed in less
than a minute. Practice on a doll and notice
how skillful you can become at alternating
between back blows and chest thrusts, holding baby sandwiched between your two
hands and flipping him from one position to
the other.

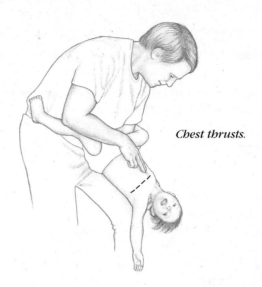

Chest thrusts.

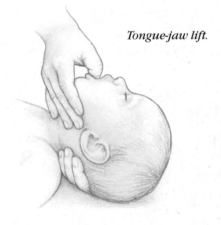

Tongue-jaw lift.

THE ABDOMINAL-THRUST (HEIMLICH) TECHNIQUE (FOR CHILDREN OVER ONE YEAR)

The Heimlich maneuver is not recommended for infants under one year of age.

If the child is unconscious. Place the child on his back on a firm surface (floor or table). Kneel or stand at the child's side or feet. (Straddling the child is not recommended when working with small children, as it encourages too much force on the thrusts.) Place the heel of one hand on the midline between the navel and ribs (being careful not to hit the tip of the breastbone, which could puncture underlying organs) and the second hand on top of the first. Depress the abdomen with up to five quick inward and upward thrusts. The smaller the child, the more gentle the maneuver. If the child does not cough up the obstruction after abdominal thrusts, open the airway using the tongue-jaw lift and, if you can see it, sweep the object out with your finger (again, no blind sweeps). If unsuccessful and the child is still not breathing, use mouth-to-mouth breathing (page 724) and repeat the abdominal thrusts.

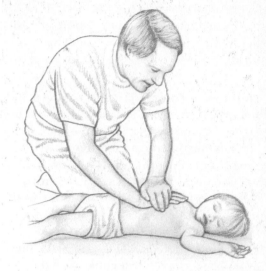

Abdominal thrusts for unconscious child.

In a conscious child. Stand behind the choking child and wrap your arms around his waist. Make a fist with one hand and place the thumb side of that fist against the child's abdomen in the midline slightly above the navel, but well below the tip of the breastbone. Grasp this fist with the other hand and press into the child's abdomen with a quick inward and upward jerk, repeating the thrust six to ten times if necessary. Be sure your fists do not touch the tip of the breastbone or the ribs.

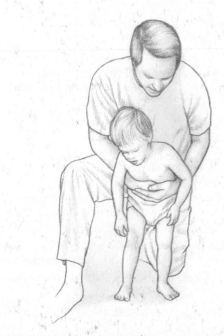

Abdominal thrusts for conscious child.

WHEN YOUR BABY ISN'T BREATHING: A STEP-BY-STEP APPROACH TO CPR

Step one: Quick assessment. If baby is pale, blue, and obviously not breathing, begin CPR, as in step two, immediately. If you are uncertain, look, listen, and feel for breathing.

Step two: Clear the mouth. Look for foreign objects, food, or gum. Carefully remove anything you find with a visible, not a blind, finger sweep. If there is vomit or any other fluid in the mouth, turn your child on one side and use gravity to clear it. If you suspect choking, apply back blows as described on page 720.

Step three: Position baby to straighten the airway. Place baby on his back, his head level with his heart. Place one hand on his head and your fingers on his chin. Clear the tongue from the back of the throat by lifting the chin up with one hand while pressing on the forehead with the other.

An infant's head should be slightly tilted upward toward the ceiling (called the sniffing position — do a practice sniff and notice how your head moves slightly upward and forward). Do not tilt an infant's head as far back as you would an adult's, as this may obstruct the airway. A towel rolled up under the neck usually maintains the correct position.

As the child gets older, the angle of backward head tilt increases slightly. Your fingers holding the chin should not press down on the throat and may be used to pull down the lower lip to keep the mouth open.

Step four: Begin mouth-to-mouth breathing.

- **Infant under one year:** Cover the baby's *mouth and nose* with your mouth. Blow into baby's mouth with just enough force to see baby's chest rise. (Blow with just the air in your cheeks, more a *puff* than a breath, not with the full force of a deep breath during exhaling. Forcing too much air in too fast may damage baby's lungs or distend the stomach and compromise breathing or trigger vomiting.) Begin with two short breaths. Watch for a chest rise during your blow.

  If baby's chest rises, you know the airway is clear and your technique is right. Continue mouth-to-mouth blowing until your baby is breathing on his own. Give a steady breath every three seconds (twenty per minute).

  If baby's chest is not rising, tighten your seal and try a few more forceful breaths. If

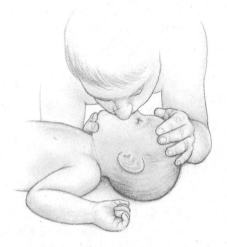

Mouth-to-mouth breathing for infants under one year.

still no chest rise, suspect airway obstruction and either reposition baby's head tilt and repeat the mouth-to-mouth procedure or immediately go to the back blow–chest thrust routine to dislodge a possible foreign body (page 720).

- **Older than one year:** In older babies and children, squeeze the nostrils between the thumb and forefinger and fit your mouth tightly around the child's lips. Form a tight seal with your lips. Then proceed as for an infant, above.

Step five: Check baby's pulse. Feeling a pulse means baby's heart is beating and you do not have to pump on baby's chest. The easiest way to find a pulse in a baby is by pressing gently between the muscles on the inner side of the upper arm, midway between the shoulder and the elbow. An alternate site in a child is the side of the neck. If baby has no pulse, go on to step six.

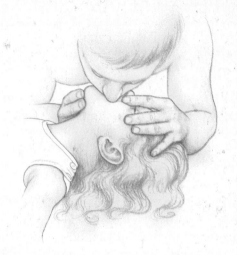

Mouth-to-mouth breathing for older babies and children.

WHEN CALLING THE PARAMEDICS

In an emergency, make sure to give the emergency medical services dispatcher the following information:

- your present location (and quick directions if place is difficult to find)
- phone number at your present location
- name and age of baby
- condition of baby
- cause of accident

If you are frozen in fear, ask another person to request instructions about what to do until the paramedics arrive.

Step six: Begin chest compressions. Place baby on a firm surface, such as the floor or a table. Open or remove shirt. Place two or three fingers on the breastbone, just below the nipple line, as described for chest thrusts, page 720. Depress the breastbone (the heart is right underneath) to a depth of *one-half to one inch* (1½ to 2½ centimeters) and at a rate of *at least one hundred per minute* — easy to time by counting "one and two and one and two and . . . ," saying "and" during the release and the number while depressing the sternum in a smooth, nonjerky rhythm.

If you are doing CPR by yourself, give baby a blow of mouth-to-mouth air after every fifth heart compression, being sure to maintain proper head position, and watch for baby's chest rising. Do not lift your fingers off the skin between strokes, except to do mouth-to-mouth breathing.

If two rescuers are working together, one compresses the chest, pausing after every five

VARIATIONS IN CHEST COMPRESSIONS WITH AGE

Newborn: You may find compressing the chest of a newborn easier if you encircle the entire chest with your two hands just below baby's armpits and compress the breastbone with the tips of your two thumbs (see illustration).

For the older child (over one year): Use the *heel* of your hand and compress deeper, one to one and a half inches (2½ to 3½ centimeters), and at a rate of one hundred strokes per minute.

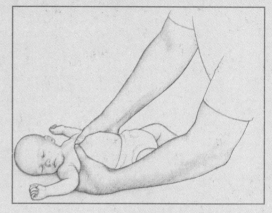

Chest compressions of newborn.

compressions to allow the second rescuer to give mouth-to-mouth breathing (such coordination is usually only practical with trained rescuers; untrained rescuers do not have to precisely coordinate heart compressions and breathing).

Continue checking for a pulse every few minutes until trained help arrives. Stop chest compressions when you feel a pulse, but continue mouth-to-mouth ventilation until baby is breathing on his own.

In review, the ABCs* of CPR are:

- **A — airway:** Position baby's head and remove obstructions to clear the airway.

The procedures for choking and CPR are those recommended by the American Academy of Pediatrics as of 2000. New research may periodically alter these recommendations so that refresher courses are necessary to learn possibly updated techniques. (See www.AskDrSears.com for updates.)

- **B — breathing:** Do mouth-to-mouth or mouth-to-nose-and-mouth breathing with baby's head properly positioned and at a rate of one breath every three seconds.

- **C — circulation:** If you do not feel a pulse or heartbeat, do chest compression at one hundred strokes per minute.

- **D — dial 911:** Call for help whenever it's practical, within a minute or two of starting CPR. (In children over eight years, dial 911 before starting CPR.)

BLEEDING

Be prepared for baby's first bleed. While most are tiny trickles needing only a sympathetic Band-Aid, knowing how to recognize and stop a hemorrhage could save your child's life.

Big Bleeds

Apply pressure. Using gauze or a clean handkerchief, use pressure over the site of bleeding for two minutes. Then, if possible, hold the bleeding site underneath cold running tap water and assess the severity of the cut. Highly vascular areas, such as the scalp, bleed profusely from only a tiny puncture wound (which heals easily with the application of pressure, a dab of antibiotic ointment, and tincture of time). The amount of bleeding depends on what type of vessel is cut. If a small vein is cut, the bleeding may only trickle and stop after two or three minutes of pressure and/or holding under cold water. If an artery has been cut, the blood will spurt; *this requires at least ten minutes of constant pressure to stop the bleeding.* If you peek, start the timer over. Then apply a pressure bandage for at least twenty more minutes, after which survey the site and seek medical attention.

Make a pressure bandage. If there is more than a cut-vein trickle, keep the pressure on for ten minutes. Instead of removing the blood-soaked pressure gauze (removing it may dislodge the clot and reopen the bleeding), apply a second fluff of gauze on top of the first. Without interrupting the pressure on the bleeding site, wrap tape around the bandage to keep pressure on the bleeding.

Calm your child. An upset child pumps more blood to the site. Be calm; take charge.

Position baby correctly. Place your child lying down and elevate the bleeding site above the level of the heart — for example, by raising the arm.

Get help. Call your doctor for further advice or take your child to the emergency room, especially if you can't stop the bleeding.

Little Bleeds

While there is no such thing as a little bleed to a child, most little people get little bleeds that can be managed easily at home.

Keep cool. Toddlers get upset at the sight of blood and the very thought of a leak in their body. If you mirror panic, you are likely to have a bloodier mess to handle.

Wash the cut. Hold the bleeding site (for example, the arm) under cold running water for a few minutes while giving reassuring "It *will be* OK" (not "It *is* OK") messages to baby. (Note: Fresh blood washes off skin and hair better with cold water than with warm.) And don't forget the adhesive bandage. Even if the bleeding has stopped, this timely patch reassures the child that his leak is fixed.

Daily care. An initial and daily cleansing under running water removes debris, germs, and dead tissue, all of which increase the chances of infection. Pat dry with clean gauze. Depending on the location and type of cut, your doctor may advise gently cleaning off the accumulating crust with half strength (half water) *hydrogen peroxide* applied twice a day with a cotton-tipped applicator. Cover with antibiotic ointment, and dress the cut according to your doctor's instructions.

Facts About Stitches

Does the cut need stitches? Stitches speed healing and minimize infection and scarring. If the wound is gaping or you can see beneath a layer of skin, it needs suturing.

As stated earlier, cuts on the scalp bleed profusely, but after the bleeding stops, you may be surprised how tiny the cut is. The same generous blood vessels that caused the initial panic also heal the wound quickly, and scalp wounds rarely become infected. These considerations and the lack of cosmetic concern make a tiny scalp cut likely to self-heal without stitches.

APPLYING STERI-STRIPS

The materials you will need are one-fourth-inch (six-millimeter) steri-strips, a cotton-tipped applicator, tincture of benzoin, and scissors.

1. Clean and dry the wound according to earlier instructions.

2. Cut steri-strips in approximately one-half- to one-inch (twelve- to twenty-five-millimeter) lengths.

3. With a cotton-tipped applicator, apply benzoin adhesive sparingly along the side of the wound, but not touching the wound, as it stings.

4. Push the edges of the wound together. If three strips are needed, apply the first across the center to hold the edges together, then another one on either side. A smaller cut will need only two strips.

WOUND GLUE VS. STITCHES

Wound glue (Dermabond) has often been a kid's best friend in the emergency room, allowing many wounds to be closed quickly and painlessly. If the wound is not too deep or ragged, the potential for scarring is no different whether you use glue or stitches.

Another profuse bleeder but self-healer is the very vascular band of tissue connecting the upper gum to the lip, called the frenum. It commonly gets cut and bleeds following a fall on the face. The frenum rarely needs stitches and heals easily following the application of pressure with gauze soaked in cold water or while baby is sucking on a popsicle.

Some tiny cuts less than a half-inch (1½ centimeters) long and not gaping can be closed with steri-strips (improved butterfly bandages — see box "Applying Steri-strips"). If you are uncertain whether or not your baby needs stitches, have your doctor or your local emergency room doctor check the cut.

The parent surgeon. If your baby needs stitches, *be sure you stay with your baby* for reassurance while your doctor performs the suturing. Tell baby exactly what to expect. Don't say it won't hurt if it will. That misstatement causes mistrust.

How to minimize scarring. Most scars occur from the way the wound is cared for rather than from how it is sutured. Try these cosmetic tips:

- Follow your doctor's instructions on wound care and the earlier suggestions for keeping cuts clean. Infections in the wound are the most common cause of scarring.

- Keep baby's appointment for suture removal. Sutures that stay in too long increase the chance for infection.

- Massage the wound after a few days. Use a moisturizing lotion containing aloe or vitamin E oil and rub it into the skin. This healing touch increases the flow of blood to the wound.

- Keep the wound out of the sun, especially a facial wound. During the first six months of healing, avoid exposure of the wound to direct sunlight. The scar may tan a much darker color than the surrounding skin, making the scar line more obvious. Use an SPF (sun protection factor) 15 or greater sunblock or a large-brimmed cap to cover or shade the wound.

HEAD INJURIES

There is no sound that sends shivers up and down your spine like the thud of a child's head meeting a hard floor. Goose eggs and scalp bleeds lead the list of doctor's phone calls about injuries. It helps to appreciate the difference between a skull injury and a brain injury. The skull acts as a protective helmet for the delicate brain, and the skull is covered with a richly vascularized scalp. The great majority of falls involve injury to the scalp only, which bleeds profusely if cut or forms a large swelling (goose egg) from broken blood vessels beneath the skin. Don't be alarmed by how quickly these large bumps appear. They go down quickly with ice packs and pressure. These bumps and bleeds are usually limited to a scalp injury and seldom indicate that the underlying brain has been injured.

The main concern after any blow to baby's head is injury to the underlying brain, which can occur in two forms: *bleeding* and *concussion.* When small blood vessels have been broken between the skull and the brain or within the brain, bleeding occurs within this space and compresses the brain. A blow to the head may also cause a concussion, meaning the brain has been "shaken up" by the fall. Pressure on the brain from bleeding or from the swelling associated with the concussion produces the outward signs of a brain injury.

▶**SPECIAL NOTE:** *Take puncture wounds to the scalp seriously. Externally these may look insignificant. But a nail, for example, may penetrate the scalp and skull and lead to a serious infection in the underlying brain. Notify your doctor.*

What to Look For — When to Worry

If baby is unconscious, but breathing and pink (no blue lips), lay her on a flat surface and call emergency medical services. If you have cause to suspect a neck injury, don't move baby but let the experts trained in neck injuries transport her. If she is not breathing, apply CPR (see technique on page 723), or if she's having a convulsion, keep her airway clear (see instructions on handling convulsions, page 731).

Sometimes, if baby is the sensitive type and prone to temper tantrums, the anger after the fall pushes baby into a breathholding spell, which may be mistaken for a convulsion. This scene naturally pushes panic buttons and gets baby rushed to the hospital. Even if this turns out to be unnecessary, it is better to be safe. I tell my patients that when in doubt, take baby and sit in the waiting area of the local hospital emergency room.

A Period of Observation

If baby is alert and conscious, walking, talking, playing, and acting just like before the fall, administer a dose of parental sympathy, apply an ice pack to the cut or bump for twenty minutes, and begin a period of observation before calling your doctor. The reason for the period of observation is that the doctor often relies more on how baby behaves *after* the injury than what happened at the time of the injury. If the brain has been injured, signs may show immediately, or they may appear slowly during the next twenty-four hours.

After the period of observation, depending on your baby's condition, you may or may not wish to call the doctor. Besides any when-to-call-the-doctor list there is an overriding inner voice treasured by mothers, which I call mother's worry signals. I have learned to

trust this monitoring system as much as the most sophisticated electronics. If it tells you something's not quite right, call your doctor to report baby's condition, seek advice, and above all tell the doctor why you are concerned. Here's what to look for over the next twenty-four hours.

Changes in Baby's Sleep Behavior

Babies normally retreat into sleep after trauma, which makes the usual admonition to "watch for a change in consciousness" an anxiety-producing instruction for the parent. If a head injury occurs near night or nap time in an already tired child, you may be confused about whether the drowsiness is due to the injury or whether it's just time for sleep to naturally overtake the child. And it may be impossible to follow the advice "Don't let baby go to sleep." Let baby fall asleep, but awaken yourself every two hours and do a baby check. Look for

- change in color from pink to pale or, even more alarming, blue
- change in breathing: periods of very shallow breathing, ten- to twenty-second periods of stop-breathing episodes

---

SIGNS OF BRAIN INJURY

If your baby shows any of the following signs after a head injury, call your doctor or take her to the hospital.

- disorientation, difficulty arousing
- unusual breathing while sleeping
- crossed eyes, unequal pupils
- persistent vomiting
- increasing paleness

- oozing of blood or watery fluid from an ear canal
- convulsions
- off balance while sitting, crawling, or walking

followed by irregular breathing, or gasping episodes (remember that newborns normally have irregular breathing)
• twitches on one side of the body involving a whole limb

If baby's color and breathing patterns are normal (no change from usual) and your parental instincts sense nothing wrong, there is no need to awaken baby unless advised to do so by your doctor. The deep sleep from a head injury is nearly always associated with shallow, irregular breathing patterns that you are unlikely to have seen before.

If, however, you are uncertain or baby's appearance sets off a "not normal" alarm, do a partial arousal. Sit or stand baby up and then put her back down. Normally a baby will fuss a bit and thrash around in the bed to resettle. If baby does not act like this, try to fully arouse her by sitting or standing her up, opening her eyes, and calling her name. If baby awakens, looks at you, fusses or smiles, and struggles to be left undisturbed, you can go back to sleep without worrying. If, on the other hand, baby does not protest, can't be awakened enough to begin fussing, is pale, shows irregular breathing, and is drooling profusely, or shows any of the signs of brain injury listed above, seek medical attention immediately.

Changes in Balance and Coordination

During the day signs of head injury are easier to observe. Watch baby's normal play. Is he doing everything the same after the fall: sitting straight, walking well, moving arms and legs normally? Or is he off balance, wobbly, dragging a leg, or becoming increasingly disoriented? In the prewalker, do you notice any change in sitting or crawling skills or in manipulative hand skills?

Vomiting

Just as some babies fall asleep after a head injury, some babies vomit, mostly from being upset at falling and hurting. Don't worry. But *persistent* vomiting over the next six to twenty-four hours is an alarming sign. Call your doctor right away. As a precaution feed the recovering faller clear liquids for a few hours. Breastfeeding is therapeutic.

Eye Signs

The eyes mirror what's going on inside the body, especially inside the brain. In fact, the back of the eye is so intimately connected with the brain that your doctor looks at the backs of the eyes for evidence of brain swelling while examining a baby following a head injury. Baby eye signs are more difficult to assess than the other signs, but here are the call-doctor cues: crossed eyes or rolling eyes, one pupil larger than the other, and behavior such as tripping or running into things that indicates baby's vision is diminished. In the older child, add complaints of seeing double and blurred vision to the worry list.

What About Skull X Rays?

Except for severe head injuries or obvious fractures, skull X rays are seldom helpful; nor is it necessary to rush a happily playing baby to the hospital for an X ray. First, try a period of observation; next, call your doctor; then comes the advice on whether or not to take baby to the hospital for X rays. A CAT scan, a series of cross-sectional X rays of the brain, has nearly replaced the plain skull X ray. In most cases if baby warrants an X ray at all, he merits a CAT scan. This technological break-

IN PRAISE OF THE SIMPLE ICE PACK

Injured babies don't take kindly to cold objects pressed against sore tissues. Cold relieves pain, lessens bleeding, and reduces swelling. But *no bare ice to bare skin, please.* This could produce frostbite damage to the tissues. You can buy instant cold packs that don't drip and place them in your medicine cabinet, or you can make your own: Put ice cubes in a sock or handkerchief. If you use a plastic bag, cover it with a thin cloth or damp washcloth. Crushed ice in a sock makes a moldable pack. You can store an ice cube in a terrycloth toy. In our freezer we have a "boo-boo bunny" on standby who has become a trusted friend for bumps and bruises and to soothe the psyche when the only damage is to baby's fragile sensitivity. Bags of frozen chopped veggies also make a handy ice pack, and sucking on a popsicle or juice bar helps swollen lips. Begin gently increasing the pressure as tolerated for as long as twenty minutes. Letting your toddler keep his hand on the ice pack helps acceptance.

through reveals much more about an injury, such as whether there is bleeding or swelling of the brain, than a simple skull X ray. On a softer note: In the life of a child, considering the many times little heads meet hard floors, injuries to the brain are uncommon.

CONVULSIONS

Convulsions (also called seizures) are caused by abnormal discharge of electrical currents in the brain, and they shake up both babies and parents. Their severity ranges from localized muscle jerks to total body shaking, called a *grand mal seizure,* which may also include falling and writhing on the ground, rolling back the eyes, frothing at the mouth, biting the tongue, and temporarily losing consciousness.

Your primary emergency goal during a convulsion is to ensure that baby's tongue or secretions do not block his airway, depriving the brain of oxygen. Most convulsions in infancy are due to fevers. These seizures are brief, self-limiting, and rarely harm baby, but may leave parents trembling. If you witness a convulsion, do the following:

- Place baby safely on the floor, facedown or on his side to allow the tongue to come forward and secretions to drain from the throat by gravity.

- Don't put any food or drink into baby's mouth during or immediately after the convulsion; nor should you try to restrain baby from shaking.

- If baby's lips are not blue and baby is breathing normally, don't worry.

- Though unlikely, if baby's lips are turning blue or he is not breathing, give mouth-to-mouth breathing after you have cleared the airway (see page 723).

- To prevent the thrashing child from bumping into furniture, clear the immediate area.

Following a convulsion, babies normally retreat into a deep sleep. Also, it's common for baby to have another convulsion within a few minutes of the first, especially if the seizure was due to fever. To prevent this recurrence, if baby feels hot immediately after the seizure, give an acetaminophen suppository (oral medications may trigger vomiting). Remove baby's clothing, and cool baby by sponge bathing with a cool towel (see discussion of fever control, page 655).

In general, it's wise to call your doctor or take baby to a hospital emergency room immediately after the convulsion. Or, depending on the circumstances, you could begin a period of observation similar to the one described earlier for a head injury. A period of observation may be appropriate if baby was previously well and the fever came on suddenly, followed by a brief convulsion, and now baby seems all right. Keep the fever controlled, and you may safely sit tight for a few hours rather than calling your doctor or rushing to the hospital at 3:00 A.M. But any convulsion not associated with a fever or occurring in a sick-appearing baby deserves immediate medical attention. It is wise to apply fever-control measures (medication and cooling) before rushing off to the hospital, since the escalating fever can bring on more seizures en route. (See also "Fever Fits," page 662.)

BURNS

Put a nine-month-old with a lightning-fast reach close to a hot cup of coffee and you have the makings of a severe burn. The degree or depth of a burn determines how painful and deforming it is. First-degree burns (such as sunburns) cause redness of the skin, are not severely painful, and need only cool water, a soothing ointment, and time. Second-degree burns cause blistering, swelling, and peeling and are very painful. Third-degree burns damage the deeper layers of the skin and are the most disfiguring.

Basic Burn Treatment

If baby gets burned, do the following:

- Immediately submerge the burned area in *cool water for at least twenty minutes.* Besides relieving pain, water cools the skin and lessens skin damage. *Do not use ice,* which increases tissue damage. If the burn is to the face, apply a cool, water-soaked towel or hold the cheek under running water. Do not put butter, grease, or powder on a burn.

- If baby's clothing is on fire, smother the flames with a towel, blanket, coat, or your own clothing.

- Quickly remove any burned or hot-water-soaked clothing, but be careful not to touch the face when pulling a hot shirt over baby's head. Cut clothes off if necessary.

- Assess the severity of the burn. If only red but not blistery, keep the area in cool water for as long as baby tolerates it. Leave the burn uncovered and observe it for change.

- If the skin becomes blistered, white, or charred, apply an antiseptic ointment and cover loosely with a clean cloth or a nonstick bandage. Call your doctor or take baby to the emergency room.

- Besides soaking the burned area in cool water, give baby acetaminophen.

Burn treatment is aimed at relieving pain and preventing infection, disfiguring, and contractures (shortening of the burned tissue while healing). Along with your doctor's advice, most home treatment of burns involves the following daily ritual.

Wash. Cleanse the burned area under lukewarm running tap water, and blot it dry with a clean towel. The water jet removes germs and dead tissue.

Apply burn cream. Keep the burned area covered with a prescription cream (a combination of silver and sulfa antibiotic) that promotes healing and prevents infection.

Cover. Your doctor will instruct you whether (and how) to keep the area covered with cream only, or you will be told to cover the burn with a nonstick pad and wrap it with gauze.

Stretch. If the burn is across an area that bends, such as the palms of the hands or joints of the fingers, stretch the area for a minute at least ten times daily to prevent contractures.

Debride. To minimize infection, your doctor may need to cut away the burned tissue several times during the course of healing (a process called debridement) or instruct you how to do this minor surgical procedure, which is as easy as trimming fingernails. *Do not break blisters,* nature's dressing, unless your doctor so advises.

With meticulous care, burned baby skin heals beautifully, without scarring unless the skin was deeply or extensively damaged.

Electrical Burns

Not only can electrical burns damage tissue even more than scalds, but the electrical current may set off abnormal heartbeats. Handling downed power lines is an extremely dangerous accident and requires immediate medical attention, even CPR. Poking an exploring finger into a light socket usually gives baby only a scary zap.

Chemical Burns (Lyes and Acids)

Immerse the burned area under cool running water for twenty minutes. Remove baby's chemical-soaked clothing, being careful not to spread the irritant to other areas of the skin. Use a scissors to cut the clothes off baby if necessary, or leave the clothing on if you can't remove it safely. For example, do not pull a bleach-soaked T shirt over a child's head. Wash the area with soap and water, but do not vigorously scrub the area, since intense scrubbing may cause more of the poison to be absorbed into the skin. If any of the substance was inhaled or swallowed, call poison control immediately and give baby the antidote recommended on the chemical's container, or give your child large amounts of water to drink. If the chemical splashed into baby's eyes, flush the eyes for twenty minutes using a steady stream of water from a pitcher, or use a bottle of eyewash from your pharmacy. (see discussion of eye injuries, page 736).

Treating Sunburn

If the skin is only slightly red and baby is not uncomfortable, no treatment is necessary. In more serious cases, try the following:

- If the skin is very red and baby is crying, immerse the burned area in cool water, or use cool water and towel compresses for fifteen minutes at least four times a day. Leave some water on the skin to cool by evaporation.

- Apply a nonpetroleum-based moisturizer lotion (aloe, for example) several times a day.

- If the skin is blistered, call your doctor for a prescription cream; consider it a second-degree burn and follow earlier suggestions for burn treatment.

- Give ibuprofen for pain and to reduce inflammation.

POISONING

The dreadful-sounding term "poisoning" refers to swallowing, inhaling, or touching any substance that harms the body. While many poisons cause no more than a brief stomach upset, some can severely damage lung and intestinal tissues; a few are fatal. (To prevent poisoning, see the home baby-proofing suggestions on pages 594–600 and the information on toxic plants and house-hold substances on 611–615.)

What to Do

If your child swallows a poison, call your local poison control center. You should have the phone number readily available. If not, call 911 or your local hospital. Give the center the following information:

- name of the substance ingested and the list of ingredients
- time and suspected amount of ingestion
- age and weight of baby
- symptoms: coughing, vomiting, behavior changes, and so on
- your telephone number

When and How to Induce Vomiting

If advised by the poison control center to induce vomiting, do the following:

- Give baby 1 tablespoon (3 teaspoons/15 milliliters) of *syrup of ipecac,* followed by 8 ounces (240 milliliters) of water or non-carbonated fruit juice. Have a large catch basin nearby or take baby outside or into the bathroom.

- To stimulate the ipecac to slosh around in the stomach, jostle or bounce baby on your knees for a few minutes.

- If vomiting does not occur within twenty minutes, repeat the dose of ipecac.

- When baby does begin to vomit, place him facedown, with his head lower than his body. Catch the vomit in the basin so the poison can be inspected.

- Observe your child for an hour or two after vomiting for any signs of poisoning.

SUN PROTECTION FOR YOUR BABY

Thin baby skin and summer sun don't mix. Besides causing sunburn, excessive sun exposure during the childhood years increases the risk of adult skin cancer. Here are ways to protect your baby from sunburn:

- Sun rays are most intense from 10:00 A.M. to 3:00 P.M. If possible, plan beach outings late in the afternoon.

- Use sun-protective clothing, such as a long-sleeved shirt and wide-brimmed hat made from sun-proof fabrics. Sun-protective clothes typically offer an SPF (sun protection factor) of at least 30 wet or dry, whereas an old hand-me-down T-shirt provides only an SPF of 6, and even less if wet.

- Place baby under a sun umbrella at the beach.

- Beware of sun rays *reflecting* off white sand. Turn baby away from this reflection.

Selecting a Sunscreen

Use a lotion or milky gel-type sunscreen rather than the clear alcohol type, which may burn baby's skin on application. Select one that offers both UVA and UVB protection (check the label), with an SPF of 15 or more. For water play, use a waterproof sunscreen and generously reapply the lotion after several dunkings. For particularly sensitive areas, such as the nose, cheeks, and ears, use an opaque zinc oxide sun block.

Some babies are sensitive to PABA, the active ingredient in many sunscreens, so use a PABA-free preparation. To determine if your baby's skin is sensitive to a sunscreen, rub a test dose on a small area of baby's arm before using it all over the body.

Because of the uncertain absorption of sunscreen through the skin of tiny babies, its use in babies under six months should be only a last resort. Use it very sparingly, only on small areas, such as the face and back of the hands. Shade and protective clothing is best for baby.

Shading Little Eyes

Baby specs may be fashionable, but are they safe? Infant eyes are more sensitive to the harmful effects of ultraviolet (UV) light than are older eyes. Little eyes need to be protected. Eye specialists believe that toy sunglasses may be worse than none at all. They simply darken the area, making baby's pupils larger and allowing more damaging light to reach the inside of the eye. Best are sunglasses labeled "100 percent UV filtration," but expect to pay a higher price for this protection, and rare is the toddler who keeps the glasses on. For infants the most practical sunshade is a wide-brimmed hat and a pair of watchful adult eyes keeping baby shaded from bright reflected light off sand, snow, or white surfaces.

Do not induce vomiting before consulting your poison control center. For some substances it may not be necessary to induce vomiting, and others may damage the lungs if aspirated and further damage the lining of the esophagus if vomited. Unless advised otherwise by your poison control center, do not induce vomiting when any of the following are ingested:

- petroleum products: gasoline, kerosene, benzine, turpentine
- polishes for furniture or cars
- strong corrosives such as lye, strong acids, drain cleaners
- cleaning products such as bleach, ammonia, toilet bowl cleaners

While it is not always necessary to induce vomiting, nearly all medicines and poisonous plants are safely vomited. For poisons for which it is dangerous to induce vomiting, your poison control center will advise you what antidotes to give. Usually it is several glasses of water or a glass of milk.

Inhaled Poisons

Nail polish, polish removers, glues, lacquers for models, varnishes, and acetone-containing hydrocarbons may be toxic to the lungs, kidneys, and brain of a developing child. To protect yourself and baby, use these substances in a well-ventilated room and definitely not in the same room with baby. If baby has inhaled toxic fumes, rush him into fresh air and observe him for severe coughing or lethargy and seek medical attention.

CALLING POISON CONTROL

A nationwide poison control phone number will connect you to the center nearest you. It is (800) 222–1222.

EYE INJURIES

Eyes are exquisitely sensitive to irritation but are quick to heal. Babies protest intrusion of their eyes by tightly squinting and rubbing, further irritating the eye. To keep dirty fingers out of hurting eyes, secure baby in a burrito wrap using a large towel, blanket, or sheet (see page 92) before trying to examine or flush out baby's eyes.

Flushing Out Little Eyes

To wash irritants from baby's eyes, it is best to have two persons, a holder and a flusher. Gently pull down the lower lid, encouraging baby to open the eyes very wide as you irrigate them with a gentle, steady stream of lukewarm water from a pitcher. Turn baby's head toward the side of the affected eye to allow the water to run across the eye and onto a towel. Continue flushing for at least fifteen minutes. If baby clamps the eyelids shut, pull down on the lower lid with your fingertip or put your index finger on the upper lid just beneath the eyebrow and another finger on the lower lid and gently pry the lids open.

Following flushing, call for medical advice. Some corrosives may irritate the cornea and promote infection. Preventive antibiotic ointment may be needed. Pain from a scratch or irritant may last for twenty-four hours. Give acetaminophen and whatever eye care your doctor advises.

Administering Eye Medicine

Eye medicines come in two forms — ointment and drops. Drops are easier to give but can sting a bit if the eyes are inflamed. Ointment requires more control and less squirming because you have to get close to the eye.

Holding baby still requires two people (or one person can "mummy" the baby in the burrito wrap) to keep baby's hands from getting in the way. If an extra pair of hands is available, have that person hold baby's head while you hold baby's body quiet enough not to have a moving target — this gets harder as baby gets older. Newborns are easy enough to handle solo. Put baby on a soft surface — couch, bed, carpet — where you can bend over her.

Hold the medicine in your dominant hand and pull down the lower eyelid to make it form a pouch into which you deliver the drops or line of ointment.

NOSE INJURIES

Be prepared for a hard fall and a flattened nose several times during the life of a growing child. Fortunately, most often both the child and the nose bounce back without deformity. The nose is beautifully designed to act as a shock absorber so that blows to the face do not injure the head. When the nose collides with a hard surface, the nose flattens as the thin nasal bones are pushed out to each side. If your baby gets a flattened nose, go through the following steps:

- Drape an ice pack over your baby's nose, gently pressing on the bulged-out swollen area on each side of the nose just below the nasal corner of the eyes. Keep the ice pack on at least twenty minutes or as long as baby tolerates it. The sooner you apply the ice pack and the longer you leave it on

after the injury, the less the swelling will be.

- Position baby upright and leaning forward to reduce blood dripping down the back of the throat.

When to Seek Medical Attention

Most flattened noses are indeed fractured, but the great majority reset themselves very easily within a couple of weeks after the injury and don't leave any cosmetic or functional impairments. There are two reasons to seek medical attention for a fractured nose: *cosmetic,* if the nose has been pushed to one side and remains crooked, and *functional,* if airflow is impaired. Observe the nose for angulation to one side or the other. With a fingertip, gently press the side of each nostril closed to see if baby can breathe normally through each nostril with his mouth closed. In a small baby you may have to try this procedure while baby is asleep. If either cosmetic or functional impairment is obvious, seek immediate medical attention. Most of the time the examining doctor will advise waiting a week or two to see if the nasal bones bounce back into a normal position. The doctor will then recheck baby's nose to see if any cosmetic or functional impairment persists and recommend treatment accordingly. Infant nasal fractures rarely need setting.

Nosebleeds

"Which finger do you use to pick your nose?" is the telling question I ask young nose pickers. (Asking, "Do you pick your nose?" is guaranteed to elicit a "no.") Bleeds from nose picking are most common during the allergy season due to the child's scratching the already inflamed nasal membranes. Central heating dries the air and irritates the lining of the nose, accounting for winter nosebleeds. A vaporizer used in baby's bedroom during the months of central heating should alleviate this cause of nosebleeds. If baby's nasal secretions get crusty during a cold, you will soon see a little fingertip inside a little nose followed by a little nosebleed. A squirt of saline nose drops and perhaps a dab of antibiotic ointment or Vaseline will loosen the crust and often prevent a nosebleed.

Here's how to stop a nosebleed:

• Sit baby on your lap, with him leaning slightly forward.

• Apply pressure by pinching the nostrils together for at least ten minutes without releasing. Most nosebleeds originate in the blood vessels lining the cartilage of the nose, called the nasal septum. For best results, apply pressure on these vessels by inserting a twisted piece of wet cotton into the bleeding nostril so that it fits snugly to fill around two-thirds of the nasal opening. Applying pinched-nostril pressure with the cotton in place transmits the pressure to the nasal septum.

• If this doesn't stop the bleeding, apply pressure to the major vessel supplying the nose, located where the upper lip joins the gum, just below the nostrils. Place a chunk of wet cotton underneath the upper lip and apply pressure with two fingers upward under the lip in the direction of the nostrils or by pressing a finger over the upper lip just below the nostrils.

• Keep your child upright to prevent blood from dripping down his throat, which may trigger vomiting or sneezing. This could dislodge the clot and cause the bleeding to resume.

• Encourage baby to keep his mouth open by holding your own mouth open, so that a sneeze or cough is not transmitted to the nose.

• Once the bleeding stops, leave the cotton in the nostril for a few hours to tamponade the bleeding, allowing a clot to form. Remove the cotton plug gently (moisten with a squirt of water if crusty), trying not to dislodge the clot and restart the bleeding. In an adult or an older child the cotton may be left in longer, as there is less of a fear of choking on the cotton.

• If these measures do not stop the nosebleed, take your child to your doctor or to the emergency room.

• To discourage the nose picker, cut baby's fingernails short, increase the humidity in his bedroom, and treat inhalant allergies.

Stuff Stuck in the Nose

Babies are pokers, and the nose is an easy place to poke. Over the years I have removed all sorts of objects from babies' noses. The most popular are beans, peas, pieces of cotton, and tiny rocks. Surprisingly, babies seldom complain of a foreign body in their nose, but suspect this if you detect a foul-smelling yellow or green discharge from *one* nostril (with a cold *both* nostrils drain and the discharge doesn't stink). To remove a foreign object from your baby's nose, try the following:

- If you can see the object, attempt to remove it with blunt-end tweezers. (The burrito wrap described on page 92 may be necessary to restrain baby's protesting arms.)

- If the object is lodged far back in the nose, compress the unblocked nostril and encourage the child to sneeze with his mouth closed. This may dislodge the obstruction.

- If the object is water soluble, such as a piece of candy, take the child into the shower and let the steam melt the candy. Or squirt some saline nasal spray into the nose to soften the object and reduce its size.

If you are unable to remove the object easily with the above measures, take your child to your doctor's office or to an emergency room where the doctor can remove the object with a special instrument. Do not allow baby to lie on his back and fall asleep with the object still in his nose, as it may be aspirated into the lungs.

INSECT STINGS AND BITES

Insects leaving their calling card in baby's skin cause two potential problems: an infection at the puncture site or an allergic reaction to the injected venom.

Removing Stingers

A bee leaves its stinger and its attached venom sac in the wound. Scrape away the protruding venom sac with a sharp knife or the edge of a credit card before removing the rest of the stinger. (Squeezing the sac with a tweezers will force more venom into the skin.) After removing the stinger with tweezers, applying ice to the sting site slows down the spread of venom and eases the pain. Wasps and hornets do not leave their stingers in the skin.

Allergic Reactions

Signs of a systemic allergic reaction are swollen hands and eyelids, wheezing, and a hivelike rash. If your baby has only localized swelling around the sting site, apply ice, give a dose of Benadryl, and wait before calling your doctor. If a concern-causing allergic reaction is going to occur, expect it to happen within an hour of the sting. If the above signs of systemic allergy occur, give your child a dose of Benadryl and take him immediately to your doctor's office or to the emergency room. The most concerning allergic sign following a sting is wheezing or difficulty breathing.

Baby's second sting may produce a more severe allergic reaction than the first. If your baby showed any of the above signs from the first bee sting, here is a wise precaution: As soon as your baby is stung, give Benadryl, apply an ice pack, and immediately go and sit in the emergency room. If no allergic signs appear within a couple of hours, then it is safe to return home.

If your child has a history of severe allergies to insect stings, ask your doctor about desensitizing the child to insect stings with a series of shots. If you are traveling and your baby has had severe reactions to stings, take along a prescription insect-sting kit that contains Adrenalin and directions on how to administer it.

Removing Ticks

Because ticks carry disease, notably the germ that causes Lyme disease (see page 712), they should be carefully and entirely removed. Here's how to remove a tick:

- Clean the area with an alcohol-soaked cotton ball.

- Using a blunt tweezers, grasp the tick as near to its mouth parts and as close to your skin as you can. Steadily pull the tick up and out, but do not squeeze or twist the tick.

- Do not attempt to pull the tick off with your fingers, as the head may break off from the body and become embedded in the skin.

- Do not use heat from a match or lit cigarette to remove the tick, as the heat may cause the tick to embed itself even farther into the skin.

- If the tick is embedded in the skin: (1) With your thumb and forefinger pinch up the fold of skin with the embedded tick head, then (2) using a scalpel or a sterilized single razor blade, carefully scrape the skin containing the head and mouth of the tick, or use a sterilized needle to break the skin and remove the head and mouth. If you are tick squeamish, ask your doctor to perform this tick extraction.

- Cleanse the bitten area thoroughly with an antiseptic.

PREVENTING DISEASES CARRIED BY TICKS

Ticks may transmit germs that cause Lyme disease or Rocky Mountain spotted fever. If you find a tick on yourself or your child, carefully remove it. There is no need to have the tick tested, or to start preventive antibiotics. The risk of disease is very small (only 3 percent even in high-risk areas), and tick-borne diseases are easily treated if recognized early. If any of these signs occur, contact your physician:

- fever within two weeks of tick bite
- rash, either at the bite site or on other areas of the body, within five weeks of the tick bite
- joint or muscle pain or fatigue
- muscle weakness in a specific area above the neck, such as a crooked smile or tongue or weakness when opening or closing one eye
- double vision

TOOTH TRAUMA

Beginning walkers and tripping toddlers often encounter table corners with their two front teeth. Most of the time these pushed-back teeth spring back and continue to survive a few more falls until surrendering their place to permanent teeth five years later. If your baby injures the gums and teeth, apply ice packs or offer a popsicle to suck on to ease the swollen gums. If the gums are bleeding, put cold water on a piece of gauze and push it between the lips and gums and hold pressure on the bleeding site. Call your dentist in case immediate realignment is necessary. If teeth have been pushed far up into the gums, the roots may be injured, and the remaining life of the tooth will be shortened (recognized by increasing darkening and loosening of the tooth). Again, consult your dentist.

Also, watch for an abscess (fever and swollen, tender gums above the injured tooth) developing at the injury site three to seven days later. If the tooth has been loosened so much that it is just hanging on for dear life and obviously won't survive, your dentist may wish to remove it immediately for fear of baby's aspirating the dislodged tooth during sleep. A knocked-out baby tooth cannot be reimplanted. If a baby tooth has been fractured leaving sharp, pointed edges, sometimes dentists recommend filing the points smooth to prevent a cut to the lip during the next fall. A permanent tooth, on the other hand, can often be reimplanted, but care of the tooth en route to the dentist is crucial. Pick up the tooth by the crown, not the root. If the tooth is very dirty, wash it off gently with water (not over an open drain), immerse the tooth in the child's saliva, and put it in a safe container for the dentist. Do not scrub the roots of the knocked-out tooth, as this may injure the roots and preclude reimplantation.

STRAINS, SPRAINS, AND FRACTURES

The four classic signs of broken bones at any age are swelling, pain, limitation of motion, and point tenderness (the site of the fracture is tender to a fingertip's touch).

First aid for common strains, sprains, and fractures can be remembered by "ICES": ice, compression, elevation, and support. All four of these measures slow down continued bleeding within the joint or muscle and shorten the recovery time. Apply an ice pack to the swollen or fractured area for at least twenty minutes. Snugly (but not constrictingly) wrap the ice pack with an elastic bandage around the affected joint or possible fracture site. Elevate the limb about six inches on a pillow or support the limb with a sling and prevent any unnecessary motion or weight bearing. If you suspect a broken bone, immobilize the limb and take your child to the emergency room.

Toddler Fractures

Mild fractures to the midshaft of the long bone of the legs occur during the frequent falls of the beginning walker. Suspect toddler fractures if your baby limps and is unwilling to bear weight on one leg. Toddlers often limp for a few hours after a fall or even from a sore on their foot or a stubbed toe. Any limp in a toddler that lasts longer than twenty-four hours merits medical attention to be sure there is not a toddler fracture or an injury to the hip joint.

Pulled Elbow

During play, or as a result of the typical tug-of-war between exploring toddler and a parent trying to keep him in tow, an arm bone may pop out of the elbow socket. Your doctor or local emergency room can usually pop a pulled elbow back into place with no particular harm done.

Appendix: Growth Charts

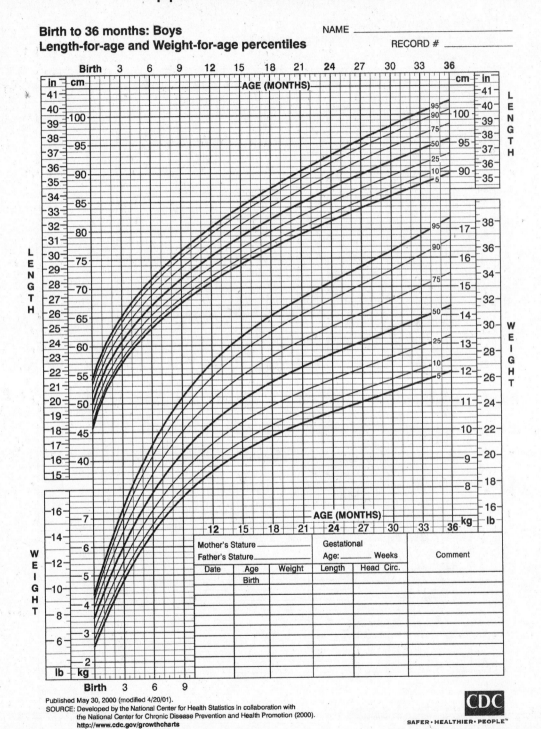

Birth to 36 months: Boys
Length-for-age and Weight-for-age percentiles

NAME _____

RECORD # _____

AGE (MONTHS)

Birth 3 6 9 12 15 18 21 24 27 30 33 36

LENGTH

WEIGHT

Mother's Stature _____
Father's Stature _____

Gestational
Age: _____ Weeks

Comment

Date	Age	Weight	Length	Head Circ.
Birth				

Published May 30, 2000 (modified 4/20/01).
SOURCE: Developed by the National Center for Health Statistics in collaboration with
the National Center for Chronic Disease Prevention and Health Promotion (2000).
http://www.cdc.gov/growthcharts

CDC
SAFER · HEALTHIER · PEOPLE™

Birth to 36 months: Girls
Length-for-age and Weight-for-age percentiles

NAME _____

RECORD # _____

AGE (MONTHS)

Birth 3 6 9 12 15 18 21 24 27 30 33 36

LENGTH

LENGTH

in — cm

WEIGHT

WEIGHT

Percentile lines: 95, 90, 75, 50, 25, 10, 5

AGE (MONTHS)

12 15 18 21 24 27 30 33 36 kg lb

Mother's Stature _____		Gestational		
Father's Stature _____		Age: _____ Weeks		Comment
Date	Age	Weight	Length	Head Circ.	
	Birth				

Birth 3 6 9

Published May 30, 2000 (modified 4/20/01).
SOURCE: Developed by the National Center for Health Statistics in collaboration with
the National Center for Chronic Disease Prevention and Health Promotion (2000).
http://www.cdc.gov/growthcharts

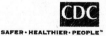

CDC

SAFER · HEALTHIER · PEOPLE™

Resources

www.AskDrSears.com

Our comprehensive website has a large volume of information on parenting and child health issues, in addition to *Baby Book* updates, answers to FAQs, valuable insights on pregnancy questions, infant and child-care issues, and nutritional tips.

Adoption Resources

Dear Birthmother, Thank You for Our Baby, by Kathleen Silber and Phyllis Speedlin, 3rd ed. (Corona, 1998)

Twenty Things Adopted Kids Wish Their Adoptive Parents Knew, by Sherrie Eldridge, (Dell, 1999)
www.adopting.com
www.adoption.com
www.adoption.org
International Adoptions:
www.cdc.gov/travel/other/adoption.htm

Attachment Parenting

The Attachment Parenting Book, by William Sears and Martha Sears (Little, Brown, 2002)

Attachment Parenting International (API), (615) 298-4344; www.attachmentparenting .org. A network of like-minded parents, API gives assistance to those forming attachment-parenting support groups and also provides educational materials, research information,

and consulting to promote attachment-parenting concepts.

Baby Carriers

The Original Babysling: (800) 421-0526; www.AskDrSears.com or www.nojo.com

Crown Crafts Infant Products: (310) 763-8100; www.crowncraftsinfantproducts.com www.AskDrSears.com. Visit our store.

Bedside Co-Sleepers

Arm's Reach Co-Sleeper: (800) 954-9353 or (818) 879-9353; www.armsreach.com

Breastfeeding

The Breastfeeding Book, by Martha Sears and William Sears (Little, Brown, 2000.)

La Leche League International (LLLI): (800) 435-8316 or (847) 519-7730; www.lalecheleague.org

International Lactation Consultant Association (ILCA): (919) 787–5181; www.ilca.org

Corporate Lactation Program by Medela: (800) 435–8316; www.medela.com

Motherwear (nursing clothing): (800) 950–2500; www.motherwear.com

Children's Books

See the following books in the Sears Children's Library, by William Sears and Martha Sears and Christie Watts Kelly, (Little, Brown, 2001 and 2002).

Baby on the Way (introducing siblings to the new arrival)

Eat Healthy, Feel Great (fun ways to teach kids about healthy nutrition)

What Every Baby Needs (explaining baby care to children)

You Can Go to the Potty (a step-by-step manual on toilet training)

Down Syndrome

The National Down Syndrome Society: www.ndss.org

Down Syndrome Quarterly Journal: www.denison.edu/dsq/

National Association for Down Syndrome: www.nads.org

Food Allergies

The Food Allergy and Anaphylaxis Network (FAAN): www.foodallergy.org

Food Allergy News for Kids: www.fankids.org

Gastroesophageal Reflux (GERD)

Pediatric/Adolescent Gastroesophageal Reflux Association (PAGER): www.reflux.org

Reflux Wedges and Slings: www.tuckerdesigns.com

Goat Milk

www.meyenberg.com

Labor Support Assistants (Professional Labor Assistants)

Doulas of North America: www.dona.org

Nutritional Information

The Family Nutrition Book: Everything You Need to Know About Feeding Your Children — From Birth Through Adolescence, by William Sears and Martha Sears (Little, Brown, 1999)

www.AskDrSears.com. (Click on "Feeding Infants and Toddlers" and "Family Nutrition")

Nutritional Analysis: www.leankids.com

Obesity

Prevention and Treatment: www.leankids.com

Omega-3 Fats

www.dhadoc.com. An informative website about the importance of brain-building omega-3 fats in infant nutrition.

Poison Control

American Association of Poison Control Centers: (800) 222-1222; www.AAPCC.org
National hotline: (800) 222-1222

Write in the number of your local poison control center here: _____

Pregnancy Resources

The Pregnancy Book, by William Sears and Martha Sears, with obstetrician Linda Hughey Holt (Little, Brown, 1997). A month-by-month guide during your pregnancy and helpful information on having a safe and satisfying birth. (See also labor support assistants.)

Recipes

www.AskDrSears.com/recipes

Relaxation Music

Soothing Moments by Livesay is available at www.AskDrSears.com.

Safety, Toys and Infant Products

U.S. Consumer Products Safety Commission: www.cpsc.gov

Juvenile Products Manufacturers Association: www.jpma.org

Sudden Infant Death Syndrome (SIDS)

SIDS: A Parent's Guide to Understanding and Preventing Sudden Infant Death Syndrome, by William Sears (Little, Brown, 1995)

SIDS Alliance: www.sidsalliance.org
www.AskDrSears.com/babybookupdates. New information about reducing the risk of SIDS.

Twins and Multiples

National Organization of Mothers of Twins Clubs: (877) 540-2200 or (615) 595-0936 or www.nomotc.org

National Organization of Fathers of Twins Club: www.nofotc.org

www.twinslist.org. A valuable resource with lots of message boards with practical tips.

Mothering Multiples: Breastfeeding and Caring for Twins or More, by Karen Gromada (La Leche League, 1999)

Index

About the Authors

William Sears, M.D., and Martha Sears, R.N., are the parents of eight children as well as the authors of several bestselling books on parenting. They are the pediatrics experts to whom American parents are increasingly turning for advice and information on all aspects of pregnancy, birth, childcare, and family nutrition. Dr. Sears was trained at Harvard Medical School's Children's Hospital in Boston and Toronto's Hospital for Sick Children, the largest children's hospital in the world. He is Associate Clinical Professor of Pediatrics at the University of California, Irvine, and has practiced pediatrics for more than thirty years. Martha Sears, a registered nurse, currently works as a parenting and breast-feeding consultant in the Sears Family Pediatric Practice.

Robert Sears, M.D., a board-certified pediatrician, earned his medical degree from Georgetown University and trained in pediatrics at Children's Hospital Los Angeles. Dr. Bob resides in Dana Point, California, with his wife, Cheryl, and their three sons. He practices with his dad and brother, Dr. Jim, in the Sears Family Pediatric Practice and is a regular contributor to www.AskDrSears.com.

James Sears, M.D., a board-certified pediatrician, graduated from St. Louis University Medical School and trained at Tod's Children's Hospital in Youngstown, Ohio. He resides in Aliso Viejo, California, with his wife, Diane, and their two children. Dr. Jim is a member of the teaching faculty at the University of California, Davis, a frequent speaker on family nutrition, and a contributor to www.AskDrSears.com.

Look for these other books in the Sears Parenting Library

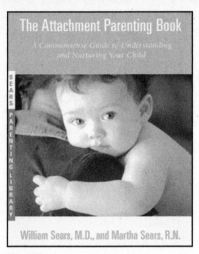

The Attachment Parenting Book
0-316-77809-5

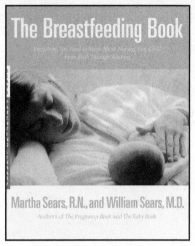

The Breastfeeding Book
0-316-77924-5

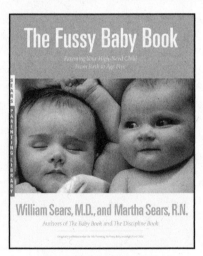

The Fussy Baby Book
0-316-77916-4

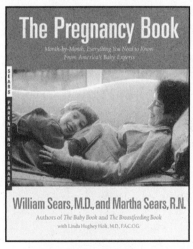

The Pregnancy Book
0-316-77914-8

The bestselling parenting guides for a new generation

Published by Little, Brown and Company
Available wherever books are sold

Look for these other books in the Sears Parenting Library

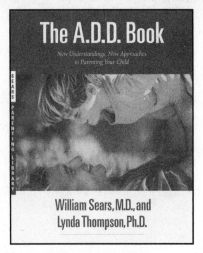

The A.D.D. Book
0-316-77873-7

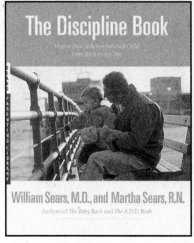

The Discipline Book
0-316-77903-2

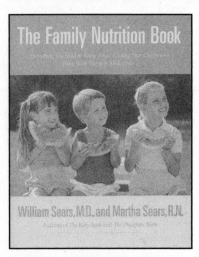

The Family Nutrition Book
0-316-77715-3

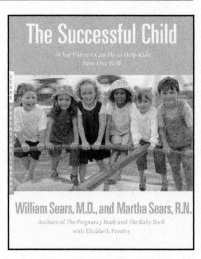

The Successful Child
0-316-77749-8

The bestselling parenting guides for a new generation

Published by Little, Brown and Company

Available wherever books are sold